Midwifery for Nurses

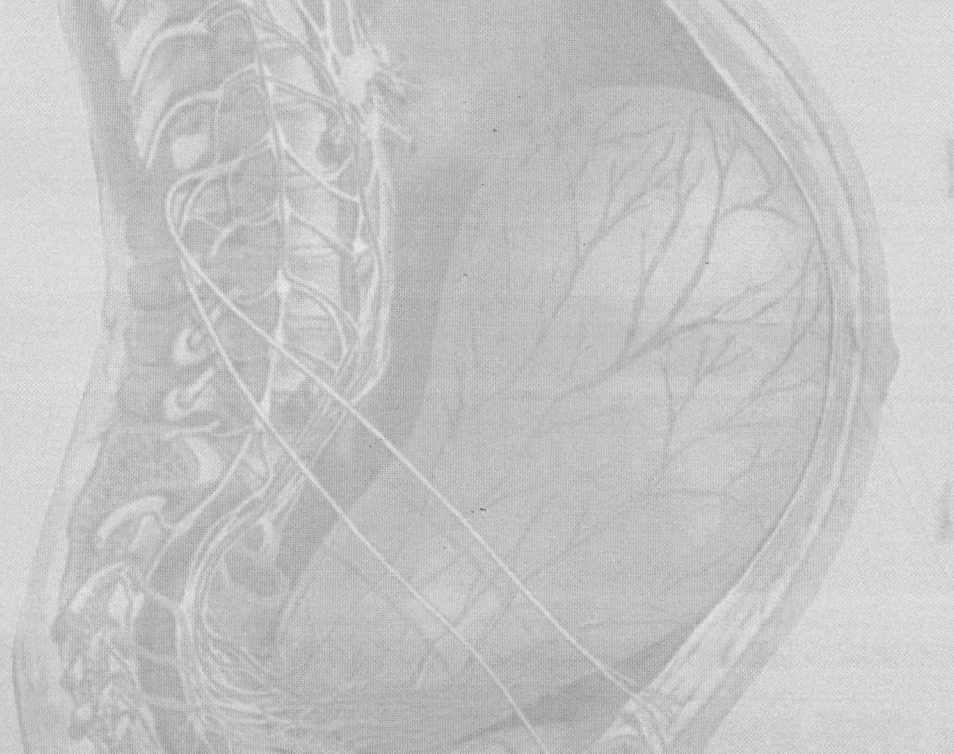

SECOND EDITION

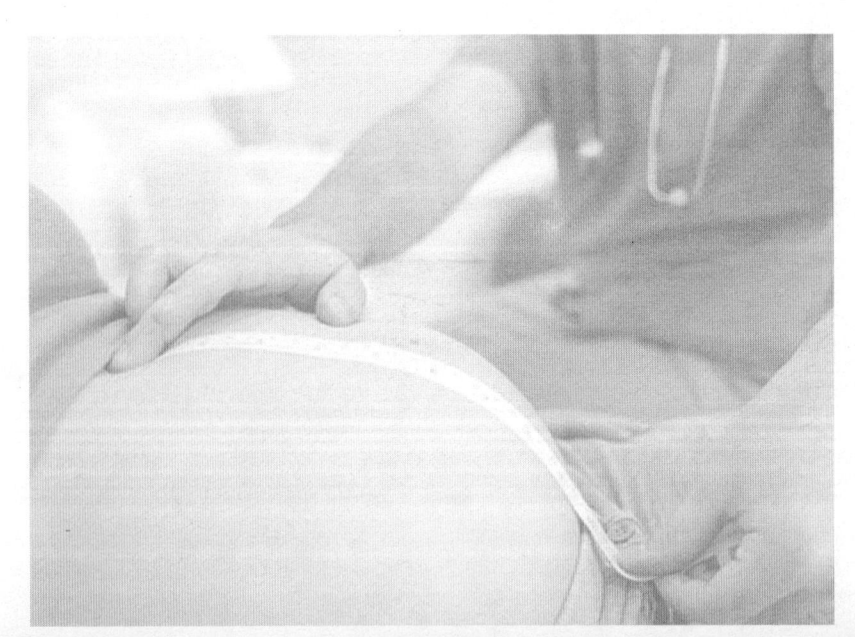

Midwifery for Nurses

SECOND EDITION

Marie Elizabeth
Principal
St. Ann's College of Nursing
Mangalore, Karnataka, India

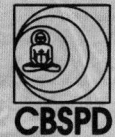

CBS Publishers & Distributors Pvt Ltd

New Delhi • Bengaluru • Chennai • Kochi • Kolkata • Lucknow • Mumbai
Hyderabad • Jharkhand • Nagpur • Patna • Pune • Uttarakhand

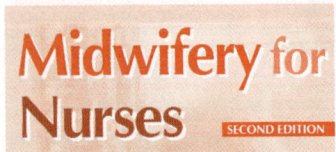

ISBN: 978-81-239-2214-0

Second Edition: 2013

Reprint: 2014, 2017, 2019, 2021, 2023, **2025**

First Edition: 2010

Published by **Satish Kumar Jain** and produced by **Varun Jain** for

CBS Publishers & Distributors Pvt Ltd

4819/XI Prahlad Street, 24 Ansari Road, Daryaganj, New Delhi 110 002, India.
Ph: 011-23266838, 23289259   Website: www.cbspd.com
                              e-mail: delhi@cbspd.com

Corporate Office: 204 FIE, Industrial Area, Patparganj, Delhi 110 092
Ph: 011-4934 4934   Fax: 011-4934 4935
                     e-mail: publishing@cbspd.com; publicity@cbspd.com

Branches

• **Bengaluru:** Seema House 2975, 17th Cross, KR Road, Banasankari 2nd Stage, Bengaluru 560 070, Karnataka, India
  Ph: +91-80-26771678/79   Fax: +91-80-26771680   e-mail: bangalore@cbspd.com
• **Chennai:** 18/8B, Subbarayan Street, Shenoy Nagar, Chennai 600 030, Tamil Nadu, India
  Ph: +91-44-42032115, 26681266   e-mail: chennai@cbspd.com
• **Kochi:** 42/1325, 1326, Power House Road, Opp KSEB, Power House, Ernakulum Kochi 682 018, Kerala, India
  Ph: +91-484-4059061-65,67   Fax: +91-484-4059065   e-mail: kochi@cbspd.com
• **Kolkata:** 147, Hind Ceramics Compound, 1st Floor, Nilgunj Road, Belghoria, Kolkata-700056, West Bengal, India
  Ph: +033-25633055, 033-25633056   e-mail: kolkata@cbspd.com
• **Lucknow:** Basement, Khushnuma Complex, 7 Meerabai Marg (Behind Jawahar Bhawan), Lucknow-226001, UP, India
  Ph: +0522-4000032   e-mail: tiwari.lucknow@cbspd.com
• **Mumbai:** PWD Shed, Gala no 25/26, Ramchandra Bhatt Marg, Next to JJ Hospital Gate no. 2, Opp. Union Bank of India, Noorbaug, Mumbai-400009, Maharashtra, India
  Ph: 022-66661880/89   e-mail: mumbai@cbspd.com

Representatives

• Hyderabad   0-9885175004   • Jharkhand   0-9811541605   • Nagpur   0-8692091830
• Patna   0-9334159340   • Pune   0-9664372571   • Uttarakhand 0-9716462459

Printed at Goyal Offset Works Pvt. Ltd., Haryana (INDIA)

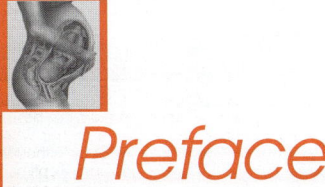

Preface

"The hands that serve are holier than the lips that pray"

—*Reiger Soll*

Second Edition

This is the thoroughly revised, completely rewritten and reorganised edition of the popular book which has won acclaim from the readers, nursing students as well as the teachers. A large number of illustrations have been redrawn to render vividness to description; whereas all the graphics now have made in two color to give clarity and ease of understanding the basics. The revision and updation of the text is likely to appeal to the readers as new information is added and colour graphics make a strong visual impact. The text retains its flavour of simplicity of expression and inherent lucidity.

First Edition

A book is an accumulation of various concepts in the vast ocean of knowledge.

This book is a compilation of the various concepts of obstetrics and gynecology, which is essential in enriching the knowledge of the nursing students in the field of obstetrics. It aims to help in moulding the nursing students to be an efficient midwife who can provide effective and safe client care.

The field of science is growing at a rapid rate and is making strides in leaps and bounds. The advent of newer technologies has helped in this and is pumping in enormous amount of information in all the fields of service. The available data are scattered in multiple formats in different print media and making it tedious and cumbersome for the students to collect the relevant data and the subject of obstetrics and gynecology is no exception considering all these problems. I have put in every effort to collect and complete all the relevant information available into one textbook that makes obstetrics and gynecology easier for the nursing students.

This book has been written in simple and lucid language that can help the nursing students grasp the subject easily. The schematic diagrams and the photographs included can be used to complement the learning process.

I dedicate this book to the nursing students in India and abroad hoping that this book will assist them in a rewarding study of this subjects.

Marie Elizabeth

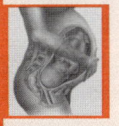

Acknowledgements

First of all I would like to thank and praise God Almighty for his grace in the completion of this book.

The preparation of this book was possible only with the help and cooperation of a number of people.

My sincere thanks to Sr. Jacintha D'Souza, Principal, Fr. Muller College of Nursing; Sr. Loredana Korah, Director of PG Education, St. Ann's College of Nursing, Mulki; and Dr. Juliana Roche, Principal, College of Nursing, KMC, Mangalore, who encouraged me to write this book.

I owe my grateful acknowledgement to Mrs. Malathi, Associate Professor, Mrs. Juliet, Ms. Anes, Ms. Natasha, Ms. Zeena, Assistant Lecturers, who have helped me to review the typed material and for their constructive suggestions and lively support to complete this task.

I am deeply appreciative of Ms. Sabitha Shenoy, Professor and Head, OBG Department, Nitte College of Nursing, and Ms. Jacintha Mariappa, Lecturer, for their wholehearted efforts in editing the typescript of the book. The reputed staff of CBS Publishers & Distributors deserve praise for this work in shaping this book.

Above all, I express my deep sense of gratitude and indebtedness to my mother and my daughters Ruma and Runa who made my path easy by their constant encouragement, prayers, support and concern at every phase of my encounter.

My sincere thanks and gratitude to all those who have helped me directly or indirectly in the successful completion of this book.

Marie Elizabeth

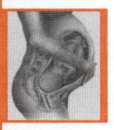

Contents

Preface   v
History   xi−xvi

1. Female Reproductive System   1

Outline   1
Introduction   1
The vulva   1
The vagina   2
The uterus   4
Uterine malformations   5
Ovaries   6
The fallopian tubes   6
Perineum   6
Pelvic floor   7
Nerve supply   9
Pelvic floor during pregnancy
   and parturition   9
Breasts   9

2. Fundamentals of Reproduction   11

Outline   11
Menstrual cycle   11
   Normal menstrual cycle   11
   Ovarian cycle   12
   Menstrual cycle   14
   Human oogenesis   15
   Ovulation   16
Fertilization   17
Development of placenta   19
   Decidua   19
   Formation of chorionic villi   20
   Further development of the placenta   23
   Placental membrane   24
   The placenta and fetal membranes   24
   The placenta at term   24
   Separation   25
   The fetal membranes   26
   Amniotic fluid   27
   Abnormalities in volume   29

Menstrual disorders   31
   1. Amenorrhoea   31
Diagnosis and investigation   32
   Primary amenorrhoea   32
   Secondary amenorrhoea   32
   Specific treatment   32
   2. Dysmenorrhoea   33
   Clinical features of primary
     dysmenorrhoea   33
   Secondary dysmenorrhoea   34
Heavy menstruation and abnormal uterine
   haemorrhage   35
   3. Metrorrhagia   35
   4. Menorrhagia   36
   5. Dysfunctional uterine bleeding
     (DUB)   36
   Metropathia haemorrhagia
     (Schroder disease)   36

3. The Fetus   40

Outline   40
Fetal circulation   40
Changes of the fetal circulation at birth   41
Fetal development   42

4. Pregnancy   45

Outline   45
Physiological changes during pregnancy   45
   Genital organs   45
   Uterus   45
   Cervix   48
   Other organs   49
   Breasts   49
   Cutaneous changes   50
   Weight gain and water metabolism   50
   Haematological changes   51
   Heart and circulation   52

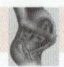
Metabolic changes 52
Systemic changes 53
Diagnosis of pregnancy 54
First trimester (first 12 weeks) 54
Second trimester (13–28 weeks) 57
Abdominal examination 57
Last trimester (29–40 weeks) 58
Chronological appearance of specific
symptoms and signs of pregnancy 60
Procedure at the first visit 61
History taking 61
Examination 63
Heart, lungs, liver and spleen 64
Procedure at the subsequent visits 65
Examination 65
Antenatal advice 65
Minor ailments in pregnancy 68
Nausea 68
Fatigue 68
Upper backache (nonpathological) 69
Leukorrhoea 69
Urinary frequency (nonpathological) 69
Heartburn 69
Flatulence 70
Constipation 70
Haemorrhoids 70
Leg cramps 71
Dependent oedema 71
Varicosities 71
Dyspareunia 72
Nocturia 72
Insomnia 72
Low back pain (nonpathological) 72
Nonpathological hyperventilation and
shortness of breath 73
Tingling and numbness of fingers 74
Supine hypotensive syndrome 74
Fetus in utero 74
Denominator 76
Methods of obstetrical examination 76
Planned parenthood 79
Antenatal exercise 83
Exercises for muscle strengthening and
relaxation 83
Do's and don'ts 84
Fetal well-being assessment 85
Prenatal fetal assessment 85
Fetal assessment during labour 85
Tests to assess fetal well-being 86

5. Fetal Skull and Maternal Pelvis   87

Outline 87
Fetal skull 87
Areas of skull 87
Sutures 87
Fontanelles 87
Anterior fontanelle 88
Posterior fontanelle 89
Sagittal fontanelle 89
Diameters of skull 89
Circumferences 90
Maternal pelvis 90
Functions 90
The normal female pelvis 91
Pelvic bones 91
Pelvic ligaments 92
The true pelvis 92
The four types of pelvis 95

6. Normal Labour   97

Outline 97
Causes of onset of labour 97
Prelabour (Syn: premonitory stage) 99
Stages of labour 100
Factors influencing labour 101
Major variables in the birth process 101
Pelvis 101
Passenger 101
Fetopelvic relationship 101
Powers: uterine contractions 102
Assessment of labour contractions 102
Events in first stage of labour 103
Uterine action 103
Mechanical factors 106
Events in second stage of labour 106
Mechanism of normal labour 108
Main movements 108
Events in third stage of labour 110
Management of normal labour 112
Antiseptics and asepsis 112
Vaginal examination in labour 113
Preliminaries 113
Indications of vaginal examination 113
Management of the first stage 114
Principles 114
Preliminaries 114
Actual management 114
Evidences of foetal distress 115
Management of the second stage 115
Immediate care of the newborn 118
Management of the third stage 120
Signs 120
Partograph 123

7. Normal Puerperium   127

Outline 127
Involution of the uterus 127

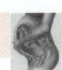

Anatomical consideration   127
Involution of other pelvic structures   128
   Vagina   128
Lochia   129
General physiological changes   130
Lactation   131
   Physiology of lactation   131
Management of normal puerperium   133
   Management of ailments   137
Postpartum exercise   137

8. Obstetric Disorders in Pregnancy   139

Outline   139
Abortion   139
   Spontaneous abortion (miscarriage)   139
   Classification of varieties   139
   Ovo-fetal factors   139
   Maternal factors (15%)   139
   Threatened abortion   141
   Inevitable abortion   143
   Complete abortion   144
   Incomplete abortion   144
   Missed abortion (silent miscarriage)   145
   Carneous mole (Syn: blood mole, fleshy
     mole or tuberous mole)   145
   Septic abortion   146
   Management   148
   Medical termination of pregnancy
     (MTP)   151
Ectopic pregnancy   152
   Tubal pregnancy   152
   Morbid anatomy   154
   Mode of termination   154
   Acute ectopic   156
   Unruptured tubes ectopic   157
   Chronic or old ectopic   157
   Diagnosis of ectopic pregnancy   158
   Subacute (chronic) ectopic   158
   Interstitial pregnancy   159
Management of ectopic pregnancy   160
   Acute   160
   Chronic ectopic   160
   Unruptured tubal pregnancy   161
   Prognosis of tubal pregnancy   162
Gestational trophoblastic diseases
   (GTDs)   162
   Hydatidiform mole (Syn: vesicular
     mole)   163
   Naked eye appearance   164
   Microscopic appearance   164
   Ovarian changes   164
   Complications   166
   Supportive therapy   168
Antepartum haemorrhage   170

Placenta praevia   170
   Confirmation of diagnosis   172
   Placentography   172
   Complications   173
   Prognosis   173
   Management   174
   Abruptio placentae   175
Multiple pregnancy   180
   Twins   180
   Sex   182
   Diagnosis   184
   Fetal   186
   Twin transfusion syndrome   186
   Antenatal management   186
   Management during labour   187
Polyhydramnios (Syn: hydramnios)   188
   Chronic polyhydramnios   189
   Abdominal examination   190
   Management   191
   Acute polyhydramnios   192
Oligohydramnios (Syn: oligoamnios)   194
Postmaturity (Syn: post-term pregnancy)   195
   Dangers   196
   Management   197
Intrauterine fetal death   198
   Management   201
Stillbirth   201
Abnormalities of placenta and cord   202
   Large placenta (more than 500 gm)   202
   Placenta succenturiata   202
   Placenta extrachorialis   203
   Placenta membranecae   203
   Placenta accreta and increta   204
   Cord abnormalities   204

9. Medical and Surgical Disorders in Pregnancy   206

Outline   206
Hypertensive disorders in pregnancy   206
   Pregnancy induced hypertension
     (PIH)   206
   Pre-eclampsia   206
   Pathophysiology   209
   Clinical types   210
   Clinical features   210
   Prognosis   213
   Prediction and prevention   213
   Management   213
   Caesarean section   217
   Eclampsia   217
   Clinical features   218
   Prognosis   219
   Management   219
Anemia in pregnancy   221

 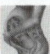

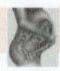
Iron deficiency anaemia 223
Specific therapy 224
Oral route 224
Parenteral therapy 224
Blood transfusion 226
Pueperium 226
Haemorrhagic anaemia 226
Sickle cell haemoglobinopathies 227
Thalassaemia in pregnancy 227
Heart disease in pregnancy 228
Management 229
Varicose veins in pregnancy 231
Diabetes mellitus In pregnancy 231
Pregnancy and diabetes 231
Gestational diabetes mellitus 232
Management 232
Obstetric management 232
Overt diabetes 233
Effects of diabetes on pregnancy 233
Hyperemesis gravidarum 238
Theories 238
Rh incompatibility 241
Manifestations of the haemolytic
disease 241
Icterus gravis neonatorum 241
Congenital anaemia of the
newborn 242
To prevent or minimise fetomaternal
bleed 244
Infections in pregnancy 244
Toxoplasmosis 244
Parasitologic considerations 244
Incidence during pregnancy 244
Risk factors 244
Transmission cycle 245
Diagnosis and treatment 245
Rubella 246
Incidence and effects during
pregnancy 246
Diagnosis and treatment 247
Cytomegalovirus (CMV) infection 247
Pregnancy and CMV infection 247
Fetal and neonatal infections 247
Diagnosis and treatment 247
Herpes simplex virus infection 248
Effect on pregnancy 248
Syphilis 248
Effects on pregnancy 249
Treatment 249
Human immunodeficiency virus (HIV)
infection and acquired immuno-
deficiency syndrome (AIDS) 250
Management 251
Nursing management 253

Parasitic and protozoal infestations in
pregnancy 253
Assessment and screening of high-risk
pregnancy 253
Risk approach of obstetric nursing
care 253
Management 255
Initial screening 260

10. Malpositions and Malpresentations 263

Outline 263
Occipitoposterior position 263
Diagnosis 264
Abdominal examination 264
Vaginal examination 264
Management of labour 268
Complications associated with
occipitoposterior positions 269
Breech presentation 271
Varieties 271
Mechanism of left sacroanterior
position 272
Prognosis 275
Antenatal management 275
Management of vaginal breech
delivery 277
Assisted breech delivery 278
Management of complicated breech
delivery 280
Arrest of the aftercoming head 282
Face Presentation 282
Mechanism of a left mentoanterior
position 283
Right mentoanterior (RMA), left
mentoposterior (RMP OR LMP) 284
Abdominal findings 285
Vaginal examination 285
Prognosis 286
Management of labour 287
Brow Presentation 287
Mechanism of labour 288
Management 288
Transverse lie 289
Diagnosis 289
Clinical course of labour 290
Unfavourable events (most
common) 291
Favourable events (very rare) 291
Management 292
Patient seen in labour 293
Unstable lie 293
Management 293
Formulation of the line of treatment 293

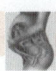
Compound presentation (Syn: complex presentation) 294
Shoulder dystocia 294
   Management 295
   Manipulative procedures 296
   Outcomes following shoulder dystocia 298
Cord prolapse 298
   Prognosis 299

11. Abnormal Labour   301

Outline 301
Preterm labour (Syn: premature labour) 301
   Management 302
   Prevention 302
   To arrest preterm labour 302
   Management of preterm labour 303
Preterm rupture of the membranes (PROM) 304
   Management 305
Obstructed labour 306
Induction of labour 307
   Preinduction scoring 308
   Methods of induction 309
   Medical Induction 309
   Surgical Induction 309
   Low rupture of the membrane (LRM) 310
   Procedures 310
   High rupture of the membranes (HRM) 310
   Stripping the membranes 311
   Combined method 311
Prolonged labour 311
Abnormal uterine action 314
   Uterine inertia (hypotonic activity) 315
   Effects on the mother and fetus 315
   Incoordinate uterine action 315
   Constriction ring 315
   General tonic contraction (Syn: uterine tetany) 316
   Precipitate labour 316
   Tonic uterine contraction and retraction 317
Amniotic fluid embolism (AFE) 318
   What causes AFE? 318
Blood coagulation disorders 320
   Disorders of blood coagulation and fibrinolysis in obstetrics 320
   Fibrinolysis 321
   Effect of pregnancy on blood coagulation and fibrinolysis systems 321
   etiology 322
   Tests for coagulation failure 323
   Treatment 323

Idiopathic thrombocytopenic purpura in pregnancy 323
Foetal distress 324
   Diagnosis 324
Shock in obstetrics 325
   Primary or initial shock 325
   Secondary or true shock 325
   Compensated (reversible) shock 326
   Progressive decompensated shock 326
   Decompensated (irreversible) shock 327
   General changes in shock (with special reference to hypovolaemic shock) 327
   Haemorrhagic shock 328
   Endotoxic shock 330
   Neurogenic shock 332
Contracted pelvis 333
   Rachitic flat pelvis 333
   Osteomalacic pelvis 333
   Asymmetrical or obliquely contracted pelvis 333
Mechanism of labour in contracted pelvis with vertex presentation 334
   Flat pelvis 334
   Diagnosis of contracted pelvis 335
   Disproportion 336
   Effects of contracted pelvis on pregnancy and labour 337
   Management of contracted pelvis (inlet contraction) 338
   Trial labour 338
Rupture of the uterus 339
   Spontaneous 339
   Scar rupture 339
   Iatrogenic or traumatic 340
   Prophylaxis 342
   Laparotomy 342
Cervical dystocia 342
Disseminated intravascular coagulation (DIC) in obstetrics 343
   Definition of DIC (minimal acceptable criteria) 343
   Chronic DIC 344
   Acute DIC 344
HELLP syndrome 346
Postpartum haemorrhage 347
Predisposing factors 348
Placenta accreta 353
   Clinical picture 354
   Velamentous insertion of the umbilical cord 356

12. Obstetric Interventions and Operations   357

Outline 357
Dilatation and evacuation 357

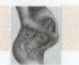

One stage operation   357
Two stage operation   358
Dangers of D and E operation   359
Hysterotomy   360
Version   361
External cephalic version   361
Actual steps   362
Internal version   363
Episiotomy   363
Steps of mediolateral episiotomy   364
Postoperative care   365
Forceps   365
Long curved obstetric forceps   366
Short curved obstetric forceps   367
Kielland's forceps   367
Ventouse   369
Caesarean section   371
Lower segment caesarean section
   (LSCS)   373
Aftercare   374
Classical caesarean section   375
Maternal and perinatal mortality   376
Symphysiotomy   378
Destructive operations   378
Craniotomy   378
Procedures   378
Actual steps   378
Decapitation   379
Procedures   379
Actual steps   379
Evisceration   380
Cleidotomy   380

13. Abnormal Puerperium   382

Outline   382
Puerperal pyrexia   382
Definition   382
Puerperal sepsis (Syn: puerperal
   infection)   382
Local infection   383
Uterine infection   383
Spreading infection   383
Investigation of puerperal pyrexia   383
Prophylaxis   384
Treatment   385
Subinvolution   385
Urinary complications in puerperium   386
Breast complications   387
Breast engorgement   387
Cracked and retracted nipple   387
Acute mastitis   388
Breast abscess   389
Failing lactation   389
Puerperal venous thrombosis and pulmonary
   embolism   389

Superficial vein thrombosis   390
Deep vein thrombosis   390
Nonsuppurative thrombophlebitis   391
Suppurative thrombophlebitis   391
Pulmonary embolism   392
Psychiatric illness in pregnancy   392
1. Postnatal 'blues'   392
2. Postnatal depression   393
3. Severe depressive illness   394
4. Puerperal psychosis   395

14. The Newborn Infant   397

Outline   397
Care and examination of the newborn   397
General appearance   397
Assessment of physical characteristics   398
Minor ailments of newborn   401
Preterm baby   402
Definition   402
Incidence   402
Features of preterm baby   402
Care of the preterm neonate   404
Kangaroo care for preterm infants   406
Intrauterine growth restriction (IUGR)   407
Problems of the newborn   410
Asphyxia neonatorum   410
Birth trauma   411
Degrees of asphyxia   411
External cardiac massage   414
Birth injuries   414
Injuries of head   414
Cephalhaematoma   414
Subaponeurotic haemorrhage   415
Scalp injuries   416
Fracture skull   416
Intracranial haemorrhage   416
Traumatic   416
Anoxic   416
Other injuries   417
Antenatal period   419
Normal delivery   419
Jaundice in newborn   420
Physiological jaundice in newborn and
   jaundice in prematurity   421
Hyperbilirubinaemia   421
Hydrops foetalis is oedematous stillborn
   baby   422
Alimentary disorders   422
Persistent mild diarrhoea   424
Vomiting   424
Convulsions (seizure) in newborn   424
Haemorrhagic disease in newborn   425

15. Pharmacology and Child Birth 427

Outline 427
Analgesics and antispasmodics in pregnancy and labour 427
   General aches, pain and discomfort 427
   Analgesics for pain relief during labour 428
Drugs used in pregnancy, labour and puerperium 428
Antiemetics in pregnancy 428
Steroids during pregnancy 428
Systemic steroids in clinical use 429
Drugs in asthma (during pregnancy) 429
Diuretics 431
Anticonvulsants 432
Tocolytics in obstetrics for the next 12 to 48 hours, at the end of which the therapy can be switched over to oral medication 432
Oxytocics in obstetrics 433
Oxytocin 434
Controlled intravenous infusion 435
Intramuscular 437
Oxytocin challenge test (OCT) 438
Oxytocin sensitivity test (OST) 438
Ergot derivatives 439
Prostaglandins (PGs) 440
Oxytocic effect 440

16. Home Birth 443

Legal issues 443
Advantages of home based antenatal care 444
Preparation for birth 444
Management of labour 445
Preparation before confinement for baby and mother 445
Requirements of baby 445
Preparation for confinement 445
Preparation and procedures for home birth 446
Postnatal visit 447

17. Complimentary and Alternative Therapies 449

Complementary and alternative therapies 449
   Historical context of complementary and alternative therapies 449
   Nursing acceptance of complementary and alternative therapies modalities 450

Selected complementary and alternative therapies 450
Acupressure 450
Acupuncture 451
Aromatherapy 452
Biofeedback 452
Hypnosis 453
Transcutaneous electrical nerve stimulation (TENS) 454
Visualization and guided imagery 455
Expressive therapy/Sound therapy 456
Hydrotherapy 456
Homeopathy 457
Massage/Touch therapy 457
Reflexology 458
Yoga 459

18. Contraception 460

Contraceptive methods 460
Physical methods 460
Chemical methods 461
Intrauterine devices (IUD) 461
Description of the devices 461
Multiload Cu 250 464
Hormonal Steroidal contraceptives 466
Combined oral contraceptives (pills) 466
How to prescribe a pill 467
Indications for withdrawal 468
Triphasic formulations of combined oral pills 469
Progestin only pill (mini pill) 470
Emergency contraception (Syn: post-coital contraception) 470
Hormones 471
Injectable steroids 471
Implant 472
Post-conceptional methods (termination of pregnancy) 472
Menstrual induction 472
Abortion 473
Miscellaneous 473
Coitus interruptus 473
Safe period (rhythm method) 473
Natural family planning methods 474
Basal body temperature (BBT) method 474
Cervical mucus method 474
Breastfeeding 474
Terminal methods or sterilization 474
Vasectomy 474
Technique 475
Female sterilization 476
Tubectomy 476
Conventional (laparotomy) 476

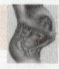

19. Instruments in Obstetrics and Gynaecology 481

Outline 481
Instruments used for the examination of a
    gynaecological and obstetric patient 481
    Sims double bladed posterior vaginal
        speculum 481
    Cusco's bivalved self-retaining
        speculum 482
    Auvard's vaginal speculum 482
    Sim's anterior vaginal wall retractor 483
    Teale's vulsellum 483
    Simpson's uterine sound 484
    Pinard's stethoscope 484
    Bouldeloque's pelvimeter 484
Instruments used in dilatation, curettage and
    evacuation operation 485
    Hegar's dilators 485
    Blakes' blunt and sharp uterine
        curette 486
    Laminaria tent 487
    Laminaria tent introducing forceps 487
    Haywood Smith's ovum forceps 487
Instruments used for
    destructive operations 488
    Simpson's modification of Oldham's
        perforator 488
    Drew Smythe's catheter 489
    Flushing curette 489
    Two-bladed Braxton-Hick's cranio
        clast 489
    Willet's scalp traction forceps 489
    Ramsbotham's decapitation saw 490
    Blond-hiedler's decapitation saw wire
        with thimble 490
    Breech hook with crochet 491
Specialized gynaecological instruments 491
    Uterine dressing forceps 491
    Uterus packing forceps 491
    Cervical punch biopsy forceps 492
    Shirodkar's cervical encirclage
        needles 493
    Green Armytage clamp 493
    Wertheim's vaginal clamp 494
Common surgical instruments 494
    Kocher's haemostatic clamp 494
    Artery forceps 494
    Needle holder 495
    Allis's tissue holding forceps 495
    Lanes's tissue holding forceps 495
    Babcock's tissue holding forceps 496
Scissors 496
    Episiotomy scissors 496
    Rampley's sponge holding forceps 496

20. Gynaecological Disorders in Pregnancy 497

Outline 497
Uterine Displacements 497
Retroversion 499
    Retroverted gravid uterus 500
Genital prolapse in pregnancy 502
Uterine fibroid in pregnancy 502
Carcinoma of cervix in pregnancy 504
Ovarian tumours in pregnancy 504

21. Social and Preventive Obstetrics 506

Outline 506
Family welfare programme in India 506
    RCH interventions 507
    Maternal mortality and morbidity and
        perinatal mortality 508
    Sudden collapse following child birth or
        abortion 509
    Factors influencing maternal
        mortality 509
    Maternal morbidity 510
    Perinatal mortality 511
Infertility and assisted reproductive
    technology 512
    Diagnostic evaluation of
        infertility 515
    Management of infertility 518
    Alternatives to child birth 521
Legal aspects in obstetrics 522
    Current legal controversies in obstetrical
        nursing 523
    The central births and death registration
        act, 1969 523
    Nurse practice acts 523
    Standard of care 524
    Agency policies 524
Menopause 527
    Advantages and disadvantages of oral
        and transdermal route of
            oestrogen 531
    Smoking 533

References 537
Bibliography 537
Journals 537
Index 539

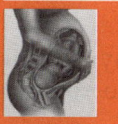

Female Reproductive System

OUTLINE

- The vulva
- The vagina
- The uterus
- Ovaries
- The fallopian tubes
- Perineum
- Pelvic floor
- Breasts

INTRODUCTION

Obstetrics is the branch of medical science which deals with childbirth and that which precedes and follows it. The nurse must acquire an understanding of the reproductive process in order to administer nursing care to the obstetric patient before and during childbirth. A knowledge of this process is also essential to caring for the mother and child following delivery.

Human life begins with the union of two cells, one from the female, called the *ovum*, and one from the male, called the *sperm*. This union of male and female cells, known as *fertilization* or *conception*, takes place within the female. She is responsible, both directly and indirectly, for the growth and development of the fertilized ovum which eventually results in the birth of a child. First examine the female reproductive system to discover how it is specially adapted for this purpose.

The female reproductive system has four basic functions:

- To produce ovarian hormones which are responsible for the female sex characteristics and 'reproductive functions'.
- To produce the ovum and deliver it to the place where conception may take place.
- To nurture and sustain the developing fertilized ovum (product of conception) until birth.
- To accomplish delivery of the product of conception.

The female reproductive system includes the external genitals, internal organs, the breasts, pelvis, and related pelvic structures.

THE VULVA

The term *vulva* applies to the external female genital organs (Fig. 1.1). It consists of the following structures:

- *The mons veneris* ('mount of Venus') or mons pubis: This is a pad of fat lying over the symphysis pubis. It is covered with pubic hair from the time of puberty.
- *The labia majora* ('greater lips'): These are two folds of fat and areolar tissue, covered with skin and pubic hair on the outer surface. They arise in the mons veneris and merge into the perineum behind.
- *The labia minora* ('lesser lips'): These are two thin folds of skin lying between the labia majora. Anteriorly they divide to

1

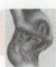

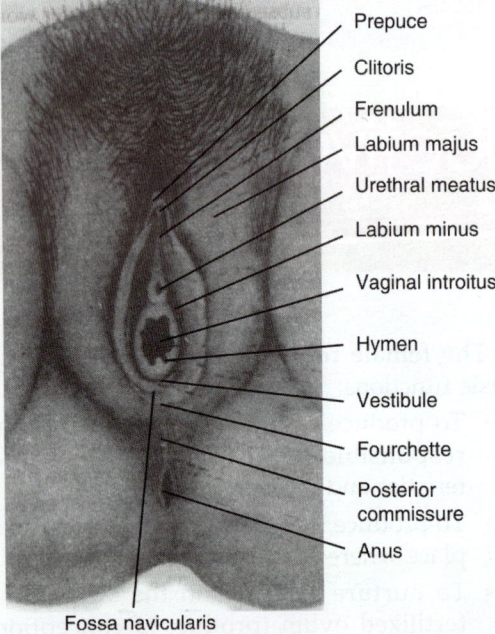

Prepuce
Clitoris
Frenulum
Labium majus
Urethral meatus
Labium minus
Vaginal introitus
Hymen
Vestibule
Fourchette
Posterior commissure
Anus

Fossa navicularis

Fig. 1.1: The virginal vulva

enclose the clitoris; posteriorly they fuse, forming the fourchette.

- *The clitoris*: This is a small rudimentary organ corresponding to the male penis. It is extremely sensitive and highly vascular and plays a part in the orgasm of sexual intercourse.
- *The vestibule:* This is the area enclosed by the labia minora in which are situated the openings of the urethra and the vagina.
- *The urethral orifice*: This orifice lies 2.5cm posterior to the clitoris. On either side lie the openings of Skene's ducts, two small blind-ended tubules 0.5 cm long running within the urethral wall.
- *The vaginal orifice*: This is also known as the introitus of the vagina and occupies the posterior two-thirds of the vestibule. The orifice is partially closed by the hymen, a thin membrane that tears during sexual intercourse or during the birth of the first child. The remaining tags of hymen are

known as the 'carunculae myrtiformes' because they are thought to resemble Myrtle berries.

- *Bartholin's glands*: There are two small glands that open on either side of the vaginal orifice and lie in the posterior part of the labia majora. They secrete mucus, which lubricates the vaginal opening.

The vulval blood supply

This comes from the internal and the external pudendal arteries. The blood drains through corresponding vein.

Lymphatic drainage

This is mainly via the inguinal glands.

Nerve supply

This is derived from branches of the pudendal nerve. The vaginal nerves supply the erectile tissue of the vestibular bulbs and clitoris and their parasympathetic fibres have a vasodilator effect.

Internal organs

The internal reproductive organs are those which lie within the pelvic cavity. They consist of the vagina, uterus, fallopian tubes, and ovaries. Also included are the supporting structures.

THE VAGINA

The vagina is a curved tubelike passage 8 to 12 centimeters long that leads from the vulva to the uterus. The lower portion of the cervix of the uterus protrudes into it. It is internally situated between the bladder and rectum. The vagina is made up of muscle and connective tissue and is capable of great distention during labor. It is lined with mucous membrane containing many folds called rugae. The secretion observed in the vagina is largely derived from the glands of the cervix. The vagina serves three important functions as a passage:

1. Introduction of the penis and reception of semen (fluid in which sperm is carried).

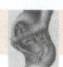

2. Discharge of menstrual flow and uterine secretions.
3. Delivery of the product of conception.

Functions

The vagina is a passage that allows the escape of the menstrual flow, receives the penis and the ejected sperm during sexual intercourse and provides an exit for the fetus during delivery.

Position

It is a canal running from the vestibular to the cervix, passing upwards and backwards into the pelvis along a line approximately parallel to the plane of the pelvic brim.

Relations

A knowledge of the relations of the vagina to other organs is essential for the accurate examination of the pregnant woman and her safe delivery.

- *Anterior:* In front of the vagina lies the bladder and the urethra, which are closely connected to the anterior vaginal wall.
- *Posterior:* Behind the vagina lies the pouch of Douglas, the rectum and the perineal body, each occupying approximately one-third of the posterior vaginal wall.
- *Lateral:* On either side of the upper two-thirds are the pelvic fascia and the ureters, which pass beside the cervix; on either side of the lower third are the muscles of the pelvic floor.
- *Superior:* Above the vagina lies the uterus.
- *Inferior:* Below the vagina lies the external genitalia.

Structure

The posterior wall is 10 cm long whereas the anterior wall is only 7.5 cm in length because the cervix projects at a right angle into its upper part.

The upper end of the vagina is known as the vault. Where the cervix projects into it, the vault forms a circular recess that is described as four arches or fornices. The posterior fornix is the largest of these because the vagina is attached

to the uterus at a higher level behind than in front. The anterior fornix lies in front of the cervix and the lateral fornices lie on either side. The vaginal walls are pink in appearance and thrown into small folds known as rugae. These allow the vaginal walls to stretch during intercourse and childbirth.

Layers

The lining is made of squamous epithelium. Beneath the epithelium lies a layer of vascular connective tissue.

The muscle layer is divided into a weak inner coat of circular fibres and a stronger outer coat of longitudinal fibres.

Pelvic fascia surrounds the vagina, forming a layer of connective tissue.

Contents

There are no glands in the vagina. It is, however, moistened by mucus from the cervix and a transudate that seeps out from the blood vessels of the vaginal wall.

In spite of the alkaline mucus, the vaginal fluid is strongly acid (pH 4.5) owing to the presence of lactic acid formed by the action of Doderlein's bacilli on glycogen found in the squamous epithelium of the lining. These lactobacilli are normal inhabitants of the vagina. The acid deteriorates the growth of pathogenic bacteria.

Blood supply

This comes from branches of the internal iliac artery and includes the vaginal artery and a descending branch of the uterine artery. The blood drains through corresponding veins.

Lymphatic drainage

This is via the inguinal, the internal iliac and the sacral glands.

Nerve supply

This is derived from the pelvic plexus. The vaginal nerves follow the vaginal arteries to supply the vaginal walls and also the erectile tissue of the vulva.

THE UTERUS

Functions

The uterus exists to shelter the fetus during pregnancy. It prepares for this possibility each month and following pregnancy it expels the uterine contents.

Position

The uterus is situated in the cavity of the true pelvis, behind the bladder and in front of the rectum. It leans forward, which is known as anteversion; it bends forwards on itself, which is known as anteflexion. When the woman is standing this results in an almost horizontal position with the fundus resting on the bladder.

Relations (Fig. 1.2)

- *Anterior:* In front of the uterus lie the utero-vesical pouch and the bladder.
- *Posterior:* Behind the uterus are the recto-uterine pouch of Douglas and the rectum.
- *Lateral:* On either side of the uterus are the broad ligaments, the uterine tubes and the ovaries.
- *Superior:* Above the uterus lie the intestines.
- *Inferior:* Below the uterus is the vagina.

Supports

The uterus is supported by the pelvic floor and maintained in position by several ligaments, of which those at the level of the cervix (Fig. 1.3) are the most important.

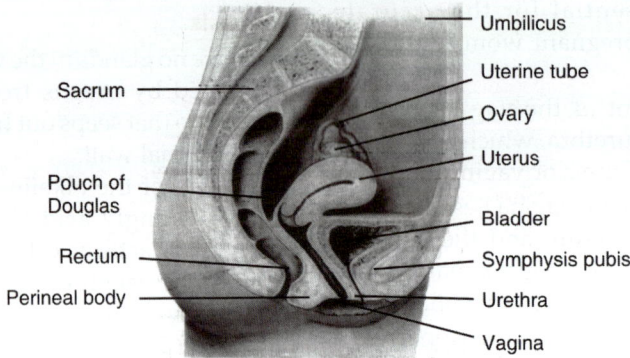

Umbilicus
Uterine tube
Ovary
Uterus
Bladder
Symphysis pubis
Urethra
Vagina
Sacrum
Pouch of Douglas
Rectum
Perineal body

Fig. 1.2: Sagittal section of the pelvis

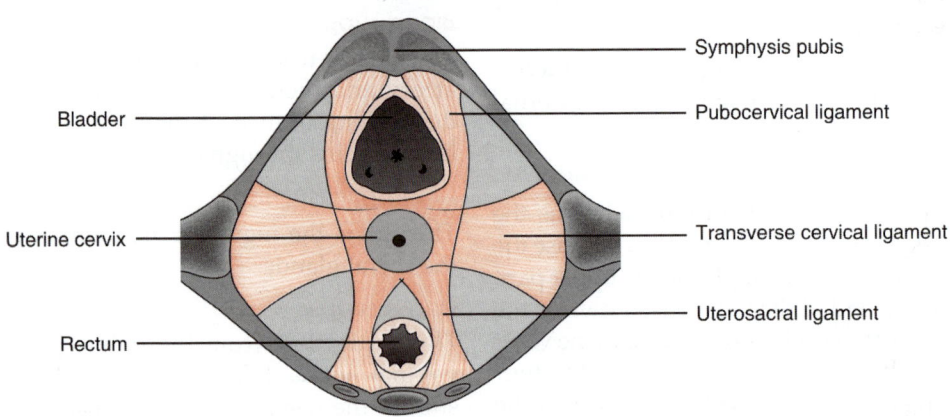

Symphysis pubis
Pubocervical ligament
Transverse cervical ligament
Uterosacral ligament
Bladder
Uterine cervix
Rectum

Fig. 1.3: Supports of the uterus, at the level of the cervix

The *transverse cervical ligaments*. These fan out from the sides of the cervix to the side walls of the pelvis. They are sometimes known as the 'cardinal ligaments' or 'Mackenrodt's ligaments'.

The *uterosacral ligaments*. These pass backwards from the cervix to the sacrum.

The *pubocervical ligaments.* These pass forwards from the cervix, under the bladder, to the pubic bones.

Uterus is the organ which carries the fetus during pregnancy. It is a hollow, pear-shaped organ with thick muscular walls, and is 2½ to middle of the pelvis between the bladder and the rectum and consists of the fundus (rounded top part), the body (middle part), and a narrow lower portion called the cervix (neck). The fundus and body make up the corpus of the uterus. The lining of the uterus is called the endometrium. The endometrium receives and nourishes the fertilized egg. During pregnancy, the uterus grows very soft and increases greatly in size to hold the growing fetus. By the end of pregnancy, the uterus becomes a thin, soft-walled muscular sac which yields to the movement of the fetus.

About half the length of the cervix projects into the vagina where the vaginal walls are attached to it. The cervix has a small round passage-way called the cervical canal; the internal os of the canal opens into the uterus, and the external os opens into the vagina.

Uterine secretions, the menstrual flow, the unfertilized ovum, the fetus during labor, and the lochial discharge (vaginal drainage during the six-week period following delivery) pass through the cervix to the vagina.

The uterine ligaments

The broad ligaments are two structures which extend from the side walls of the uterus to the pelvic walls. The ovaries and fallopian tubes are attached to these ligaments. The round ligaments of the uterus, attached to the side walls of the uterus, pass through the broad ligaments to reach the mons veneris. These ligaments help to support the pelvic organs. The uterosacral ligaments extend from the posterior cervical portion of the uterus to the sacrum and support the cervix.

UTERINE MALFORMATIONS (Fig. 1.4)

Embryological development of the uterus

The female genital tract is formed in early embryonic life when a pair of ducts develop. These paramesonephric or Müllerian ducts come together in the midline and fuse into a Y-shaped canal. The open upper ends of this structure lead into the peritoneal cavity and the infused portions become the uterine tubes. The fused lower portion forms the uterovaginal area, which further develops into the uterus and vagina.

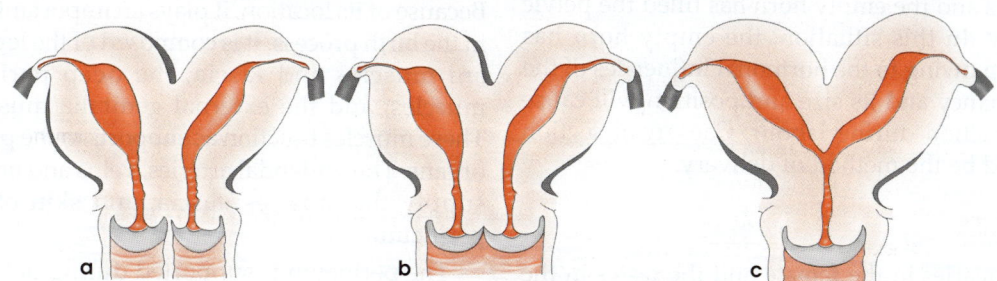

Fig. 1.4: Uterine malformations. **a.** Double uterus with duplication of the body of the uterus, cervix and vagina, **b.** Duplication of uterus and cervix with single vagina, **c.** Duplication of uterus with single cervix and vagina

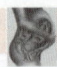

Types of uterine malformation

Various types of structural abnormality can result from failure of fusion of the Mullerian ducts. Three of these abnormalities can be seen in Fig. 1.4. A double uterus with an associated double vagina will develop where there has been complete failure of fusion. Partial fusion results in various degrees of duplication. A single vagina with a double uterus is the result of fusion at the lower end of the ducts only. A bicornuate uterus (one with two horns) is the result of incomplete fusion at the upper portion of the uterovaginal area. In rare cases, one Mullerian duct regresses and the end result is a uterus with one horn termed a unicornuate uterus.

Effect of abnormality on pregnancy

When pregnancy occurs in the woman with an abnormal uterus, the outcome depends on the ability of the uterus to accommodate the growing fetus. A problem exists only if the tissue is insufficient to allow the uterus to enlarge for a full-term fetus lying longitudinally.

If there is insufficient hypertrophy, the possible difficulties are abortion, premature labour and abnormal lie of the fetus. In labour, poor uterine function may be experienced.

Minor defects of structure cause little problem and might pass unnoticed with the woman having a normal outcome to her pregnancy. Occasionally problems arise when a fetus is accommodated in one horn of a double uterus and the empty horn has filled the pelvic cavity. In this situation, the empty horn has grown owing to the hormonal influences of the pregnancy and its size and position will cause obstruction during labour. Caesarean section would be the method of delivery.

OVARIES

The ovaries in the female and the testes in the male are similar in embryologic origin. The ovaries are two small, almond-shaped organs located on each side of the uterus. They are the female gonads or sex glands. About 1 million ova (eggs) are present at birth. Many ova degenerate, until puberty when approximately 400,000 remain. During the course of a woman's reproductive life, only about 400 ova mature enough to be fertilized.

During the reproductive years, the ovaries act in concern with the uterus. Sac like structures are in various stages of maturity; as they mature they are called follicles. During each menstrual cycle, one follicle matures into what is called a Graafian follicle, which contains the ovum that is released each month.

THE FALLOPIAN TUBES

The two fallopian tubes, or oviducts, extend outward from the upper corners of the uterus to the abdominal cavity. They are about the diameter of a drinking straw and are largely muscular structures. The distal portion of the tube curves around the ovary in such a way that the fingerlike projections cup over the ovary but are not actually attached to it (Fig. 1.5). Their function is to carry the ovum along the canal by peristaltic action from the ovary to the uterus. Conception usually takes place in the outer third of the fallopian tube.

PERINEUM

The perineum is the region of the genital area that lies between the vagina and the anus. Because of its location, it plays an important role in the birth process. It is composed of the levator ani muscles and fascia, the deep perineal muscles, and the external genitalia muscles. These muscles function as supports to the pelvic organs. The pudendal arteries, veins and nerves supply the muscles, fascia, and skin of the perineum.

The perineum is supported during delivery of the infant's head and shoulders because it stretches significantly during the infant's birth

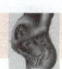

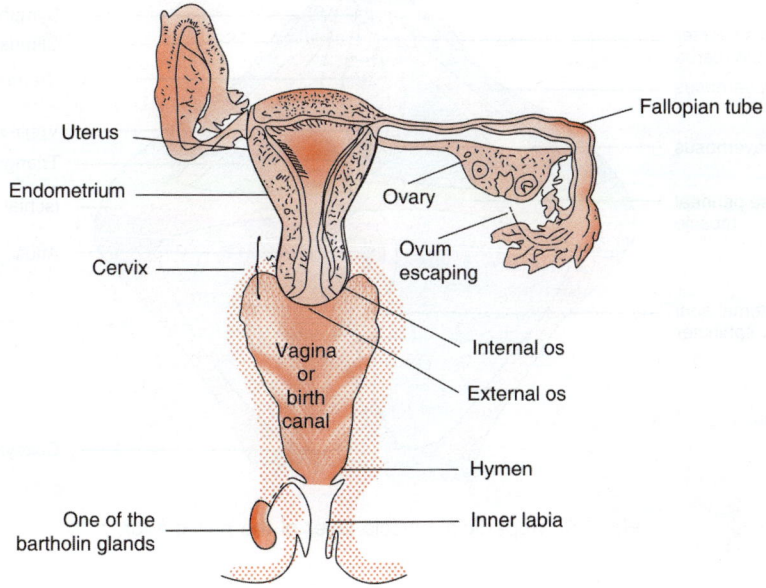

Fig. 1.5: Internal female reproductive organs

and may tear. An episiotomy (incision) on the perineal area may be performed to prevent tears in the underlying muscles or tissues; the episiotomy is repaired (sutured) immediately after delivery.

PELVIC FLOOR

The pelvic floor is formed by the soft tissues that fill the outlet of the pelvis. The most important of these is the strong diaphragm of muscle slung like a hammock from the walls of the pelvis. Through it pass the urethra, the vagina and the anal canal.

Functions

The pelvic floor supports the weight of the abdominal and pelvic organs. Its muscles are responsible for the voluntary control of micturition and defecation and play an important part in sexual intercourse. During childbirth it influences the passive movements of the fetus through the birth canal and relaxes to allow the exit of the fetus from the pelvis.

Muscle layers

The superficial layer: This layer is composed of five muscles (Fig. 1.6).

- The *external anal sphincter* encircles the anus and is attached behind by a few fibres to the coccyx.

- The *transverse perineal muscles* pass from the ischial tuberosities to the centre of the perineum.

- The *bulbocavernosus muscles* pass from the perineum forwards around the vagina to the corpora cavernosa of the clitoris just under the pubic arch.

- The *ischiocavernosus muscles* pass from the ischial tuberosities along the pubic arch to the corpora cavernosa.

- The *membranous sphincter of the urethra* is composed of muscle fibres passing above and below the urethra and attached to the pubic bones. It is not a true sphincter since it is not circular, but it acts to close the urethra.

 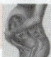

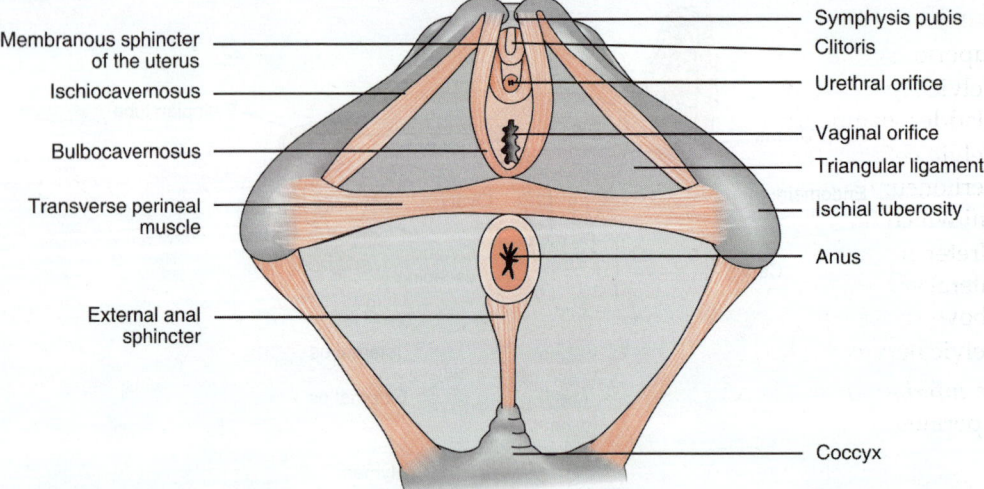

Membranous sphincter of the uterus

Ischiocavernosus

Bulbocavernosus

Transverse perineal muscle

External anal sphincter

Symphysis pubis

Clitoris

Urethral orifice

Vaginal orifice

Triangular ligament

Ischial tuberosity

Anus

Coccyx

Fig. 1.6: Superficial muscle layer of the pelvic floor

The deep layer (Fig. 1.7): This layer is composed of three pairs of muscles, which together are known as the levator ani muscles. They are so called because they lift or elevate the anus. Each levator ani muscle (left and right) consists of the following:

- The pubococcygeus muscle passes from the pubis to the coccyx, with a few fibres crossing over in the perineal body to form its deepest part.
- The iliococcygeus muscle passes from the fascia covering the obturator internus muscle (the white line of pelvic fascia) to the coccyx.
- The ischiococcygeus muscle passes from the ischial spine to the coccyx, in front of the sacrospinous ligament.

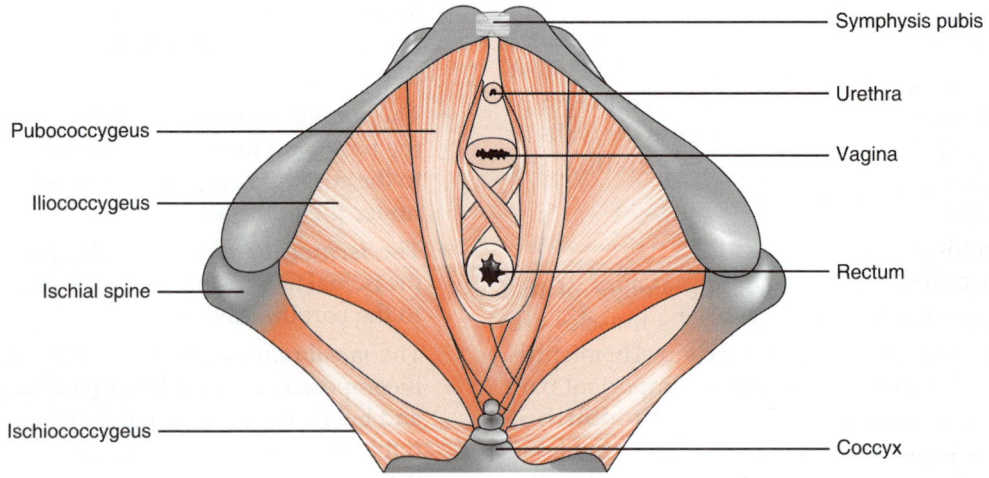

Pubococcygeus

Iliococcygeus

Ischial spine

Ischiococcygeus

Symphysis pubis

Urethra

Vagina

Rectum

Coccyx

Fig. 1.7: Deep muscle layer of the pelvic floor

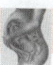

Structures in relation to pelvic floor

The superior surface is related to the following:

1. Pelvic organs from anterior to posterior are bladder, vagina, uterus and rectum.
2. Pelvic cellular tissues between the pelvic peritoneum and upper surface of the levator ani which fill all the available spaces.
3. Ureter lies on the floor in relation to the lateral vaginal fornix. The uterine artery lies above and the vaginal artery lies below it.
4. Pelvic nerves

The inferior surface is related to the anatomical perineum.

NERVE SUPPLY

It is supplied by the 4th sacral nerve, inferior rectal nerve and a perineal branch of pudendal nerve S2, 3, 4.

Functions

1. To support the pelvic organs - The pubovaginalis which forms a 'U' shaped sling, supports the vagina which in turn supports the other pelvic organs, bladder and uterus. Weakness or tear of this sling during parturition is responsible for prolapse of the organs concerned.
2. To maintain intra abdominal pressure by reflexly responding to its changes.
3. Facilitates anterior internal rotation of the presenting part when it presses on the pelvic floor.
4. Puborectalis plays an ancillary role to the action of the external anal sphincter.
5. Ischiococcygeus helps to stabilise the sacroiliac and sacrococcygeal joints.
6. To steady the perineal body.

PELVIC FLOOR DURING PREGNANCY AND PARTURITION

During pregnancy levator muscles hypertrophy, become less rigid and more distensible. Due to water retention, it swells up and sags down. In the second stage, the pubovaginalis and puborectalis relax and the levator ani is drawn up over the advancing presenting part in the second stage. Failure of the levator ani to relax at the crucial moment may lead to extensive damage of the pelvic structures. The effect of such a displacement is to elongate the birth canal which is composed solely of soft parts below the bony outlet. The soft canal has got deep lateral and posterior walls and its axis is in continuation with the axis of the bony pelvis.

BREASTS

The breasts, or mammary glands, are considered accessory organs of reproduction because of their functional relationship to reproduction, that is, to secrete milk for the infant (Fig. 1.8). The process is called lactation. The nipple, in the center of the breasts, is surrounded by a pigmented areola, which darkens during pregnancy. Montgomery's glands (Montgomery's tubercles) are small sebaceous glands in the areola that secrete a substance that lubricates and protects the breasts during lactation (when the infant sucks). Each breast is divided into a number of lobes (15 to 20), which can be visualized as a tree-like structure. They are separated by adipose and fibrous tissue. Beginning at the nipple are 10 to 20 branch like structures called lobes. Branching off from each lobe are 20 to 40 lobules; each lobule branches further, dividing into 20 to 80 sac like structures called alveoli. These sac like structures have a lining that contains tiny secretory cells called acini, which secrete milk. Surrounding the alveolar cells are contractile cells called myoepithelial cells, which contract the alveolus and eject milk into the reservoir called the lactiferous ducts. It is from these ducts that the infant, by sucking, gets milk through the nipple.

During pregnancy, high levels of estrogen and progesterone produced by the placenta inhibit milk secretion. After the expulsion of the placenta, there is an abrupt change in estrogen

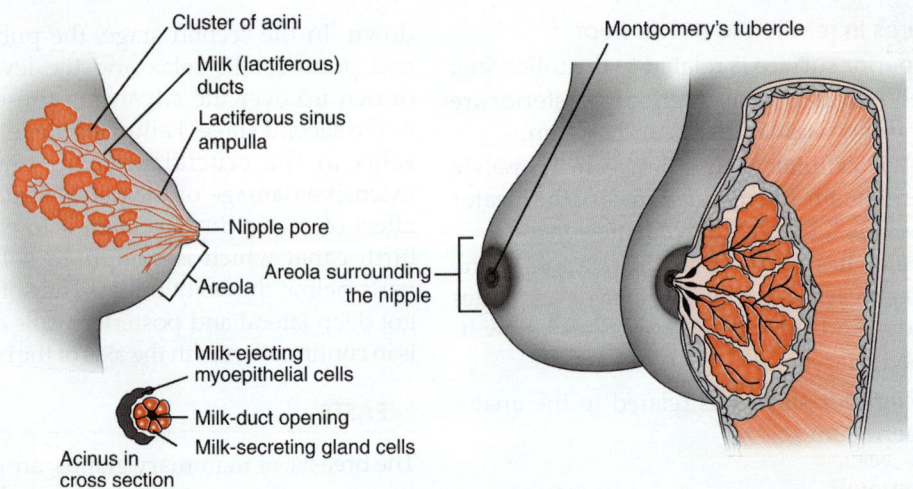

Cluster of acini
Milk (lactiferous) ducts
Lactiferous sinus ampulla
Nipple pore
Areola
Areola surrounding the nipple
Milk-ejecting myoepithelial cells
Milk-duct opening
Milk-secreting gland cells
Acinus in cross section
Montgomery's tubercle

Fig. 1.8: Position and anatomy of mammary glands and milk-producing structures

and progesterone levels. This allows a hormone called prolactin to be released from the anterior pituitary gland when the infant sucks. Prolactin stimulates the acini cells to produce milk. Infant sucking also affects the release of the hormone oxytocin from the posterior pituitary. Oxytocin stimulates the contraction of the myoepithelial cells, which causes the ejection of milk from the alveoli into the ductal system.

The size of the breasts depends on the amount of fatty tissue deposited in the breasts. Breast size does not indicate the amount of milk the breasts will produce.

Blood supply

Arterial supply
- Lateral thoracic branches of the axillary artery
- Internal mammary
- Inter costal arteries

Veins
The veins follow the courses of arteries.

Lymphatics
- *Lateral hemisphere*—anterior axillary nodes
- *Upper convexity*—infra clavicular group.
- *Medial convexity*—mediastinal glands (cross connection between the two breasts). There is no contralateral drainage of lymph, until and unless there is ipsilateral obstruction.
- *Inferior convexity*—mediastinal glands.

Nerve supply
The nerve supply is from fourth, fifth and sixth intercostal nerves.

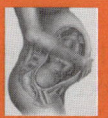

2

Fundamentals of Reproduction

OUTLINE

- Menstrual cycle
- Gametogenesis
- Ovulation
- Fertilization
- Development

MENSTRUAL CYCLE

NORMAL MENSTRUAL CYCLE

The menstrual cycle is a predictable event that normally occurs monthly. The typical menstrual cycle is influenced by follicle maturation, ovulation and corpus luteum formation and ends with menstrual bleeding. The changes that occur in the uterus depend on the changes occurring simultaneously in the ovaries. In this unique pattern of events, the development of endometrium, occurs at the precise time of the month that the ovum develops in maturity.

For understanding the physiology, the menstrual cycle may be divided into four phases, the menstrual phase, the proliferative phase, the secretory phase and the ischemic phase (Fig. 2.1).

The *menstrual phase* is the cyclic uterine bleeding after ovulation in response to cyclic changes. The first day of menstruation (menses) is the beginning of the menstrual cycle. Many of the endometrial cells are sloughed off and discarded and other cells of the endometrium begin to regenerate. The menstrual discharge is dark red and has a distinctive odor. Menstruation occurs when the ovum is not fertilized and begins *about 14 days after ovulation* in a 28 day cycle and lasts 3 to 5 days. Estrogen levels are low during this part of the cycle, and the cervical mucus is scanty, viscous and opaque.

The *proliferative phase* begins when the endometrial cells enlarge. Blood vessels become more prominent and dilated. The endometrium increases in thickness and gradually reaches its peak just before the time of ovulation. The cervical mucus is more prominent as the level of estrogen increases. The cervical mucus becomes thin, clear and alkaline, making the cervical mucosa more favourable to spermatozoa (i.e., enhancing sperm's motility). As ovulation nears, the mucus increases in elasticity, called *spinnbarkeit*. The mucus will stretch more and form a ferning pattern, which is a useful aid in determining the time of ovulation. The proliferative phase of the uterus coincides with the follicular phase of the ovarian cycle.

During the secretory phase some estrogen is secreted, but the phase is dominated by progesterone secretion. Progesterone causes the endometrial cells to become thicker, dilated and tortuous. The coiling of spiral arteries becomes intensified. The endometrial glands (cells) secrete fluids that contain an increased amount of glycogen in preparation for the fertilized ovum.

If fertilization of the ovum does not occur, the ischemic phase begins. The corpus luteum begins to degenerate, resulting in a fall in both estrogen and progesterone secretion. Vascular changes occur, including the rupture of small blood vessels and the constriction of spiral arteries, causing a deficiency of blood necessary for the endometrium. Small pools of blood soon form and break through the endometrial surfaces. This indicates the beginning of another menstrual phase (Table 2.1).

OVARIAN CYCLE

The ovarian cycle has two phases, the follicular phase and the luteal phase, in a 28-day cycle.

During the follicular phase (days 1 to 14), the development of the ovarian follicles occurs. The ovary is under the influence of the follicle stimulating hormone (FSH) and the luteinizing hormone (LH) secreted by the anterior pituitary gland. Their function is to stimulate ovarian follicles to grow, develop, and produce estrogen. Each month, one of the primordial follicles is activated by FSH and begins to grow and mature. Its cells produce a fluid (follicular fluid) high in estrogen content. The structure grows and propels itself toward the surface of the ovary as it continues to develop. At maturity, it is

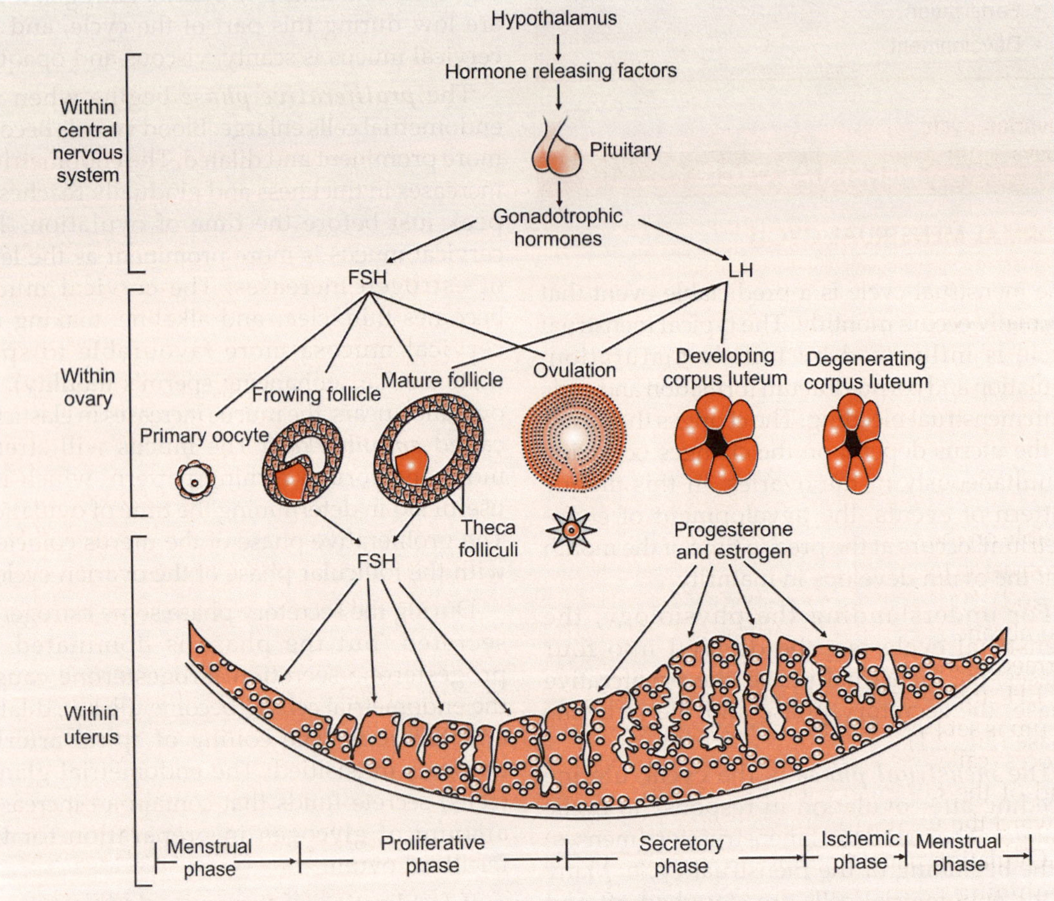

Fig. 2.1: Female reproductive cycle. (FSH - follicle stimulating hormone, LH - luteinizing hormone)

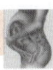

Table 2.1: Facts about the female reproductive cycle

Menstrual phase (days 1–5)	Endometrium is shed Estrogen levels are low Cervical mucus is scanty, viscous, and opaque
Proliferative phase (days 6–14)	Endometrium thickness increases Estrogen levels increase Cervical mucus at ovulation is thinner, watery, and alkaline. Cervical mucus increases in elasticity, called spinnbarkeit and shows ferning pattern. Cervical mucus is more favorable to sperm
Secretory phase (days 15–26)	Estrogen levels decrease and progesterone dominates Endometrial cells become thicker, dilated and tortuous Glycogen is secreted by endometrial glands in preparation for the fertilized ovum.
Ischemic phase (days 27–28)	Both estrogen and progesterone levels fall Spiral arteries undergo vasoconstriction, causing a deficiency of blood necessary for endometrium. Blood pools and escapes through the endometrial surfaces (beginning of next menstrual phase).
Ovarian cycle follicular phase (days 1–14)	Ovarian follicle (ovum) matures under the influence of two hormones: Follicle stimulating hormone (FSH) and luteinizing hormone (LH). In beginning, more than one follicle starts maturing; eventually one outgrows the other. Follicle(s) secretes estrogen, which accelerates maturation. Estrogen produced affects the uterine lining (endometrium). Ovulation occurs, with a surge of LH.
Luteal phase (days 15–28)	After the rupture of the follicle, the ovum leaves; corpus luteum develops under LH influence and produces high levels of estrogen and progesterone. Increased estrogen and progesterone levels suppress the growth of other follicles.

visible on the surface of the ovary as a blisterlike protrusion (approximately the, size of a printed period). At this stage of maturity, the follicular membrane surrounding the ovum and fluid is termed a Graafian follicle. Following an upsurge of LH, the Graafian follicle ruptures and the ovum is set free from the surface of the ovary, a process called ovulation. It is swept into the open end of the fallopian tube to begin its journey toward the uterus for implantation (nidation).

Ovulation usually occurs 14 days before the beginning of the next menstrual cycle. The timing of ovulation is important because the ovum must be fertilized by a sperm within the fertile time. Ova are considered to be fertile for about 24 hours after ovulation (Fig. 2.2). Sperm may survive for up to 72 hours.

The luteal phase (days 15 to 28) begins at about day 15 of the cycle. After the rupture of the graafian follicle and the release of the ovum, the cells of the empty follicle become larger and fill with the corpus luteum. Under the influence of LH, the corpus luteum begins to produce increased amounts of estrogen and progesterone. The increased progesterone level suppresses the growth of other follicles in the ovary.

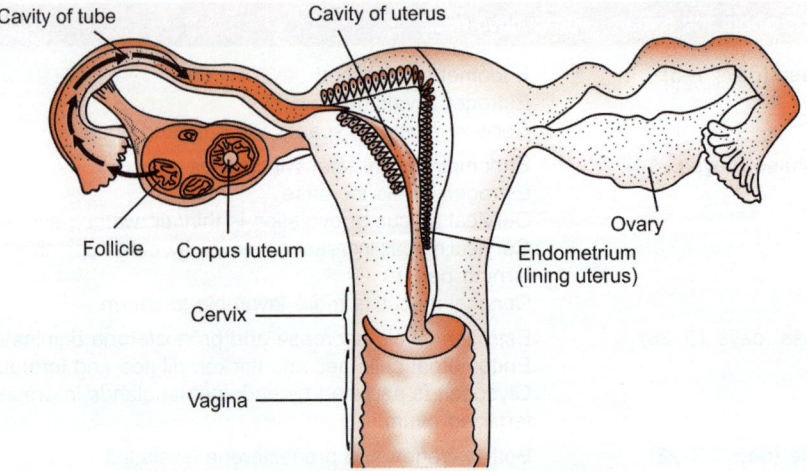

Fig. 2.2: Ovulation: release of the ovum from the follicle

MENSTRUAL CYCLE (Refer Table 2.1)

If fertilization of the ovum does not occur, the size of the corpus luteum decreases. At this time, the LH level becomes so low that it can no longer support the corpus luteum. As the corpus luteum degenerates, its secretion of estrogen and progesterone rapidly decreases. As a result, the endometrium (lining of the uterus) starts to shed, menstrual flow starts and a new cycle begins.

Structure of mature ovum

A fully mature ovum is the largest cell in the body and is about 130 microns in diameter. It consists of cytoplasm and a nucleus with its nucleolus which is eccentric in position and contains 23 chromosomes (23 X). During fertilization, the nucleus is converted into a female pronucleus. The ovum is surrounded by a cell membrane called *vitelline membrane.*

There is an outer transparent envelope the *zona pellucida.* The zona pellucida is penetrated by tiny channels which are thought *to be important for the transport of the materials from the granulosa cells to the oocyte.* In between the vitelline membrane and the zona pellucida, there is a narrow space called

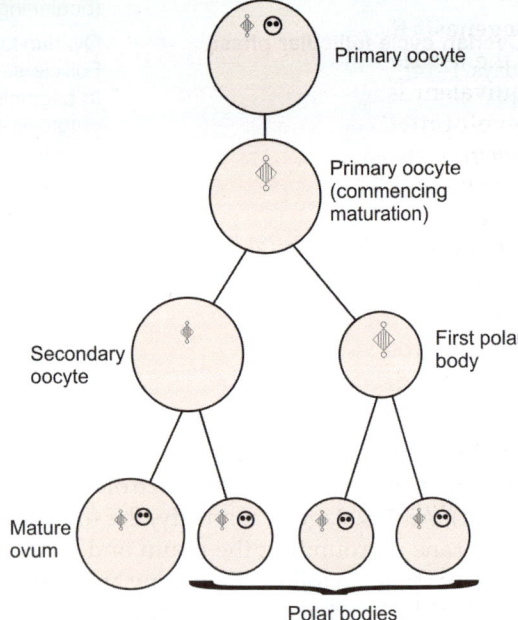

Fig. 2.3: Diagram showing the reduction in number of the *chromosomes* in the process of maturation of the *ovum*

perivitelline space, which accommodates the *polar bodies.* The human oocyte after its escape from the follicle retains a covering of granulosa cells known as the *corona radiata* (Fig. 2.4).

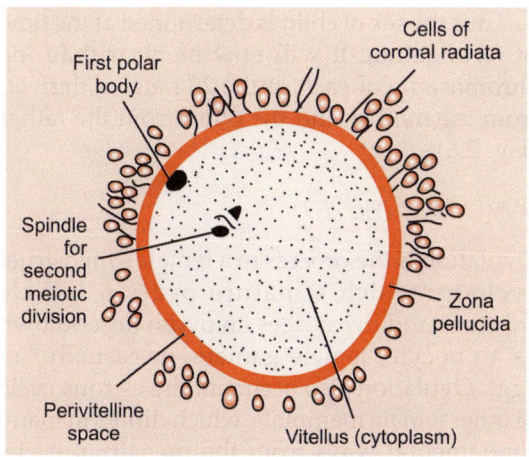

Fig. 2.4: Structure of the ovum at the time of ovulation

HUMAN OOGENESIS

Oogenesis the creation of an *ovum* (egg cell). It is the female form of *gametogenesis*. The male equivalent is *spermatogenesis*. It involves the development of the various stages of the *immature ovum*.

At the start of the menstrual cycle, some 12–20 primary follicles begin to develop under the influence of elevated *FSH* to form secondary follicles. The primary follicles have formed from primordial follicles, which developed in the ovary at around 10–30 weeks after conception. By around day 9 of the cycle, only one healthy secondary follicle remains, with the rest having undergone *cellular atresia*. The remaining follicle is called the dominant follicle and is responsible for producing large amounts of *oestradiol* during the late follicular phase. Oestradiol production depends upon co-operation between the *theca* and *granulosa cells*. On day 14 of the cycle, an *LH surge* occurs, which itself is triggered by the positive feedback of oestradiol. This causes the secondary follicle to develop into a tertiary follicle, which then ovulates some 24–36 hours later. An important event in the development of the tertiary follicle occurs when the primary oocyte completes the first meiotic division, resulting in the formation of a *polar body* and a secondary oocyte. The empty follicle then forms a *corpus luteum*.

Oocytogenesis

Oogenesis starts with the process of developing *oogonia*, which occurs via the transformation of *primordial follicles* into primary *oocytes*, a process called *oocytogenesis*. Oocytogenesis is complete either before or shortly after birth.

Structure of mature spermatozoon

The spermatozoon has a head, a neck, a middle piece and a principal piece or tail (Fig. 2.5). An axial filament passes through the middle piece and extends into the tail.

The head of the human spermatozoan is covered by a cap like structure called the acrosomic cap.

The neck is narrow and it contains a funnel shaped basal body and a spherical centriole.

The axial filament begins just behind the centriole. It passes through the middle piece and most of the tail.

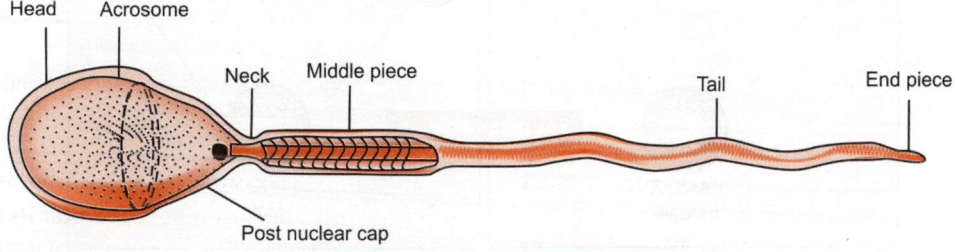

Fig. 2.5: Structure of a mature spermatozoon

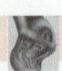

Spermatogenesis is the process by which male primary germ cells undergo division, and produce a number of cells termed spermatogonia, from which the primary spermatocytes are derived. Each primary spermatocyte divides into two secondary spermatocytes, and each secondary spermatocyte into two spermatids or young spermatozoa. These develop into mature spermatozoa, also known as sperm cells. Thus, the primary spermatocyte gives rise to two cells, the secondary spermatocytes, and the two secondary spermatocytes by their subdivision produce four spermatozoa.

Spermatozoa are the mature male gametes in many sexually reproducing organisms. Thus, spermatogenesis is the male version of gametogenesis.

Sex determination

However, we have seen that spermatozoa are of two types. Half of them have 22 + X chromosomes and the other half of them have 22 + Y chromosomes. We speak of these as 'X-bearing' or 'Y-bearing' spermatozoa. An ovum can be fertilized by either type of spermatozoon. If the sperm is X-bearing, the zygote has 44 + X + X chromosomes and the offspring is a girl (Fig. 2.6). If the sperm is Y-bearing, the zygote has 44 + X + Y chromosomes and the offspring is a boy.

Thus the sex of child is determined at the time of fertilization. It will now be clear that one chromosome of each of the 23 pairs is derived from the mother and the other from the father (Fig. 2.6).

OVULATION (Fig. 2.7)

Ovulation is the process in a female's menstrual cycle by which a mature ovarian follicle ruptures and discharges an ovum (also known as an oocyte, female gamete, or casually, an egg). Ovulation also occurs in the estrous cycle of other female mammals, which differs in many fundamental ways from the menstrual cycle. The time immediately surrounding ovulation is referred to as the ovulatory phase or the periovulatory period

Ovulation is the release of a single, mature egg from a follicle that developed in the ovary. It usually occurs regularly, around day 14 of a 28-day menstrual cycle. Once released, the egg is capable of being fertilized for 12 to 48 hours before it begins to disintegrate. Although there are several days of the month in which a woman is fertile, she is most fertile during the days around ovulation.

Ovulation occurs when a mature egg is released from the ovary into the abdominal cavity.

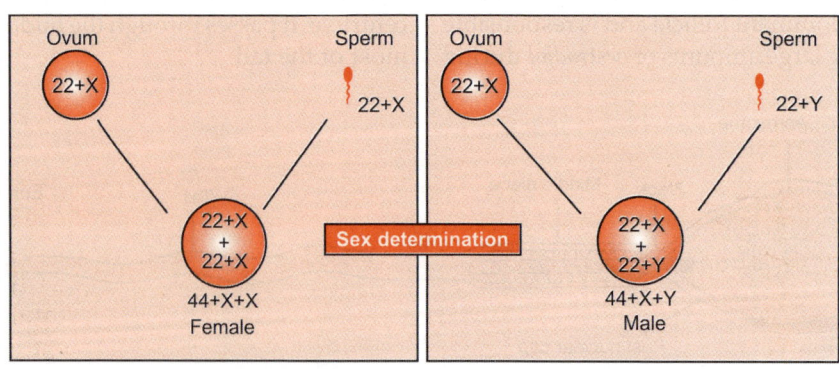

Fig. 2.6: Scheme to show how the sex of the child is determinated

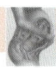

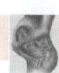

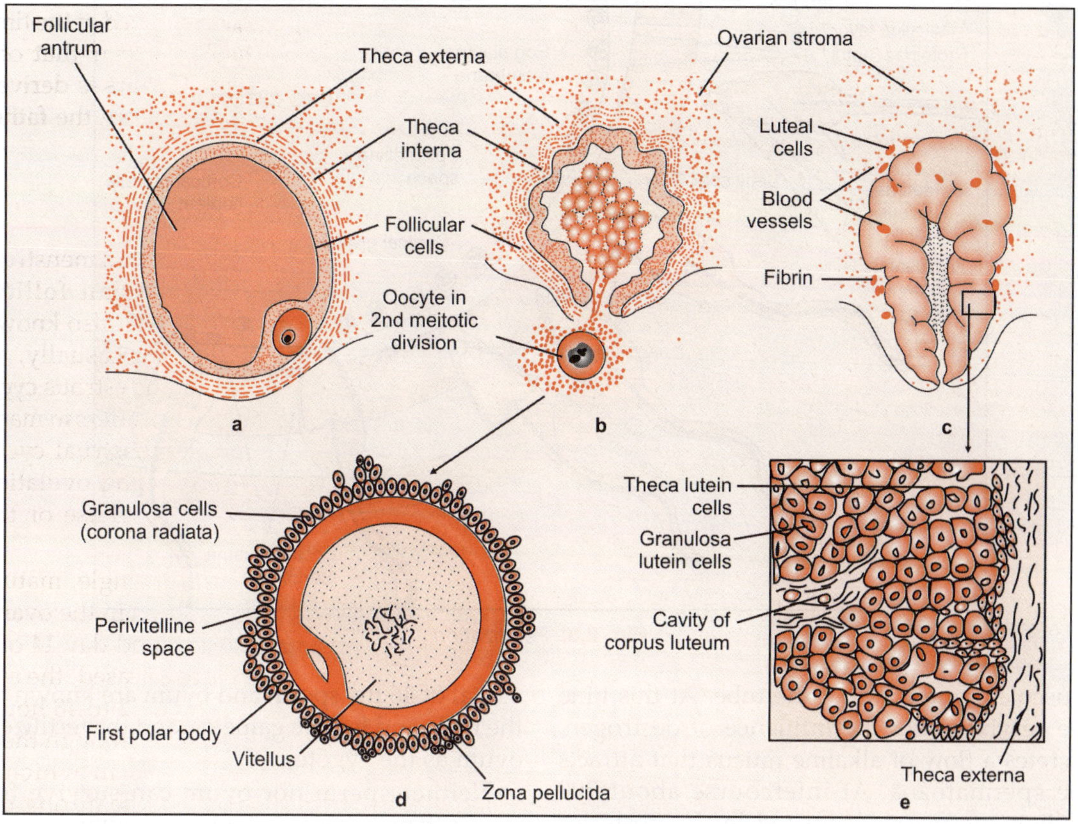

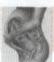

Fig. 2.7: Schematic diagram showing: **a.** Mature Graafian follicle on the verge of ovulation, **b.** Ovulation with discharge of secondary oocyte surrounded by cumulus oophorus, **c.** Formation of corpus luteum, **d.** Secondary oocyte after first maturation division with formation of first polar body, **e.** Microscopic structure of corpus luteum

The process of ovulation is controlled by the hypothalamus of the brain and through the release of hormones secreted in the anterior lobe of the pituitary gland, luteinizing hormone (LH) and follicle stimulating hormone (FSH). In the pre-ovulatory phase of the menstrual cycle, the ovarian follicle will undergo a series of transformations called cumulus expansion, which is stimulated by FSH. After this is done, a hole called the stigma will form in the follicle, and the ovum will leave the follicle through this hole. Ovulation is triggered by a spike in the amount of FSH and LH released from the pituitary gland. During the luteal (post-ovulatory) phase, the ovum will travel through the fallopian tubestoward the uterus. If fertilized by a sperm, it may perform implantation there 6–12 days later.

FERTILIZATION (Fig. 2.8)

Following ovulation, the ovum, which is about 0.15 mm in diameter, passes into the uterine tube and is moved along towards the uterus. The ovum, having no power of locomotion, is wafted along by the cilia and by the peristaltic

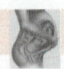

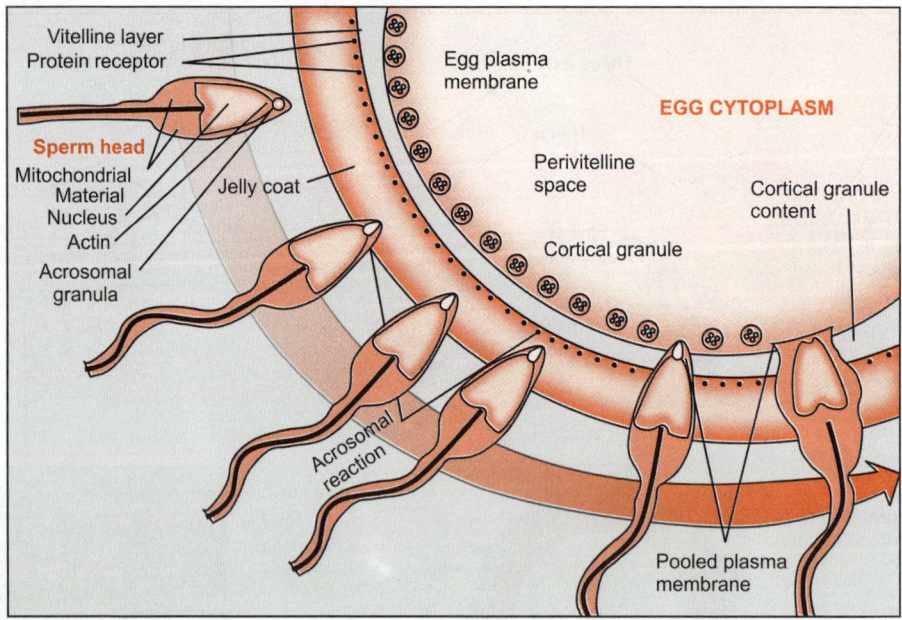

Fig. 2.8: Fertilization

muscular contraction of the tube. At this time the cervix, under the influence of oestrogen, secretes a flow of alkaline mucus that attracts the spermatozoa. At intercourse about 300 million sperm are deposited in the posterior fornix of the vagina. Those that reach the loose cervical mucus survive to propel themselves towards the uterine tubes while the reminder are destroyed by the acid medium of the vagina. More will die on the journey through the uterus and only thousands reach the uterine tube where they meet the ovum, usually in the ampulla. It is only during this journey that the sperm finally become mature and capable of releasing the enzyme hyaluronidase, which allows penetration of the zona pellucida and the cell membrane surrounding the ovum. Many sperm are needed for this to take place but only one will enter the ovum. After this, the membrane is sealed to prevent entry of any further sperm and the nuclei of the two cells fuse. The sperm and the ovum each contribute half the complement of chromosomes to make

a total of 46 the sperm and ovum are known as the male and female gametes, and the fertilized ovum as the zygote.

Neither sperm nor ovum can survive for longer than 2 or 3 days and fertilization is most likely to occur when intercourse takes place not more than 48 hours before or 24 hours after ovulation. It therefore follows that conception will take place about 14 days before the next period is due.

Development of the fertilized ovum

When the ovum has been fertilized, it continues its passage through the uterine tube and reaches the uterus 3 or 4 days later. During this time segmentation or cell division takes place and the fertilized ovum divides into 2 cells, then into 4, then 8, 16 and so on until a cluster of cells is formed known as the **morula** (mulberry). These divisions occur quite slowly, about once every 12 hours. Next, a fluid cavity, or blastocele, appears in the morula, which now becomes known as the **blastocyst.** Around the outside

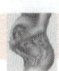

Table 2.2: Morula and Implantation

Morula

A morula (Latin, morus: mulberry) is an embryo at an early stage of embryonic development, consisting of cells (called blastomeres) in a solid ball contained within the zona pellucida.

The morula is produced by embryonic cleavage, the rapid division of the zygote. Once the zygote has divided into 32 cells, it begins to resemble a mulberry, hence the name morula (Latin, morus: mulberry). Within a few days after fertilization, cells on the outer part of the morula become bound tightly together. This process is known as compaction. The cells of the morula then secrete a viscous liquid, causing a central cavity to be formed, forming a hollow ball of cells known as the blastocyst.

Implantation

Implantation (human embryo), an event that occurs early in human pregnancy in which the human embryo adheres to the wall of the uterus

Table 2.3: Important events following fertilization

0 hour	–	Fertilization
30 hours	–	2 cell stage (blastomeres)
40–50 hours	–	4 cell stage
72 hours	–	12 cell stage
96 hours	–	16 cell stage, morula enters the uterine cavity
5th day	–	Blastocyst
6–7th day	–	Zona pellucida disappears, interstitial implantation occurs.
9th day	–	Lacunar period, endometrial vessels-tapped.
10–11th day	–	Implantation completed
13th day	–	Primary villi
16th day	–	Secondary villi
21st day	–	Tertiary villi
21–22nd day	–	Fetal heart, fetoplacental circulation

of the blastocyst there is a single layer of cells known as the trophoblast; the remaining cells are clumped together at one end forming the inner cell mass. The trophoblast will form the placenta and chorian, while the inner cell mass will become the fetus, amnion and umbilical cord. On its journey, the ovum is nourished by glycogen from the goblet cells of the uterine tubes and later the secretory glands of the uterus.

When the blastocyst first tumbles into the uterus, it lies free for 2 or 3 more days. The trophoblast, especially the part which lies over the inner cell mass, then becomes quite sticky and adheres to the endometrium. It begins to secrete substances that digest the endometrial cells, allowing the blastocyst to become embedded in the endometrium. Embedding, sometimes known as nidation (nesting), is normally complete by the 11th day after ovulation and the endometrium closes over it completely, the only evidence of the presence of the blastocyst being a small bulge on the surface.

DEVELOPMENT OF PLACENTA

The process of implantation is supported by proteolytic enzymes produced by the trophoblast. The uterine mucosa also aids the process.

In some animals like rabbit, cow, dog, monkey, etc., the blastocyst remains in the uterine cavity. This is called central implantation. In others (e.g. rat), the blastocyst comes to lie in a uterine crypt or recess. This is called *eccentric implantation*.

DECIDUA

After the implantation of the embryo, the uterine endometrium is called the *decidua.* When the morula reaches the uterus, the endometrium is in the secretory phase. The stromal cells enlarge, become vacuolated, and store glycogen and lipids. This change in the stromal cells is called the *decidual reaction.*

The portion of the decidua where the placenta is to be formed (i.e. deep to the developing blastocyst) is called the *decidua basalis* (Fig. 2.9). The part of the decidua that separates the embryo from the uterine lumen is called the *decidua capsularis*, while the part lining the rest of the uterine cavity is called the *decidua parietalis.* The decidua basalis consists predominantly of large decidual cells which contain large amounts of lipids and glycogen (that presumably provide a source of nutrition for the embryo). The decidua basalis is also referred to as the decidual plate, and is firmly united to the chorion.

At the end of pregnancy, the decidua is shed off, along with the placenta and membranes.

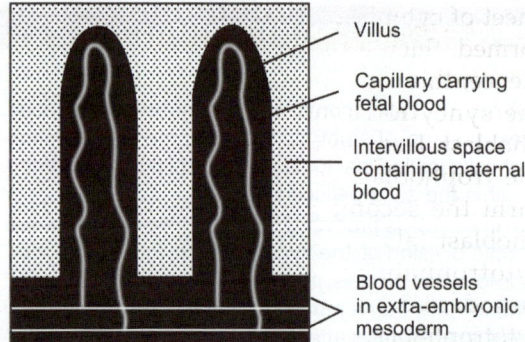

Fig. 2.10: Scheme to show that fetal blood circulating through capillaries of villi is in close relation to maternal blood in the transverse space

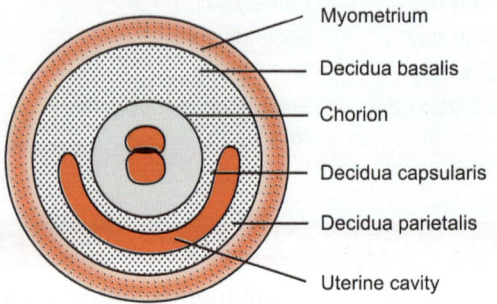

Fig. 2.9: Subdivisions of decidua

FORMATION OF CHORIONIC VILLI

The essential functional elements of the placenta are very small finger-like process or villi. These villi are surrounded by maternal blood. In the substance of the villi, there are capillaries through which the fetal blood circulates. Exchanges between the maternal and fetal circulations take place through the tissues forming the walls of the villi (Fig. 2.10).

The villi are formed as off shoots from the surface of trophoblast, along with the underlying extra-embryonic mesoderm, constitutes the chorion (the villi), the arising from it, are called chorionic villi.

The chorionic villi are first formed all over the trophoblast and grow into the surrounding decidua (Fig. 2.11). Those related to the decidua

capsularis are transitory. After sometime they degenerate. This part of the chorion becomes smooth and is called the *chorion laevae*.

The part of the chorion that helps form the placenta is called the *chorion frondosum*.

The essential features of the formation of chorionic villi are as follows:

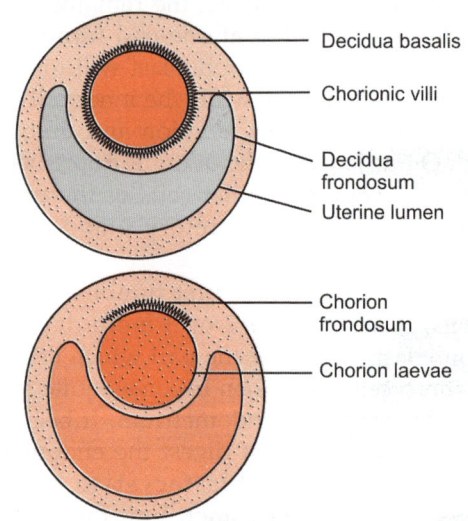

Fig. 2.11: Two stages in the formation of chorionic villi

The trophoblast is at first made up of a single layer of cells (Fig. 2.12). As these cells multiply, two distinct layers are formed. One continuous

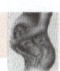

sheet of cytoplasm containing many nuclei is formed. Such a tissue is called a syncytium. Hence, this layer of the trophoblast is called the syncytiotrophoblast or plasmodiotrophoblast. Deep to the syncytium, the cells of the trophoblast retain their cell walls and form the second layer called the cytotrophoblast (also called Langhan's layer). The cytotrophoblast rests on extra-embryonic mesoderm. All these elements (syncytium, cytotrophoblast and mesoderm) take part in forming chorionic villi.

Details of the process of villus formation are as follows:

1. The syncytiotrophoblast grows rapidly and becomes thick. Small cavities called *lacunae* appear in this layer (Fig. 2.12c). Gradually, the lacunae increase in size. At first they are irregularly arranged (Fig. 2.12d), but

gradually they come to lie radially around the blastocyst. The lacunae are separated from one another by partitions of syncytium, which are called *trabeculae*. The lacunae gradually communicate with each other, so that eventually one large space is formed. Each trabeculas is now surrounded all round by this lacunar space (Fig. 2.13).

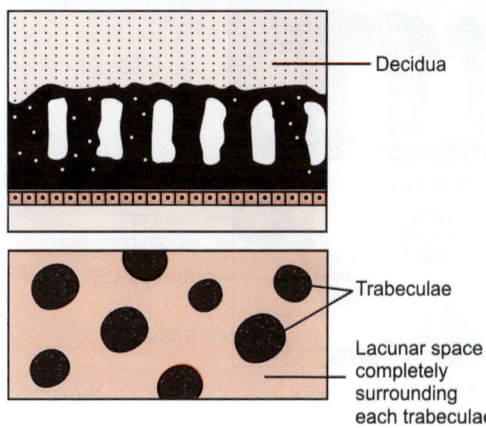

Fig. 2.13: Formation of chorionic villi

2. The syncytiotrophoblast (in which these changes are occurring) grows into the endometrium. As the endometrium is eroded, some of its blood vessels are opened up and blood from them fills the lacunar space (Fig. 2.14).

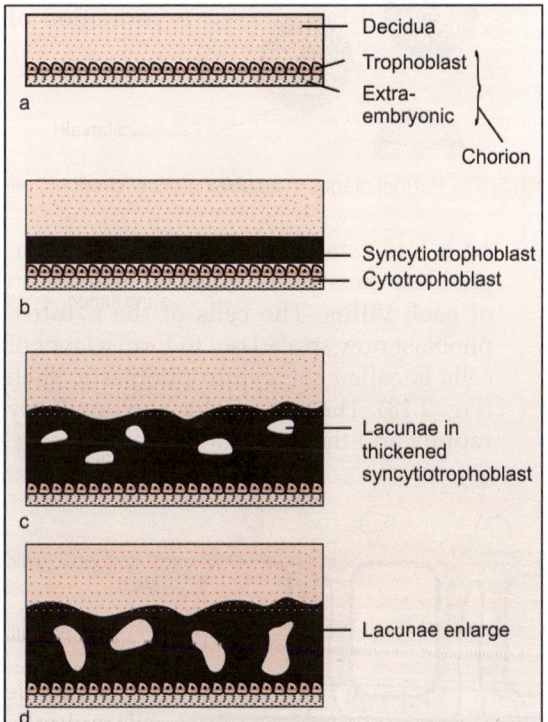

Fig. 2.12: Early stages in formation of chorionic villi

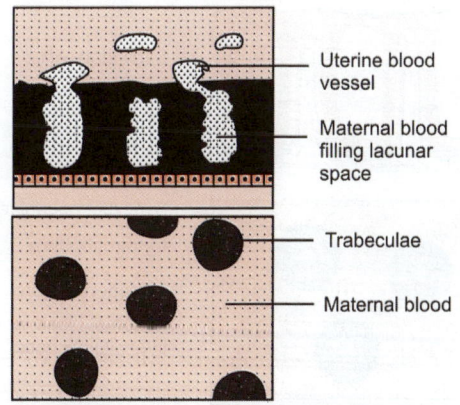

Fig. 2.14: Further stages in establishment of chorionic villi

3. Each trabeculas is, initially made up entirely of syncytiotrophoblast. Now the cells of the cytotrophoblast begin to multiply ad grow into each trabeculas. The trabeculas is now called a primary villus (Fig. 2.15) and the lacunar space is now called the *intervillous space*.

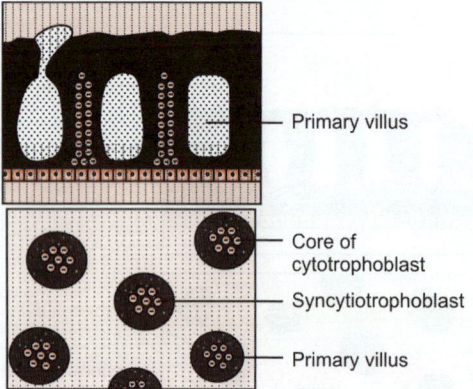

— Primary villus

— Core of cytotrophoblast

— Syncytiotrophoblast

— Primary villus

Fig. 2.15: Further stages in establishment of chorionic villi

4. Extra-embryonic mesoderm invades the centre of each primary villus (Fig. 2.16). This structure is called a *secondary villus.*
5. Soon thereafter, blood vessels can be seen in the mesoderm forming the core of each

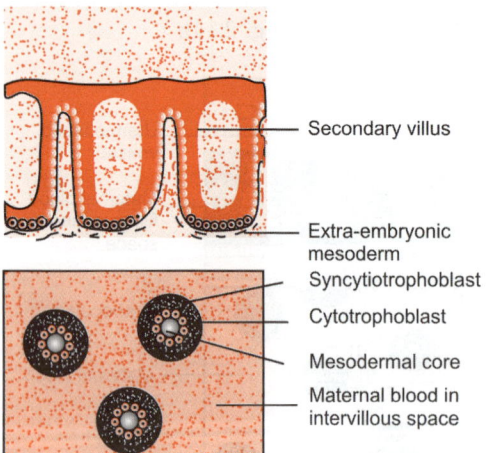

— Secondary villus

— Extra-embryonic mesoderm
— Syncytiotrophoblast

— Cytotrophoblast

— Mesodermal core
— Maternal blood in intervillous space

Fig. 2.16: Further stages in establishment of chorionic villi

villus. With their appearance, the villus is fully formed and is called a tertiary villus (Fig. 2.17). The blood vessels of the villus establish connections with the circulatory system of the embryo. Fetal blood now circulates through the villi, while maternal blood circulates through the intervillous space.

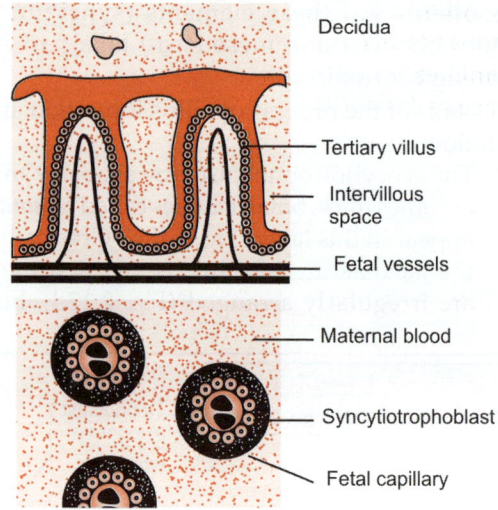

Decidua

— Tertiary villus

— Intervillous space

— Fetal vessels

— Maternal blood

— Syncytiotrophoblast

— Fetal capillary

Fig. 2.17: Further stages in establishment of chorionic villi

6. At a later stage, however, the cytotrophoblast emerges through the syncytium of each villus. The cells of the cytotrophoblast now spread out to form a layer of cells is called the cytotrophoblastic shell (Fig. 2.18). The cells of this shell multiply rapidly and the placenta increases in size.

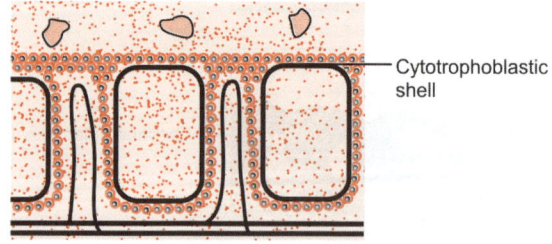

—Cytotrophoblastic shell

Fig. 2.18: Formation of cytotrophoblastic shell

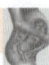

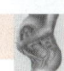

The villi that are first formed (as described above) are attached on the fetal side (Fig. 2.19) to the embryonic mesoderm and on the maternal side to the cytotrophoblastic shell. They are, therefore, called anchoring villi. Each anchoring villus consists of a stem (**truncus chorii**); this divides into a number of branches (**rami chorii**) which in turn divide into finer branches (**ramuli chorii**). The ramuli are attached to the cytotrophoblastic shell. The anchoring villi give off numerous branches which grow into the intervillous space as free villi.

FURTHER DEVELOPMENT OF THE PLACENTA

The placenta now becomes subdivided into a number of lobes, by septa that grow into the intervillous space from the maternal side (Fig. 2.20). Each such lobe of the placenta is often called a **maternal cotyledon.** These lobes generally number 15 to 20. Each lobe contains a number of anchoring villi and their branches. One such villus and its branches constitute a fetal cotyledon. The fully formed placenta has 60 to 100 such fetal cotyledons. The placenta now forms a compact mass and is disc-shaped (Fig. 2.21).

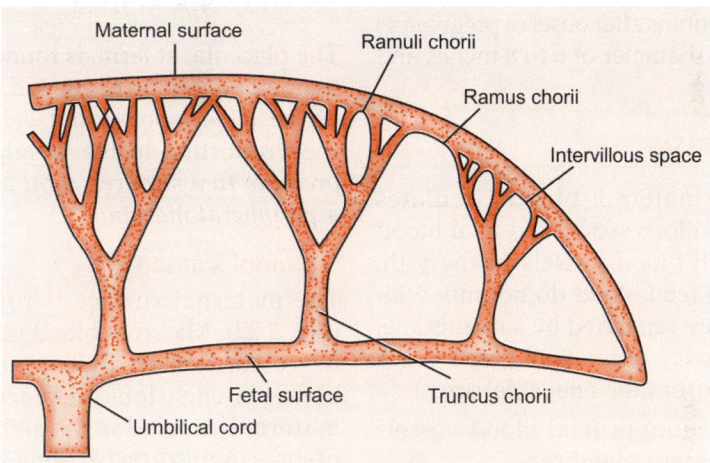

Fig. 2.19: Arrangement of anchoring villi and intervillous space within the placenta

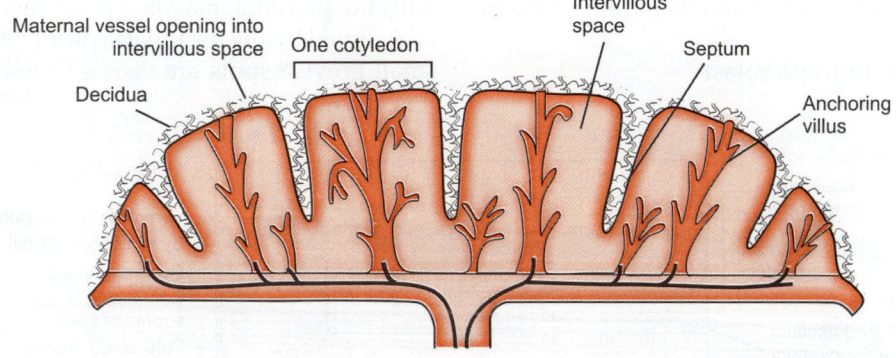

Fig. 2.20: Structure of a fully formed placenta. Each lobe (labelled cotyledon) contains a number of anchoring villi but only one is shown here for the sake of simplicity

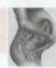

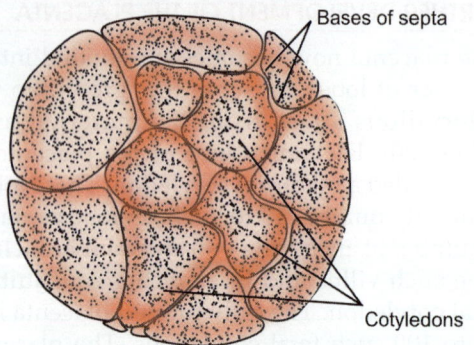

Fig. 2.21: Placenta after shedding, viewed from the maternal aspect

At full term (9 months after onset of pregnancy) the placenta has a diameter of 6 to 8 inches and weighs about 500 g.

PLACENTAL MEMBRANE

In the placenta, maternal blood circulates through the intervillous space, and fetal blood circulates through blood vessels in the villi. The maternal and fetal blood do not mix with each other. They are separated by a membrane, made up of the layers of the wall of the villus (Fig. 2.22). These (from the fetal side) are:

- The endothelium of fetal blood vessels and its basement membrane.
- Surrounding mesoderm (connective tissue)
- Cytotrophoblast and its basement membrane.
- Syncytiotrophoblast

These structures constitute the *placental membrane or barrier.*

THE PLACENTA AND FETAL MEMBRANES

Development of placenta is completed by 12th week. Until the end of the 16th week, the placenta grows both in thickness and circumference due to growth of the chorionic villi with accompanying expansion of the intervillous space. Subsequently, there is little increase in thickness but it increases circumferentially till term.

THE PLACENTA AT TERM

The placenta, at term, is round flat mass with a diameter of about 20 cm and 2.5 cm thick at its centre. It feels spongy and weighs about 500 gm, the proportion to the weight of the baby. *It presents two surfaces, fetal and maternal, and a peripheral margin.*

Maternal surface

The maternal surface is rough and spongy (Fig. 2.23). Maternal blood gives it a dull dark red colour. It is sub divided into number of lobes by septa each lobe of placenta is called as maternal cotyledons which are limited by fissures. A thin greyish, somewhat shaggy layer which is the *remnant of the decidua basalis* (compact and spongy layer) and has come away with the placenta, may be visible. Each fissure is occupied by the decidual septum. Numerous small greyish spots are visible. These are due

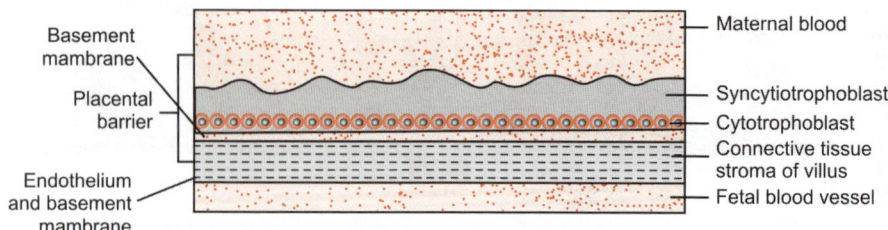

Fig. 2.22: Schematic diagram showing layers of placental barrier

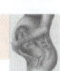

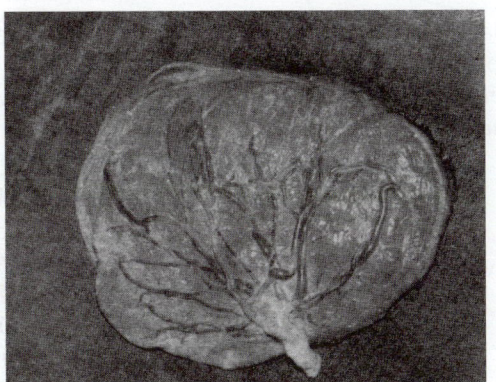

Fig. 2.23: Fetal surface of the placenta showing attachment of the umbilical cord with ramification of the umbilical vessels

to deposition of calcium in the degenerated areas and are of no clinical significance. The maternal portion of the placenta amounts to less than one fifth of the total placenta. *Only the decidua basalis and the blood in the inter-villous space are of maternal origin.*

Fetal surface

The fetal surface is covered by the smooth and glistening amnion with the umbilical cord attached at or near its centre. Branches of the umbilical vessel's are visible beneath the amnion as they radiate from the insertion off the cord (Fig. 2.24). The amnion can be peeled of from the underlying chorion except at the insertion

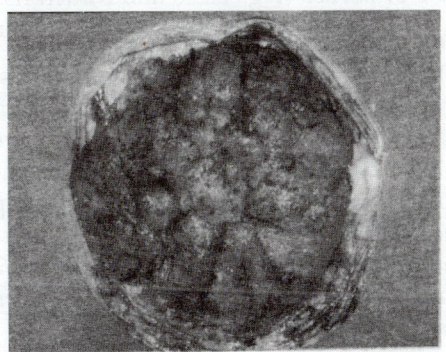

Fig. 2.24: Maternal surface of the placenta showing shaggy look with cotyledons limited by fissures

of the cord. *At term, about four-fifths of* the placenta is of fetal origin.

Margin

Peripheral margin of the placenta is limited by the fused basal and chorionic plates and is continuous with the chorion laeve and amnion.

Attachment

The placenta is usually attached to the upper part of the body of the uterus encroaching to the fundus adjacent to the anterior or posterior wall with equal frequency. *The attachment to the uterine wall is effective due to* anchoring villi.

SEPARATION

Placenta separates after the birth of the baby and *the line of separation is through the decidua spongiosum.*

Placental function

1. Transfer of nutrients and waste products between the mother and fetus. In this respect it attributes to the following functions:
   - Respiratory
   - Excretory
   - Nutritive
   - Endocrine
2. Produces or metabolises the hormones and enzymes necessary to maintain the pregnancy
3. Barrier function
4. Immunological function

Foetal respiratory function

By simple diffusion across placental membrane, oxygen goes to foetal circulation (at a rate of 5ml/kg/min) from maternal sinus and carbon dioxide diffuses out.

Foetal excretory function

Placenta acts as a foetal kidney by excreting small amounts of creatinine, urea, uric acid.

Nutritive function

The fetus obtains its nutrients from the maternal blood and when the diet is

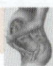

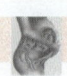

inadequate, then only, depletion of maternal tissue storage occurs. Thus, to avoid maternal tissue storage depletion, a diet rich in essential foods is needed during pregnancy. Foetus require amino acid for building tissue, glucose, lipids, calcium, phosphorus, vitamin, water, electrolyte are transferred through the maternal sinus to fetal circulation.

Endocrine function

Insulin, steroids from the adrenals, thyroid, chorionic gonadotrophin or placental lactogen cross the placenta at a very slow rate, so that their concentration in fetal plasma are appreciably lower than in maternal plasma. Neither parathormone nor calcitonin crosses the placenta.

Enzymatic function

Numerous enzymes are elaborated in the placenta, mentioning only few of them are:
- Diamine oxidase which inactivates the circulatory pressure (or pressor) amines
- Oxytocinase which neutralises the oxytocin
- Phospholipase A which synthesises arachidonic acid, etc.

Barrier function

Fetal membrane has long been considered as a protective barrier to the fetus against noxious agents circulating in the maternal blood.

Maternal infection during pregnancy by virus (rubella, chicken pox, measles, mumps, poliomyelitis), bacteria (*Treponema pallidum, Tubercle bacillus*) or protozoa (*Toxoplasma gondii*, malaria parasites) may be transmitted to the fetus across the so called alleged placental barrier and affect the fetus in utero. Similarly, *almost any drug used in pregnancy can cross the placental barrier and may have deleterious effect on the fetus.*

Immunological function

The fetus and the placenta contain paternally determined antigens, foreign to the mother but fails to inherit all the mother's antigens. In spite of this, there is no evidence of graft rejection.

Placenta probably offers immunological protection against rejection. *The exact mechanism is yet speculative but the interest has centered on the following:*
- Fibrinoid and sialomucin coating of trophoblast may suppress the trophoblastic antigen.
- Placental hormones, proteins steroids and chorionic gonadotrophin, although have got weak immunosuppressive effect, may be responsible for producing sialomucin.
- Nitabuch's layer which intervenes between the decidua basalis and the cytotrophoblast probably inactivates the antigenic property of the tissue.

THE FETAL MEMBRANES

It consists of two layers—*outer chorion and the inner amnion.*

Chorion

It is thicker than amnion, friable and shaggy on both the sides. Internally, it is attached to the amnion by loose areolar tissue and remnant of primitive mesenchyme. Externally, it is covered by vestiges of trophoblastic layer and the decidual cells of the fused decidua capsularis and parietalis which can be distinguished microscopically. *The term chorion contains no vessels or nerves* (Figs 2.25a and b).

Amnion

It is the inner layer of the fetal membranes. Its internal surface is smooth and shiny and is in contact with liquor amnii. The outer surface consists of a layer of connective tissue and is apposed to the similar tissue on the inner aspect of the chorion from which it can be peeled off. *The amnion can also be peeled off from the fetal surface of the placenta except at the insertion of the umbilical cord.*

Functions

1. Contribute to the formation of liquor amnii.

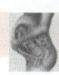

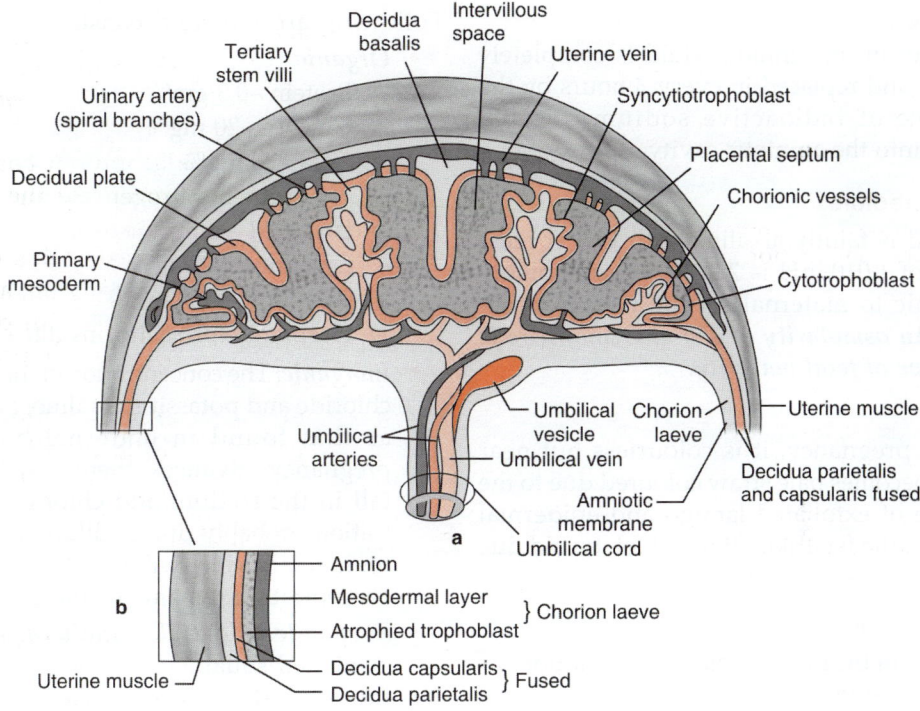

Fig. 2.25: Schematic view of **a.** Structure of placenta at term **b.** Structure of the membranes in relation to decidua

2. Intact membranes prevent ascending uterine infection.
3. Facilitate dilatation of the cervix during labour.
4. Has got enzymatic activities for steroid hormonal metabolism.
5. Rich source of glycerophospholipids containing arachidonic acid precursor of prostaglandin F_2 and $F_{2\alpha}$.

AMNIOTIC FLUID

It is a colourless fluid in early pregnancy and at term it becomes clear pale or straw colour in which fetus flots.

Amniotic fluid origin

- As a transudate from the maternal serum across the fetal membranes or from maternal circulation in the placenta.
- As a transudate across the umbilical cord or from fetal circulation in the placenta or secretion from the amniotic epithelium.
- Contribution from the fetal urine: *The fetus drinks about 400 ml of liquor every day at term* and equal amount is excreted in the urine.
- Secretion from the tracheobronchial tree and across the fetal skin before the skin becomes keratinised at 20th week.

Volume

Amniotic fluid measures about 30 ml at 10 weeks, 300 ml at 20 weeks, 600 ml at 30 weeks, 1000 ml at 38 weeks, 800 ml at 40 weeks, 200 ml at 42 weeks.

 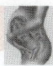

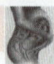

Circulation

The water in the amniotic fluid is completely changed and replaced in every 3 hours by the clearance of radioactive sodium injected directly into the amniotic cavity.

Physical features

The fluid is faintly alkaline with low specific gravity of 1.010, pH is 7.2. It becomes highly hypotonic to maternal serum at term pregnancy. *An osmolarity of 250 m Osmol/litre is suggestive of fetal maturity.*

Colour

In early pregnancy, it is colourless but near term, it becomes pale straw coloured due to the presence of exfoliated lanugo and epidermal cells from the fetal skin. It may look turbid due to the presence of vernix caseosa.

Abnormal colour

Deviation of the normal colour of the liquor has got clinical significance.

- *Meconium stained (green)* is suggestive of fetal distress in presentations other than the breech or transverse. Depending upon the degree and duration of the distress, it may be thin or thick or pea souped (thick with flakes). Thick with presence of flakes suggests chronic fetal distress.

- *Golden colour* in Rh incompatibility is due to excessive haemolysis of the fetal RBC and production of excess bilirubin.

- *Greenish yellow (saffron)* in post maturity.

- *Dark coloured* in concealed accidental hemorrhage is due to contamination of blood.

- *Dark brown (tobacco juice)* amniotic fluid is found in I.U.D.

Composition

The composition includes:
1. Water 98–99%
2. Solid (1–2%)

Following are the solid constituents:

- *Organic*
  - Protein –0.3 gm%
  - Glucose –20 mg%
  - Urea –30 mg%
  - Non-protein nitrogen –30 mg%
  - Uric acid –4 mg%
  - Creatinine –2 mg%
  - Total lipids –50 mg%
  - Hormones (prolactin, insulin and renin)

- *Inorganic:* The concentration of the sodium, chloride and potassium is almost the same as that found in maternal blood. As pregnancy advances, there may be slight fall in the sodium and chloride concentration probably due to dilution by hypotonic fetal urine, whereas the potassium concentration remains unaltered.

- *Suspended particles include:* Lanugo, exfoliated squamous epithelial cells from the fetal skin, vernix caseosa, cast off amniotic cells and cells from the respiratory tract, urinary bladder and vagina of the fetus.

Functions

Its main function is protective to the fetus.

During pregnancy

1. It acts as a shock absorber, to protect fetus from injury.
2. Maintains an even temperature
3. The fluid distends the amniotic sac and thereby allows for growth and free movement of the fetus and prevents adhesion between the fetal parts and amniotic sac.
4. Its nutritive value is negligible because of small amount of protein and salt content.

During labour

1. The amnion and chorion are combined to form a hydrostatic wedge which helps in dilatation of the cervix.

2. During uterine contraction, it prevents marked interference with the placental circulation so long as the membranes remain intact.
3. It flushes the birth canal at the end of first stage of labour and by its aseptic and bactericidal action protects the fetus and prevents ascending infection to the uterine cavity.

Clinical importance of liquor amnii study

During pregnancy

1. Foetal well being is determined by adequate liquor volume appropriate for duration of pregnancy.
2. Foetal maturity is determined by foetal lung surfactants (phospholipids)—lecithin and sphingomyelin obtained in liquor amnii by amniocentesis.
3. Foetal diseases. Excess bilirubin in liquor amnii can detect affected foetus by rhesus (Rh) blood group isoimmunization.
4. Foetal malformations. During 16–18 weeks cell culture of amniotic fluid obtained by amniocentesis can identify chromosomally defective babies (e.g. Down syndrome). Enzyme deficiency in cultured amniotic cells and amniotic fluid can identify inherited metabolic error in foetus.
5. Amniotic fluid excess alpha-foetoprotein (AFP) can identify foetus with open neural tube defects (anencephaly).

During labour

1. In premature rupture of membranes liquor amnii obtained by amniocentesis can identify infection.
2. Foetal hypoxia is identified by presence of meconium during labour. Clear liquor amnii ensures foetal well-being.

ABNORMALITIES IN VOLUME

Oligohydramnios (decreased amounts of amniotic fluid)

1. Less than 500 ml between 32 and 36 weeks
2. Common causes
   a. Amniotic leakage
   b. Abnormalities of the fetal kidneys (e.g. renal agenesis)
3. Primary oligohydramnios is associated with fetal abnormalities
   a. Renal agenesis
   b. Polycystic kidneys
   c. Urinary tract obstructions
4. Oligohydramnios that occurs during or before the second trimester usually results in a poor pregnancy outcome
   a. Compression of the fetus
   b. Fetal death is due to respiratory insufficiency and a lack of lung development.

Hydramnios (increased amounts of amniotic fluid)

1. Excess 2 liters of liquid between 32 and 36 weeks
2. Is often associated with poor fetal outcomes because of
   a. Preterm delivery
   b. Fetal malpresentation
   c. Cord prolapse
3. Hydramnios that occurs during or before second trimester spontaneously resolve in 45% of the cases, resulting in normal outcomes
4. Pathogenesis is usually unclear
   a. Is possibly caused by defective regulation of fluid transfer across the amniochorion.
   b. Occurs in Rh sensitized pregnancies, monozygotic multiple pregnancy, and gestational or insulin dependent diabetes mellitus.
   c. Occurs with fetal gastrointestinal obstructions or atresias.

The umbilical cord

Umbilical cord or funis is a long cord like structure that connects the foetal umblicus with foetal surface of placenta.

Development

It is developed from body stalk of mesodermal tissue stretching between embryonic disc and chorion. By sixth week amniotic cavity gradually engulfs embryo, amnitoic membranes form the covering membrane of body stalk and amnioectodermal junction converges on ventral aspect of foetus. Thus umbilical cord is formed. Mesoderm forms Wharton's jelly.

Structures

The constituents of the umbilical cord when fully formed are as follows (Fig. 2.26).

1. *Covering* of amnion showing stratified cubical cells at term like epidermis.
2. *Wharton's jelly:* It consists of elongated cells in a gelatinous fluid formed by mucoid degeneration of the extra embryonic mesodermal cells. It is rich in mucopolysaccharides and has got protective function to the umbilical vessels.
3. *Blood vessels:* Initially, there are 4 vessels— 2 arteries and 2 veins. The arteries are derived from the internal iliac arteries of the fetus and carry the venous blood from the fetus to the placenta. Of the two umbilical veins, *the right one disappears by the 4th month, leaving behind* one vein which carries oxygenated blood from the placenta to the fetus. Umbilical vein is larger than umbilical artery. *Presence of a single umbilical artery is often associated with fetal congenital abnormalities.*
4. *Remnant of the umbilical vesicle (yolk sac)* and its vitelline duct: Remnant of the yolk sac may be found as a small yellow body near the attachment of the cord to the placenta or on rare occasion, the proximal part of the duct persists as Meckel's diverticulum.
5. *Allantois:* A blind tubular structure may occasionally present near the fetal end which is continuous inside the fetus with its *urachus and bladder.*
6. *Obliterated extraembryonic coelom:* In the early period, intra embryonic coelom is

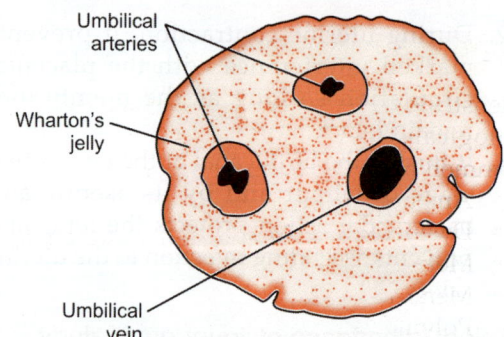

Fig. 2.26: Cross section of a term umbilical cord

continuous with extraembryonic coelom along with herniation of coils of intestine (midgut). The condition may persist as congenital umbilical hernia or exomphalos.

Naked eye characteristics

It is about 50 cm in length with an usual variation of 30–100 cm. Its diameter average 1.5 cm with variation of 1–2.5 cm. Its thickness is not uniform but presents nodes or swelling at places. These swellings *(false knots)* may be due to dilatation of the umbilical veins or local collection of Wharton's jelly.

Attachment

In the early period, the cord is attached to the ventral surface of the embryo close to the caudal extremity but as the coelom closes and the yolk sac atrophies, the point of attachment is moved permanently to the centre of the abdomen at fourth month. It usually attaches to the fetal surface of the placenta somewhere between the centre and the edge of the placenta called *eccentric insertion.* The attachment may be *central, marginal* or even on the chorion laeve at a varying distance away from the margin of the placenta, called *velamentous insertion*.

Functions

1. Life line between placenta and foetus supplying oxygen and nutrients to foetus and disposing waste products.
2. Exchange of fluid and electrolytes between *umbilical vessels and the amniotic fluid.*

MENSTRUAL DISORDERS

Menstrual disorders are the commonest gynecological problem among the women. The common menstrual disorders are:

- Amenorrhoea
- Dysmenorrhoea
- Metrorrhagia
- Menorrhagia
- Polymenorrhoea

1. AMENORRHOEA

Definition

Amenorrhoea is a symptom of absence of menses. This is not a disease but symptom of a disease.

Aetiology

Physiological amenorrhoea is caused by pregnancy, sometimes during lactation, after menopause and before menarche; pregnancy is the commonest cause of amenorrhoea.

Pathological amenorrhoea

I. Primary
II. Secondary

Primary amenorrhoea menarche does not appear in a girl who completed 18 year's age. The causes are grouped as:

1. Endocrinal

1. Hypothalamic

- obesity (>70 kg)
- Environmental change
- Anorexia nervosa in adolescents.
- Kallman's syndrome due to lack of hypothalamic GnRh—primary amenorrhoea, sexual infantilism and anosmia (loss of smell)
- Hydrocephalus
- Head injury, meningitis

2. Pituitary

- *Pituitary dwarf*
  - *Empty sella syndrome*—deficient pituitary tissue

- Pituitary tumours (adenoma) as in acromegaly (growth hormone, tumour) Cushing syndrome
- Hyperprolactinaemia
- *Ovarian*
- Polycystic ovarian syndrome
- Testicular feminisation syndrome-gonad is testes, external genitalia female, uterus absent, there is androgen insen-sitivity to end organ tissues
- ovarian tumours—arrhenoblastoma

3. Thyroid—hypo or hyperthyroidism
4. Adrenal—Congenital adrenogenital syndrome, adrenal tumours
5. Pancreas—Juvenile diabetes mellitus

I. **Nutrition:** Gross under nutrition in childhood and adolescence may cause amenorrhoea

II. **Drugs and disease**

Anabolic hormones GnRh analogue, Depoprovera in precocious puberty, testosterone, antipsychotic, antiepileptic drugs systemic diseases—tuberculosis of lungs, lymph nodes, bone, severe anaemia and other serious illness.

III. **Chromosomal** (a) Turner's syndrome (45×0)—streak gonad, absent breast, infantile uterus, primary amenorrhoea.

IV. **Uterovaginal atresia**

- Cyptomenorrhoea due to imperforate hymen
- Endometrial tuberculosis can be the cause in developing countries.
- Pregnancy is rarely encountered.

Secondary amenorrhoea common

This is cessation of menses for 3 months or more following normal menstrual cycles.

Causes are grouped as

I. **Endocrinal**
  - Hypothalamic
  - Anxiety, mental tension, environmental changes
  - Obesity

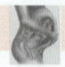

- Weight loss as in athletes
- Pituitary
- Cushing syndrome
- Cromegaly
- **Prolactinoma:** Microadenoma of pituitary causing hyperprolactinaemia—amenorrhoea—galactorrhoea syndrome.
1. **Ovarian**
   - Polycystic ovarian syndrome. This can also cause secondary amenorrhoea.
   - Premature menopause (premature ovarian failure).
   - Ovarian tumour—androgen producing arrhenoblastoma.
   - Oophorectomy and radiation to ovary.
2. **Thyroid:** Hypothyroidism or hyperthyroidism
3. **Pancreas:** Maturity onset diabetes mellitus.
4. **Adrenal hyperplasia or neoplasia**
II. **Nutrition:** Gross under nutrition and severe anaemia.
III. **Drugs and systemic diseases:** Drugs—progestogen, androgen, GnRh analogue, antipsychotic drugs, antiepilepsy drugs, etc. systemic diseases like tuberculosis, mental diseases.
IV. **Uterovaginal:** Pregnancy is the commonest cause. Endometrial tuberculosis hysterectomy, radiation.

DIAGNOSIS AND INVESTIGATION

PRIMARY AMENORRHOEA

Clinical

The first step is to diagnose pregnancy as a cause of amenorrhoea. Thereafter, all nonendocrinal causes are excluded to find out endocrinal amenorrhoea. Hormones are tested as detailed under secondary amenorrhoea.

SECONDARY AMENORRHOEA

Clinical

First step is to exclude pregnancy. Non-endocrinal causes are clinically excluded. Finally endocrinal secondary amenorrhoea shows clinical signs.

Hormones tested: Serum FSH, LH, TSH, prolactin testosterone.

Treatment of amenorrhoea in general

Patient's education is given to woman that she will get back her menses in most situations. As such amenorrhoea has no ill effects on her health. Same education is given for secondary amenorrhoea.

Primary health care is the first line treatment for amenorrhoea—both primary and secondary.

In malnourished girl with anaemia, she can have spontaneous menses by six months on weight gain, correction of anaemia by adequate food, afternoon rest, boiled water, deworming and iron folic acid (Autrin) capsule a day for 4 months. In obese 5–10 kg weight loss on nonfat diet, exercise and walking brings menses.

SPECIFIC TREATMENT

Primary amenorrhoea

- Treat the cause.
- For uterine hypoplasia, primary health care and cyclical oestrogen—progestogen therapy may help
- **Agenesis:** Imperforate hymen is opened by hymenotomy in young girl; thereafter, she gets regular menses.
- Turner's syndrome is treated by giving oestrogen (Premarin 0.625 mg or Lynoral 0.05 mg) daily at bed time for years together for development of secondary sex, character starting at 12 year.
- Testicular feminization syndrome is left till full growth is achieved after puberty. Thereafter, bilateral gonadectomy is done to avoid gonadal malignancy. Fertility and menses cannot be restored in Müllerian atresia, gonadal atresia and intersex.
- Drug amenorrhea is treated by stopping the drugs if possible.

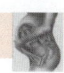

- Anorexia nervosa, other endocrines disorders, anaemia, tuberculosis are referred to physician.

Secondary amenorrhoea

- Progestogen challenge test in oestrogenic woman. Commonly oestrogenic woman (serum oestradiol above 40 pg/ml) gets secondary amenorrhoea due to hypothalamic cause when all other organic causes are excluded. Tablet Medroxyprogesterone acetate (Modes) 10 mg while taken thrice daily by mouth for 7 days brings menses within 7–10 days. Repeat cycles can be given for one week starting from 16th day of menses × 6 cycles. Anxiolytic drug—alprazolam (Restyl) 0.5 mg is taken daily at bed time for one month by anxious woman. Meditation (doing puja) is advised to practice daily for 1 hour.
- Hypothyroidism is treated by eltroxine. Hyperthyroidism is referred to physician. Maturity onset diabetes mellitus is referred to physician. On treatment she may get menses.
- Adrenal cortical hyperplasia or neoplasia is referred to physician/surgeon. Premature menopause is treated by HRT for many years. She rarely gets menses.

Prognosis

- Primary amenorrhoea cannot be successfully treated except in girls who have delayed puberty and specific cause in others which could be removed.
- Secondary amenorrhoea without any identifiable cause can have a spontaneous cure rate of 50% within 1 year. Longer the period of amenorrhoea, poorer becomes coming back to spontaneous menses.

2. DYSMENORRHOEA

Definition

Dysmenorrhoea is means painful menses incapacitating the woman.

Incidence

Probably 5–10 percent girls in their late teens and women in early twenties suffer from dysmenorrhoea.

Types

1. Primary spasmodic dysmenorrhoea signifies lower abdominal pain due to menstruation and of uterine origin. No obvious pelvic lesion is found to cause pain
2. Membranous dysmenorrhoea is a variety of primary spasmodic dysmenorrhoea where there is casting of big pieces of endometrium. This is said to run in families
3. Secondary dysmenorrhoea means pain associated with menstruation and is due to pelvic lesions, e.g. endometriosis (severe pelvic pain) adenomyosis, chronic pelvic inflammatory disease (PID), uterine fibroid.
   - **Primary**—occurs in the absence of organic disease
   - **Secondary**—occurs as a result of organic disease

It can be categorized into
- **Mild:** No interference with normal activities
- **Moderate:** Some interference with normal activities
- **Severe:** Interference with majority of everyday activities

Aetiology of primary dysmenorrhoea

1. Excess prostaglandins (PG_2 and PGE_2) are released from secretory endometrium to cause spasm of uterine muscles during menses.
2. Psychological: Girls with anxiety has low pain threshold and suffers more from primary dysmenorrhoea.

CLINICAL FEATURES OF PRIMARY DYSMENORRHOEA

Symptoms

1. Patient is young, usually 18–24 years, rare after 30 years

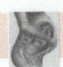

2. Painful menses usually occur years after menarche.
3. Pain starts 1–2 hours before the onset of menses, continues for first 12–24 hours and then gradually gets less and ceases on stoppage of menses.
4. Pain is colicky and cramplike at the hypogastric region and radiates to the thighs there may be low backache.
5. Menses are regular and ovulatory. The intermenstrual period is free from any pain.
6. Constitutional symptoms—nausea, vomiting, diarrhoea (prostaglandin effect) headache, sometimes fainting due to severe pain may occur during painful menses.

Signs
1. Patient may be in poor state of health often thin and anxious state of mind.
2. Per abdomen—nothing abnormal is detected.
3. Vaginal pelvic examination in a unmarried girl can be made by right index finger per vagina or rectum where uterus and adnexa are felt normal. Instead of this painful pelvic examination, pelvic USG (TAS) is done.

Diagnosis
- Typical history of painful menses.
- Routine laboratory testing is done on Hb%, postmeal blood glucose and routine urine analysis.

SECONDARY DYSMENORRHOEA

Clinical features
Symptoms
- Patient is around 30 years
- Lower abdominal pain associated with menses.
- Pain starts 3–5 days before the start of menses, persists during menses and lasts for days after menses in endometriosis, pain can be at times very severe, not relieved by analgesic.
- There can be associated dyspareunia and menorrhagia.

- In adenomyosis there can be menstrual pain with menorrhagia.
- Fibroid can also have pelvic pain in menses.
- In pelvic inflammatory disease, pain appears before and during menses in lower abdomen.

Diagnosis
- Clinical
- Pelvic USG

Treatment
- Primary dysmenorrhoea
- Girl is assured that she will get relief of pain on treatment.
- Application of hot water bag on hypogastrium helps to reduce pain during dysmenorrhoea.

Drugs
A. **First line of drug**
1. **Aspirin** (acetyl salicylic acid—antiprostaglandin) is the first line of drug for pain relief. Tablet aspirin (Disprin 350 mg, Ecosprin 325 mg) is taken orally twice daily with food for painful days during menses × 6 cycle. Tab Gelusil MPS is also taken along with aspirin twice daily to prevent gastric irritation. Tablet Alprazolam (Restyl 0.5 mg) is given at bed time daily during painful days of menses.
2. **If aspirin cannot be tolerated**, nonsteroidal anti-inflammatory drug (NSAID)—antiprostaglandin—mefenamic acid (ponstan) 250 mg for girl below 60 kg or 500 mg for girl above 60 kg) capsule is taken thrice daily with food for 2–3 painful days for 6 cycles.
B. **Second line of drug oral contraceptive (OC)**—(Mala D, Ovral L, Triquilar) one tab, at bed time daily from 5th day of menses × 21 days for 6 cycles. OC causes anovulation, less endometrial PG production thus relieves dysmenorrhoea. Ponstan can be combined with OC.

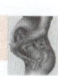

In case of intolerable dysmenorrhoea with vomiting, tab Norethisterone (Primolut N) 5 mg twice daily with food continuously starting from 5th day of menses × 6 months. If small menses appear during the therapy, tab. Primolut N is taken thrice daily × 5 days • returning to one tab twice daily till course is completed. Following 6 months amenorrhoea on stoppage of Primolut N she gets back her menses with no or less pain but no vomiting during menses.

3. **Mid-menstrual pain (Mittelschmerz)** (ovulation pain) It is the pelvic pain occurring near about the middle of the menstrual cycle at the time of ovulation. The pain recurr regularly in succeeding intermediate menstrual cycles.

Cause

Painful ovulation

Clinical features

- The woman suffers from dull aching pelvic pain for about 12 hours regularly at the mid menstrual period, generally between 11 and 18 days of the cycle.
- The site of pain is at hypogastrium or one or other iliac fossa. The pain is almost always referred to the same site and does not change. There may be associated watery vaginal discharge or even scanty vaginal bleeding during pain.

Treatment

- Analgesics tablet Aspirin is given as in primary dysmenorrhoea for pain as spontaneous cure often happens.
- Oestrogen—progestogen oral contraceptive pill therapy can be useful to make the cycle anovular and painless for 6 cycles.

HEAVY MENSTRUATION AND ABNORMAL UTERINE HAEMORRHAGE

Polymenorrhoea (epimenorrhoea)

This means too frequent menstruation at regular intervals of two weeks but less than 3 weeks.

Such cyclical bleeding can be normal in amount but when becomes heavy, the condition is called epimenorrhagia.

Aetiology

a. Endocrine disorders—anovulation
b. Systemic disorders—malnutrition and mental anxiety.
c. Pelvic disorders—chronic pelvic inflammatory disease, chocolate cyst of the ovary.

Clinical features

- It may occur at any time during the menstruating life, but can temporarily develop at premenopause, after abortion and childbirth.
- The menstrual loss may be normal or profuse.
- This disorder spontaneously gets corrected.

Treatment

1. The general health of the women is improved, and anaemia is corrected.
2. Hormonal treatment should not be done for a recent case; in persistent cases producing anaemia, hormone therapy is useful. Six months cycle control is made by oral contraceptive tablet for 21 days from 5th day of menses. Pelvic USG by TVS is done to exclude any pelvic pathology.

3. METRORRHAGIA

- This means intermenstrual irregular uterine bleeding (metrostaxis). However, in practice, the term is used for any irregular bleeding per vagina.

Aetiology

- Carcinoma of cervix or that of the endometrium
- Uterine or cervical polypus—commonly mucous and submucous fibroid polypi
- Dysfunctional uterine haemorrhage
- Any ulcer on the cervix
- Tuberculosis of cervix or endometrium
- Disturbed early pregnancy haemorrhage, e.g. abortion and tubal gestation

- Breakthrough bleeding in oral contraceptive
- Post-IUCD bleeding.

Where the term is used for irregular vaginal haemorrhage, the vaginal and vulval growths, vaginitis, vaginal ulcer are the causes of metrorrhagia.

Treatment: The cause is investigated and appropriately treated.

4. MENORRHAGIA

Means excessive menstrual loss in amount or duration or both causing (more than 80 ml) blood loss. Menotaxis means prolonged menstruation in duration.

Aetiology

I. Pelvic causes
- Uterine fibroid
- Pelvic inflammatory disease, e.g. chronic salpingo-oophoritis, chronic endometritis (tubercular)
- Pelvic endometriosis, adenomyosis
- Endometrial polyps
- Carcinoma of the endometrium
- Uterine malformation, e.g. double uterus
- Intrauterine contraceptive device (IUCD)

II. Endocrinal disorders
- Dysfunctional uterine bleeding
- Polycystic ovarian syndrome (PCOS)
- Hypothyroidism.

III. Systemic diseases
a. **Blood disorders** (haematological)— purpura, leukaemia, some cases of moderate anaemia.
b. **General disease**
- Chronic hypertension
- Heart disease with chronic congestive failure
- Chronic nephritis
- Under nutrition
- Emotional disturbances like mental anxiety, sorrow, sexual excesses, etc.

IV. Drugs—prolonged taking of aspirin

5. DYSFUNCTIONAL UTERINE BLEEDING (DUB)

Definition

This is excessive menses more than 80 ml where no organic cause (systemic, haematological or pelvic) can be detected. The nature of bleeding is one of menorrhagia, polymenorrhoea, metrorrhagia and continuous bleeding preceded by amenorrhoea (metropathic bleeding).

Incidence

Dysfunctional uterine haemorrhage constitutes about 15–20 percent of all gynaecological admissions in an institution.

Aetiology

Dysfunctional uterine bleeding is due to
- Anovulation (85%) particularly during adolescent and premenopause, anovulatory DUB is painless.
- Mental anxiety

Histology

Endometrial pattern in DUB shows:
1. Proliferative endometrium in secretory phase (anovulation)
2. Secretary endometrium (ovulatory)
3. Endometrial hyperplasia and adenomatous hyperplasia, cystic glandular hyperplasia (metropathia) due to chronic anovulation.

METROPATHIA HAEMORRHAGIA (SCHRODER DISEASE)

Bleeding is painless. This is commonly seen in premenopause and adolescence. Chronic anovulation and prolonged oestrogen effect causes cystic glandular hyperplasia in endometrium and myohyperplasia in uterus.

Pathology of metropathia

1. The ovary, either one or both ovaries are more or less enlarged and contain unruptured cystic follicles with absence of active corpus luteum.
2. The uterus. This becomes uniformly but mildly enlarged due to myohyperplasia.

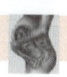

The endometrium becomes markedly overgrown, thick, vascular and polypoidal. Microscopically, there is hyperplasia of all elements of the endometrium. The glands increase in number but may vary in size, some of them become dilated and cystic, this dysparity gives rise to the characteristic 'Swiss cheese pattern' (cystic glandular hyperplasia). The interstitial tissue becomes abundant, cellular, vascular and compact. There is no secretory change in the endometrium. This type of haemorrhage comprises about one-fourth to one-third of all cases of dysfunctional uterine haemorrhage.

Clinical classification of DUB
1. Adolescent group during 11–19 years
2. Maturity group (20–40 years)
3. Perimenopausal group above 40 years.

Clinical features
History
- DUB is common in parous, adolescent and premenopausal woman. Special attention in history is given to various groups as:
- Adolescent group—haematological disorders (bleeding from nose, gum ecchymosis due to purpura, leukemia, etc.) endocrine disorders (hypothyroidism).
- Maturity group childbirth, abortion, MTP in particular, anemia, anxiety, liver dysfunction and drug taking.
- Perimenopausal group menorrhagia without any systemic or pelvic causes as under causes of menorrhagia.

Symptoms
- Menorrhagia is the key symptom.
- Menorrhagia is considered when more than 10 pads or clean cloth used in slum and villages are changed with passage of clots with progressively developing anemia.
- Menorrhagia can be regular or irregular or polymenorrhoea or metropathic bleeding-

short period of amenorrhoea with prolonged bleeding.
- Symptoms due to anemia—weakness, breathlessness on exertion.

Signs
- Patient is anemic.
- Head to foot thorough clinical examination shows no other systemic diseases.
- In maturity and perimenopause, pelvic exam, shows cervix is normal, uterus is felt normal sized or just bulky parous size as in metropathia, clear fornices. Bilateral palpable ovaries (cystic) can be felt in metropathia. In adolescent, one index finger vaginal examination is more certain to exclude pelvic pathology.

Investigations
These are directed to eliminate all other causes of menorrhagia when uterus is normal, ovaries not enlarged except in metropathia. Basic blood tests are done in all cases.
- Blood haemoglobin, total and differential white cells, ABO-Rh group, postmeal blood glucose, serum TSH and routine urine analysis.
- For haematological disorders specially in adolescent group (in 5%)—blood for platelet count, bleeding and coagulation time are done.
- Hormone tests are FSH, LH, prolactin, testosterone.
- Cytology PAP stain cervical scrape cytology and endometrial brush or aspiration cytology are done in women aged over 35 years to exclude neoplasia.
- Ultrasonography pelvic TVS, color Doppler sonography is very useful to exclude pelvic lesion in sexually active group. TAS is done in adolescent group.
- Dilatation and curettage (D and C) this when properly done is diagnostic and curative as well particularly for irregular menorrhagia, continuous bleeding in perimenopausal group.

- In regular menorrhagia in maturity group D and C is avoided. In adolescent group this is almost always avoided.
- Hysteroscopy is done to exclude endometrial polyp and other pathology in elderly patient.

Diagnosis

Both clinical and investigations as detailed above can diagnose DUB when all other causes are excluded and uterus ovaries remain normal.

Table 2.4: Specific treatment for DUB menorrhagia

1. **Adolescent group menorrhagia with blood disorders is referred to haematologist**
   Medical treatment: Progestogen is effective to counter oestrogenic menses with prolonged bleeding. Prolonged menses is controlled by tab. Primolut N (norethisterone enanthate)—5 mg t.d. × 7 days • one tab bd × 13 days. Then 2nd, 3rd, 4th course or more. Primolut N is given one tab b.d. × 20 days from 5th day of menses. In regular menorrhagia primolut N four courses are given as above. On improvement of health and concurrent anaemia she gets normal menses.
   For hypothyroidism (serum TSH above 10 U/ml tab. Eltroxine 0.1 mg is given before breakfast daily.
   Surgical treatment D and C (dilatation and curettage) is seldom done when USG report suggests uterine polyp, product of conception or in suspected endometrial tuberculosis.

2. **Maturity group medical treatment**
   Emergency treatment for heavy flooding in menses on 3rd or 4th day—inj. Aquaviron (free testosterone) 50 mg. 25 mg × 2 ampules IM gluteal daily × 3 days. This stops bleeding.
   On stoppage of bleeding:
   1. Tab Primolut N one tab b.d. × 20 days course is given. Further 3 courses of Primolut N of 20 days is given to control menorrhagia from 5th day of menses. This 20 days course is also given for regular menorrhagia × 4 courses.
   2. **For regular menorrhagia** in ovulatory group, oral contraceptive course of 21 days from 5th day of menses × 1 year.
   3. **Ponstan 250 mg** (for wt. below 60 kg) or 500 mg (above 60 kg) capsule t.d. is orally given for 3–4 days of heavy menses × 4–6 menses. This can be combined with OC.
      Alternatively Levonorgestrel IUCD releasing 20 g hormone daily to endometrium can be fitted for regular menorrhagia for 5 years.
   4. For intractible menorrhagia inj. Depoprovera (medroxyprogesterone) 150 mg i.m. gluteal 6 weekly × 1 year can cause amenorrhoea and spotting.
   5. In infertility with menorrhagia, clomiphene citrate courses are given.
   (a) Ponstan is given during menses for menorrhagia.
   (b) GnRh analogue—decapeptyl 3.75 mg IM every 28 days can be given for 6 months. The drug causes hypogonadal amenorrhoea. The drug is unaffordable in India for its very high cost.
      Surgical treatment D and C is needed in irregular menorrhagia (not controlled by hormone) and incomplete abortion.

3. **Perimenopausal group**
   Surgical treatment (D and C) is the first line therapy. While doing D and C uterine cavity is explored by small polypectomy forceps removing endometrial polyps from fundus, cornu and corpus. Thereafter, hard D and C two rounds of curetting is routinely done. This is diagnostic and curative.

Medical treatment
In case of recurrence of menorrhagia following D and C Primolut N or Danazol 100 or 200 mg b.d. for 6 months or low dose OC combined with Ponstan for 6 cycles along with haematinics can control menorrhagia.
   If menorrhagia recurs, total hysterectomy either abdominal or vaginal gives cure of menorrhagia.

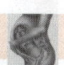

Management of DUB

- Primary health care is given in all cases. Patient's education is given that she will have control of heavy menses or cured by surgery.
- For anxiety she does meditation (prayer) daily and takes restyl 0.5 mg at bed time daily × 30 days.
- Standard diet chart is handed over to patients and she follows it. For thin, weight gain to 5–10 kg by adequate food. Boiled water is always taken and also daily walking a mile.

- For overweight and obese, reduction of 5–10 kg weight is valuable by avoiding extra rice, potato, sweets, butter, ghee, cold drinks she also takes boiled water and walk a mile daily.
- Deworming drug is taken as a routine. Tab Nemocid (pyrantel pamoate) 250 mg 3 tabs At bed time single dose (one after another) is taken. Haematinic is taken as a routine— iron folic acid (Autrin) one capsule twice daily with food when Hb% below 10 gm% × 1 month one capsule daily for 3 months.

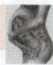

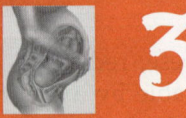

3

The Fetus

OUTLINE

- Fetal circulation
- Changes of the fetal circulation at birth
- Fetal development

FETAL CIRCULATION

The circulation in the fetus is essentially the same as in the adult except for the following:

1. The source of oxygenated blood is not the lung but the placenta.

2. Oxygenated blood from the placenta comes to the fetus through the umbilical vein which joins the left branch of the portal vein. A small portion of this blood passes through the substance of the liver to the inferior vena cava. But the greater part passes directly to the inferior vena cava through the ductus venosus. A sphincter mechanism in the ductus venosus controls blood flow.

3. The oxygen-rich blood reaching the right atrium through the inferior vena cava is directed by the valve of the inferior vena cava towards the foramen ovale.

   a. Most of it passes through the foramen ovale into the left atrium (75%).

   b. The rest of it gets mixed up with the blood returning to the right atrium through the superior vena cava and passes into the right ventricle (25%).

4. From the right ventricle, the blood (mostly deoxygenated) enters the pulmonary trunk. Only a small portion of this blood reaches the lungs and passes through it to the left atrium. The greater part is short-circuited by the ductus arteriosus into the aorta.

5. The left atrium receives

   a. Oxygenated blood from the right atrium.

   b. A small amount of deoxygenated blood from the lungs.

The blood in this chamber is, therefore, fairly rich in oxygen. This blood passes into the left ventricle and then into the aorta. Some of this oxygen-rich blood passes into the carotid and subclavian arteries to supply the brain, the head and neck and the upper extremities. The rest of it gets mixed up with

---

Box 3.1: Structures in fetal circulation

- **Placenta and vessels:** Vessels necessary for oxygenation and exchange of waste products.

- **Umbilical vein:** One vein that carries oxygenated blood from the placenta to the fetus.

- **Umbilical arteries:** Two arteries that carry deoxygenated blood from the fetus to the placenta.

- **Foramen ovale:** Opening between the right and left atria of the heart.

- **Ductus arteriosus:** Fetal blood vessel connecting the pulmonary artery and the aorta.

- **Ductus venosus:** Fetal blood vessel connecting the umbilical vein with the vena cava.

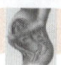

poorly oxygenated blood from the ductus arteriosus. Thus, mixed blood is distributed to the viscera and lower extremities.

The deoxygenated blood leaves the body by way of two umbilical arteries to reach the placenta where it is oxygenated and gets ready for recirculation (Fig. 3.1).

CHANGES OF THE FETAL CIRCULATION AT BIRTH

The haemodynamics of the fetal circulation undergoes profound changes soon after birth due to:

1. Cessation of the placental blood flow.
2. Initiation of respiration.

The following changes occur in the vascular system

1. *Closure of the umbilical arteries:* Functional closure is almost instantaneous preventing even slight amount of the fetal blood to drain out. Actual obliteration takes about 2–3 months.
2. *Closure of the umbilical vein:* The obliteration occurs a little later than the arteries, allowing a little extra volume of blood (80–100 ml) to be received by the fetus from the placenta. The ductus venosus collapses and the venous pressure of the inferior vena cava falls and so also the right atrial pressure. After obliteration, the umbilical vein forms the **ligamentum teres** and the ductus venosus becomes **ligamentum venosum.**

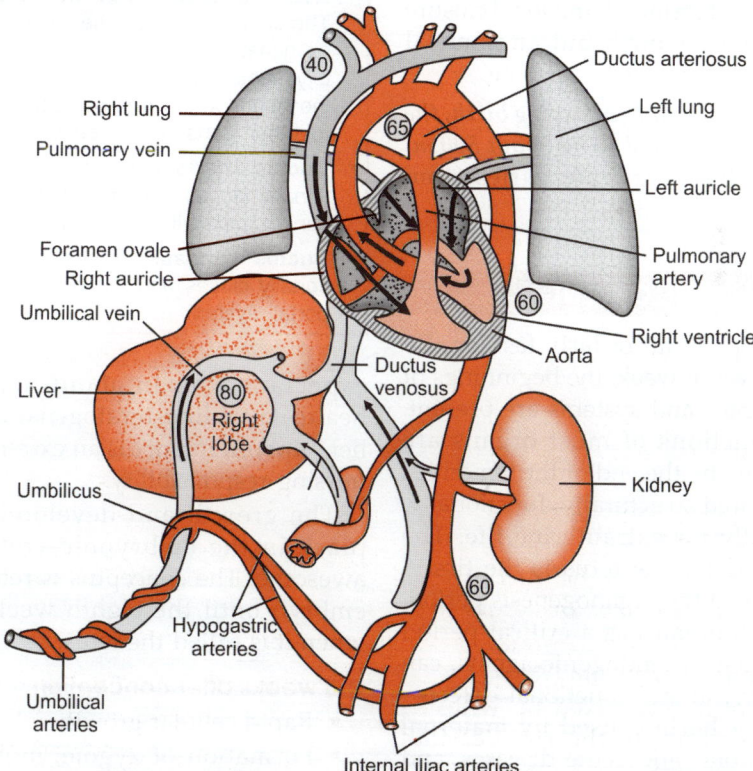

Fig. 3.1: Fetal circulation. Number inside the circle indicates the percentage saturation of O_2

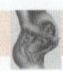

3. *Closure of the ductus arteriosus:* Within few hours of respiration, the muscle wall of the ductus arteriosus contracts probably in response to rising oxygen tension of the blood flowing through the duct. The effects of the variation of the O_2 tension on the ductus arteriosus are thought to be mediated through the action of prostaglandins. Prostaglandin antagonists, given to the mother, may lead to the premature closure of the ductus arteriosus. Whereas functional closure of the ductus may occur soon after the establishment of pulmonary circulation, the anatomical obliteration takes about 1–3 months and becomes **ligamentum arteriosum.**

4. *Closure of the foramen ovale:* This is caused by an increased pressure of the left atrium combined with a decreased pressure on the right atrium. Functional closure occurs soon after birth but anatomical closure occurs in about 1 year time.

Within one or two hours following birth, the cardiac output is estimated to be about 500 ml per minute and the heart rate varies from 120–140 per minute (Fig. 3.2).

FETAL DEVELOPMENT

The fetus develops in an orderly fashion. By the end of the seventh week, the beginnings of all the major organs and systems are present. At first, the functions of most organs are minimal; however, by the end of the 9 months, the fetus is prepared structurally, functionally, and metabolically for extrauterine life. The most critical time for the fetus is the first 8 weeks; this is called the organogenesis period. In addition, each organ has a critical period when insults, such as teratogenic agents, can easily cause physical and functional defects . The potential for harm caused by maternal malnutrition, chronic and acute diseases, and drugs continues until birth. Teaching the

---

Box 3.2: Circulatory changes after birth

- **Umbilical vessels:** The umbilical vessels are cut; to receive oxygen the infant must use the lungs.
- **Lungs:** Aeration occurs; blood is circulated through the lungs.
- **Pattern of blood flow:** Blood flow pattern changes to that of a mature circulation (as the infant begins to breathe).
- **Circulation to lungs:** As the infant inflates the lungs, pressure is released on the blood vessels of the lungs.
- **Line of least resistance:** As the blood vessels open in the lungs, blood is no longer diverted through the ductus arteriosus; rather, following the line of least resistance, blood enters the lungs.
- **Increased pressure:** The change of blood flow increases the pressure in the left atrium, which causes the foramen ovale to close.
- **Heart functions with two separate pumps:** The right side of the heart receives non-oxygenated blood and pumps it to the lungs. The oxygenated blood is directed to the left side of the heart, where it is pumped through the aorta to other parts of the body.
- **Ductus arteriosus:** The ductus arteriosus functionally closes; therefore non-oxygenated blood cannot mix with oxygenated blood.
- **Ductus venosus:** The ductus venosus functionally closes and the blood flows through the portal system.

---

expectant woman about maintaining her health (avoiding teratogens) and protecting her "unborn infant" is an extremely important nursing responsibility.

The growth and development that take place in the embryonic—fetal period are awesome. The conceptus is referred to as the embryo until the eighth week of gestation, when it is called the fetus.

0–3 weeks after conception
- Rapid cellular growth
- Formation of zygote, morula-blastocyst and trophoblast

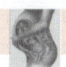
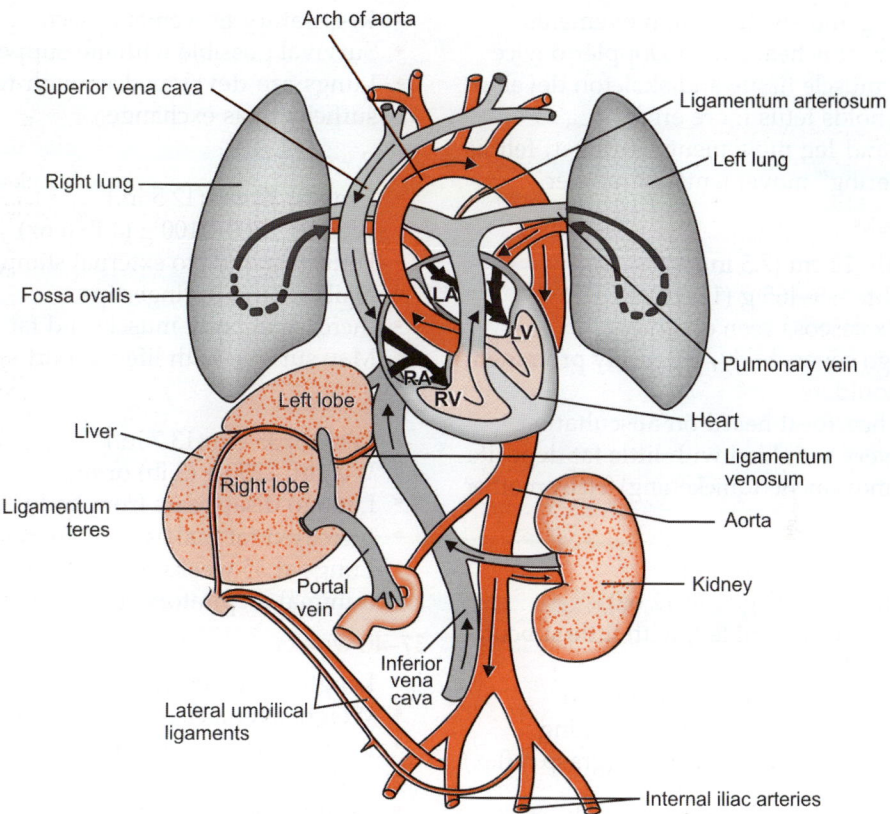

Fig. 3.2: Change in fetal circulation afterbirth

- Primitive central nervous system
- Primitive cardiovascular system formed.

4–8 weeks
- Beginning uteroplacental circulation
- At 8 weeks, embryo is approximately 3 cm (1–2 in.) in length
- Rapid cell division
- Rapid head growth; facial features develop
- Paddle-shaped hands and webbed fingers
- All major organs laid down in primitive form
- Heart capable of pumping small amounts of blood
- Early movements seen on ultrasound
- Development easily disturbed by teratogens (drugs, viruses, radiation).

9–12 weeks
- Fetus approximately 6–8 cm (2–3 in.) in length
- Eyelids fused
- Fetal circulation is functioning
- Kidneys begin to pass urine
- Amniotic fluid swallowed
- Blood cells produced in spleen
- Moves freely (not felt by mother)
- Fetal heart tones can be detected by electronic Doppler device.

13–16 weeks
- Fetal length: 9 cm (3.6 in.)
- Rapid skeletal development
- Lanugo or fine hair especially on head
- Meconium in gut (black tarry stools, known as meconium in the intestines).

- Sucking and swallowing movements
- Heartbeat is heard with Doppler device
- More muscle tissue and skeleton development holds fetus more erect.
- Arm and leg movements stronger, felt as "fluttering" movements by mother.

17–20 weeks

- Length: 19 cm (7.5 in.)
- Weight: 435–465 g (15–16 oz)
- Vernix caseosa seen on body
- Lanugo covers body, especially prominent on shoulders
- Fetal heartbeat heard on auscultation
- Skin very wrinkled with little fat deposits
- Fetal movements (quickening) felt by mother

21–24 weeks

- Length: 26 cm (10.2 in.)
- Weight: 780–820 g (1 lb 12 oz)
- Skin red and wrinkled, with little subcutaneous fat
- Eyebrows and eyelids are formed
- Most organs capable of functioning
- Fetus has a hand grasp reflex (grasp reflex)
- Periods of sleep and activity
- Responds to sound; has a startle reflex

25–28 weeks

- Length: 30 cm (11.8 in.)
- Weight: 1200–1250 g (2 lb 12 oz)
- Eyelids reopen; eyebrows and eyelashes present

- Respiratory movements seen
- Survival possible with life-support system
- Lungs are developed enough to provide sufficient gas exchange

29–32 weeks

- Length: 32 cm (12.5 in.)
- Weight: 1800–2100 g (4 lb 6 oz)
- Fetus responds to external stimuli (noises)
- Nails extend to fingertips
- Increase in body muscle and fat
- May survive with life-support system

33–36 weeks

- Length: 35 cm (13.7 in.)
- Weight: 2250 g (5 lb) or more
- Lanugo disappears from body
- Increased fat makes body more rounded
- Lungs at 35 weeks ready for survival with minimal respiratory difficulty

37–40 weeks

- Length averages 51 cm (20 in.)
- Weight averages 3200 g (7 lb 1 oz) or more
- Lanugo almost gone, except on shoulders and upper back
- Vernix caseosa mainly seen in skin folds and creases
- Body organs mature; eyes and extremities functional
- Body plump; good skin turgor
- Testes fully descended
- Fetus ready to be born

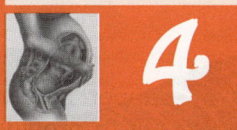

4

Pregnancy

OUTLINE

- Physiological changes during pregnancy
- Diagnosis of pregnancy
- Antenatal care
- Minor ailments of pregnancy
- Fetus in utero
- Planned parenthood
- Antenatal exercise
- Fetal well being assessment

PHYSIOLOGICAL CHANGES DURING PREGNANCY

Physiologic alterations do occur in the mother during pregnancy to enable her to provide and maintain a healthy environment for satisfactory fetal growth, without compromising her own health. During pregnancy, there is progressive anatomical and physiological changes not only confined to the genital organs but also to all systems of the body. This is principally a phenomenon of maternal adaptation to the increasing demands of the growing fetus.

GENITAL ORGANS

Vulva

Vulva becomes oedematous and hyperaemic, superficial varicosities may appear especially in multiparae. Labia minora are pigmented and hypertrophied.

Vagina

Vaginal walls become hypertrophied, oedematous and more vascular. Increased blood supply of the venous plexus surrounding the walls gives the bluish colouration to the mucosa *(Jacquemier's sign)*. The length of the anterior vaginal wall is increased.

Secretion

The secretion becomes copious, thin and curdy white, due to marked exfoliated cells and bacteria. The pH becomes acidic (3.5–6) due to more conversion of glycogen into lactic acid by the *Lactobacillus acidophilus* consequent on high oestrogen level. The acidic pH prevents multiplication of pathogenic organisms.

Cytology

There is preponderance of *navicular cells in cluster* (small intermediate cells with elongated nuclei).

UTERUS

There is enormous growth of the uterus during pregnancy. The uterus which, in non-pregnant state, weighs about 50 gm and measures about 7.5 cm in length, *at term, weighs 900–1000 gm and measures 35 cm in length.* Changes occur in all the parts of the uterus body, isthmus and cervix.

Body of the uterus

There is increase in growth and enlargement of the body of the uterus.

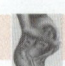
Enlargement: The enlargement of the uterus is affected by the following factors:

Changes in the muscles

1. *Hypertrophy and hyperplasia:* Not only the individual muscle fibre increases in length and breadth but there is limited addition of new muscle fibres also. These occur under the influence of the hormones–oestrogen and progesterone limited to the first half of pregnancy but pronounced up to 12 weeks.

2. *Stretching:* The muscle fibres further elongate beyond 20 weeks due to distension by the growing foetus. The wall becomes thinner and, at term, measures about 1.5 cm or less. The uterus feels soft and elastic in contrast to firm feel of the nongravid uterus.

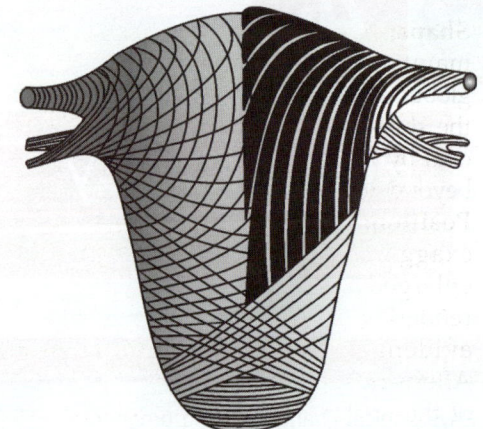

Fig. 4.1: Schematic presentation of the longitudinal oblique and circular muscle fibres of the pregnant uterus

Arrangement of the muscle fibres: Three distinct layers of muscle fibres are evident:

1. *Outer longitudinal:* It follows a hood-like arrangement over the fundus; some fibres are continuous with the round ligaments.

2. *Inner circular:* It is scanty and has sphincter like arrangement around the tubal orifices and internal os.

3. *Intermediate:* It is the thickest and strongest layer arranged in criss cross fashion.

   - *There is simultaneous increase in number and size* of the supporting fibrous and elastic tissues (Figs 4.1 and 4.2).

Vascular system: Whereas in the non-pregnant state, the blood supply to the uterus is mainly through the uterine and least through the ovarian but in the pregnant state, the latter carries as much blood as the former. There is marked spiralling of the arteries, reaching the maximum at 20 weeks, thereafter, they straighten out and become dilated. Veins are very much dilated which have got no valves. Numerous lymphatic channels are opened up. The vascular changes are most pronounced at the placental site.

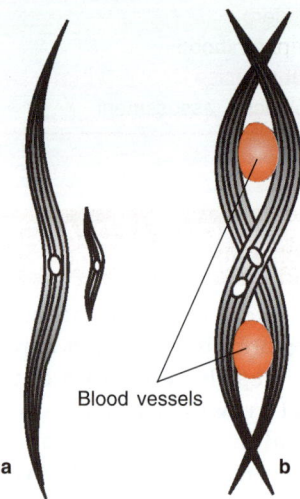

Blood vessels

a   b

Fig. 4.2: a. Marked elongation of the muscle fibres during pregnancy, **b.** Blood vessels in between interlacing muscle fibres

The enlargement is neither symmetrical one. *The fundus enlarges more than the body.* It is evident by the low down attachment of the round ligaments or insertion of the uterine end of the fallopian tubes at term.

Weight: The increase in weight is due to increased growth of the uterine muscles, connective tissues and vascular channels.

Relation

- **Shape:** Non-pregnant pyriform shape is maintained in early months. It becomes globular at 12 weeks. As the uterus enlarges, the shape once more becomes pyriform or oval by 28 weeks and changes to spherical beyond 36th week.
- **Position:** Normal anteverted position is exaggerated upto 8 weeks. Thus, the enlarged uterus may lie on the bladder rendering it incapable of filling, clinically evident by frequency of micturition. Afterwards, it becomes erect, the long axis of the uterus confirms more or less to the axis of the inlet. As the term approaches, especially in multiparae with lax abdominal wall, there is a tendency of anteversion. But in primigravidae with good tone of the abdominal muscles, it is held firmly against the maternal spine.

Lateral obliquity: As the uterus enlarges to occupy the abdominal cavity, it usually rotates on its long axis to the right (dextrorotation). This is due to the occupation of the rectosigmoid in the left posterior quadrant of the pelvis. This makes the anterior surface of the uterus to turn to the right and brings the left cornu closer to the abdominal wall. *The cervix, as a result, is deviated to the left side (levo-rotation), bringing it closer to the ureter.*

Contractions (Braxton-Hicks): The contractions are irregular, infrequent, spasmodic and painless without any effect on dilatation of the cervix. In abdominal pregnancy, Braxton-Hicks contraction is not felt.

Endometrium: The changes of the endometrium of the non-pregnant uterus are as follows:

The well developed decidua differentiates into three layers.

1. *Superficial compact layer* consists of compact mass of decidual cells, gland ducts and dilated capillaries. The greater part of the surface epithelium is either thinned out or lost.

2. *Intermediate spongy glands,* decidual cells and blood vessels. *It is through this layer that the cleavage of placental separation occurs.*

3. *Thin basal layer* contains the basal portion of the glands and is apposed to the uterine muscle. Regeneration of the mucous coat occurs from this layer following parturition.

After the interstitial implantation of the blastocyst into the compact layer of the decidua, the different portions of the decidua are renamed as,

1. *Decidua basalis or serotina:* the portion of the decidua capsularis or reflexa—the thin superficial compact layer covering the blastocyst.

2. *Decidua capsularis or reflexa:* the thin superficial compact layer covering the blastocyst.

3. *Decidua vera or parietalis:* the rest of the decidua lining the uterine cavity outside the site of implantation. Its thickness progressively increases to maximum of 5–10 mm at the end of the second month and, thereafter, regression occurs with advancing pregnancy so that beyond 20th week, it measures not more than 1 mm.

Isthmus

There are important structural and functional changes in the isthmus during pregnancy.

During the first trimester, isthmus hypertrophies and elongates to about 3 times its original length. It becomes softer. With advancing pregnancy beyond 12 weeks, it progressively unfolds from above, downwards until it is incorporated into the uterine cavity. The circularly arranged muscle fibres in the region function as a sphincter in early pregnancy and thus help to retain the fetus within the uterus. Incompetency of the sphincteric action leads to mid trimester abortion and the encircled operations done to rectify the defect are based on the principle of

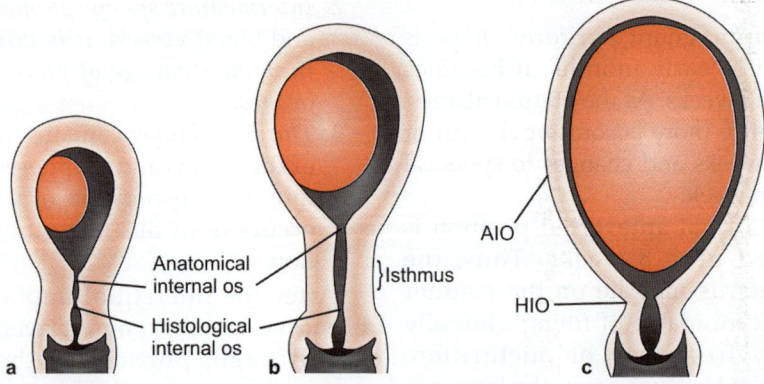

Fig. 4.3: Elongation and formation of the lower uterine segment. **a.** at 8 weeks, **b.** at 12 weeks, **c.** at 16 weeks

restoration of the retentive function of the isthmus (Fig. 4.3).

CERVIX

Stroma: **There is hypertrophy and hyperplasia** of the elastic and connective tissues. **Fluids accumulate** inside and in between the fibres. **Vascularity** is increased specially beneath the squamous epithelium of the portio vaginalis which is responsible for its bluish colouration. There is marked hypertrophy and hyperplasia of the glands which occupy about half the bulk of the cervix. **All these lead to marked softening of the cervix (Goodell's sign)** which is evident as early as 6 weeks. It begins at the margin of the external os and then spreads upwards. Not only it provides diagnostic aid in pregnancy but also the changes in the cervix facilitate its dilatation during labour.

Epithelium: There is marked proliferation of the endocervical mucosa with downward extension beyond the squamocolumnar junction (Fig. 4.4).

This gives rise to clinical appearance of erosion cervix. **Sometimes, the squamous cells also become hyperactive and the mucosal changes simulate basal cell hyperplasia or carcinoma in situ.** These changes are hormone

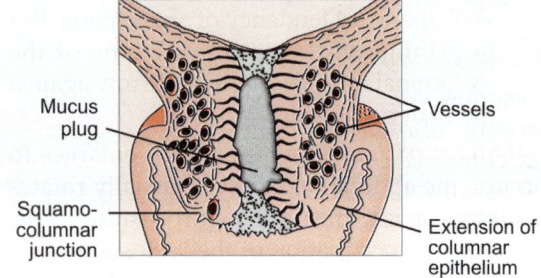

Fig. 4.4: Changes of the cervix during advanced pregnancy

induced (oestrogen) and regress spontaneously after delivery.

Secretion: The secretion is copious and tenacious—physiological leucorrhoea of pregnancy. This is due to the effect of progesterone. The mucus not only fills up the glands but also forms a thick plug effectively sealing the cervical canal. Microscopic examination shows fragmentation or crystallization (beading).

Anatomical: The length of the cervix remains unaltered but becomes bulky. The cervix is directed posteriorly but after the engagement of the head, directed in line of vagina. There is no alteration in the relation of the cervix. There is unfolding of the isthmus; beginning 12 weeks onwards and takes part in the formation of the lower uterine segment. Variable amount of

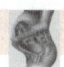
effacement is noticed near term in primi-gravidae. In multiparae, the canal is slightly dilated.

OTHER ORGANS

Fallopian tube

At term, its attachment to the uterus is placed at the lower end of the upper one-third, because of marked growth of the fundus. The total length is somewhat increased. The tube becomes congested. Epithelium becomes flattened and patches of decidual reaction are observed.

Ovary

There is persistence and growth of the corpus luteum which reaches its maximum at 8th week when it measures about 2.5 cm and becomes cystic. It looks bright orange, later on becomes yellow and finally pale. Regression occurs following decline in the secretion of hCG from the placenta. Colloid degeneration occurs at 12th week which later becomes calcified at term. Hormones, oestrogen and progesterone secreted by the corpus luteum, maintain the environment for the growing ovum before the action is taken over by the placenta. The hormones not only control the formation and maintenance of decidua of pregnancy, but also inhibit ripening of the follicles. *Thus, both the ovarian and uterine cycles of the normal menstruation remain suspended.*

Decidual reaction : There may be patchy sheet of decidual cells on the outer surface of the ovary. These are metaplastic changes due to high hormonal stimulation. The same stimulus may also produce luteinisation of partially developed follicles.

BREASTS

The changes in the breasts are best evident in a primigravida. In multipara who has once lactated, the changes are not clearly defined.

Size

Increased size of the breasts becomes evident even in early weeks. This is due to marked hypertrophy and proliferation of the ducts (oestrogen) and the alveoli (oestrogen and progesterone) which are marked in the peripheral lobules. There is also hypertrophy of the connective tissue stroma. Myoepithelial cells become prominent. Vascularity is increased which results in appearance of bluish veins running under the skin. Quite often, the **axillary tail** (prolongation of the breast tissue under cover of the pectoralis major) becomes enlarged and painful. There may be evidence of striation due to stretching of the cutis.

Nipples and areola

The nipples become larger, erectile and deeply pigmented. Variable number of sebaceous glands (5–15) which remain invisible in the non-pregnant state in the areola, become hyper-trophied are called *Montgomery's tubercles.* These are placed surrounding the nipples. Their secretion keeps the nipple and the areola moist

> **Box 4.1:** Breast changes in chronological order
>
> - **3–4 weeks:** Pricking, tingling sensation due to increased blood supply particularly around nipple.
> - **6–8 weeks:** Increase in size, painful, tense and nodular due to hypertrophy of the alveoli. Delicate, bluish surface veins become visible just beneath the skin.
> - **8–12 weeks:** Montgomery's tubercles become more prominent on the areola. These hypertrophic sebaceous glands secrete sebum, which keeps the nipple soft and supple. The pigmented area around the nipple (the primary areola) darkens and may enlarge and become more erectile.
> - **16 weeks:** Colostrum can be expressed. The secondary areola develops with further extension of the pigmented area that is after mottled in appearance.
> - **Late pregnancy:** Colostrum may leak from the breasts, progesterone causes the nipple to become more prominent and mobile.

and healthy. An outer zone of less marked and irregular pigmented area appears in second trimester and is called *secondary areola.*

Secretion

Secretion can be squeezed out of the breast at about 12th week which, at first, becomes sticky. Later on, by 16th week, it becomes thick and yellowish. *The demonstration of secretion in the breast of a woman who has never lactated, is an important sign of pregnancy.* However, in parous woman, it is of least diagnostic significance.

CUTANEOUS CHANGES

Pigmentation

The distribution of pigmentary changes is selective.

1. **Face** (chloasma gravidarum or pregnancy mask): It is an extreme form of pigmentation around the cheek, forehead and around the eyes. It may be patchy or diffuse; disappears spontaneously after delivery.
2. **Breast:** The changes are already described.
3. **Abdomen**
   - **Linea nigra:** It is a brownish black pigmented area in the midline stretching from the xiphisternum to the symphysis pubis. The pigmentary changes are probably due to melanocyte stimulating hormone from the anterior pituitary. However, oestrogen and progesterone may be related to it as similar changes are observed in women taking oral contraceptives. The pigmentation disappears after delivery.
   - **Striae gravidarum:** These are slightly depressed linear marks with varying length and breadth found in pregnancy. They are predominantly found in the abdominal wall below the umbilicus, sometimes, over the thighs and breasts. *These represent the scar tissues in the deeper layer of the cutis.* Initially, these

are pinkish but after the delivery, the scar tissues contract and obliterate the capillaries and they become glistening white in appearance and are called *Striae Albicans.* Thus, in multiparae, both pinkish and white striae are visible. Apart from the mechanical stretching of the skin, increase in aldosterone production during pregnancy is the responsible factor. Controlled weight gain during pregnancy and massaging the abdominal wall by lubricants like olive oil, may be helpful in reducing their formation. *Apart from pregnancy, it may form in cases of generalized oedema, marked obesity or in Cushing's syndrome.*

WEIGHT GAIN AND WATER METABOLISM

Weight gain

The total weight gain during the course of a singleton pregnancy averages 11 kg (24 lb). This has been distributed to 1 kg in first trimester and 5 kg in second and third trimester. The total weight gain, at term, is distributed approximately as follows:

1. Reproductive weight gain—6 kg
   - Fetus—3.3 kg, placenta—0.6 kg and liquor—0.8 kg,
   - Uterus—0.9 kg and breasts—0.4 kg.
2. Net maternal weight gain—6 kg
   - Increase in blood volume—1.3 kg
   - Increase in extracellular fluid—1.2 kg
   - Accumulation of fat (mainly) and protein—3.5 kg

Importance of weight checking

Single weight checking is of little value except to identify the weight or underweight patient. Periodic and regular weight checking is of importance to detect abnormality.

- Rapid gain in weight of more than 0.5 kg (1 lb) a week or more than 2 kg (5 lb) a month in later months of pregnancy may

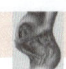

be the early manifestation of preeclampsia and need for careful supervision.

- Stationary or falling weight is one of the suggestive feature of intrauterine growth retardation or intrauterine death of the foetus.

HAEMATOLOGICAL CHANGES

Blood volume

During pregnancy, there is increased vascularity of the enlarging uterus with the interposition of uteroplacental circulation. *The blood volume is markedly raised during pregnancy.* The blood volume starts to increase from about 10th week, expands rapidly thereafter to *maximum 40% above the nonpregnant level at 30–32 weeks.* The level remains almost static till term.

Plasma volume

Plasma volume increases during pregnancy. The rate of increase almost parallels to the blood volume but *the maximum is reached to the extent of 50%. Total plasma volume increases to the extent of 1.25 litres.* The increase is greater in multigravida, in multiple pregnancy and with large baby.

RBC and haemoglobin

The RBC volume is increased to the extent of 20–30%. The total increase in volume is about 350 ml, the amount to be regulated by the increased demand of oxygen transport during pregnancy.

The disproportionate increase in plasma and RBC volume produces a state of haemodilution during pregnancy (Table 4.1).

Leucocytes

Neutrophilic leucocytosis occurs to the extent of 10–15,000/cu.mm and even to 20,000/cu.mm in labour. The increase is due to rise in the number of mature and immature neutrophils.

Total protein

Total plasma protein increases from the normal 180 gm (nonpregnant) to 230 gm at term. *The normal albumin : globulin ratio of 1.7:1 is diminished to 1:1.*

Blood coagulation factors

Fibrinogen level is raised by 50% from 200–400 mg% in non-pregnant to 300–600 mg% in pregnancy. *ESR gives a much higher value* (four fold increase) during pregnancy. *As such, ESR has got little diagnostic value in pregnancy.* There is increase in activities of clotting factors like X, IX, VIII, VI and II. The level of the factors XI and XIII are slightly decreased. The clotting time does not show any significant change. These are all effective to control blood and haemostasis after the separation of placenta.

	Non-pregnant	Pregnancy near term	Total increment	Change
Blood volume (ml)	4000	5500	1500	+30–40%
Plasma volume (ml)	2500	3750	1250	+40–50%
Red cell volume (ml)	1400	1750	350	+20–30%
Total Hb (gm)	475	560	85	+18–20%
Haematocrit (whole body)	38%	32%		Diminished

Table 4.1: Principal blood changes during pregnancy

 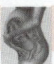

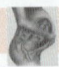

HEART AND CIRCULATION

Anatomical changes

Due to elevation of the diaphragm consequent to the enlarged uterus, *the heart is pushed upwards and outwards* with slight rotation to left. There is no evidence of hypertrophy or dilatation of the heart.

Cardiac output

The cardiac output starts to increase from 10th week of pregnancy, reaches its peak 40% at about 24–30 weeks. In the nonpregnant state, the cardiac output measures 4.5 litres per minute which rises to 6.1 liters, 6.1 liters and 6.26 liters per minute in first, second and third trimester respectively.

Blood pressure

In spite of increased cardiac output, the blood pressure remains almost within normal values (systolic 110–120 mm Hg. Diastolic 65–80 mm Hg). *This is due to diminished peripheral vascular resistance affected by high level of progesterone.*

Venous pressure

Femoral venous pressure is markedly raised especially in the later months. *It is due to pressure exerted by the gravid uterus on the common iliac veins, more on the right side due to dextrorotation of the uterus.*

Supine hypotension syndrome
(postural hypotension)

During late pregnancy, the gravid uterus produces a compression effect on the inferior vena cava when the patient is in supine position. This, however, results in opening up of the collateral circulation by means of paravertebral and azygos veins. In some cases (10%), when collateral circulation fails to open up, the venous return of the heart may be seriously curtailed. This results in production of hypotension, tachycardia and syncope. *The normal blood pressure is quickly restored by turning the patient to lateral position.* The augmentation of the venous during uterine contraction prevents the manifestation from developing during labour.

Regional distribution of blood flow

Uterine blood flow is increased from 50 ml per minute in non-pregnant state to about 750 ml near term.

METABOLIC CHANGES

General metabolic changes

Total metabolism is increased due to the needs of the growing uterus and the fetus. Basal metabolic rate is increased to the extent of 30% higher than that of the average for the non-pregnant women.

Protein metabolism

There is a positive nitrogenous balance throughout pregnancy. As the conversion of amino acid to urea is depressed, the blood urea level falls to 15–20 mg%.

Carbohydrate metabolism

Transfer of increased amount of glucose from mother to the fetus is needed throughout pregnancy. Insulin secretion is increased due to hyperplasia and hypertrophy of beta cells of pancreas.

Fat metabolism

There is increased absorption of fat in later months of pregnancy. An average of 3–4 kg of fat is stored during pregnancy mostly in the abdominal wall, breasts, hips and thighs. Plasma lipids increase appreciably during the later half of pregnancy due to increased oestrogen level. The activity of lipoprotein lipase is increased (Table 4.2).

Iron metabolism

Iron is absorbed in ferrous form from duodenum and jejunum and is released into the circulation as transferrin. Iron is transported actively across the placenta to the fetus. Iron requirement, during pregnancy, is considerable

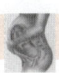

Table 4.2: Changes in lipid metabolism

	Non-pregnant	Pregnancy near term	Change
Total lipid (mg/100 ml)	650	1000	+ 50%
Cholesterol (mg/100 ml)	180	260	+ 40%
Phospholipid (mg/100 ml)	250	350	+ 40%
Triglycerides (mg/100 ml)	80	160	+ 50%

and is mostly limited to the second half of the pregnancy especially to the last 12 weeks. *Total iron requirement during pregnancy is estimated approximately 1000 mg.*

SYSTEMIC CHANGES

Respiratory system

With the enlargement of the uterus, especially in the later months, there is elevation of the diaphragm and breathing becomes diaphragmatic. Both the transverse diameter and the circumferences of the thoracic cage are increased. Mucosa of the upper respiratory tract shows hyperaemia and congestion. A state of hyperventilation occurs during pregnancy, leading to *increase in tidal volume.*

Urinary system

Kidney: There is dilatation of renal pelvis. *Renal plasma flow* is increased by 25–50%, maximum in the first trimester. *Glomerular filtration rate (GFR)* is increased by 50% all throughout pregnancy. *Renal function test* is augmented. Renal tubules fail to reabsorb glucose, uric acid, amino acids, water soluble vitamins and other substances completely. This is mainly due to increased GFR.

Ureter: **Ureters become atonic** due to high progesterone level. *Dilatation* of the ureter above the pelvic brim with stasis is marked on the right side especially in primigravidae. It is due to dextrorotation of the uterus pressing the right ureter against the pelvic brim and also due to pressure by the right ovarian vein which crosses the right ureter at right angle. *The stasis is marked between 20 and 24 weeks.* There is marked hypertrophy of the muscle and the sheath of the ureter especially the pelvic part probably due to oestrogen. *There is elongation, kinking and outward displacement of the ureters.*

Bladder: There is marked congestion with hypertrophy of the muscles and elastic tissues of the wall. In late pregnancy, the bladder mucosa becomes oedematous due to venous and lymphatic obstruction, especially in primigravidae following early engagement. Increased frequency of micturition is noticed at 6–8 weeks of pregnancy which subsides after 12 weeks. It is due to the anteverted uterus irritating the fundus of the bladder. *In late pregnancy, frequency of micturition once more reappears due to* pressure on the bladder as the presenting part descends down the pelvis. Stress incontinence may be an annoying symptom in late pregnancy due to urethral sphincter weakness.

Alimentary system

The gums become congested and spongy and may bleed to touch. *Muscle tone and motility of the entire gastrointestinal tract* are diminished due to high progesterone level. *Cardiac sphincter* is relaxed and regurgitation of acid gastric content into the oesophagus may produce chemical oesophagitis and heart burn. Atonicity of the gut leads to constipation, while diminished peristalsis facilitates more absorption of food materials.

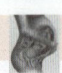
Liver and gallbladder

There is marked atonicity of the gall bladder. This, together with high blood cholesterol level during pregnancy, favours stone formation.

Nervous system

Nausea, vomiting, mental irritability and sleeplessness are probably due to some psychological background. Melancholia and real psychosis may develop in a susceptible individual having a family history. There may be generalised neuritis probably due to vitamin B$_1$ (thiamine) deficiency.

Compression of the median nerve underneath the carpal ligament over the wrist joint, leading to pain and paraesthesia in the hands and arm *(carpal tunnel syndrome)*, may appear in the later months of pregnancy.

Calcium metabolism and locomotor system

During pregnancy there is increase in the demand of calcium by the growing fetus to the extent of 28 gm, two-third of which is required in the last trimester.

Daily requirement of calcium during pregnancy averages 1–1.5 gm.

DIAGNOSIS OF PREGNANCY

Duration of pregnancy

The duration of pregnancy has traditionally been calculated by the clinicians in terms of 10 lunar months or 9 calendar months and 7 days or 280 days or 40 weeks, *calculated from the first day of the last menstrual period. This is called menstrual or gestational age.*

FIRST TRIMESTER (FIRST 12 WEEKS)

Subjective symptoms

The following are the presumptive symptoms of early months of pregnancy:

Amenorrhoea: During the reproductive period in an otherwise healthy individual having previous normal periods, is likely due to pregnancy unless proved otherwise. However, cyclic bleeding may occur up to 12 weeks of pregnancy, until the decidual space is obtained by the fusion of decidua vera with decidua capsularis.

Morning sickness: Is inconsistently present in about 50% cases, more often in the first pregnancy than in the subsequent one. *It usually appears soon following the missed period and rarely lasts beyond the 3rd month.* Its intensity varies from nausea on rising from bed to loss of appetite or even vomiting. But it usually does not affect the health status of the mother.

Frequency of micturition is quite troublesome symptom during 8–12th weeks of pregnancy. It is due to:

1. Resting of the bulky uterus on the fundus of the bladder because of exaggerated anteverted position of the uterus
2. Congestion of the bladder mucosa
3. Stretching of the bladder base due to backward displacement of the cervix.

Breast discomfort: In the form of feeling of fullness and 'pricking sensation' is evident as early as 6–8th week especially in primigravidae.

Fatigue: Is a frequent symptom which may occur early in pregnancy.

Objective signs

Breast changes: Are valuable only in primigravidae, as in multiparae, the breasts are enlarged and often contain milk for years. The breast changes are evident between 6 and 8 weeks (Fig. 4.5).

The nipple and the areola (primary) become more pigmented especially in dark women. Montgomery's tubercles are prominent. Thick yellowish secretion (colostrum) can be expressed as early as in 12th week.

Per abdomen: Uterus remains a pelvic organ until 12th week, it may be just felt per abdomen as a suprapubic bulge.

Pelvic changes: The pelvic changes are diverse and appear at different periods.

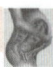

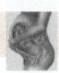

6th week, size of a cricket ball at 8th week and size of a fetal head by 12th week. The pyriform shape of the non-pregnant uterus becomes globular by 12th weeks. The uterus becomes acutely anteverted between 6 and 8 weeks. There may be asymmetrical enlargement of the uterus if there is lateral implantation. This is called *Piskacek's sign. The pregnant uterus feels soft and elastic.*

5. **Hegar's sign:** It is present in two-thirds of cases. *It can be demonstrated between 6 and 10 weeks,* a little earlier in multiparae (Fig. 4.6). *This sign is based on the fact that.*

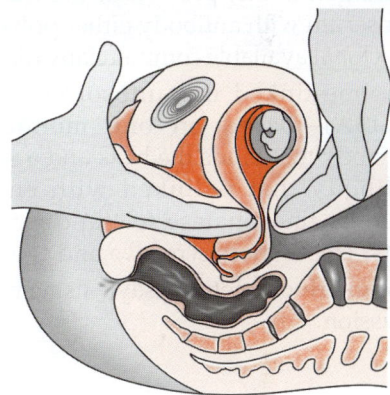

Fig. 4.6: Demonstration of Hegar's sign

- Upper part of the body of the uterus is enlarged by the growing ovum.
- Lower part of the body of the uterus is empty and extremely soft.
- The cervix is comparatively firm. Because of variation in consistency, on bimanual examination, the abdominal and vaginal fingers seem to appose below the body of the uterus.

6. **Palmer's sign:** Regular and rhythmic uterine contraction can be elicited during bimanual examination as early as 4–8 weeks. Palmer in 1949, first described it and it is a valuable sign when elicited (Fig. 4.7).

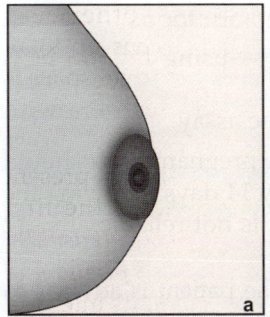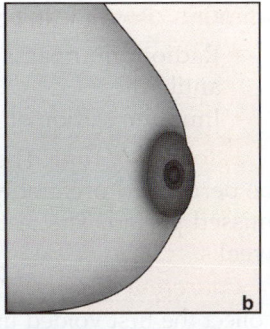

Fig. 4.5: Breast changes during pregnancy. **a.** Pronounced pigmentation of the primary areola and nipple, **b.** Appearance of secondary areola, development of Montgomery's tubercles and increased vascularity

1. **Jacquemier's or Chadwick's sign:** It is the dusky hue of the vestibule and anterior vaginal wall visible at about 8th week of pregnancy. The discolouration is due to local vascular congestion.
2. **Vaginal sign**
   - Apart from the bluish discolouration of the anterior vaginal wall
   - The walls become softened
   - Copious nonirritating mucoid discharge appears at 6th week.
   - There is increased pulsation, felt through the lateral fornices at 8th week called Osiander's sign. Similar pulsation is, however, felt in acute pelvic inflammation.
3. **Cervical signs**
   - Cervix becomes soft as early as 6th week *(Goodell's sign),* a little earlier in multiparae. The softening is pronounced surrounding the external os and also in the upper part. The pregnant cervix feels like the lips of the mouth.
   - On speculum examination, the bluish discolouration of the cervix is visible. It is due to increased vascularity.
4. **Uterine signs**
   - *Size, shape and consistency:* The uterus is enlarged to the size of hen's egg at

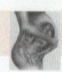

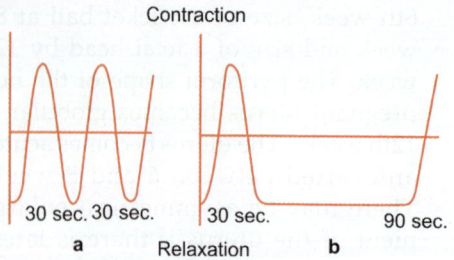

Fig. 4.7: Graphic representation of Palmer's sign. a. At 4–8th week, b. At 10th week

Immunological tests (Fig. 4.8)

Principle: Pregnancy tests depend on detection of the antigen (hCG) present in the maternal urine or serum with antibody either polyclonal or monoclonal available commercially (Fig. 4.9).

- Enzyme-linked immunosorbent assay (ELISA)—based on one monoclonal antibody that binds the hCG and a second antibody that is linked with enzyme alkaline phosphatase to 'sandwich' the hCG. This is more sensitive and specific.
- Immunofluorometric assay—using photon emission.

Immuno assays with radioisotopes

- Radioimmunoassay—using I^{125} ido hCG antibodies
- Immuno radiometric assay.

Selection of time: The pregnancy test should be performed preferably 14 days following the missed period. The test is not reliable after 12 weeks.

Collection of urine: The patient is advised to collect the first voided urine in the morning in a clean container **(not to wash with soap)**. The urine should be sent to the laboratory so that the test could be performed within 12 hours.

Radioimmunoassay: This is more sensitive method and can be employed to detect the presence of hCG in the serum as early as 8–9 days after ovulation, probably on the day of blastocyst implantation.

Were based on the classic discovery of Aschheim and Zondek in 1927. All these tests are obsolete now-a-days.

Sonography (Fig. 4.10)

The characteristic small white gestational ring is as early as 5th week of pregnancy. The other ultrasonic observations are: fetal pole at 6th

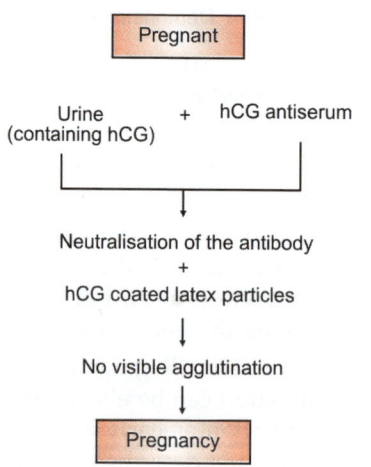

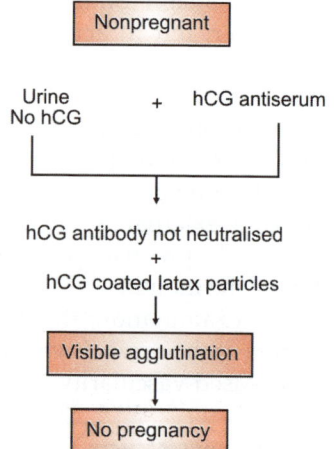

Fig. 4.8: Schematic representation of the principles employed in immunological test to confirm pregnancy

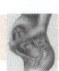

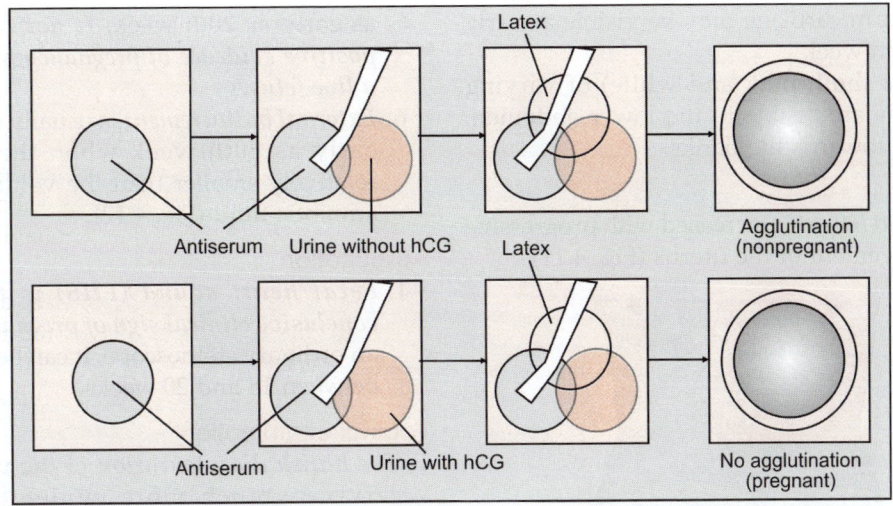

Fig. 4.9: Diagrammatic representation of the technique of the immunological tests of pregnancy (LAI)

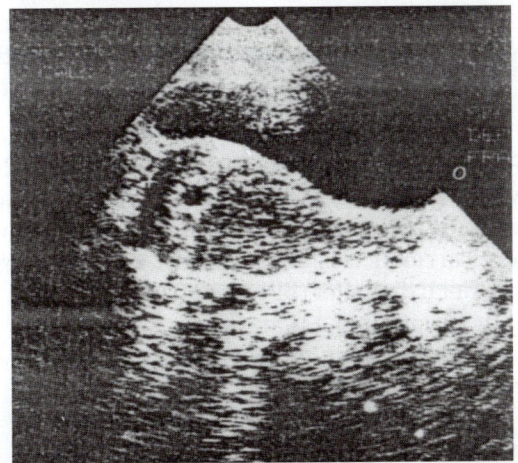

Fig. 4.10: Gestational ring at 5th week

week, yolk sac at 6th week, cardiac pulsation at 7th week and embryonic movements at 8th week of gestation.

SECOND TRIMESTER (13–28 WEEKS)

Symptoms

The subjective symptoms such as nausea, vomiting and frequency of micturition usually subside, while amenorrhoea continues.

The new features that appear are

1. **Quickening:** *(Feeling of life) denotes the perception of active fetal movement by the women.* It is usually felt about the 18th week, about 2 weeks earlier in multiparae.
2. **Progressive enlargement** of the lower abdomen by a mass.

General examination

1. **Chloasma:** Pigmentation over the forehead and cheek may appear at about 24th week.
2. **Breast changes**
   - Breasts are more enlarged with prominent veins under the skin.
   - Secondary areola specially demarcated in primigravidae, usually appears at about 20th week.
   - Montgomery's tubercles are prominent and extend to the secondary areola.
   - Colostrum becomes thick and yellowish by 16th week.
   - Variable degree of striae may be visible with advancing weeks.

ABDOMINAL EXAMINATION

Inspection

1. Linear pigmented zone *(linea nigra)* extending from the symphysis pubis to

 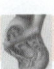

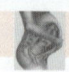

ensiform cartilage may be visible as early as 20th week.

2. *Striae* (both pink and white) of varying degree are visible in the lower abdomen, more towards the flanks.

Palpation

1. *Fundal height* is increased with progressive enlargement of the uterus (Fig. 4.11).

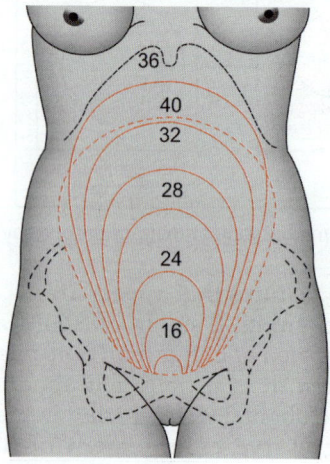

Fig. 4.11: The level of fundus uteri at different weeks

The height of the uterus is midway between the symphysis pubis and umbilicus at 16th week, at the level of umbilicus at 24th week and at the junction of the lower third and upper two-thirds of the distance between the umbilicus and ensiform cartilage at 28th week.

2. *The uterus feels soft and elastic* and becomes ovoid in shape.

3. *Braxton-Hicks contractions* are evident, the features of which have been mentioned before.

4. *Palpation of fetal parts* can be made distinctly by 20th week. The findings are of value not only to diagnose pregnancy but also to identify the presentation and position of the fetus in later weeks.

5. *Active fetal movements* can be felt at intervals by placing the hand over the uterus

as early as 20th week. *It not only gives positive evidence of pregnancy but also of a live fetus.*

6. *External ballottement* is usually elicited as early as 20th week when the fetus is relatively smaller than the volume of the amniotic fluid (Fig. 4.12).

Auscultation

1. *Fetal heart sound (FHS) is the most conclusive clinical sign of pregnancy.* With an ordinary stethoscope, it can be detected between 18 and 20 weeks.

Vaginal examination

1. *The bluish discolouration* of the vulva and cervix is much more evident, so also softening of the cervix.

2. *Internal ballottement* can be elicited between 16 and 28 weeks. The fetus is so small before 16th week and too large to displace after 28th week (Figs 4.13a to c).

Investigations

Sonography: Routine sonography at 18–20 weeks permits a detailed survey of fetal anatomy, placental site and the integrity of the cervical canal. Gestational age is determined by biparietal diameter (BPD) and femur length (FL) with variation of ±10 days.

Radiologic evidence of fetal skeletal shadow may be visible *as early as 16th week.*

LAST TRIMESTER (29–40 WEEKS)

Symptoms

1. *Amenorrhoea* persists

2. *Enlargement of the abdomen* is progressive which produces some mechanical discomfort to the patient such as palpation or dyspnoea following exertion.

3. *Lightening:* At about 38th week, especially in primigravida, a sense of relief of the pressure symptoms is obtained due to engagement of the presenting part.

4. *Frequency of micturition* reappears.

5. *Fetal movements* are more pronounced.

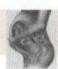

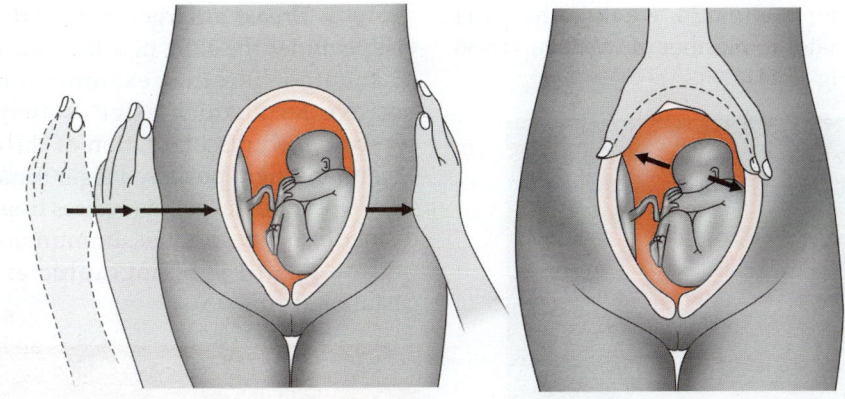

Fig. 4.12: External ballottement

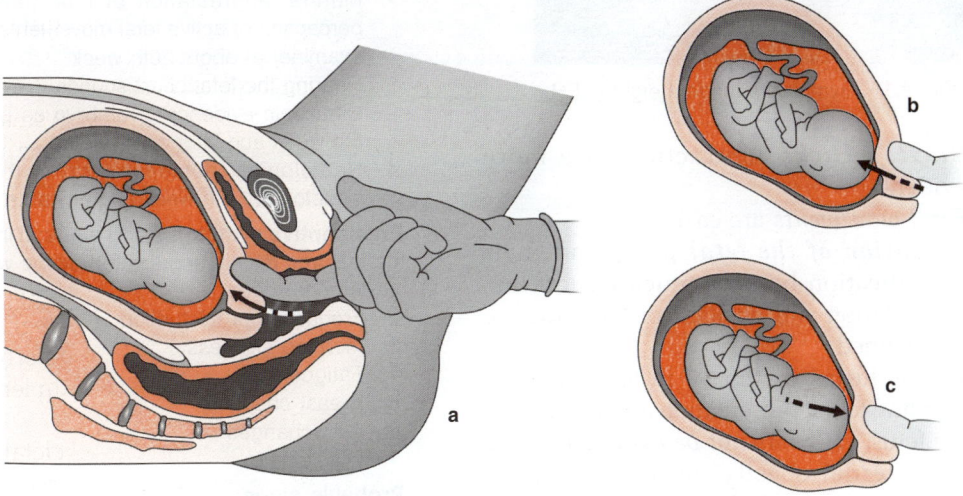

Fig. 4.13: Steps (a, b, c) showing how to elicit internal ballottement

Signs

- *Cutaneous changes* are more prominent with increased pigmentation and striae.
- *Uterine shape* is changed from cylindrical to spherical beyond 36th week.
- *Fundal height*: The distance between the umbilicus and the ensiform cartilage is divided into three equal parts. The fundal height corresponds to the junction of the upper and middle third at 32 weeks, up to level of ensiform cartilage at 36th week and it comes down to 32 week level at 40th week because of engagement of the presenting part. *If the head is floating, it is 32 weeks pregnancy and if the head is engaged, it is 40 weeks pregnancy.*
- *Symphysis fundal height (SFH).* The upper border of the fundus is located by the ulnar border of the left hand and this point is marked. The distance between the upper border of the symphysis pubis up to the marked point is measured by a tape in

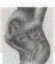

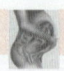

centimeter. After 24 weeks, the SFH approximates to number of weeks up to 36 weeks (Fig. 4.14).

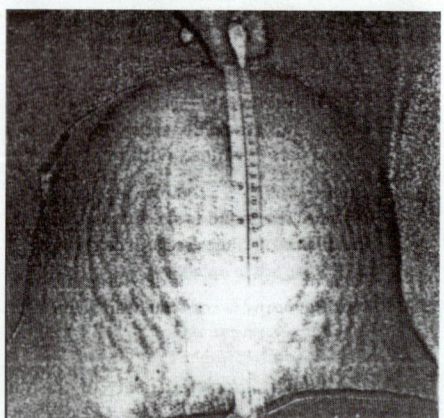

Fig. 4.14: Symphysis fundal height (SFH)

- *Braxton-Hicks* contractions are more evident.
- *Fetal movements* are easily felt.
- *Palpation of the fetal parts* and their identification become much easier. Lie, presentation and position of the fetus are determined.
- *FHS* is heard distinctly in areas corresponding to the presentation and position of the fetus. **FHS may not be audible in cases** of maternal obesity, polyhydramnios, occipitoposterior and certainly in IUD.
- *Sonography*: Gestational age estimation by BPO, FL, AC and HC are less accurate (variation ±3 weeks). Fetal growth assessment can be made provided accurate dating scan has been done in first or second trimester.

CHRONOLOGICAL APPEARANCE OF SPECIFIC SYMPTOMS AND SIGNS OF PREGNANCY

At 6–8 weeks

Symptoms: Amenorrhoea, morning sickness, frequency of micturition, fatigue, breast discomfort.

Signs: Breast enlargement, engorged veins visible under the skin, nipples and areola more pigmented. Internal examination reveals–positive Jacquemier's sign, softening of the cervix, bluish discolouration of the cervix and Osiander's sign, positive Hegar's and Palmer's sign. Uterine enlargement varies from hen's egg to medium size orange. Immunological tests will be positive. Sonographic evidence of gestational ring.

> **Box 4.2:** Summary of diagnosis of pregnancy

- **Positive or absolute sign**
  1. Manual appreciation of fetal parts and perception of active fetal movements by the examiner at about 20th week.
  2. Hearing the fetal heart sounds.
  3. Ultrasonic evidence of embryo as early as 6th week and later on the fetus.
  4. Radiological demonstration of the fetal skeleton at 16th week and onwards.
- **Presumptive symptoms and signs:** It includes the features mainly appreciated by the women.
  1. Amenorrhoea
  2. Frequency of micturition
  3. Morning sickness
  4. Fatigue
  5. Breast changes
  6. Skin changes
  7. Quickening
- **Probable signs**
  1. Abdominal enlargement
  2. Braxton-Hicks contractions
  3. External ballottement
  4. Outlining the fetus
  5. Changes in the size, shape and consistency of the uterus
  6. Jacquemier's sign
  7. Softening of the cervix
  8. Osiander's sign
  9. Internal ballottement
  10. Immunological test

At 16th week

Symptoms: Except amenorrhoea, all the previous symptoms disappear.

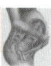

Signs: **Breast changes**—pigmentation of primary areola and prominence of Montgomery's tubercles, colostrum can be expressed.

Uterus: Midway between symphysis pubis and umbilicus, Braxton-Hicks contractions, uterine souffle, internal ballottement X-ray shows fetal shadow. Sonographic diagnosis.

At 20th week

Symptoms: Amenorrhoea, quickening (18th week).

Signs: Appearance of secondary areola (20 weeks), uterus at the level of umbilicus at 24 weeks, Braxton-Hicks contractions, external ballottement (20th week), fetal parts (20 weeks), fetal movements (20 weeks), FHS (20 weeks), internal ballottement (16–28 weeks). X-ray shows fetal shadow, sonographic diagnosis. Antenatal care.

Antenatal care comprises

- Careful history taking and examinations (general and obstetrical).
- Advice given to the pregnant woman.

Aims and objectives

1. To screen the 'high-risk' cases.
2. To prevent or to detect and treat at the earliest any untoward complications.
3. To ensure continued medical surveillance and prophylaxis.
4. To educate the mother about the physiology of pregnancy and labour by demonstrations, charts and diagrams (mother craft classes), so that fear is removed and psychology is improved.
5. To discuss with the couple about the place, time and mode of delivery, provisionally and care of the newborn.
6. To motivate the couple about the need of family planning and also appropriate advice to couple seeking medical termination of pregnancy.

The objective is to ensure a normal pregnancy with delivery of a healthy baby from a healthy mother.

The criteria of a normal pregnancy are delivery of a single baby in good condition between 38 and 42 weeks by dates, with fetal weight of 2.5 kg or more and with no maternal complication. As such, a normal pregnancy is a retrospective term.

PROCEDURE AT THE FIRST VISIT

Objectives

1. To assess the health status of the mother and fetus; to screen out the 'at risk' pregnancy and to formulate the plan of subsequent management.
2. To obtain a base line information against which the subsequent changes are assessed and which are of importance in the determination of the gestational age.

HISTORY TAKING

Vital statistics

Name: ....

Date of first examination: ....

Address: ....

Age: A woman having her first pregnancy at the age of 30 or above is called *elderly primigravida.*

Gravida denotes a pregnant state both present and past, irrespective of the period of gestation. *Parity* denotes a state of previous pregnancy beyond the period of viability.

Terminology

A *nullipara* is one who has never completed a pregnancy to the stage of viability. She may or may not have aborted previously.

A *nulligravida* is one who is not now and never has been pregnant.

A *primipara* is one who has delivered one viable child.

A *primigravida* is one who is pregnant for the first time.

A *multigravida* is one who has previously been pregnant. She may have aborted or have delivered a viable baby.

Multipara is one who has delivered two or more children.

A *parturient* is a woman in labour.

A *puerpera* is a woman who has just given birth.

Duration of marriage

This is relevant when dealing with pregnancy in comparatively advanced age to note the fertility or fecundity. A pregnancy long after marriage without taking recourse to any method of contraception, is called low fecundity and soon after marriage is called high fecundity. A woman with low fecundity is unlikely to conceive frequently.

Religion: ....

Occupation: It may be helpful in interpreting symptoms due to fatigue or occupational hazards.

Occupation of the husband: A fair idea about the socioeconomic condition of the patient can be assessed. This knowledge is of value

1. To anticipate the complications likely to be associated with low social status such as anaemia, pre-eclampsia, prematurity, etc.
2. To give reasonable and realistic antenatal advice.
3. During family planning guidance.

Period of gestation: The duration of pregnancy is to be expressed in terms of completed weeks. A fraction of a week of more than 3 days is to be considered as completed week. *In calculating the weeks of gestation* in early part of pregnancy, counting is to be done from the first day of last menstrual period (LMP) and in later months of pregnancy, counting is to be done from expected date of delivery (EDD).

Complaints: Categorically, the genesis of the complaints are to be noted stating the mode of onset, progress and duration. Even if there is no complaint, enquiry is to be made about the sleep, appetite, bowel habit and urination.

History of present pregnancy: The important complications in different trimesters of the present pregnancy are to be noted carefully. These are hyperemesis and threatened abortion in first trimester; features of pyelitis in second trimester and anaemia, pre-eclampsia and antepartum haemorrhage in the last trimester. Number of previous antenatal check up, if any, has to be noted. Any medication or radiation exposure in early pregnancy, or medical-surgical events during pregnancy should be enquired.

Obstetrical history: This is only related with multigravidae. The previous obstetric events are to be recorded chronologically as per the proforma given in the table. To be relevant, enquiry is to be made whether she had antenatal and intranatal care before (Table 4.3).

The obstetrical history is to be summed up as

No. of living children: ....

Boys: .... Girls: ....

Health status of the baby: ....

Immunisation: ....

Last issue: ....

The sex of children is needed when permanent sterilisation is to be considered. An unduly long gap between the last and the present pregnancy requires careful supervision during pregnancy and labour. *The minimum spacing* between one birth and subsequent pregnancy should be 2 years. It is adequate to replenish about 1000 mg of iron depletion due to childbirth and lactation by a balanced diet. However, in the underprivileged sector, *it should be at least 3 years.*

Menstrual history: Cycle, duration, amount of blood flow and first day of the last menstruation period (LMP) are to be noted. From the LMP, the expected date of delivery (EDD) has to be calculated. The first day of the

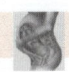

Table 4.3: Obstetrical history

No.	Year and date	Pregnancy events	Labour events	Methods of delivery	Puerperium	Baby • Wt. and Sex • Condition at birth • Duration of breastfeeding • Immunisation
1.	1984 January	Abortion at 8 week	-------------	MTP	Uneventful	-------------
2.	1987 April	Well covered antenatally. Uneventful	Uneventful	Spontaneous vaginal	Uneventful	Boy, average wt. Cried at birth. Breastfed—8 months
3.	1991	- do-	- do-	- do-	- do-	Girl average wt. Cried at birth. Breastfed—6 months Both the babies fully immunised.

menstruation, being the important event, can be remembered precisely while the last day of the period is often tailed off and hence may be forgotten.

Calculation of the expected date of delivery (EDD): This is done according to **Naegele's formula (1812)** by adding calendar months 9 and 7 days, to the first day of the last period. Alternatively, one can count back 3 calendar months from the first day of the last period and then add 7 days to get the expected date of delivery; the former method is commonly employed.

Example: The patient had her first day of last menstrual period on 1st January. By adding 9 calendar months it comes to 1st October and then add 7 days, i.e. 8th October, which becomes the expected date of delivery.

Past medical history: Relevant history of past medical illnesses is to be elicited.

Past surgical history: Previous surgery, general or gynaecological, if any, is to be enquired.

Family history: Family history of hypertension, diabetes, tuberculosis, blood dyscrasias, known hereditary disease, if any, or twinning is to be enquired.

Personal history: Contraceptive practice prior to pregnancy, smoking or alcohol habits, if any, are to be enquired. LMP may have a withdrawal bleed following pill usage. The first ovulation may be delayed for 4 to 6 weeks. If pregnancy occurs, the estimated date of confinement may be understated by 2 or more weeks. Smoking or alcohol abuse has got some relation with low birth weight of the baby. Previous history of blood transfusion, corticosteroid therapy, any drug allergy and immunisation against tetanus or prophylactic administration of anti-D immunoglobulin are to be enquired.

EXAMINATION

General

Build: Obese/average/thin

Nutrition: Good/average/poor

Height: Short stature is likely to be associated with a small pelvis.

Thus, in primigravidae the height is to be measured to screen out the short stature. While an arbitrary measurement of 5 ft. is considered as short stature in western countries, it is 4"–7" in India considering the low average height.

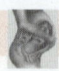

Weight: Weight should be taken in all cases in an accurate weighing machine. Repeat weight checking in subsequent visit should preferably be done in the same weighing machine. The importance of weight checking has already been discussed.

Pallor: The sites to be noted are lower palpebral conjunctiva, dorsum of the tongue and nail beds.

Jaundice: The sites to be noted are bulbar conjunctiva, under surface of the tongue, hard palate and skin.

Tongue, teeth, gums and tonsils: Evidences of malnutrition are evident from glossitis and stomatitis. Evidence of any source of infection in the mouth is to be eradicated least there be a chance of autogenous infection in puerperium.

Neck: Neck veins, thyroid gland or lymph glands are looked for any abnormality. Slight physiological enlargement of the thyroid gland occurs during pregnancy in 50% of cases.

Oedema of legs

Both the legs are to be examined. The sites for evidence of oedema are over the medial malleolus and anterior surface of the lower one-third of the tibia. The area is to be pressed with the thumb for at least 5 seconds. Varicosity in the legs, if any, is to be noted.

Causes of oedema in pregnancy

1. Physiological
2. Pre-eclampsia
3. Anaemia and hypoproteinaemia
4. Cardiac failure
5. Nephrotic syndrome

Physiological oedema: The cause of physiological oedema is due to increased venous pressure of the inferior extremities by the gravid uterus pressing on the common iliac veins. *The features of the physiological oedema are:*

1. Slight degree (ankle oedema), usually confined to one leg, more on the right.

2. Unassociated with any other pre-eclampsia features such as hypertension or protei-nuria.

3. Disappears on rest alone.

Pulse

BP: Disappearance of sounds (Korotkoff 5) rather than muffling of sounds (Korotkoff 4) is the best representation of diastolic pressure during pregnancy.

HEART, LUNGS, LIVER AND SPLEEN

Breasts: Examination of the breasts is manda-tory not only to note the presence of pregnancy changes but also to note the nipples (cracked or depressed) and skin condition of the areola. The purpose is to correct the abnormality, if any, so that there will be no difficulty in breast feeding immediately following delivery.

Obstetrical examination

Abdominal: Tone of the abdominal muscles, presence of any incisional scar or presence of herniation and skin condition of the abdomen are to be looked for. Fundus of the uterus is just palpable above the symphysis pubis at 12 weeks.

Vaginal: Examination is done in the ante-natal clinic when the patient attends the clinic for the first time before 12 weeks. It is done,

1. To diagnose the pregnancy
2. To corroborate the size of the uterus with the period of amenorrhoea
3. To exclude any pelvic pathology

Internal examination is, however, omitted in cases with previous history of abortion, occasional vaginal bleeding in present preg-nancy or specially valuable pregnancy.

Ultrasound examination: (where available) has replaced routine internal examination at present. It is more informative and without any known adverse effect.

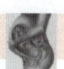

PROCEDURE AT THE SUBSEQUENT VISITS

General check up is done at interval of 4 weeks up to 28 weeks; at interval of 2 weeks up to 36 weeks and thereafter weekly till the expected date of delivery. Ideally this should be more flexible depending on the need, and the convenience of patient. In the developing countries, as per **WHO recommendation,** the visit may be curtailed to at least 3; first in second trimester between 16 and 20 weeks, second at 28–32 weeks and the third at 36 weeks.

Objectives

1. **To assess**
   - Fetal well being
   - Lie, presentation, position and number of fetuses
   - Growth restriction, pre-eclampsia, anaemia, polyhydramnios, etc.
   - To organize specialist antenatal clinics for patients with problems like cardiac disease and diabetes.
2. **To select time for** amniocentesis or chorion villus biopsy when indicated.

History: *To note*

1. Appearance of any new complaints
2. Date of quickening.

EXAMINATION

General: In each visit the following are recorded:
1. Weight
2. Pallor
3. Oedema legs
4. Blood pressure

Abdominal examination

1. To note the height of the fundus above the symphysis pubis. From the 20th week, the symphysis—fundus height increases by about 1 cm per week.
2. **In the second trimester,** to identify the fetus by external ballottement, fetal movements, palpation of fetal parts and auscultation of fetal heart sounds.

3. **In the third trimester** abdominal palpation will help to identify fetal lie, presentation, position, growth pattern, volume of liquor and also any abnormality. Examination also helps to detect whether the presenting part is engaged or not. Girth of abdomen is measured at the level of umbilicus. The girth increases by about 2.5 cm per week beyond 30 weeks and, at term, measures about 95–100 cm.

Vaginal examination

Vaginal examination in the later months of pregnancy (beyond 37 weeks) with an idea to assess the pelvis is not informative. Pelvic assessment is best done with the onset of labour or just before induction of labour. *Any history of vaginal bleeding contraindicates vaginal examination.*

ANTENATAL ADVICE

Principles

1. **To impress the patient** about the importance of regular check up.
2. **To maintain or improve,** if necessary, the health status of the woman to the optimum till delivery by judicious advice regarding diet, drugs, and hygiene.
3. **To improve and tone up** the psychology and to remove the fear of the unknown by talking sympathetically to the patient and explaining the principal changes and events likely to occur during pregnancy and labour.

Diet

The diet during pregnancy should be adequate to provide for:
1. The maintenance of maternal health
2. The needs of the growing fetus
3. The strength and vitality required during labour
4. Successful lactation

During pregnancy, there is increased calorie requirement due to increased growth of the

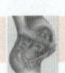

maternal tissues, fetus, placenta and increased basal metabolic rate. *The increased calorie requirement is to the extent of 300 over the non-pregnancy state during second half of pregnancy.* The increased demand is to be compensated by exogenous supply of diet or drugs especially when the majority of women remain active during pregnancy.

The pregnancy diet ideally should be light, nutritious, easily digestible and rich in protein, minerals and vitamins. In terms of figures, the following are the daily requirement during pregnancy. It is not an absolute recommendation but simply a guide (Table 4.4).

The diet should consist of, in addition to the principal food, at least half litre, if not, 1 litre of milk (1 litre of milk contains about 1 gm of calcium), one egg, plenty of green vegetables and fruits as available. The amount of salt should be of sufficient amount to make the food tasty. At least, half of the total protein should be first class containing all the amino-acids and majority of the fat should be animal type which contains vitamins A and D.

Dietetic advice should be given with due consideration to the socioeconomic condition, food habits and taste of the individual.

Supplementary nutritional therapy: As previously mentioned, there is negative iron balance during pregnancy and the dietetic iron is not enough to meet the daily requirement especially in the second half of the pregnancy. Thus, supplementary iron therapy is needed for all pregnant mothers from 20 weeks onwards. Above 10 gm% of haemoglobin, 1 tab. of ferrous sulphate (Fersolate) containing 60 mg of elemental iron is enough. The dose should be proportionately increased with lower haemoglobin level to 2–3 tablets a day. *3 tablets provide 45 mg of absorbable iron.* As the essential vitamins are either lacking in the foods or are destroyed during cooking, supplementary vitamin tablet, containing the following, is to be given daily from 20th week onwards ascorbic acid—50 mg, folic acid—1 mg, thiamine—2 mg, riboflavin—2 mg and nicotinic acid—15 mg.

Table 4.4: Recommended daily nutrients for woman weighing 50 kg

	Non-pregnant	Pregnancy Second half	Lactation
Kilocalories	2200	2500	2900
Protein	50 gm	60 gm	70 gm
Calcium	500 mg	1000 mg	1500 mg
Iron	18 mg	40 mg	30 mg
Vitamin A	5000 I.U.	6000 I.U.	8000 I.U.
Vitamin D	400 I.U.	400 I.U.	400 I.U.
Thiamine	1.1 mg	1.5 mg	
Riboflavin	1.1 mg	1.5 mg	
Nicotinic acid	14 mg	15 mg	Almost same as in
Ascorbic acid	45 mg	60 mg	pregnancy
Folic acid	0.5 mg	1 mg	
Vitamin B$_{12}$	2 mg	2 mg	

To be supplemented

Antenatal hygiene

In otherwise uncomplicated cases, the following advice is to be given:

Rest and sleep: The patient may continue her usual activities throughout pregnancy. However, hard and strenuous work should be avoided especially in the first trimester and the last 6 weeks.

There is individual variation of the amount of sleep required. However, on an average, the patient should be in bed for about 10 hours (8 hours at night and 2 hours at noon) especially in the last 6 weeks. In late pregnancy, lateral posture is more comfortable.

Bowel: There is a tendency of constipation during pregnancy which may be related to backache and abdominal discomfort. Regular bowel movement may be facilitated by regulation of diet taking plenty of fluids, vegetables and milk or prescribing mild laxative like milk of magnesia or cremaffin (pink) 4 teaspoons at bed time or Isogel (Isafgul) 2 teaspoons at bed time to be taken with warm milk.

Bathing: The patient should take daily bath **but be careful against slipping in the bathroom** due to imbalance.

Clothing, shoes and belt: The patient should wear loose but comfortable garments. High heel shoes should better be avoided in advanced pregnancy when the centre of balance alters.

Dental care: The dentist should be consulted at the earliest, if necessary. This will facilitate extraction or filling of the caries tooth, if required, comfortably in the 2nd trimester, the best time for such procedure.

Care of the breasts: If the nipples are anatomically normal, nothing is to be done beyond ordinary cleanliness. If the nipples are retracted, correction is to be done in the later months by manipulation or by using shields.

Coitus: Coitus should be avoided during the first trimester preferably during the time of missed periods and also during the last 6 weeks for fear of abortion in the former and introduction of infection and premature labour in the latter period.

Travel: Travel by vehicles having jerks are better to be avoided especially in first trimester and the last 6 weeks. The long journey is preferably to be limited to the second trimester. Rail route is preferably to bus route. Travel in pressurised aircraft offers no risk.

Smoking and alcohol: In view of the fact that smoking is injurious to health, it is better to stop smoking not only during pregnancy but even thereafter. Heavy smokers have smaller babies and there is also more chance of abortion. Similarly, alcohol consumption is to be drastically curtailed or avoided, if possible, so as to prevent fetal maldevelopment or growth retardation.

Immunisation

Fortunately, most of life threatening epidemics are a rarity even in the developing countries. In the developing countries immunisation in pregnancy is a routine for tetanus; others are given when epidemic occurs or travelling to an endemic zone or for travelling overseas.

Tetanus: *Immunisation against tetanus not only protects the mother but also the neonates.* In unprotected women, 0.5 ml tetanus toxoid is given intramuscularly at 6 weeks interval for 2 doses, the first one to be given between 16 and 24 weeks. Women who are immunised in the past, a booster dose of 0.5 ml IM is given in the last trimester.

General advice

The patient should be persuaded to attend for antenatal check up positively on the schedule date of visit. She is instructed to report to the physician even at an early date if some untoward symptoms arise such as intense headache, disturbed sleep with restlessness, urinary troubles, epigastric pain, vomiting and scanty urination.

 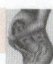

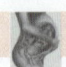
She is advised to come to hospital for consideration of admission in the following circumstances:

- Painful uterine contractions at interval of about 10 minutes or earlier and continued for at least an hour—suggestive of onset of labour.
- Sudden gush of watery fluid per vaginam—suggestive of premature rupture of the membranes.
- Active vaginal bleeding, however slight it may be.

MINOR AILMENTS IN PREGNANCY

Not all women experience all of the following common discomforts of pregnancy but many women experience a few to a great number of them. Relief from these discomforts can make a significant difference in how a woman views her pregnancy experience. In so far as is known or commonly accepted, the physiologic, anatomic and psychologic bases for each discomfort are given to stimulate your thinking of further possible relief measures. Relief measures are predicted on the causes of the discomfort and are geared towards symptomatic management.

NAUSEA

Nausea, with or without vomiting, is known as morning sickness but frequently occurs during the day or evening. It is more apt to occur when the stomach is empty, so it is usually worse in the morning. The cause of morning sickness is not really known, although a number of ideas have been advanced. These include hormonal changes of pregnancy, gastric overloading, slowed peristalsis, enlarged uterus, and emotional factors. Nausea is a common problem occurring in over half of pregnant women so common, in fact, that it is a presumptive sign of pregnancy. Nausea eases as the first trimester ends, about the same time the uterus is

becoming an abdominal organ. Persistent nausea and vomiting beyond the first trimester may indicate a severe emotional problem, hyperemesis gravidarum, or hydatidiform mole.

The relief measures for morning sickness are numerous. The relief measures are as follows:

1. Small, frequent meals, even as often as every 2 hours, as these are more apt to be retained than three large meals a day.
2. Dry crackers before getting up in the morning.
3. Something sweet to eat or drink (e.g. fruit, fruit juices), before going to bed at night and before getting up in the morning.
4. Avoidance of foods with strong or offensive odors.
5. Restriction of fats in her diet.
6. Reassurance that nausea will end sometime during the fourth month of pregnancy.
7. Considerate, understanding, loving treatment of the woman with special attention to the little things that are important to her.
8. Vitamin B_6, 50 mg b.i.d. po
9. Medication—opinion varies because of possible teratogenic effects of any drugs on the embryo or fetus during this period of time.

FATIGUE

Fatigue occurs during the first trimester for no known reason. One idea is that it is due to the initial fall in the basic metabolic rate early in the pregnancy but why this happens is not clear. Fortunately, it is a limited discomfort, usually disappearing by the end of the first trimester. It can have the effect of increasing the intensity of the psychological responses the woman is having during this time.

The relief measures are to reassure the woman of its normality and spontaneous remission by the second trimester. It will help

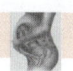

her to have frequent rest periods, if possible, during the day until this passes.

UPPER BACKACHE (NONPATHOLOGICAL)

Upper backache is first noticeable during the first trimester due to the increase in size and resulting heaviness of the breasts, which is one of the presumptive signs of pregnancy. This enlargement may produce muscular strain if the breasts are not adequately supported.

The relief measure, then, is a well-fitting and supportive brassiere. By decreasing breast mobility, a snug, supportive bra also reduces the discomfort of breast tenderness resulting from their enlargement.

LEUKORRHOEA

Leukorrhoea is a profuse, thick, excessive vaginal secretion that begins during the first trimester. The secretion is acidic because of the conversion of an increased amount of glycogen in the vaginal epithelial cells by Doderlein's bacilli into lactic acid. While this serves the function of providing a protection to the mother and fetus against possible harmful infection, it does provide a medium which fosters the growth of the organisms responsible for vaginitis. The productivity of the cervical glands in secreting an increased amount of mucus at this time to form the cervical mucus plug may also contribute to leukorrhoea. Relief measures are close attention to bodily cleanliness in the area and a frequent change of soft, cotton-crotch panties.

URINARY FREQUENCY (NONPATHOLOGICAL)

Urinary frequency as a nonpathological discomfort of pregnancy often occurs at two different times during the antepartal period. Frequency during the first trimester is due to the increased weight in the fundus of the uterus, with the softening of the isthmus (Hegar's sign) causing increased anteflexion of the enlarging uterus, which exerts direct pressure on the bladder. This is relieved as the uterus continues to enlarge and rises out of the pelvis to become an abdominal organ while the bladder remains a pelvic organ. Urinary frequency during the third trimester occurs most often in primigravidas, after lightening has occurred. The effect of lightening is that the presenting part descends into the pelvis and causes direct pressure against the bladder. The pressure makes the woman feel the need to void. The enlarging uterus or the presenting part also takes up space in the pelvic cavity, thereby allowing less room for distention of the bladder before the woman feels the need to void.

The only relief measures are an explanation of why this is happening and a decrease in fluid intake before bedtime so that the woman is not disturbed with many trips to the bathroom when she is trying to sleep.

HEARTBURN

Heartburn is a discomfort that may start toward the end of the second trimester and extend through the third trimester. Heartburn is another word for regurgitation or the reflux of acidic gastric contents into the lower esophagus by reversed peristalsis. The gastric contents are acidic by virtue of the hydrochloric acid in the stomach. This causes the material to burn the throat and taste bud. The causes of heartburn are thought to be as follows:

1. Relaxation of the cardiac sphincter of the stomach due to the effects of increased amounts of progesterone
2. Decreased gastrointestinal motility resulting from smooth muscle relaxation which is probably due to increased amounts of progesterone and to uterine pressure

Relief measures

1. Small, frequent meals, avoiding overloading of the stomach.

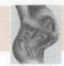

2. Good posture, to give more room for the stomach to function.
3. Avoidance of fats with meals.
4. Avoidance of beverages with meals since this tends to inhibit gastric juices—a dry diet without breadstuffs has helped some women.
5. Avoidance of very cold foods with meals, to inhibit gastric juices.
6. Drinking cultured milk rather than sweet milk has helped some women.
7. Drinking milk and/or eating ice cream has helped some women.
8. Antacid preparations such as maalox, gelusil, amphojel, and milk of magnesia.

FLATULENCE

Increased flatulence is thought to be due to decreased gastrointestinal motility. This probably results both from the effect of increased progesterone on relaxing smooth muscle and from the displacement of and pressure upon the intestines by the enlarging uterus.

The only relief measures are to encourage a regular pattern of daily bowel movements and to avoid gas-forming foods.

CONSTIPATION

Women previously without a problem of constipation may develop this problem during the second or third trimester. This is thought to be due to decreased peristalsis as a result of relaxation of the smooth muscle of the large bowel in the presence of increased amounts of progesterone. The displacement and compression of the bowel by the enlarging uterus or presenting part may also contribute to decreased motility in the gastrointestinal tract and thus to constipation. One of the common side effects of iron medication is constipation; this compounds the problem for a large percentage of pregnant women.

Following is the list of relief measures for constipation:

1. An adequate fluid intake defined as a minimum of eight glasses per day.
2. Prunes or prune juice—prunes are a natural mild laxative.
3. Adequate rest-this may require rest periods during the day.
4. Warm liquids, e.g. water, tea, upon rising.
5. Foods in the diet which contain roughage, bulk, and natural fiber, e.g. lettuce, celery, bran.
6. Establishment of regular and good bowel habits.
7. General exercise, good posture, good body mechanics, and daily exercise of contracting the lower abdominal muscles. All of these measures facilitate venous circulation, thereby preventing congestion in the large intestines.
8. Mild laxatives, stool softeners, and/or glycerin suppositories if indicated.

HAEMORRHOIDS

Haemorrhoids often are preceded by constipation. Therefore, all the reasons for constipation have the potential of leading to the development of haemorrhoids. Progesterone also causes relaxation of the vein walls and of the large bowel. In addition, the enlarging uterus causes increasing pressure especifically in the haemorrhoidal veins as well as generally interfering with venous circulation and causing congestion in the pelvic veins.

There are a number of relief measures for haemorrhoids. Some solely give comfort and others both numb and reduce the haemorrhoids.

1. Avoidance of constipation—prevention is the most effective measure.
2. Avoidance of straining during defecation.
3. Sitz baths the heat of the water not only gives comfort but also increases circulation.
4. Witch hazel compresses—for reduction.
5. Ice bag—for reduction.
6. Epsom salt compresses—for reduction.

7. Reinsertion of the haemorrhoids into the venous pressure.
8. Bed rest with hips and lower extremities elevated.
9. Analgesic ointments and/or topical anesthetics.

LEG CRAMPS

The physiologic basis for leg cramps is not clear. For a number of years, leg cramps were thought to be due to inadequate or impaired calcium intake or an imbalance in the calcium-phosphorus ratio in the body, but these are no longer stated in current literature. Another school of thought is that the enlarged uterus exerts pressure either on the pelvic blood vessels, thereby impairing circulation, or on the nerves as they course through the obturator foramen on their way to the lower extremities. Relief measures are as follows:

1. Have the woman straighten her affected leg and point her heel, i.e. dorsiflex her foot. If she is in bed she needs strong, steady pressure against the bottom of her foot, either someone's hand or the foot-board of the bed, to push against; if she is standing the floor serves this function. This measure is nearly guaranteed to instantly alleviate an acute leg cramp.
2. General exercise and a habit of good body mechanics to improve circulation.
3. Leg elevation periodically throughout the day.
4. A diet which includes both calcium and phosphorus.

DEPENDENT OEDEMA

Dependent pedal oedema is the result of impaired venous circulation and increased venous pressure in the lower extremities. These circulatory disturbances are caused by pressure of the enlarging uterus on the pelvic veins when sitting or standing and on the inferior vena cava when supine. Any constrictive clothing that inhibits venous return from the lower extremities adds to the problem. Dependent edema is generally evidenced in the ankles and feet and must be carefully differentiated from edema associated with preeclampsia/eclampsia. Relief measures include the following:

1. Avoidance of constrictive clothing
2. Elevation of the legs periodically throughout the day
3. Positioning on the side when lying down

VARICOSITIES

A number of factors may contribute to the development of varicosities during pregnancy. Varicose veins are more apt to occur in women who have a familial tendency or congenital predisposition. Varicosities may result from impaired venous circulation and increased venous pressure; in the lower extremities; these changes are caused by pressure of the enlarging uterus on the pelvic veins when sitting or standing and on the inferior vena cava when supine. Any constrictive clothing inhibiting venous return from the lower extremities or prolonged periods of standing add to the problem. Progesterone-induced relaxation of the vein walls and valves and surrounding smooth muscle also contributes to the development of varicosities.

Varicosities during pregnancy are most pronounced in the legs and/or vulva. Relief measures specific to vulvar varicosities are so noted in the following listing:

1. Use of support hose, ace bandages, or elastic stockings—whichever is used, they should be put on after elevation of the legs and before arising.
2. Avoidance of constrictive clothing, e.g. knee-high or ankle hose, round garters.
3. Avoidance of long periods of standing.
4. Rest periods with the legs elevated periodically throughout the day.
5. Lying in the right-angle position several times daily.

 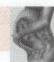

6. Assuming the incline position several times daily (for vulvar varicosities).
7. Keeping the legs uncrossed when sitting.
8. Sitting whenever possible, preferably with legs elevated, rather than standing.
9. Maintaining good posture and good body mechanics, and walking to facilitate increased circulation.
10. Providing physical support for vulvar varicosities with a foam rubber pad held in place with a sanitary belt.

DYSPAREUNIA

Pain during sexual intercourse may stem from a number of causes during pregnancy. Physiologic changes may be responsible, such as pelvic/vaginal congestion resulting from impaired circulation due to pressure of the enlarging uterus or the presenting part. Physical problems may be posed by an enlarged abdomen or may be encountered in late pregnancy when the presenting part descends into the true pelvis. Psychologic factors may cause dyspareunia because of misconceptions and fears such as hurting the baby when there is no indication for this concern. Appropriate relief measures depend on the causes.

1. Positional changes will alleviate problems with an enlarged abdomen.
2. Accessible congestion may be reduced with ice, but this treatment imposes its own discomforts.
3. Explanation and discussion of misconceptions and fears with substitution of facts and knowledge may be immensely helpful and reassuring.
4. Education of both partners in alternative ways of sexually satisfying each other may be welcomed.

NOCTURIA

Venous return from the extremities is facilitated when the woman lies in a recumbent lateral position, since the uterus is no longer pressing against the pelvic vessels and inferior vena cava. When the woman lies in this position while sleeping at night, the result is a reversed diurnal pattern, which yields increased urinary output. The only relief measures consist of whatever comfort she derives from an explanation of why this is happening and reduction of fluids after the evening meal so her intake during this time does not add to the problem.

INSOMNIA

Insomnia may be due to any number of causes such as concerns, anxieties, or excited anticipation of an event the next day, akin to insomnia in the nonpregnant state. The pregnant woman, however, has additional, physical, reasons for insomnia. These include the discomfort of the enlarged uterus, the associated discomforts, the enlarging uterus and pregnancy cause, and fetal movement, especially if the fetus is active. The relief measures for insomnia are time-honored and may or may not be effective. For many women, they are at least something to do.

1. Warm bath
2. Warm drink (milk, tea with milk) before going to bed
3. Nonstimulating activity prior to going to bed
4. Use of relaxation positions
5. Use of the technique of progressive relaxation.

LOW BACK PAIN (NONPATHOLOGICAL)

Low back pain is backache in the lumbosacral region. This usually increases in intensity as the pregnancy progresses because it results from a shift in the woman's centre of gravity and thus in her posture; these changes are produced by the weight of the enlarging uterus. Unless the woman pays deliberate attention to her posture she will walk with a sway back from increasing

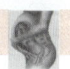

lordosis. This curvature strains the back muscles and causes the ache or pain.

The problem is exaggerated if the woman's abdominal muscles are lax; they fail to give any support to the heavy enlarged uterus. This causes the uterus to sag, a condition that increases the curvature of the back still further. Weakness of the abdominal muscles is more common in grand multiparas who have not exercised and regained their abdominal muscle tone after each pregnancy. Primigravidas usually have excellent muscle tone because their muscles have not been stretched before. Low back pain, thus, generally increases in severity with parity.

Backache may also result from excessive bending, walking without rest periods, and lifting, especially if any or all of these are done while tired. Such activities add strain to the back. Proper body mechanics for lifting are essential to avoid this type of muscular strain. There are two principles to be followed:

1. Stoop, rather than bend, to lift an object, (e.g. toddler, groceries) so that the legs (thighs), rather than the back, bear the weight and strain.

2. Have the feet spread apart and one foot slightly in front of the other when stooping so that there is a broad base for balance when arising from the stooped position.

Relief measures for low back pain

1. Good posture.

2. Proper body mechanics for lifting.

3. Avoiding excessive bending, lifting, or walking without rest periods.

4. Pelvic rocking.

5. Supportive low-heeled shoes—high heels are unstable and further exaggerate the problem of the center of gravity and lordosis.

6. For resting or sleeping:

- A hard mattress
- Positioning with pillows to straighten the back and alleviate pulling and strain.

7. If the problem is severe, external abdominal support is advisable, e.g. a maternity girdle or an abdominal binder.

NONPATHOLOGICAL HYPERVENTILATION AND SHORTNESS OF BREATH

It is thought that the increased amount of progesterone during pregnancy acts directly on the respiratory center to lower the levels of carbon dioxide and increase the oxygen levels. Increased oxygen level benefits the fetus. The increased metabolic activity which occurs with pregnancy, causes an increase in carbon dioxide levels, hyperventilation lowers the level of carbon dioxide. Women may experience this effect of progesterone early in the second trimester.

Shortness of breath is largely a discomfort of the third trimester. During this time, the uterus has enlarged to the point of pressing and the diaphragm elevates approximately 4 centimeters during pregnancy. Although, there is some widening of the transverse diameter of thoracic cage it is not sufficient to compensate for the elevation of the diaphragm, and a decrease in both the functional residual capacity and the residual volume of the air results. This, combined with the pressure being exerted on the diaphragm possibly decreasing still further the functional residual volume, causes a feeling of slight difficulty (or awareness of difficulty) in breathing and shortness of breath. Many women tend to respond to this by hyperventilating.

The relief measures for hyperventilation are as follows:

1. Explain its physiologic basis.

2. Encourage the woman to deliberately regulate the speed and depth of her respirations at normal rates when she is aware of hyperventilating.

 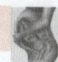

3. Alleviate shortness of breath as a causative factor (described below).

The relief measures for shortness of breath are geared toward providing more room for abdominal contents, thereby reducing the pressure on the diaphragm and facilitating lung functioning. These are as follows:

1. Have the woman periodically stand up and stretch her arms above her head and take a deep breath.
2. Encourage good posture—no slumping of shoulders.
3. Teach the woman to do intercostal breathing.
4. Instruct her to do the same stretching when in bed as when standing.
5. Explain the reasons for shortness of breath; alleviation of anxieties or fears will reduce a response of hyperventilation.

TINGLING AND NUMBNESS OF FINGERS

The change in the center of gravity resulting from the enlarged and heavy uterus may cause the woman to assume a posture in which her shoulders are too far back and her head is anteflexed in an effort to counterbalance her heavy front and curved back. This posture is thought to cause compression of the median and ulnar nerves in the arm, which would cause tingling and numbness of the fingers. Hyperventilation may also cause finger tingling and numbness, but most women do not hyperventilate enough as a result of pregnancy to have this effect. Relief measures include explaining scrupulous attention to good posture. Some women obtain relief simply by lying down.

SUPINE HYPOTENSIVE SYNDROME

Supine hypotensive syndrome causes the woman to feel faint, she may pass out if the problem is not immediately alleviated. Supine hypotensive syndrome occurs when the woman lies in a supine position (such as for sleep or an examining table) because the full weight of the enlarged uterus and its contents is on the inferior vena cava and other vessels of the venous system. Venous return from the lower half of the body is inhibited, which in turn reduces the amount of blood filling the heart and subsequently lowers cardiac output. Supine hypotensive syndrome is actually obvious arterial hypotension. In addition, the aorta, which also results in deleterious changes in arterial pressure.

Supine hypotensive syndrome is alleviated immediately by simply having the woman either turn on her side up. Reassurance and explanation are essential since she is likely to be frightened.

The fetus lies inside the uterus in a closed sac filled with liquor amnii. It has enough freedom of movement until the later months of pregnancy, when it becomes relatively fixed. Till then, periodic examination is essential to note its lie, presentation, position and attitude. Incidental idea can be gained about the size of the fetus or amount of liquor amnii.

Lie

The lie refers to the relationship of the long axis of the fetus to the long axis of the centralized uterus or maternal spine, the commonest lie being longitudinal (99.5%). The lie may be transverse or oblique; sometimes, the lie is unstable until labour sets in, when it becomes either longitudinal or transverse (Fig. 4.15).

Presentation

The part of the fetus which occupies the lower pole of the uterus is called the presentation of the fetus. Accordingly, the presentation may be cephalic (96.5%), podalic (3%) or shoulder and other (0.5%). When more than one part of the fetus are present, it is called *compound presentation.*

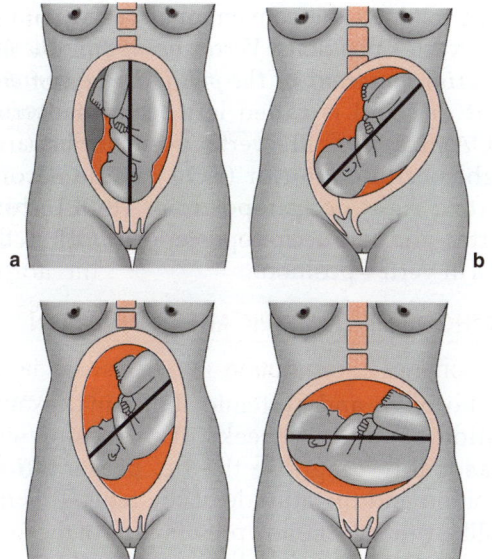

Fig. 4.15: Figure showing fetal lie. The fetus seems to lie in oblique position in relation to the maternal spine but remains in longitudinal lie in relation to uterine axis (Fig. 4.15b). Correction of the uterine obliquity rectifies apparent oblique lie of the fetus (Fig. 4.15a)

Presenting part

The presenting part is defined as the part of the presentation which overlies the internal os and is felt by the examining finger through the cervical opening. Thus, in cephalic presentation, the presenting part may be vertex (commonest), brow or face, depending upon the degree of flexion of the head (Fig. 4.16).

Similarly, the fetal legs in a breech presentation may be flexed (complete breech), extended (frank breech) or a foot may present (footling). However, the term presentation and presenting part are often used synonymously and expressed more commonly in clinical practice according to the latter definition (Table 4.5).

Attitude

The relation of the different parts of the fetus to one another is called attitude of the fetus. The universal attitude is that of flexion. During the later months, the head, trunk and limbs of the fetus maintain the attitude of flexion on all joints

Lie		Presentation		Presenting part of cephalic	
Longitudinal	(99.5%)	Cephalic (96.5%)		Vertex (96%)	
Transverse		Breech (3%)		Brow	
Oblique	(0.5%)	Shoulder (0.5%)	}	Face	} (0.5%)
Unstable					

Table 4.5: Preponderance of lie, presentation and presenting part

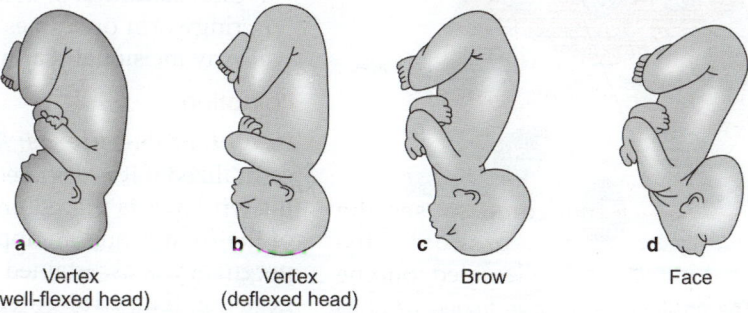

a	b	c	d
Vertex (well-flexed head)	Vertex (deflexed head)	Brow	Face

Fig. 4.16: Varieties of cephalic presentations in different attitude

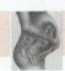
and form an ovoid mass that corresponds approximately to the shape of uterine ovoid. The characteristic flexed attitude is, however, modified by the amount of liquor amnii. There may be exceptions to this universal attitude and extension of the head may occur (deflexed vertex, brow or face presentation, according to the degree of extension), or the legs may become extended in breech. The course of labour in such circumstances may be modified accordingly.

DENOMINATOR

It is an arbitrary bony fixed point on the presenting part which comes in relation with the various quadrants of the maternal pelvis. *The following are the denominators of the different presentations*—occiput in vertex, mentum in face, frontal eminence in brow, sacrum in breech and acromion in shoulder.

Position

It is the relation of the denominator to the different quadrants of the pelvis. For descriptive purpose, the pelvis is divided into equal segments of 45° to place the denominator in each segment. Thus, theoretically, there are 8 positions with each presenting part (Fig. 4.17).

Anterior, posterior, right or left position is referred in relation to the maternal pelvis, with the mother in erect position. However, some

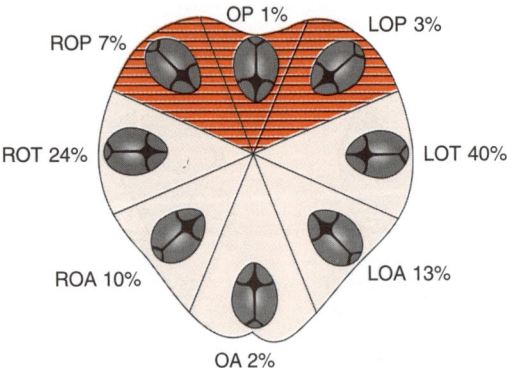

Fig. 4.17: The position and relative frequency of the vertex at the onset of labour

have retained the conventional description of four vertex positions. *Vertex occupying the left anterior quadrant of the pelvis is the commonest one* and is called left occipitoanterior (LOA). This is the first vertex position. Similarly, right occipitoanterior (ROA) is the second vertex; right occipitoposterior (ROP), third vertex and left occipitoposterior (LOP) is the fourth vertex position.

METHODS OF OBSTETRICAL EXAMINATION

Abdominal examination

A thorough and systemic abdominal examination beyond 28 weeks of pregnancy can reasonably diagnose the lie, presentation, position and the attitude of the fetus. It is not unlikely that the lie and presentation of the fetus might change, especially in association with excess liquor amnii and hence periodic check up is essential.

Preliminaries: The patient is asked to evacuate the bladder. She is then made to lie in dorsal position with the thighs slightly flexed. Abdomen is fully exposed. The examiner stands on the right side of the patient.

Inspection: To note:
1. Whether the uterine ovoid is longitudinal or transverse or oblique
2. Contour of the uterus—fundal notching, convex or flattened anterior wall, cylindrical or spherical shape
3. Undue enlargement of the uterus
4. Skin condition of abdomen for evidence of ringworm or scabies
5. Any incisional scar mark on the abdomen.

Palpation

Height of the uterus: The uterus is to be centralized if it is deviated. The ulnar border of the left hand is placed on the uppermost level of the fundus and an approximate duration of pregnancy is ascertained in terms of weeks of gestation (Fig. 4.18). Alternatively, the SFH can be measured with a tape.

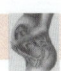

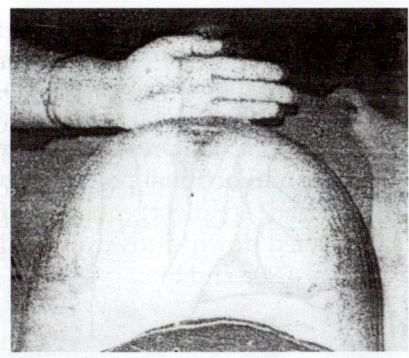

Fig. 4.18: To note the height of the uterus. Linea nigra and striae gravidarum are also visible

There are conditions where the height of the uterus may not correspond with the period of amenorrhoea. *The conditions where the height of the uterus is more than the period of amenorrhoea are*

1. Mistaken date of the last menstrual period
2. Twins
3. Polyhydramnios

4. Big baby
5. Pelvic tumours—ovarian or fibroid
6. Hydatidiform mole
7. Concealed accidental haemorrhage.

The condition where the height of the uterus is less than the period of amenorrhoea are:

1. Mistaken date of the last menstrual period
2. Scanty liquor amnii
3. Fetal growth retardation and
4. Intrauterine fetal death.

Obstetric grips (Fig. 4.19): Palpation should be conducted with utmost gentleness. Clumsy and purposeless palpation is not only uniformative but also may cause undue uterine irritability. **During Braxton-Hicks contraction or uterine contraction in labour, palpation should be suspended.**

1. **Fundal grip:** The palpation is done facing the patient's face. The whole of the fundal area is palpated using both hands laid flat on it to find out which pole of the fetus is lying in the fundus.

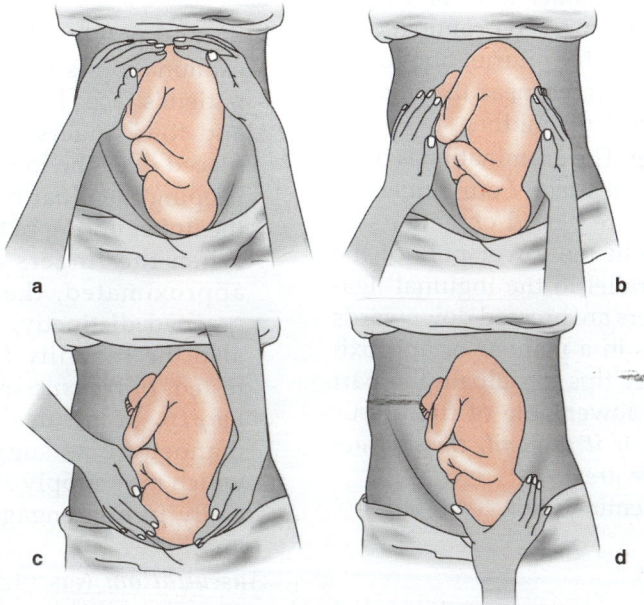

Fig. 4.19: Obstetric grips. **a.** Fundal grip, **b.** Lateral grip, **c.** First pelvic grip, **d.** Second pelvic grip

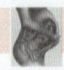

- Broad, soft and irregular mass suggestive of breech
- Smooth, hard and globular mass suggestive of head. *In transverse lie,* neither of the fetal poles is palpated in the fundal area.

2. **Lateral or umbilical grip:** The palpation is done facing the patient's face. The hands are to be placed flat on either side of the umbilicus to palpate one after the other, the sides and front of the uterus *to find out the position of the back, limbs and the anterior shoulder.* The back is suggested by smooth curved and resistant feel. The 'limb side' is comparatively empty and there are small knob like irregular parts. After the identification of the back, it is essential to note its position whether placed anteriorly or towards the flank or placed transversely. Similarly, the disposition of the small parts, whether placed to one side or placed anteriorly occupying both the sides, is to be noted. *The position of the anterior shoulder is to be sought for.* It forms a well-marked prominence in the lower part of the uterus above the head. It may be placed near the midline or well away from the midline.

3. **First pelvic grip:** The examination is done facing the patient's feet. Four fingers of both the hands are placed on either side of the midline in the lower pole of the uterus and parallel to the inguinal ligament. The fingers are pressed downwards and backwards in a manner of approximation of finger tips to palpate the part occupying the lower pole of the uterus (presentation). *If it is head, the characteristics to note are:*
- Precise presenting parts
- Attitude
- Engagement.

To ascertain the presenting part, the greater mass of the head (cephalic prominence) is carefully palpated and its relation to the limbs and back is noted. *The attitude* of the head is inferred by noting the relative position of the sincipital and occipital poles. *The engagement* is ascertained noting the presence or absence of the sincipital and occipital poles or whether there is convergence or divergence of the finger tips when pushed downwards over the lower abdomen (Figs 4.20a and b).

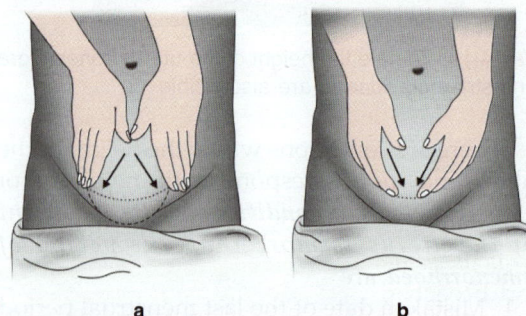

Fig. 4.20: Abdomen palpation to determine engagement of the head. **a.** Divergence of fingers—engaged head, **b.** Convergence of fingers—not engaged

4. **Second pelvic grip (Pawlik's grip):** The examination is done facing towards the patient's face. The over stretched thumb and four fingers of the right hand are placed over the lower pole of the uterus keeping the ulnar border of the palm on the upper border of the symphysis pubis. When the fingers and the thumb are approximated, the presenting part is grasped distinctly, if not engaged, and also the mobility from side to side is tested. *In transverse lie, Pawlik's grip is empty.* Some use this grip as third manoeuvre as suggested by Leopold, which may supply all informations especially in non-engaged head (Figs 4.21a and b).

Auscultation: Auscultation of distinct fetal heart sounds (FHS) not only helps in the diagnosis of a live baby but also its location of

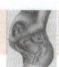

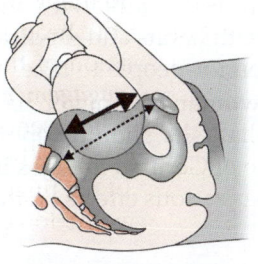 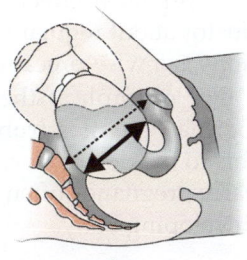

a   **b**

Fig. 4.21: The relationship of the biparietal diameter to the pelvic brim and that of lower pole of the head to the ischial spines. **a.** Non-engaged head, **b.** Engaged head

maximum intensity can resolve doubt about the presentation of the fetus.

The fetal heart sounds are best audible through the back (left scapular region) in vertex and breech presentation where the convex portion of the back is in contact with the uterine wall. However, in face presentation, the heart sounds are heard through the fetal chest.

Engagement

When the greatest horizontal plane has passed of the pelvic brim, the head is said to be engaged.

If the head fails to engage in primigravidae even at 38th week, the causes are sought for.

Causes

1. Deflexed head placing the larger diameter to engage
2. Cephalopelvic disproportion due to contracted pelvis, big head or combination of both
3. Polyhydramnios
4. Poor formation or yielding of lower uterine segment—preventing the head to sink into the pelvis.
5. Hydrocephalus
6. Placenta praveia
7. Pelvic tumours—ovarian or fibroid
8. High pelvic inclination
9. Functional—when no cause can be detected (20%).

PLANNED PARENTHOOD

Most parents start getting ready for the arrival of a baby as soon as the doctor confirms the woman's pregnancy. This gives them seven or eight months at the most to make all the preparations. It is enough time for meeting the baby's needs. But meeting the family's needs is another thing. This unit is about preparing families for a new baby. The earlier the preparation begins, the better chance a family will have to learn to accept, love and understand its new member.

Figures show that first babies usually arrive nine months to two years after marriage. Second, third and later babies most often arrive a year to a year and a half after the last child's birth.

This means that couples have barely adjusted to their new roles as husband and wife and have hardly settled in their new home when they begin to prepare for a new family member.

To be or not to be a parent

One of the most important preparations for parenthood is deciding whether one really wants to be a parent. In the past, marriage and parenthood went hand in hand. It was assumed that when people married they wanted and expected to have children.

Today, this is no longer true. With the modern methods of contraception, means of preventing pregnancy and the legalizing of abortion, people can decide not only if they want to be parents but also when they want to have their children.

In complicated or difficult cases, however, most feel that such advice should come from someone who specializes in the study of genes and heredity, a geneticist. Doctors and medical centres can refer a couple to a heredity clinic for counselling.

Long range preparation for parenthood

Even though a couple may not plan to become parents for several years, they can and should begin some preparation for the parental role. This preparation should include three important areas. They are: physical well being, psychological health and financial security.

Physical preparation

Some physical conditions affect the kind of reproductive cells, men and women produce and also affect the developing baby. These include glandular imbalance, chronic diseases, such as diabetes, anemia and venereal diseases.

A physical check up and a talk with the doctor about regular health habits and medications is a wise precaution for people to take.

For example if the woman has never had German measles (rubella), she should report this to the doctor. A case of German measles in early pregnancy often has serious effects on the developing baby.

Psychological preparation

An attitude is a feeling towards people, situations and roles that affects the way a person

---

Box 4.3: Conditions affecting prenatal development

Maternal nutrition: The unborn child's nourishment comes from the maternal bloodstream through the placenta. The mother's diet must contain sufficient proteins, fats and carbohydrates to keep the child healthy.

Vitamin deficiency: Deficiency of vitamins B_6, B_{12}, D, E and K is especially likely to interfere with the normal pattern of prenatal development.

Maternal health: Maternal health conditions that are known or believed to have the greatest effect on the unborn child, include endocrine disorders, infectious diseases (especially rubella and the venereal diseases), prolonged or wasting diseases and pronounced under or overweight.

Rh factor: Incompatibility between the maternal and paternal blood types causes damage to the cells of the fetus. This leads to physical or mental complications often serious enough to result in death or permanent injury to the child.

Drugs: Too little is known, to date, about which drugs are safe for a pregnant woman to use and which may be damaging to her unborn child. Pregnant women are strongly advised to take no drugs without their doctor's knowledge or consent.

X-ray and radium: There is medical evidence, though not conclusive at this time, that the use of X-ray and radium for therapeutic purposes in pregnant women tends to be damaging to the unborn child. This damage may take the form of birth defects, miscarriages or stillbirths. The use of X-ray for diagnostic purposes—to determine the size and position of the fetus in the uterus toward the end of pregnancy does not affect the fetus.

Alcohol: There is little evidence that use of an alcohol by a pregnant woman will damage her unborn child so long as it is used sparingly. If used frequently and heavily, it is likely to damage the child's physical and mental development.

Tobacco: Smoking is most damaging to the unborn child when the mother inhales. Even when she does not inhale, there is some evidence that maternal smoking affects the fetal heart rate and the chemical content of the fetal blood.

Parental age: Before 21 years of age, the female reproductive apparatus is not fully mature and the hormones needed for reproduction have not reached their optimum levels. After 29 years, hormonal activity gradually decreases. There is no evidence that paternal age affects the unborn child's development.

Maternal emotions: In mild maternal stress, fetal activity and fetal heart rate increase. Severe and prolonged maternal stress lead to "blood-borne anxieties" which affect postnatal as well as prenatal development.

Uterine crowding: In multiple births, crowding may limit fetal activity, which is important for normal development.

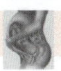

reacts. Psychological preparation means developing attitudes. If a person's attitude toward something is favorable, the person will react positively and adjust well to it.

There are many factors that affect attitudes. They differ for different people and depend on a person's temperament, interests and experiences. However, there are three factors that affect attitudes so often that they can be thought of as almost universal among people today. They are knowledge about a situation, experience in dealing with it, and mental flexibility toward it.

Financial preparation

Having a baby is an added family expense. Saving some money regularly from the family income in preparation for the baby is a wise policy for a couple to follow.

Many women who work give up their jobs as pregnancy progresses. Even if a woman just takes a temporary leave from the job, the reduced income comes at the same time as the

---

Box 4.4: Factors influencing parental attitudes

Desire to have children: Some people want many children, other want a few or none. Some feel that a marriage is incomplete without children and others feel that children are an obstacle to vocational success or upward mobility.

Physical state during pregnancy: If the mother-to-be feels well and has few discomforts even when discomforts are common, she will likely have a more favorable attitude than the mother-to-be who has many discomforts.

Emotional state during pregnancy: For many women, pregnancy is a time of depression, anxiety and worry about childbirth, having a deformed child, or her adequacy for motherhood; for others, it is a time of joyful anticipation.

Maternal dreams and fantasies: The fears, doubts and anxieties mothers-to-be experience, are often intensified by dreams and fantasies just as are they happy emotional states.

Early experiences with children: Parents-to-be who expected to assume responsibilities for the care of younger siblings in their youth, tend to have less favourable attitudes toward having children than those who never had these experiences.

Attitudes and experiences of friends: Friends who have had unfavourable experiences in their homes and who are unhappy in their parental roles, can and do influence the attitude of parents-to-be unfavourably.

Concept of a dream child: If parents have a highly romanticized concept of the child-to-be, it is likely to lead to disappointment and resentment when the child does not conform to this concept.

Social class of parents: Many adults from the lower classes tend to regard parenthood as the "inevitable payment for sex relations" while those from middle and upper classes regard it as the "fulfillment" of marriage.

Economic status of family: If financial conditions are strained, parental attitudes toward the arrival of a child are likely to be adversely affected.

Age of parents: Older parents, in general, welcome their parental roles more wholeheartedly than younger parents.

Maternal interests and aspirations: Women whose major aspirations are to be good mothers have more favourable attitudes toward their children-to-be than women whose interests center mainly on social or vocational activities.

Mass media: Different mass media-books, magazines, movies, radio and television, tend to present a romanticized picture of children and parenthood. Women, as a rule, tend to be more influenced by these media than men.

added financial burden. This often dampens the anticipated pleasure of parenthood.

Immediate areas of preparation

All parents-to-be will have to make some preparation for the arrival of a baby. Those families that already have one or more children will prepare differently from those expecting a first baby. The preparation explained below are some of the most important.

Confirming the pregnancy

A woman who has fairly regular menstrual periods and who has had sexual intercourse during the preceding month, has reason to suspect that she is pregnant if she skips a menstrual period. If the next menstrual period is also skipped, she has reason to assume that she is pregnant. This is the time to consult a doctor, to make sure.

When the doctor's examination and tests show that pregnancy has begun there are many things a woman may want to know. Doctors usually give their patients printed instruction about diet, rest and exercise. They also usually give personal advice to fit each woman's needs. It is essential that the woman follows her doctor's advice very carefully.

Selecting a pediatrician

If the family doctor is caring for the woman during pregnancy and child-birth, the same doctor will probably take care of the baby. However, shortly after the visit to an obstetrician, the mother should consult a pediatrician.

Choosing a hospital

Doctors usually send their patients to the hospital where they are on staff. If her doctor is one on the staff of more than one hospital, the mother-to-be may be able to choose where she will have her baby. If that is the case, the hospital's location and childbirth policies will probably determine the choice. Some hospitals let the father be in the labor and delivery rooms to share with the mother the experience of childbirth.

Some hospitals let newborn babies be in the rooms with their mothers rather than in the nursery. This is usually called rooming in. It gives the mother chance to learn how to take care of her baby while she is in the hospital under the guidance of a nurse. On the other hand, with rooming in, the mother has less time to rest and regain her strength before going home.

Budgeting expenses for the baby

No matter how careful parents-to-be are in spending money, they will find that having a baby is an expense that often taxes the family budget.

Besides the costs of medical and hospital care, there is the cost of equipment for the baby. Equipment for a new baby can be expensive. It is less costly when some of it is made at home, bought second hand or borrowed from friends and relatives.

When a new baby is the second, third or later-born of the family, new equipment is usually not needed. However, it is a good idea to check the equipment used for the last baby, clean it up, and fix any damages to make it comfortable and safe.

Choosing a name for the baby

A child's name should be given careful consideration. When selecting a name, parents must keep in mind that the name they choose will be the baby's name, and not theirs. It is the label by which the child will be known throughout life. Once it is legally registered a name cannot be changed without parental or court approval.

Parents should consider how the name they select will affect the child's personal and social adjustments. The name may be a source of constant teasing, embarrassment or irritation for the child, or it may make a favorable impression on other people and thus increase the child's self-confidence.

Because it is not possible to know whether the baby will be a girl or a boy, it is important to select a name for both. Most doctors can tell, as pregnancy goes on, whether there will be one or more babies. If more than one baby is expected, combinations of names have to be chosen. In the case of twins, for example names should be chosen for a new boy and a girl, two girls and two boys.

Arranging for help

Few women are strong enough to do their usual household duties right after they return home from the hospital. Many new fathers arrange to be at home to help out when the baby arrives. Other new parents may get help from neighbours, friends and relatives.

When there are older children, arrangements must be made for their care when the mother is in the hospital. If the father is unable to care for them, a friend or relative might be able to do so. If not, parents have no choice but to hire outside help. Here again is an expense that adds to the cost of having a baby.

Arrangements for help should be made several months before the baby is due. This is not easy when friends and relatives have their own families, homes and jobs to take care of and when domestic help is scarce. The matter is also complicated by the fact that the exact date for arrival of a baby is difficult to predict. An early or later arrival may mean that the help will not be available. That is why, two sets of plans should be made.

Learning to be a new parent

While some new parents are lucky enough to have a friend, relative or paid caretaker to help them with the baby's care, most are not. They have to face this responsibility alone. It is often a terrifying experience for a couple to be parents of a first baby.

To avoid being unprepared, parent-to-be should try to take a course in infant care. Such a course is offered by the prenatal clinics of most hospitals and is open to anyone who wants to enroll. In the course, people are shown how to feed, clothe and diaper new babies as well as how to place them in comfortable positions.

In this course, everyone has a chance to care for the "baby" under a watchful eye of the nurse. Such a course gives new parents confidence about handling their babies. Books or pamphlets, written by doctors and nurse telling how to take care of new baby, are also helpful to new parents.

Being ready

At a routine checkup late in pregnancy, the doctor is able to determine the size and position of the unborn baby in the mother's body. On the basis of this examination, the doctor forecasts the approximate date of baby's arrival. It is a good idea, at this time for the mother-to-be to pack a bag for her stay in the hospital. She can also make some last-minute preparation for the baby or arrange for someone else to make them while she is in the hospital.

As pregnancy reaches its final stages, the doctor explains in detail what the warning signals of birth are and tells the woman exactly what to do when they begin. The mother-to-be knows that her baby is on the way because of periodic pains known as labor. As a rule, babies rarely arrive in the world without warning, even in the easiest birth. If everything is ready, the woman will have no cause to fear that the baby will arrive before she can reach the hospital.

ANTENATAL EXERCISE

Exercises for muscle strengthening and relaxation

Tailor sitting: The woman sits cross-legged on the floor to strengthen thigh and pelvic muscles (Figs 4.22 and 4.23).

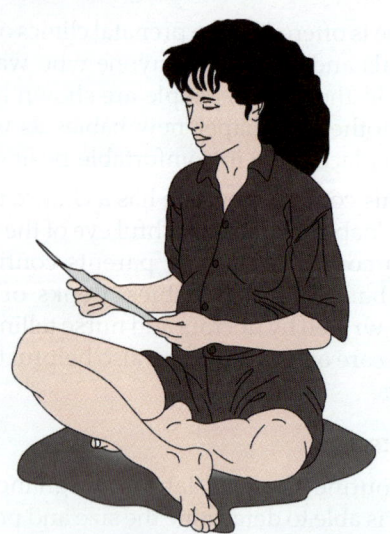

Fig. 4.22: Tailor sitting strengthens the thighs and stretches perineal muscles

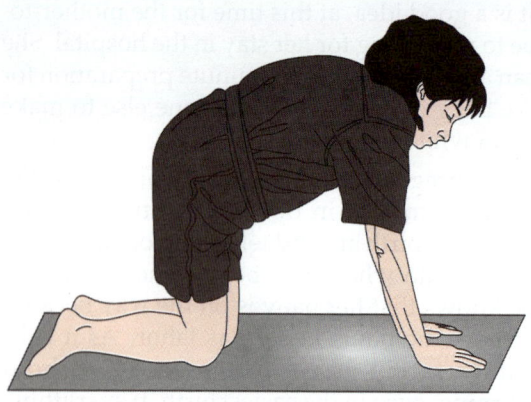

Fig. 4.23: Pelvic rocking is helpful in relieving backache during pregnancy and labour. The woman hollows her back and then arches it

Pelvic tilt: Seated with knees bent and arms in back for support, the woman arches lower back then relaxes to neutral position. This exercise strengthens back and abdominal muscles. The exercise can also be done in a lying or standing position. Perform abdominal muscle contractions during pelvic tilt while standing, lying or sitting to strengthen rectus abdominous muscles.

Straight-leg-lift: In a sitting position with one knee bent and one leg extended with foot flexed, the woman lifts the extended leg up a comfortable distance from the floor (inhaling), then lowers the leg slowly to the floor (exhaling). This is repeated with the other leg. This exercise promotes venous return.

Foot rotation: Seated with leg straight, the woman rotates first one foot, then the other. Movements promote venous return.

Shoulder circling: The fingertips are placed on the shoulders, then brought forward and up during inhalation, back and down during exhalation. Movements lessen backache.

Kegel's exercises (perineal muscle tightening): The woman contracts the pubococcygeal muscle, which surrounds the vagina and urinary meatus. This perineal exercise strengthens muscle tone and elasticity.

Relaxation: The woman relaxes body muscle groups starting from head to toe. She relaxes all the body parts including face and hands (Fig. 4.24).

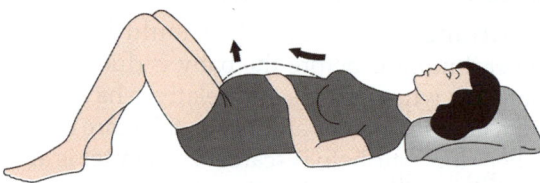

Fig. 4.24: Abdominal breathing aids relaxation and lifts up abdominal wall off uterus

DO'S AND DON'TS

- Consult with health care provider before starting exercise programmes.
- The goal of the exercise programme should be maintenance of fitness.
- Concentrate on non-weight bearing exercise, such as swimming and cycling.
- Decrease high impact activities as third trimester approaches.
- Avoid activities that require balance and coordination.

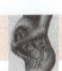
- Avoid activities that involve holding breath.
- Avoid excessive intensity and sweating during exercise.
- Do not exercise in supine position after first trimester.
- Do not use hot tubs that raise body temperature above 38°C.
- Prepare joints by warming up before exercise.
- Wear a supportive bra and appropriate shoes. Be aware of changes in centre of gravity.
- Heart rate should not go above 140 beats/minute.
- Prevent dehydration by taking fluids liberally before, during, after exercise.
- Avoid becoming overly warm.
- Recognize warning signs that indicate the need to stop exercise.

FETAL WELL-BEING ASSESSMENT

PRENATAL FETAL ASSESSMENT

Diagnostic techniques and nursing considerations

A variety of tests can be used to assess fetal well being during pregnancy. These tests include diagnostic ultrasound, Doppler ultrasound blood flow, chronic villus sampling, amniocentesis, percutaneous umbilicus blood sampling, non-stress test (NST), contraction stress test (CST), biophysical profile (BPP), vibroacoustic stimulation test, and maternal assessments of fetal movements.

FETAL ASSESSMENT DURING LABOUR

Intermittent fetal heart monitoring during labour

Fetal monitoring during labour is an integral part of nursing care. Intrapartum fetal monitoring is surveillance used to identify the health status of the fetus showing signs associated with

---

Box. 4.5: Nursing diagnoses

- Anxiety, related to anatomic and physiologic changes associated with pregnancy.
- Fatigue, related to physical adjustments associated with pregnancy.
- Knowledge deficit, related to increased nutrition needs of pregnancy.
- Risk for fluid volume deficit, related to nausea and vomiting.
- Body image disturbance, related to weight gain during pregnancy.
- Sleep pattern disturbances, related to physical discomforts.
- Risk for maternal urinary tract infection, related to pressure of uterus on bladder.
- Risk for Infection, related to invasive procedures.
- Activity intolerance related to maternal physical changes
- **Nutrition:** less than body requirements, altered, related to nausea and vomiting.
- Anxiety related discomforts of pregnancy.
- Body image disturbance related to anatomic and physical changes.
- Constipation related to delayed emptying time of the gastrointestinal tract.
- Fear related to exposure to harmful chemicals.
- Physical mobility, impaired, related to unsteadiness in gait.
- Knowledge deficit related to physical adjustment during pregnancy.
- Self-care deficit to lack of information about potential harm to fetus.

---

compromise. During labour, uterine contractions compress the spiral arteries, temporarily stopping maternal blood flow into intervillous spaces. Between contractions, during the period of relaxation, fresh oxygenated maternal blood reenters the intervillous spaces and waste products drain out. Because of this, fetal wellbeing during labor is measured by the response of fetal heart rate (FHR) to uterine contractions.

Low-risk technology is a method of fetal monitoring that used intermittent auscultation of FHR by a Doppler and hand-held ultrasound device or a fetoscope between, during and immediately after uterine contractions. The FHR is assessed at 30 minutes intervals during the first stage of labour and at 15 minutes intervals during the second stage of labour. In addition, the FHR is assessed after the contraction, and an increase or decrease in FHR is documented.

TESTS TO ASSESS FETAL WELL-BEING

Ultrasound imaging: High frequency waves are used to visualize internal organs or tissues within the body, e.g. fetus, placenta or moving object as beating fetal heart, also called ultrasonography. A transvaginal probe or abdominal transducer is used, abdominal ultrasound requires a full bladder for better visualization (have the woman drink 1 to 2 quarts of water before the examination). Procedure is noninvasive, painless and lasts about 20 minutes.

Doppler ultrasound blood flow: Method of noninvasively studying blood flow in maternal and fetal circulations. A hand-held ultrasound device is used.

Chorionic villus sampling: A first trimester alternative to amniocentesis for placental diagnosis of some conditions. Small amount of the developing placenta (chorionic villi) is obtained to analyze fetal cells at 10 to 12 weeks gestation.

Amniocentesis: Performed to obtain amniotic fluid containing fetal cells. Under direct visualization of ultrasound, a thin needle is inserted through the abdominal and uterine wall to withdraw into a syringe amniotic fluid (with cast-off cells). Sufficient fluid must be present for the test to be done (15 to 17 weeks gestation and 10 to 14 weeks for some disorders).

Tests for fetal lung maturity: Foam stability index (FSI or 'shake test'). If ring of bubbles persist for 15 minutes after shaking solution, test is termed positive indicating surfactant is present and lungs are mature.

Non-stress test (NST): Assessment of fetal well-being by evaluating the ability of the fetal heart to accelerate (speed up) in association with fetal movement (FM) by using an electronic fetal monitor. Accelerations occur either spontaneously or in association with FM. An external electronic monitor is applied while the woman is in a semi-Fowler's or left-lateral position. Conduction gel is put over the abdomen. Two belts are applied on the woman's abdomen. One belt and a device detect fetal heart rate (FHR) and the other belt detects contraction. The woman is given a marker to press, which records the time of movement on a strip on which the FHR is recorded. The test is continued for 40 minutes, or until the criterion for reactivity is met. Because almost all accelerations are accompanied by FM, the movement need not be recorded for the test to be reactive.

Contraction stress test (CST): Evaluation of the FHR response to mild uterine contractions by using an electronic fetal monitor. Contractions are induced by intravenous oxytocin (Pitocin) infusion or by self stimulation of the nipples, which causes the woman's pituitary gland to release oxytocin. The woman must have at least three contractions of at least 40 seconds duration in a 10 minutes period for interpretation of the CST test.

Biophysical profile (BPP): Method used to evaluate the condition of the fetus, using five observations. Biophysical variables include fetal breathing movements, gross fetal movements (movements of body), FHR variability and reactivity (the NST), and the volume of amniotic fluid (amniotic fluid index [AFI]).

Maternal assessment of fetal movement (kick counts): Simple but valuable method for monitoring fetus. It should be encouraged after 28 weeks' gestation, with women setting aside a consistent time to do the "kick counts." Mother should count:the number of fetal movements for 30 to 60 minutes three times a day. Other protocols may be used.

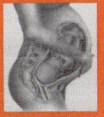

5

Fetal Skull and Maternal Pelvis

OUTLINE

- Fetal skull
- Maternal pelvis

FETAL SKULL

Fetal skull is the most important part of the fetus because it is the most common presenting part, it is the largest and least compressible and once born, generally, ensures smooth delivery of the rest of the body.

Fetal skull is to some extent compressible, and made mainly of thin pliable tabular (flat) bones forming the vault.

AREAS OF SKULL

The skull is arbitrarily divided into several zones of obstetrical importance (Fig. 5.1). These are:

- **Vertex:** It is a quadrangular area bounded anteriorly by the bregma and coronal sutures behind by the lambda and lambdoid sutures and laterally by lines passing through the parietal eminences.
- **Brow:** It is an area bounded on one side by the anterior fontanelle and coronal sutures and on the other side, by the root of the nose and supra-orbital ridges of either side.
- **Face:** It is an area bounded on one side by root of the nose and supraorbital ridges and on the other, by the junction of the floor of the mouth with neck.

Sinciput is the area lying in front of the anterior fontanelle and corresponds to the area of brow and the occiput is limited to the occipital bone.

Flat bones of the vault are united together by non-ossified membranes attached to the margins of the bones. These are called sutures and fontanelles.

SUTURES (Fig. 5.2)

- *The sagittal or longitudinal suture* lies between two parietal bones.
- *The coronal sutures* run between parietal and frontal bones on either side.
- *The frontal suture* lies between two frontal bones.
- *The lambdoid sutures* separate the occipital bone and the two parietal bones.

Importance

1. It permits gliding movement of one bone over the other during moulding of the head, a phenomenon of significance while the head passes through the pelvis during labour.
2. Digital palpation of sagittal suture during internal examination in labour gives an idea of the manner of engagement of the head (asynclitism or synclitism), degree of internal rotation of the head and degree of moulding of the head.

FONTANELLES

Wide gap in the suture line is called fontanelle.

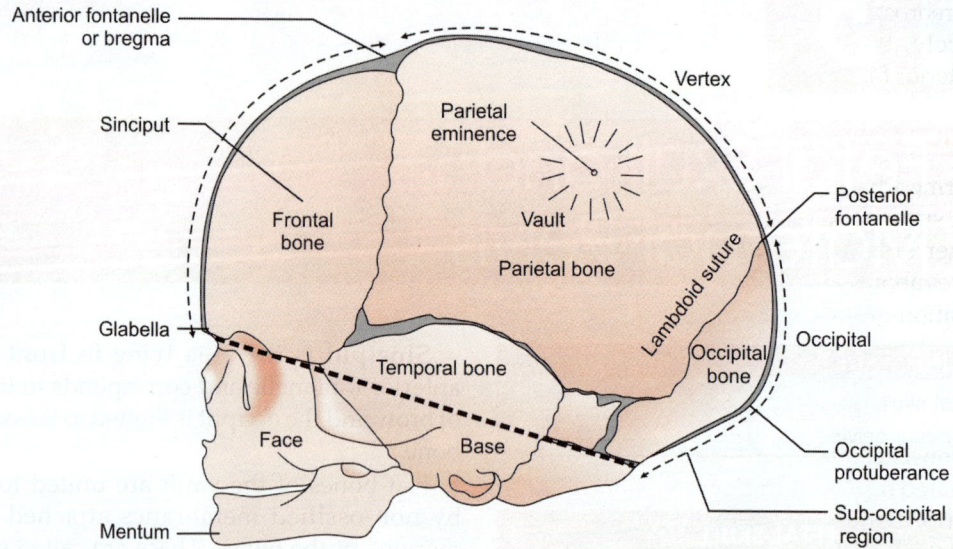

Fig. 5.1: Fetal skull showing different regions and landmarks of obstetrical significance

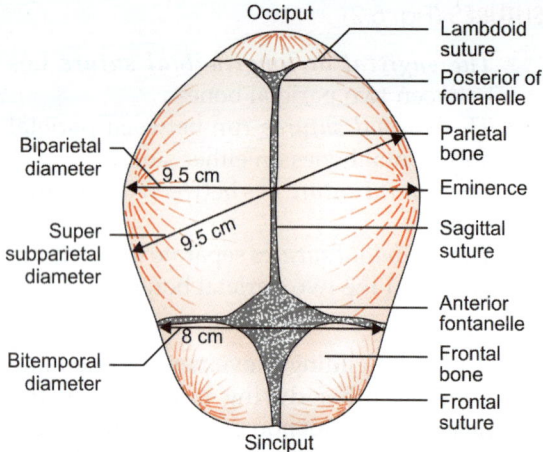

Fig. 5.2: Fetal skull showing important sutures, fontanelles and diameters of obstetric significance

Of the many fontanelles (6 in number), two are of obstetric significance:
1. Anterior fontanelle or bregma
2. Posterior fontanelle or lambda

ANTERIOR FONTANELLE

It is formed by joining of the four sutures in the midplane. The sutures are, anteriorly frontal, posteriorly sagittal and on either side, coronal. The shape is like a diamond. Its anteroposterior and transverse diameters measure approximately 3 cm each. The floor is formed by a membrane and it becomes ossified 18 months after birth. It becomes pathological, if it fails to ossify even after 24 months.

Importance

- Fetal skull showing different regions and landmarks of obstetrical significance. Its palpation through internal examination denotes the degree of flexion of the head.
- It facilitates moulding of the head.
- As it remains membranous long after birth, it helps in accommodating the marked brain growth; the brain becoming almost double its size during the first year of life.
- Palpation of the floor reflects intracranial status—depressed in dehydration, elevated in raised intracranial tension.
- Collection of blood and exchange transfusion, on rare occasion, can be performed through it via the superior longitudinal sinus.

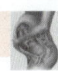

- Cerebrospinal fluid can be drawn, although rarely, through the lateral angle of the anterior fontanelle from the lateral ventricle.

POSTERIOR FONTANELLE

It is formed by junction of three suture lines sagittal suture anteriorly and lambdoid suture on either side. It is triangular in shape and measures about 1.2 × 1.2 cm (½" × ½"). It denotes the position of the head in relation to maternal pelvis.

SAGITTAL FONTANELLE

It is inconsistent in its presence. When present, it is situated on the sagittal suture at the junction of anterior two-thirds and posterior one-third. It has got no clinical importance.

DIAMETERS OF SKULL

The engaging diameter of the fetal skull depends on the degree of flexion present. *The anteroposterior diameters of the head which may engage, are listed in Table 5.1.*

The transverse diameters which are concerned with the mechanism of labour are (Fig. 5.3):

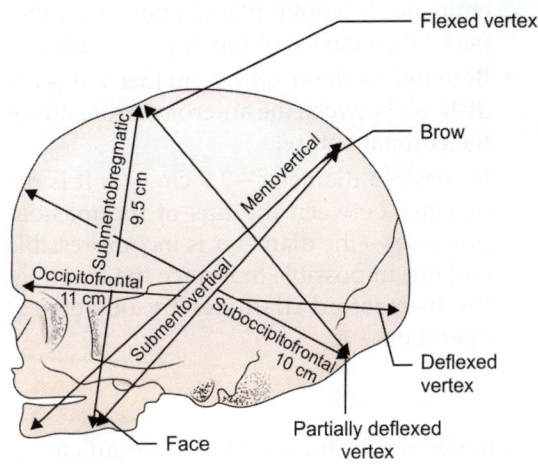

Fig. 5.3: The important diameters of the fetal skull

Table 5.1: The anteroposterior diameter of the head		
Diameters	**Attitude of the head**	**Presentation**
1. Suboccipitobregmatic—9.5 cm (3¾") extends from the nape of the neck to the centre of the bregma.	Complete flexion	Vertex
2. Suboccipitofrontal—10 cm (4") extends from the nape of the neck to the anterior end of the anterior fontanelle or centre of the sinciput.	Incomplete flexion	Vertex
3. Occipitofrontal—11.5 cm (4½") extends from the occipital eminence to the root of the nose (glabella).	Marked deflexion	Vertex
4. Mentovertical—14 cm (5½") extends from the mid point of the chin to the highest point on the sagittal suture.	Partial extension	Brow
5. Submentovertical—11.5 cm (4½") extends from junction of floor of the mouth and neck to the highest point on the sagittal suture.	Incomplete extension	Face
6. Submentobregmatic—9.5 cm (3¾") extends from junction of floor of the mouth and neck to the centre of the bregma.	Complete extension	Face

- Biparietal diameter—9.5 cm (3 ¾"): It extends between two parietal eminences—whatever may be the position of the head, this diameter nearly always engages.
- Super-subparietal—8.5 cm (3½"): It extends from a point placed below one parietal eminence to a point placed above the other parietal eminence of the opposite side.
- Bi-temporal diameter—8 cm (3¼"): It is the distance between the anteroinferior ends of the coronal suture.
- Bi-mastoid diameter—7.5 cm (3"): It is the distance between the tips of the mastoid processes—the diameter is incompressible and it is impossible to reduce the length of the bi-mastoid diameter by obstetrical operation.

CIRCUMFERENCES

Circumference of the plane of the diameter of engagement differs according to the attitude of the head.

Circumferences of the head in different attitudes (Table 5.2)

Moulding (Fig. 5.4)
It is the alteration of the shape of the forecoming head while passing through the resistant birth

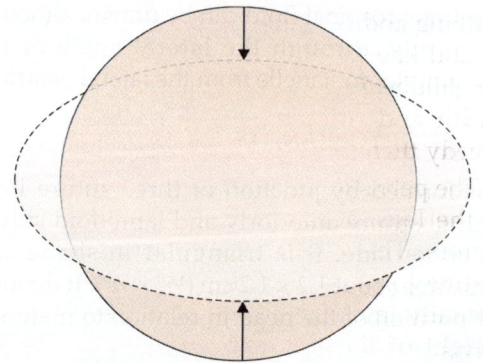

Fig. 5.4: Diagrammatic representation showing principle of moulding of the head

passage during labour. There is, however, very little alteration in size of the head, as volume of the content inside the skull is incompressible although small amounts of cerebrospinal fluid and blood escape out in the process. During normal delivery, an alteration of 4 mm in skull diameter commonly occurs.

MATERNAL PELVIS

FUNCTIONS

The primary function of the pelvic girdle is to allow movement of the body, especially

Table 5.2: Circumference of the head in different attitudes

Attitude of the head	Plane of engagement	Circumference
Complete flexion	Biparietal—suboccipitobregmatic shape—almost round	7.5 cm (11")
Deflexed	Biparietal—occipitofrontal Shape—oval	34 cm (13½")
Incomplete extension	Biparietal—mentovertical Shape—bigger oval	37.5 cm (15")
Complete extension	Biparietal—submentobregmatic Shape—almost round	27.5 cm (11")

* Conversion of the centimetres into inches is approximate.

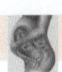

walking and running. It permits the person to sit and kneel. The woman's pelvis is adapted for childbearing, and, because of its increased width and rounded brim, women are less speedy than men.

The pelvis transmits the weight of the trunk to the legs, acting as a bridge between the femurs. This makes it necessary for the sacroiliac joint to be immensely strong and virtually immobile. The pelvis also takes the weight of the sitting body onto the ischial tuberosities.

The pelvis affords protection to the pelvic organs and, to a lesser extent, to the abdominal contents. The sacrum transmits the cauda equina and distributes the nerves to the various parts of the pelvis.

THE NORMAL FEMALE PELVIS

The female pelvis (Fig. 5.5), because of its characteristics, gives rise to no difficulties in childbirth, provided the fetus is of normal size. A knowledge of pelvic anatomy, needed for the conduct of labour as one of the ways to estimate the progress made, is by assessing the relation-ship of the fetus to certain pelvic landmarks. A midwife must be competent to recognise a normal pelvis in order to be able

to detect deviations from normal and refer them to the doctor.

PELVIC BONES

There are four pelvic bones:

- Two innominate (nameless) or hip bones
- One sacrum
- One coccyx

Innominate bones

Each innominate bone (Fig. 5.6) is composed of three parts:

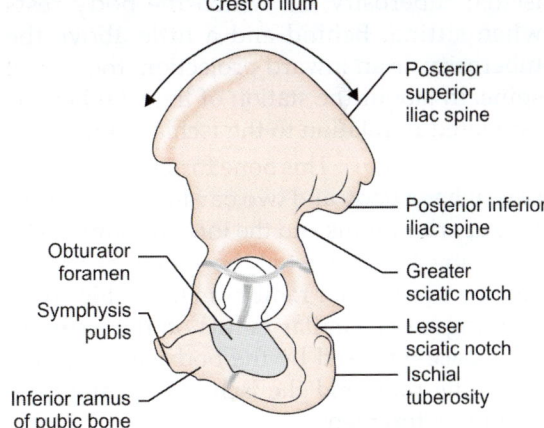

Fig. 5.6: Innominate bone showing important landmarks

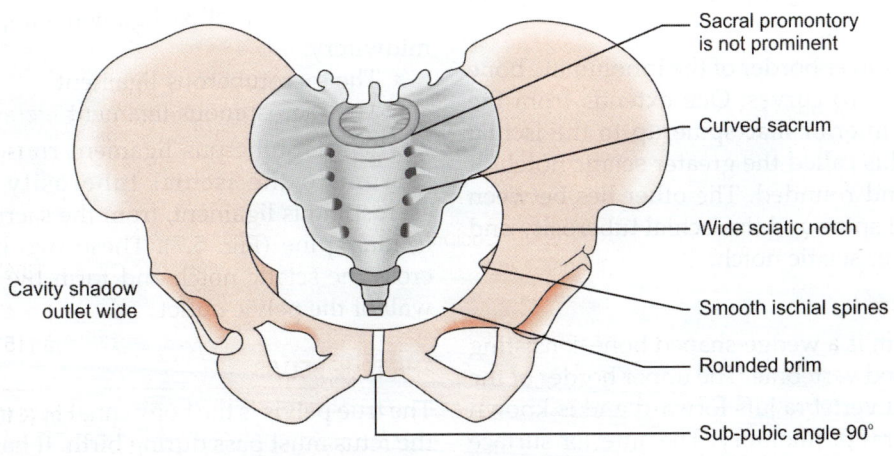

Fig. 5.5: Normal female pelvis

The ilium: The ilium is the large flared-out part. When the hand is placed on the hip it rests on the iliac crest, which is the upper border. At the front of the iliac crest can be felt a bony prominence known as the anterior superior iliac spine.

A short distance below it is the anterior inferior iliac spine. There are two similar points at the other end of the iliac crest, namely the posterior superior and the posterior inferior iliac spines. The concave anterior surface of the ilium is the iliac fossa.

The ischium: The ischium is the thick lower part. It has a large prominence known as the ischial tuberosity, on which the body rests when sitting. Behind and a little above the tuberosity, is an inward projection, the ischial spine. In labour the station of the fetal head is estimated in relation to the ischial spines.

The pubic bone: This bone forms the anterior part. It has a body and two oar-like projections, the superior ramus and the inferior ramus. The two pubic bones meet at the symphysis pubis and the two inferior rami form the pubic arch/ merging into a similar ramus on the ischium. The space enclosed by the body of the pubic bone, the rami and the ischium is called the obturator foramen.

The innominate bone contains a deep cup to receive the head of the femur. This is termed the acetabulum.

On the lower border of the innominate bone are found two curves. One extends from the posterior inferior iliac spine up to the ischial spine and is called the greater sciatic notch. It is wide and rounded. The other lies between the ischial spine and the ischial tuberosity and is the lesser sciatic notch.

The sacrum

The sacrum is a wedge-shaped bone consisting of five fused vertebrae. The upper border of the first sacral vertebra juts forward and is known as the sacral promontory. The anterior surface of the sacrum is concave and is referred to as the hollow of the sacrum. Laterally, the sacrum extends into a wing or ala.

The coccyx

The coccyx is a vestigial tail. It consists of four fused vertebrae, forming a small triangular bone.

Pelvic joints

There are four pelvic joints:
- One symphysis pubis
- Two sacroiliac joints
- One sacrococcygeal joint.

The symphysis pubis: The symphysis pubis is formed at the junction of the two pubic bones, which are united by a pad of cartilage.

The sacroiliac joints: These are the strongest joints in the body. They join the sacrum to the ilium and, thus, connect the spine to the pelvis.

The sacrococcygeal joint: This joint is formed where the base of the coccyx articulates with the tip of the sacrum.

PELVIC LIGAMENTS

Each of the pelvic joints is held together by ligaments:
- Interpubic ligaments at the symphysis pubis
- Sacroiliac ligaments
- Sacrococcygeal ligaments.

There are two other ligaments important in midwifery:
- The sacrotuberous ligament
- The sacrospinous ligament.

The sacrotuberous ligament runs from the sacrum to the ischial tuberosity and the sacrospinous ligament, from the sacrum to the ischial spine (Fig. 5.7). These two ligaments cross the sciatic notch and form the posterior wall of the pelvic outlet.

THE TRUE PELVIS

The true pelvis is the bony canal through which the fetus must pass during birth. It has a brim/ a cavity and an outlet.

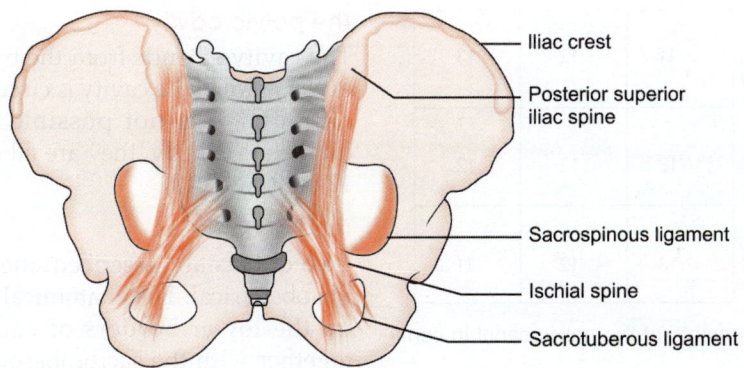

Fig. 5.7: Posterior view of the pelvis to show ligaments

The pelvic brim

The brim (Fig. 5.8) is round except where the sacral promontory projects into it. The promontory and wings of the sacrum form its posterior border, the iliac bones, its lateral borders and the pubic bones, its anterior border.

Landmarks

- Sacral promontory (1)
- Sacral ala or wing (2)
- Sacroiliac joint (3)
- Iliopectineal line, which is the edge formed at the inward aspect of the ilium (4)

- Iliopectineal eminence, which is a roughened area formed where the superior ramus of the pubic bone meets the ilium (5)
- Superior ramus of the pubic bone (6)
- Upper inner border of the body of the pubic bone (7)
- Upper inner border of the symphysis pubis (8).

Diameters of the brim

Three diameters are measured (Figs 5.9 and 5.10)

The anteroposterior diameter: This diameter is a line from the sacral promontory to the upper

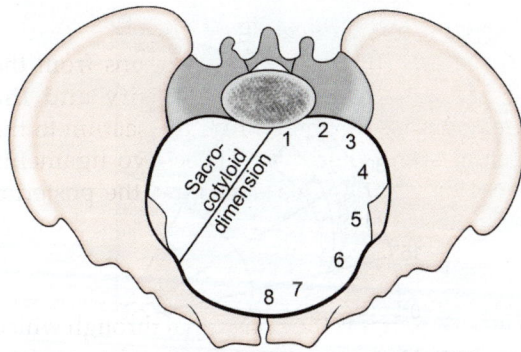

Fig. 5.8: Brim or inlet of female pelvis

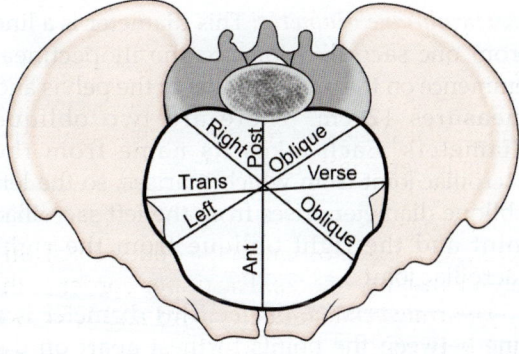

Fig. 5.9: View of pelvic inlet showing diameters

 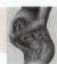

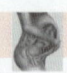
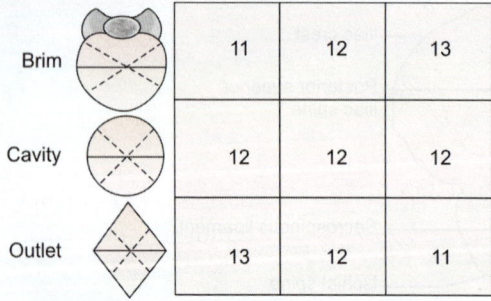

Brim		11	12	13
Cavity		12	12	12
Outlet		13	12	11

Fig. 5.10: Measurements of the pelvic canal in centimetres

border of the symphysis pubis. When the line is taken to the uppermost point of the symphysis pubis it is called the anatomical conjugate and measures 12 cm; when it is taken to the posterior border of the upper surface, which is about 1.25 cm lower, it is called the obstetrical conjugate and measures 11 cm. The reason for this is that the obstetrical conjugate represents the available space for passage of the fetus. The term true conjugate may be used to refer to either of these measurements and the midwife should take care to establish which is meant.

The diagonal conjugate is also measured anteroposteriorly from the lower border of the symphysis to the sacral promontory. It may be estimated on vaginal examination as part of a pelvic assessment and should measure 12–13 cm.

The oblique diameter: This diameter is a line from one sacroiliac joint to the iliopectineal eminence on the opposite side of the pelvis and measures 12 cm. There are two oblique diameters. Each takes its name from the sacroiliac joint from which it arises, so the left oblique diameter arises from the left sacroiliac joint and the right oblique from the right sacroiliac joint.

The transverse diameter: This diameter is a line between the points furthest apart on the iliopectineal lines and measures 13 cm.

The pelvic cavity

The cavity extends from the brim above to the outlet below. The cavity is circular in shape and although it is not possible to measure its diameters exactly, they are all considered to be 12 cm (Fig. 5.10).

The pelvic outlet

Two outlets are described: the anatomical and the obstetrical. The anatomical outlet is formed by the lower borders of each of the bones together with the sacrotuberous ligament. The obstetrical outlet is of greater practical significance because it includes the narrow pelvic strait through which the fetus must pass.

This outlet is diamond-shaped. Its three diameters are as follows:

The anteroposterior diameter: This is a line from the lower border of the symphysis pubis to the sacrococcygeal joint. It measures 13 cm. As the coccyx may be deflected backwards during labour, this diameter indicates the space available during delivery.

The oblique diameter: This is said to be between the obturator foramen and the sacrospinous ligament, although there are no fixed points. The measurement is taken as being 12 cm.

The transverse diameter: This is a line between the two ischial spines and measures 10–11 cm.

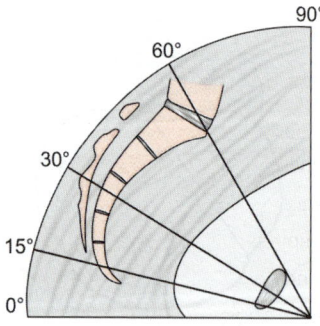

Fig. 5.11: Median section of the pelvis showing the inclination of the planes and the axis of the pelvic canal

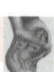

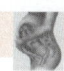

The false pelvis

This is the part of the pelvis situated above the pelvic brim. It is formed by the upper flared-out portions of the iliac bones.

Pelvic inclination

When a woman is standing in the upright position, her pelvis is on an incline. The anterior superior iliac spines are immediately above the symphysis pubis in the same vertical plane. The brim is tilted and if the line joining the sacral promontory and the top of the symphysis pubis were to be extended, it would form an angle of 60° with the horizontal floor. Similarly, if a line joining the centre of the sacrum and the centre of the symphysis pubis were to be extended, the resultant angle with the floor would be 30°. The angle of inclination of the outlet is 15° (Fig. 5.11). When the woman is in the recumbent position the same angles are made with the vertical, which should be kept in mind when carrying out an abdominal examination.

Pelvic planes

These are imaginary flat surfaces at the brim, cavity and outlet of the pelvic canal at the levels of the lines.

Axis of the pelvic canal

A line drawn exactly half-way between the anterior wall and the posterior wall of the pelvic canal would trace a curve known as the curve of Carus.

THE FOUR TYPES OF PELVIS (Table 5.3)

Classically, pelves have been described as falling into four categories according to the shape of the brim.

The gynaecoid pelvis

This is the ideal pelvis for childbearing. Its main features are the rounded brim, the general forepelvis (the part in front of the transverse diameter), straight side walls, a shallow cavity with a broad, well-curved sacrum, blunt ischial spines, rounded sciatic notch and a sub-pubic angle of 90°. It is found in women of average build and height with a shoe size of 4 or larger.

The android pelvis

This is so called because it resembles the male pelvis. Its brim is heart shaped with a narrow forepelvis, and has a transverse diameter that is towards the back. The side walls converge, making it a funnel shape with a deep cavity and a straight sacrum. The ischial spines are prominent and the sciatic notch is narrow. The sub-pubic angle is less than 90°. It is found in short and heavily built women who have a tendency to be hirsute.

Table 5.3: Features of the four types of pelvis

Features	Gynaecoid	Android	Anthropoid	Platypelloid
Brim	Rounded	Heart-shaped	Long oval	Kidney-shaped
Forepelvis	Generous	Narrow	Narrowed	Wide
Side walls	Straight	Convergent	Divergent	Divergent
Ischial spines	Blunt	Prominent	Blunt	Blunt
Sciatic notch	Rounded	Narrow	Wide	Wide
Sub-pubic angle	90°	< 90°	> 90°	> 90°
Incidence	50%	20%	25%	5%

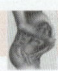

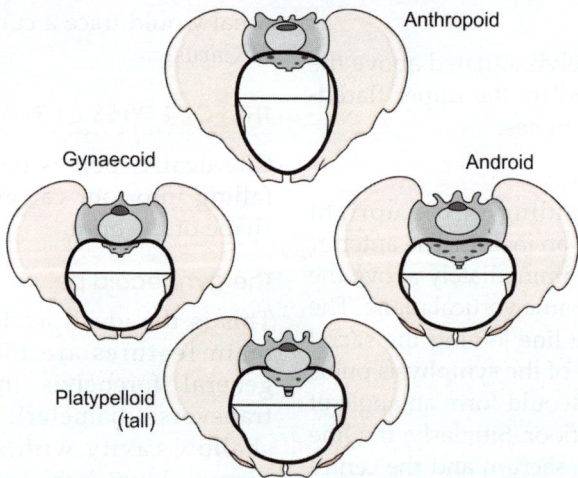

Fig. 5.12: Characteristic inlet of the four types of pelvis

The anthropoid pelvis

It has a long, oval brim in which the antero-posterior diameter is longer than the transverse. The side walls diverge and the sacrum is long and deeply concave. The ischial spines are not prominent and the sciatic notch is very wide, as is the sub-pubic angle. Women with this type of pelvis tend to be tall, with narrow shoulders. Labour does not usually present any difficulties, but a direct occipito-anterior or direct occipito-posterior position is often a feature and the position adopted for engagement may persist to delivery.

The platypelloid pelvis

This flat pelvis (Fig. 5.12) has a kidney-shaped brim in which the anteroposterior diameter is reduced and the transverse increased. The side walls diverge, the sacrum is flat and the cavity shallow. The ischial spines are blunt, and the sciatic notch and the sub-pubic angle are both wide.

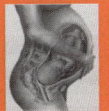

6

Normal Labour

OUTLINE

- Causes of onset of labour
- Factors influencing labour
- Events in first, second and third stage of labour
- Management of the first, second and third stage of labour
- Partograph

DEFINITION

Series of events that take place in the genital organs in an effort to expel the viable products of conception out of the womb through the vagina into the outer world is called labour. It may occur prior to 37 completed weeks, when it is called preterm labour.

Normal labour (eutocia)

Labour is called normal if it fulfils the following criteria:

1. Spontaneous in onset and at term
2. With vertex presentation
3. Without undue prolongation
4. Natural termination with minimal aids
5. Without having any complications affecting the health of the mother and/or the baby.

Abnormal labour (dystocia)

Any deviation from the definition of normal labour is called abnormal labour.

CAUSES OF ONSET OF LABOUR

The precise mechanism of initiation of labour is still obscure. Advancement of chemico-hormonal technology and inferences obtained from animal experiments, however, put forth the following hypotheses:

- *Uterine distension:* Stretching effect on the myometrium by the growing size of the fetus and liquor amnii can explain the onset of labour at least in twins or polyhydramnios.

- *Fetoplacental contribution:* It has been postulated that, due to unknown factors, fetal pituitary is stimulated prior to onset of labour →release of ACTH →stimulates fetal adrenals→increased cortisol secretion →accelerated production of oestrogen and prostaglandins from the placenta. *The probable modes of action of oestrogen are:*

  – Increase the release of oxytocin from maternal pituitary.

  – Promotes the synthesis of receptors for oxytocin in the myometrium and decidua.

  – Accelerates lysosomal disintegration inside the decidual cells resulting in increased prostaglandin synthesis.

  – Stimulates the synthesis of myometrial contractile protein, actomyosin, through activation of adenosine triphosphatase.

  – Increases the excitability of the myometrial cell membranes.

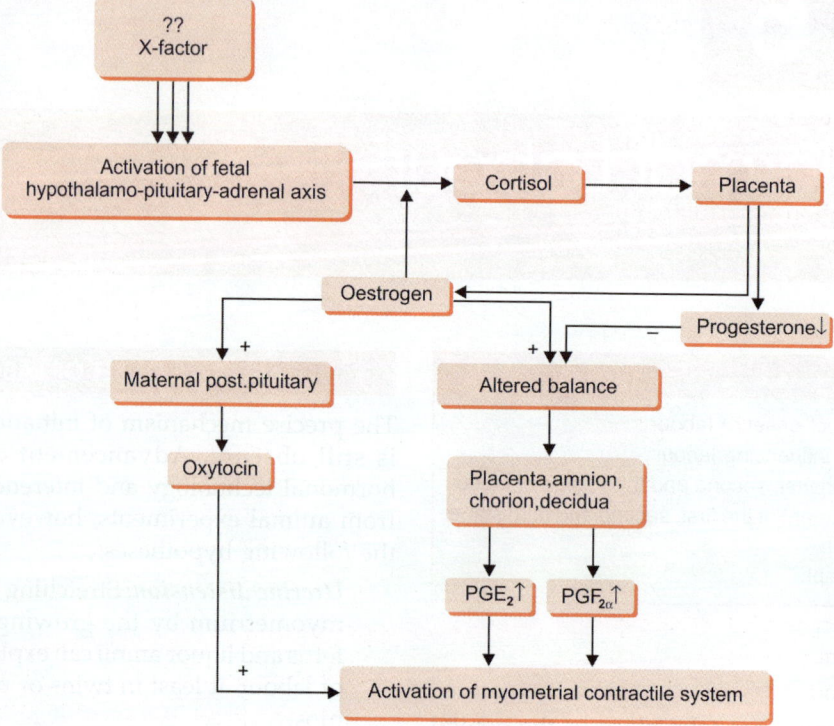

Fig. 6.1: Possible mechanism in initiation of labour

- *Progesterone:* The alteration in the oestrogen: progesterone ratio rather than in the absolute concentration of progesterone which is linked with prostaglandin synthesis.
- *Prostaglandins:* Prostaglandins have attracted much attention in recent years as the possible factors which initiate and maintain labour.

The major sites of synthesis of prostaglandins are placenta, fetal membranes, decidual cells and myometrium. *Synthesis is triggered by*

- Rise in oestrogen level, altered oestrogen, progesterone balance, mechanical stretching in late pregnancy, increase in oxytocin receptors especially in the decidua vera, infection, vaginal examination, separation or rupture of the membranes.

Biochemical examination involved in the synthesis of prostaglandins

- *Oxytocin:* It is probable that myometrial contraction is more dependent on its own readiness to respond to oxytocin. There is no conclusive proof that oxytocin level is increased prior to labour. There is, however, increase in oxytocin receptors especially in the decidua vera which in turn stimulates prostaglandin synthesis. Vaginal examination and amniotomy cause rise in maternal plasma oxytocin level (Ferguson reflex). *Oxytocin level reaches the maximum* at the moment of birth.
- *Neurologic factor:* Although labour may start in denervated uterus, labour may also be initiated through nerve pathways. Both α and β adrenergic receptors are present in the myometrium, oestrogen causing the

α receptors and progesterone the β receptors to function predominantly. The contractile response is initiated through the a receptors of the post ganglionic nerve fibres in and around the cervix and the lower part of the uterus. This is based on observation of the onset of labour following stripping or low rupture of membranes.

False pain

It is found more in primigravidae than in parous women. It usually appears prior to the onset of true labour pain, by one or two weeks in primigravidae and by a few days in multiparae. The woman feels pain and discomfort in the abdomen and these are mistaken for labour pain.

False pain has got the following features

1. Dull in nature and usually confined to the lower abdomen and groin.
2. Continuous and unrelated with hardening of the uterus.
3. Without any effect on dilatation of the cervix.
4. Usually relieved by enema and administration of a sedative.

PRELABOUR (SYN: PREMONITORY STAGE)

The premonitory stage may begin two or three weeks before the onset of true labour in primigravidae and a few days before in multiparae. The features are inconsistent and may consist of the following:

- *Lightening:* Few weeks prior to the onset of labour especially in primigravidae, the presenting part sinks into the true pelvis. It is due to active pulling up of the lower pole of the uterus around the presenting part. This diminishes the fundal height and hence minimizes the pressure on the diaphragm. The mother experiences a sense of relief from the mechanical cardio-respiratory embarrassment. There may be frequency of micturition or constipation due to mechanical factor, pressure by the engaged presenting part. *It is a welcome sign,* as it rules out cephalopelvic disproportion and other conditions preventing the head from entering the pelvic inlet (Figs 6.2a and b).

- *Cervical changes:* Variable days prior to the onset of labour the cervix becomes ripe. *A ripe cervix is* soft, less than 1.5 cm

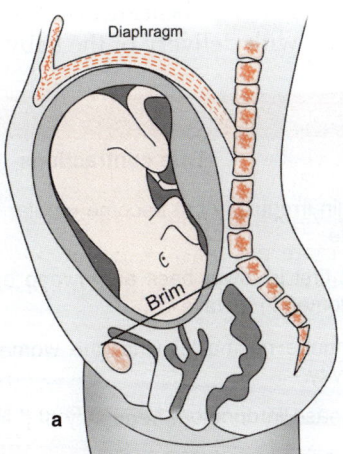 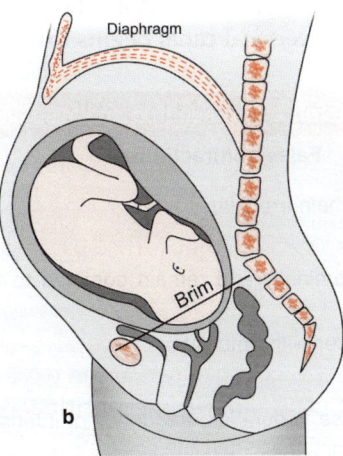

Fig. 6.2: Showing phenomenon of lightening. **a.** Before and **b.** After lightening

in length, admits a finger easily and is dilatable.

• *Appearance of false pain*

True labour pains

The features of true labour pains are:

• Painful uterine contractions (labour pains) at regular intervals
• Contraction with increasing intensity and duration
• "Show"
• Progressive effacement and dilatation of the cervix
• Formation of the "bag of waters" (Table 6.1).

Labour pains: Throughout pregnancy, painless Braxton-Hicks contractions with simultaneous hardening of the uterus occur. These contractions change their character, become more powerful, intermittent and are associated with pain.

Show: With the onset of labour, there is profuse cervical secretion. Simultaneously, there is slight oozing of blood from rupture of capillary vessels of the cervix and from the raw decidual surface caused by separation of the membranes due to stretching of the lower uterine segment. *Expulsion of cervical mucus plug, mixed with blood is called show.*

Dilatation of internal OS: With the onset of labour pain, the cervical canal begins to dilate.

Formation of bag of waters: Due to stretching of the lower uterine segment, the membranes are detached easily because of its loose attachment to the poorly formed decidua. With the dilatation of the cervical canal, the lower pole of the fetal membranes becomes unsupported and tends to bulge into the cervical canal. As it contains liquor which has passed below the presenting part, it is called "bag of waters".

STAGES OF LABOUR

Conventionally, events of labour are divided into three stages:

• **First stage:** It starts from the onset of true labour pain and ends with full dilatation of the cervix. It is, in other words, the "cervical stage" of labour. Its average duration is 12 hours in primigravidae and 6 hours in multiparae.
• **Second stage:** It starts from the full dilatation of the cervix (not from the rupture of the membranes) and ends with expulsion of the fetus from the birth canal. It has got two phases:
  1. *The propulsive phase* starts from full dilatation up to the descent of the presenting part to the pelvic floor.
  2. *The expulsive phase* is distinguished by maternal bearing down efforts and ends with delivery of the baby.

Table 6.1: Difference between true and false labour contractions

False contractions	True contractions
Begin and remain irregular	Begin irregularly but become regular and predictable.
Felt first abdominally and remain confined to the abdomen.	Felt first in lower back and sweep around to the abdomen in a wave.
Often disappear with ambulation	Continue no matter what the woman's, level of activity.
Do not increase in duration, frequency or intensity.	Increase in duration, frequency and intensity.
Do not achieve cervical dilatation.	Achieve cervical dilatation

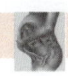

Its average duration is 2 hours in primigravidae and 30 minutes in multiparae.

- **Third stage:** It begins after expulsion of the fetus and ends with expulsion of the placenta and membranes (afterbirths). Its average duration is about 15 minutes in both primigravidae and multiparae. The duration is, however, reduced to 5 minutes in active management.

- **Fourth stage:** It is the stage of observation for at least one hour after expulsion of the afterbirths. During this period, general condition of the patient and the behaviour of the uterus are to be carefully watched.

FACTORS INFLUENCING LABOUR

MAJOR VARIABLES IN THE BIRTH PROCESS

Four factors are significant in the process of labour:

1. Pelvis (size and shape of pelvis)
2. Passenger (fetus) size and position
3. Powers (effectiveness of contractions)
4. Psyche (preparation, previous experience)

These are known as the four P's. An ideal labour is one in which the bony pelvis is adequate, the fetus is of average size and the strength of the uterine contractions increases sufficiently to cause the cervix to fully efface and dilate. The woman's psyche, her ability to relax and concentrate on muscle groups, as well as maintain a low level of anxiety, also plays a role in the normal progress of her labour.

PELVIS

Estimation of the adequacy of the pelvis is important and is part of the prenatal physical examination. The pelvic curve must be negotiated by the fetus during the birth process. If the pelvic anteroposterior (AP) diameter is shortened by the sacral promontory or narro-

wed by the transverse diameter from protrusion of the ischial spines or by the presence of a narrow pubic arch, the fetus will have difficulty coming through the birth canal. Pelvic measurements are an important part of prenatal care to determine adequacy of the pelvis for the birth process. An X-ray pelvimetry may be needed when the measurements are questionable.

PASSENGER

Fetal head

The fetal head is engineered to withstand the pressure of uterine contractions and descent through the birth canal. Great pressure is exerted on the fetal head during labour, and even stronger pressure is applied to the head after the rupture of membranes because the amniotic fluid no longer serves as a cushion between the fetal head and the bony canal.

Fetal bony skull

The bones in the fetal skull are thin and poorly ossified. The skull is made up of small, slightly curved little bones, connected by very flexible elastic membranous tissues (sutures). This construction allows an overlap and reduction of the fetal head circumference necessary to squeeze through the fetal head elongates. The bones of the head may overlap at the suture lines as the head passes through the birth moulding canal; this overlapping is called moulding.

FETOPELVIC RELATIONSHIP

Fetal attitude

It is the relation of the fetal parts to one another. The normal attitude of the fetus is one of flexion. The fetus is flexed with head on chest, arms and legs folded, and legs drawn up onto the abdomen. Changes in fetal attitude, particularly in flexion or extension of head, cause the fetus to present larger or smaller diameters of the fetal head to maternal pelvis. Extension of the fetal head, especially full extension in which chin or face presents, makes vaginal birth difficult and sometimes impossible.

Fetal lie

It is the relationship of the longitudinal axis of the fetus to the longitudinal axis of the mother. The ideal is a parallel relationship in which the long axis of the fetus and mother are the same. In rare instances, the fetus lies crosswise in the uterus (transverse lie), which necessitates a caesarean section.

Fetal presentation

It is determined by the body part of the fetus that is lowest in the mother's pelvis. A cephalic, breech or shoulder presentation may occur. Cephalic (head first) presentation is the most common, occurring in about 95% of all births, and labour most often proceeds normally. If the head is flexed, it is referred to as a vertex presentation. Breech presentation occurs in approximately 3% of all births. In the breech presentation, the presenting parts may be either the buttocks (complete or frank breech) or one or both feet (footling breech). The rarest type of presentation is the transverse (or oblique), which occurs in approximately 1% of births. These are referred to as malpresentations and do not proceed normally.

Fetal position

It is a more specific indication of the fetopelvic relationship, is the relationship of some designated point on the presenting part to the four quadrants of the maternal pelvis, anterior, posterior, left side and right side. If the reference point is directed towards the transverse diameter of the maternal pelvis, it is referred to as a transverse position.

Station

It is the relationship of the presenting part of the fetus to an imaginary line drawn between the ischial spines of the maternal pelvis. Station defines the progression of (usually) the fetal head down toward the pelvic floor. It is measured in centimeters above or below the ischial spines. When the presenting part is above the ischial spines, it is at minus station, with −5 at the inlet. When the presenting part is 1 or 2 cm below the spines, it is at +1 or +2 station. Station +4 is at the outlet. When the presenting part is level with the spines, it is said to be at 0 station, in this case the head is referred to as engaged. Before the head becomes engaged, it is said to be floating.

POWERS: UTERINE CONTRACTIONS

During labor, the contractions begin in the top of the uterus (fundus) and spread throughout the uterus in approximately 15 seconds. Because each contraction starts at the top, in the assessment of contractions, the nurse is able to ascertain the beginning of the contraction by placing her or his hands on the fundus.

A unique property of the uterine muscle is its ability to retain some of the shortening achieved during the contraction. This ability is called *retraction* or *brachystasis*. When the myometrium cells contract, the fibers of both the fundus and the body of the uterus shorten. When the contraction ends and the muscles relax, the fibers do not return to their original size but remain shorter than before the contraction. This continued shortening of the muscle fibers in the upper portion of the uterus results in a progressive decrease in the size of the uterine cavity and a thickening of the muscle tissue of the upper portion. These changes supply the force needed to advance the fetus.

ASSESSMENT OF LABOUR CONTRACTIONS

Uterine contractions are the important source of power that

- Produces cervical effacement and dilatation
- Causes the fetus to engage and rotate
- Causes the fetus to be delivered
- Detaches and expels the placenta (afterbirth)

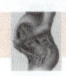

Therefore, to assess the progress of labour, it is important to know the type of contractions the woman is experiencing. The characteristics of labour contractions include the frequency, duration, and intensity.

The frequency of contractions is determined by the amount of time between the beginning of one contraction and the beginning at the next. The frequency of contractions increases as labour progresses.

The duration of a contraction is the time between the onset of the contraction to its end. Contractions may last only 15 seconds at the beginning of labour but last longer as labour advances. Toward the end of labour, the contractions usually last at least 45 seconds, and during transition (the last phase of stage 1), contractions last 60 to 90 seconds.

The intensity of a contraction is the strength of the contraction. A rough estimation is made by palpation of the fundus to determine the firmness of the uterus during a contraction. Intensity of the contraction is described as mild, moderate, or strong. During a contraction, if the uterus has little firmness and can be easily indented with the fingertips, the contraction is a mild one. In a moderate contraction, the fundus of the uterus is firmer, but it is possible to indent it. In a strong contraction, the fundus of the uterus is very firm, and indentation is difficult.

The contraction pattern of frequency, duration, and intensity should be recorded by the nurse at least every hour during the beginning of labour and more frequently as labour progresses. This information is valuable in evaluating the normal progress of labour.

Psyche

The psyche is recognized as part of the labour process. For example, anxiety and fear can decrease a pregnant woman's ability to cope with pain in labour. Maternal catecholamine, stress hormones secreted when the woman is anxious or fearful, are known to inhibit uterine contractility and placental blood flow. However, relaxation augments the natural process of labour.

Prenatal care and classes provide preparations for the mother to cope with the labour process. The nursing responsibilities during labour include using strategies to reduce anxiety and promote relaxation.

Culture, expectations, past experiences, language barriers, and availability of a support person are factors that influence a woman's ability to cope with the experience of labour and delivery.

EVENTS IN FIRST STAGE OF LABOUR

The length of labour varies widely and is influenced by parity, birth interval, psychological state, presentation and position of the fetus, maternal pelvic shape and size and the character of uterine contractions.

UTERINE ACTION

Fundal dominance (Fig. 6.3)

Each uterine contraction starts in the fundus near one of the cornua and spreads across and downwards. The contraction lasts longest in the fundus where it is also most intense, but the peak is reached simultaneously over the whole uterus and the contraction fades from all parts together. This pattern permits the cervix to dilate and the strongly contracting fundus to expel the fetus.

Polarity

Polarity is the term used to describe the neuromuscular harmony that prevails between the two poles or segments of the uterus throughout labour. The upper pole contracts strongly and retracts to expel the fetus, the lower pole contracts slightly and dilates to allow expulsion to take place. If polarity is disorganized, the progress of labour is inhibited.

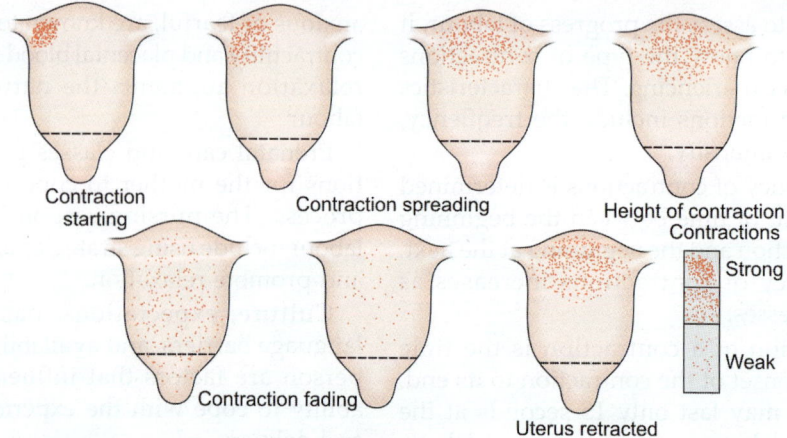

Contraction
starting

Contraction spreading

Height of contraction
Contractions

Strong

Weak

Contraction fading

Uterus retracted

Fig. 6.3: Series of diagrams to show fundal dominance during uterine contractions

Contraction and retraction

Uterine muscle has a unique property. During labour, the contraction does not pass off entirely, but muscle fibres retain some of the shortening of contraction instead of becoming completely relaxed (Fig. 6.4). This is termed retraction. It assists in the progressive expulsion of the fetus, the upper segment of the uterus becomes gradually shorter and thicker and its cavity diminishes.

Formation of upper and lower uterine segments

By the end of pregnancy, the body of the uterus is described as having divided into two segments, which are anatomically distinct (Fig. 6.5). The upper uterine segment, having been formed from the body of the fundus, is mainly concerned with contraction and retraction, it is thick and muscular. The lower uterine segment is formed of the isthmus and the cervix, and is about 8–10 cm in length. The lower segment is prepared for distension and dilatation.

The retraction ring

A ridge forms between the upper and lower uterine segments, this is known as the 'retraction' or 'Bandl's ring' (Fig. 6.6). It is customary to use the former term to describe the physiological retraction ring and to reserve the term

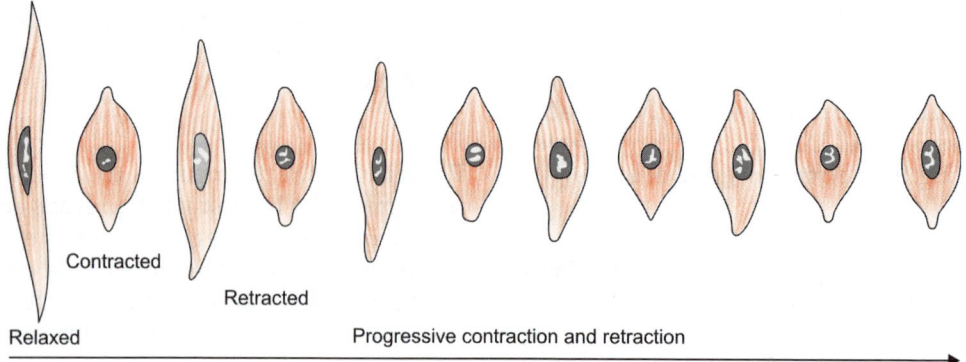

Contracted

Retracted

Relaxed

Progressive contraction and retraction

Fig. 6.4: Diagram to show how uterine muscle retains some shortening after each contraction

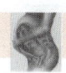

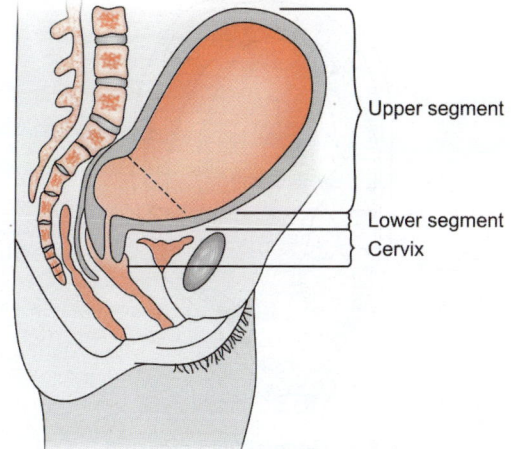

Fig. 6.5: Birth canal before labour begins

Bandl's ring for an exaggerated degree of the phenomenon that becomes visible above the symphysis pubis in mechanically obstructed labour when the lower segment thins abnormally.

The physiological ring gradually rises as the upper uterine segment contracts and retracts and the lower uterine segment thins out to accommodate the descending fetus. Once the cervix is fully dilated and the fetus can leave the uterus, the retraction ring rises no further.

Cervical effacement

Effacement refers to the inclusion of the cervical canal into the lower uterine segment. The muscle fibres surrounding the internal os are drawn upwards by the retracted upper segment and the cervix merges into the lower uterine segment.

Effacement may occur late in pregnancy, or it may not take place until labour begins. In the nulliparous woman, the cervix will not usually dilate until effacement is complete, whereas in the parous woman, effacement and dilatation may occur simultaneously and a small canal may be felt in early labour.

Cervical dilatation

Dilatation of the cervix is the process of enlargement of the os uteri from a tightly closed aperture to an opening large enough to permit passage of the fetal head. Dilatation is measured in centimeters and full dilatation at term equates to about 10 cm.

Dilatation occurs as a result of uterine action and the counter pressure applied by either the intact bag of membranes of the presenting part, or both. A wellflexed fetal head closely applied to the cervix favours efficient dilatation.

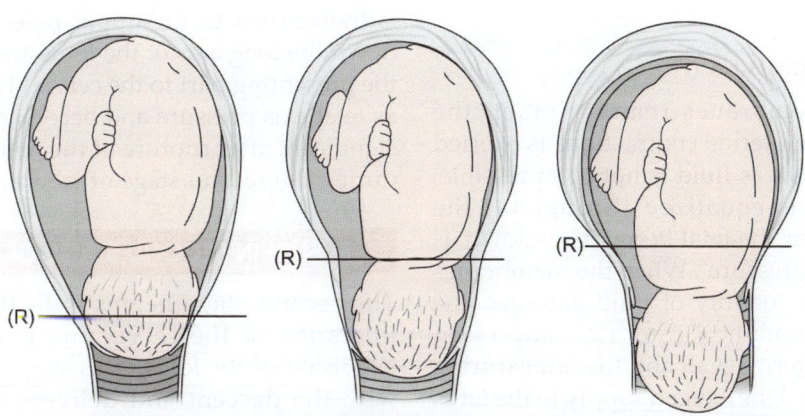

Fig. 6.6: Retraction ring between the upper and lower uterine segments

Show

As a result of the dilatation of the cervix, the operculum, which formed the cervical plug during pregnancy, is lost. The woman may see a bloodstained mucoid discharge a few hours before, or within a few hours after, labour starts. The blood comes from ruptured capillaries in the parietal decidua where the chorion has become detached from the dilating cervix. Referred to as 'show'.

MECHANICAL FACTORS

Formation of the forewaters

As the lower uterine segment forms and stretches, the chorion becomes detached from it and the increased intrauterine pressure causes this loosened part of the fluid sac to bulge downwards into the internal os, to a depth of 6–12 mm. The well-flexed head fits snugly into the cervix and cuts off the fluid in front of the head from that which surrounds the body. The former is known as *forewaters* and the latter, the *hindwaters.*

The effect of separation of the forewaters prevents the pressure that is applied to the hindwaters during uterine contractions from being applied to the forewaters. This may help keep the membranes intact during the first stage of labour and be a natural defence against infection.

General fluid pressure (Fig. 6.7)

While the membranes remain intact, the pressure of the uterine contractions is exerted on the fluid and, as fluid is not compressible, the pressure is equalized throughout the uterus and over the fetal body; it is known as 'general fluid pressure'. When the membranes rupture and a quantity of fluid emerges, the placenta and umbilical cord are compressed between the uterine wall and the fetus during contractions and the oxygen supply to the fetus is diminished.

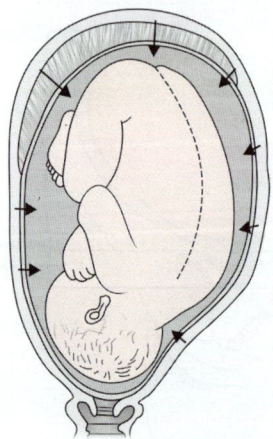

Fig. 6.7: General fluid pressure

Rupture of the membranes

The optimum physiological time for the membranes to rupture spontaneously is at the end of the first stage of labour after the cervix becomes fully dilated and no longer supports the bag of forewaters. The uterine contractions are also applying increasing force at this time. Occasionally, the membranes do not rupture even in the second stage and appear at the vulva as a bulging sac covering the fetal head as it is born, this is known as the *caul.*

Fetal axis pressure (Fig. 6.8)

During each contraction, the uterus rises forward and the force of the fundal contraction is transmitted to the upper pole of the fetus, down the long axis of the fetus and applied by the presenting part to the cervix. This is known as fetal axis pressure and becomes much more significant after rupture of the membranes and during the second stage of labour.

EVENTS IN SECOND STAGE OF LABOUR

The second stage begins with the complete dilatation of the cervix and ends with the expulsion of the fetus. This stage is concerned with the descent and delivery of the fetus through the birth canal.

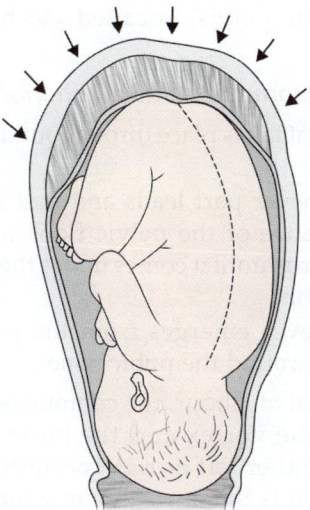

Fig. 6.8: Fetal axis pressure

The events result from a continuation of the same forces which have been at work during the first stage of labour but activity is accelerated once the cervix has become fully dilated (Fig. 6.9).

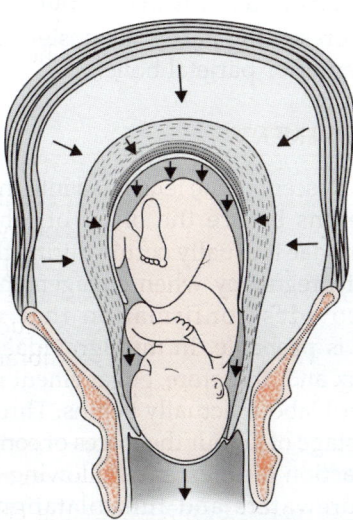

Fig. 6.9: Diagram showing the expulsive forces in the second stage. Increased intra-abdominal pressure augments the downward expulsive force of uterine contraction.

Uterine action

Contractions become stronger and longer but may be less frequent, allowing both mother and fetus a recovery period during the resting phase. The membranes often rupture spontaneously at the onset of the second stage. The consequent drainage of liquor allows the hard, round fetal head to be directly applied to the vaginal tissues and aid distension. Fetal axis pressure increases flexion of the head which results in smaller presenting diameters.

The contractions become expulsive and as the fetus descends further into the vagina, pressure from the presenting part stimulates nerve receptors in the pelvic floor and the woman experiences the need to push. This reflex may initially be controlled to a limited extent but becomes increasingly compulsive, overwhelming and involuntary during each contraction. The mother's response is to employ her secondary powers of expulsion by contracting her abdominal muscles and diaphragm.

Soft tissue displacement

As the hard fetal head descends, the soft tissues of the pelvis become displaced. Anteriorly, the bladder is pushed upwards into the abdomen where it is at less risk of injury during fetal descent. This results in the stretching and thinning of the urethra so that its lumen is reduced. Posteriorly, the rectum becomes flattened into the sacral curve and the pressure of the advancing head expels any residual faecal matter. The levator ani muscles dilate, thin out and are displaced laterally, and the perineal body is flattened, stretched and thinned. The fetal head becomes visible at the vulva, advancing with each contraction and receding during the resting phase until crowning takes place and the head is born. The shoulders and body follow with the next contraction, accompanied by a gush of amniotic fluid. The second stage culminates in the birth of the baby.

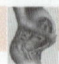

Recognition of the commencement of the second stage of labour

The transition from the first to the second stage is not always clinically apparent. Several of the signs are presumptive and not a reliable index that this stage has been reached.

Presumptive signs and differential diagnoses and expulsive uterine contractions

It is possible for a woman to feel a strong desire to push before the cervix is fully dilated, especially if the fetus is in an occipitoposterior position, the rectum is full or the woman is highly parous.

Rupture of the forewaters: This may occur at any time during labour.

Dilatation and gaping of the anus: Deep engagement of the presenting part and premature maternal effort may produce this sign during the latter part of the first stage.

Appearance of the presenting part

Excessive moulding may result in the formation of a large caput succedaneum which can protrude through the cervix prior to full dilatation. Similarly, a breech presentation may be visible when the cervix is only 7–8 cm dilated.

Show: This must be distinguished from bleeding due to partial separation of the placenta or that caused by ruptured vasa praevia.

Congestion of the vulva: Enthusiastic premature pushing may also cause this.

Confirmatory evidence

Confirmation of the onset of second stage can only be established by performing a vaginal examination. No cervix can be felt on examination.

MECHANISM OF NORMAL LABOUR

Definition

The series of movements that occur on the head in the process of adaptation during its journey through the pelvis, is called mechanism of labour.

Principles common to all mechanisms

- Descent takes place throughout the mechanism.
- Whichever part leads and first meets the resistance of the pelvic floor will rotate forwards until it comes under the symphysis pubis.
- Whatever emerges from the pelvis will pivot around the pubic bone.

At the onset of labour, the commonest presentation is the vertex and the most common position, either left or right occipitoanterior; therefore, it is this mechanism which will be described. When these conditions are met, the way that the fetus is normally situated can be described as follows:

- The lie is longitudinal
- The presentation is cephalic
- The position is right or left occipitoanterior
- The attitude is one of good flexion
- The denominator is the occiput
- The presenting part is the posterior part of the anterior parietal bone.

MAIN MOVEMENTS

Descent: Descent of the fetal head into the pelvis often begins before the onset of labour. In primigravidae it usually occurs during the latter weeks of pregnancy when engagement of the head provides confirmation that vaginal delivery is probable. In multigravidae muscle tone is lax and, therefore, engagement may not occur until labour actually begins. Throughout the first stage of labour the forces of contraction and retraction aid descent. Following rupture of the forewaters and full dilatation of the cervix, maternal effort speeds progress.

Flexion: This increases throughout labour. The fetal spine is attached nearer the posterior part of the skull; pressure exerted down the fetal

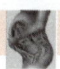

axis will be more forcibly transmitted to the occiput than the sinciput. The effect is to increase flexion which results in smaller presenting diameters which will negotiate the pelvis more easily. At the onset of labour, the suboccipitofrontal diameter, 10 cm, is presenting, with greater flexion the suboccipitobregmatic diameter, 9.5 cm, presents. The occiput becomes the *leading part.*

Internal rotation of the head: During a contraction the leading part is driven downwards onto the pelvic floor. The slope of the pelvic floor determines the direction of rotation. *The muscles are gutter-shaped and slope down anteriorly,* so whichever part of the fetus first meets the lateral half of this slope will be directed forwards and towards the centre. In a well-flexed vertex presentation, the occiput leads and meets the pelvic floor first and rotates anteriorly through one-eighth of a circle. This causes a slight twist in the neck of the fetus as the head is no longer in direct alignment with the shoulders. The anteroposterior diameter of the head now lies in the widest (anteroposterior) diameter of the pelvic outlet, facilitating an easy escape (Figs 6.10a and b).

Crowning: The occiput slips beneath the subpubic arch and crowning occurs when the head no longer recedes between contractions and the widest transverse diameter (biparietal) is born. If flexion is maintained, the suboccipitobregmatic diameter, 9.5 cm, distends the vaginal orifice.

Extension of the head: Once crowning has occurred the fetal head can extend, pivoting on the suboccipital region around the pubic bone. This releases the sinciput, face and chin which sweep the perineum and are born by a movement of extension. The suboccipitofrontal diameter, 10 cm, distends the vaginal outlet (Fig. 6.11a)

Restitution: The twist in the neck of the fetus which resulted from internal rotation, is now corrected by a slight untwisting move-

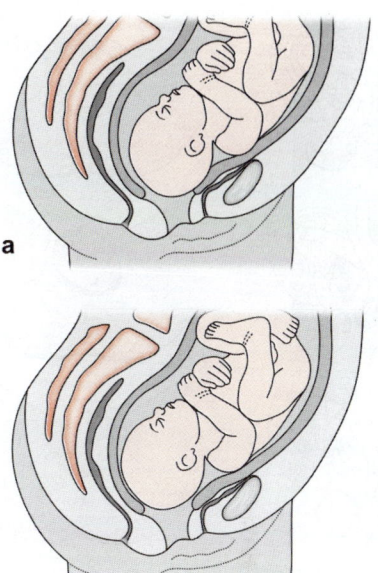

Fig. 6.10: a. Internal rotation of the head begins, **b.** Upon completion, the occiput lies under the symphysis pubis

ment. The occiput moves one-eighth of a circle towards the side from which it started (Fig. 6.11b).

Internal rotation of the shoulders: The shoulders undergo a similar rotation to that of the head to lie in the widest diameter of the pelvic outlet, namely anteroposterior. The anterior shoulder is the first to reach the levator ani muscle and therefore rotates anteriorly to lie under the symphysis pubis. This movement can be clearly seen as the head turns at the same time **(external rotation of the head).** It occurs in the same direction as restitution and the occiput of the fetal head now lies laterally (Fig. 6.11c).

Lateral flexion

The shoulders are born sequentially. The anterior shoulder slips beneath the sub-pubic arch and the posterior shoulder passes over the perineum. This enables a smaller diameter to distend the vaginal orifice than if both shoulders

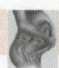

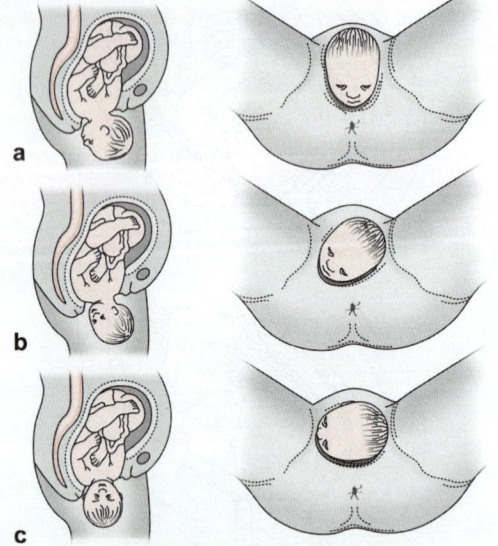

Fig. 6.11: **a.** Birth of the head, **b.** Restitution, **c.** External rotation

were born simultaneously. The remainder of the body is born by lateral flexion as the spine bends sideways through the curved birth canal (Fig. 6.12).

EVENTS IN THIRD STAGE OF LABOUR

The third stage of labour comprises the phase of placental separation, its descent to the lower segment and finally its expulsion with the membranes.

Placental separation

At the beginning of labour, the placental attachment roughly corresponds to an area of 20 cm (8″) in diameter. During the second stage, there is slight but progressive diminution of the surface area following successive retractions, which attains its peak immediately following the birth of the baby.

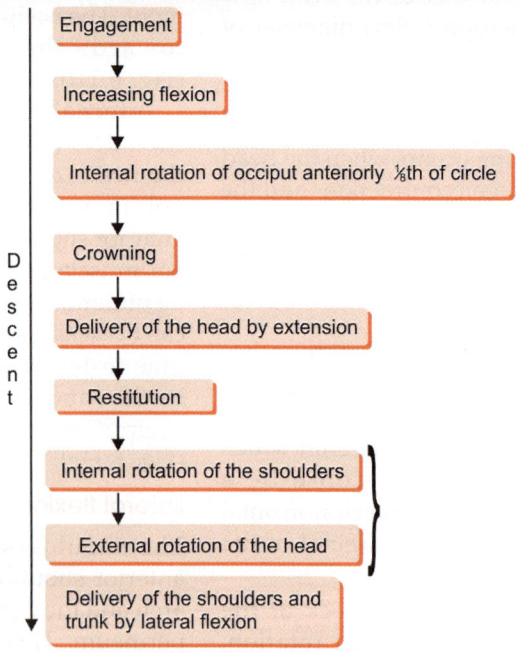

Diameter of engagement: Available transverse diameter of the inlet.
Engaging diameter of the head: Sub-occipitobregmatic 9.5 cm (3·¾″)

Engagement

Increasing flexion

Internal rotation of occiput anteriorly ⅛th of circle

Crowning

Delivery of the head by extension

Restitution

Internal rotation of the shoulders

External rotation of the head

Delivery of the shoulders and trunk by lateral flexion

Descent

Fig. 6.12: Summary of mechanism of labour

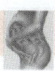

After the birth of the baby, the uterus measures about 20 cm (8") vertically and 10 cm (4") antero-posteriorly, the shape becomes discoid. The wall of the upper segment is much thickened while the thin and flabby lower segment is thrown into folds. The cavity is much reduced to accommodate only the afterbirths (Fig. 6.13).

Mechanism of separation: Marked retraction reduces effectively the surface area at the placental site to about its half. A shearing force is instituted between the placenta and the placental site which brings about its ultimate separation. **There are two ways of separation of placenta.**

1. *Central separation (Schultze):* Detachment of placenta from its uterine attachment starts at the centre resulting in opening up of few uterine sinuses and accumulation of blood behind the placenta (retroplacental haematoma). With increasing contraction, more and more detachment occurs which is facilitated by weight of the placenta and retroplacental blood until whole of the placenta gets detached.

2. *Marginal separation (Mathews-Duncan):* Separation starts at the margin as it is mostly unsupported. Marginal separation is found more frequently (Fig. 6.14).

Separation of the membranes: The membranes which are attached loosely in the active part are thrown into multiple folds. Those attached

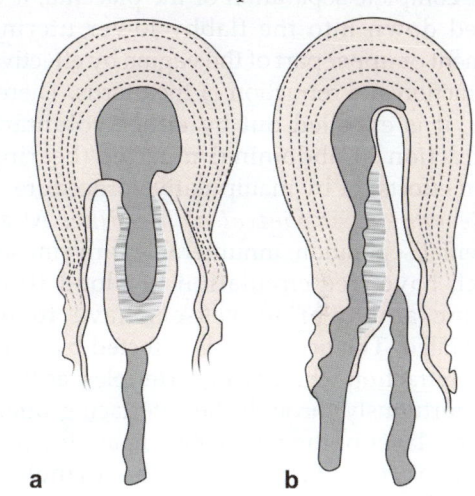

a   **b**

Fig. 6.14: Types of separation of the placenta. **a.** Schultze method, **b.** Mathews-Duncan method

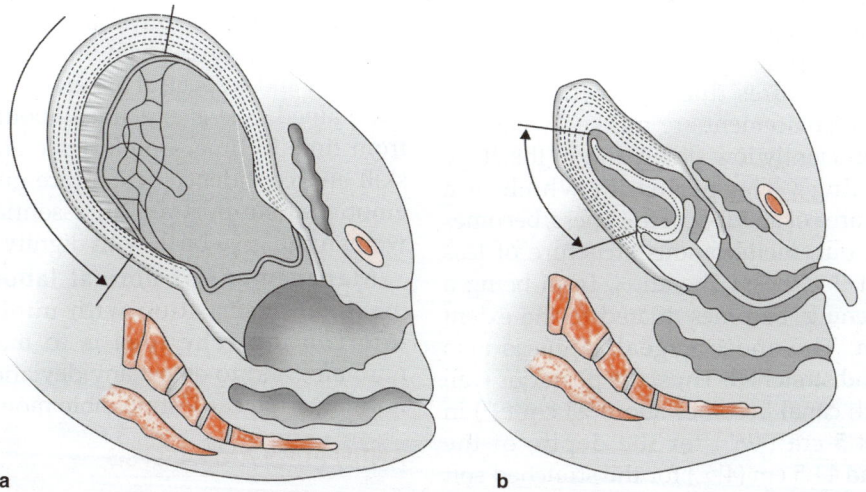

a   **b**

Fig. 6.13: Diagram showing area of placental site before and after the delivery of the baby. **a.** Before the delivery of the baby, **b.** After the delivery of the baby. Note the reduction of the surface area of the placental site resulting in buckling of the placenta. P.S. = Placental surface

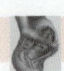
to the lower segment are already separated during its stretching. The separation is facilitated partly by uterine contraction and mostly by weight of the placenta as it descends down from the active part.

Expulsion of placenta

After complete separation of the placenta, it is forced down into the flabby lower uterine segment or upper part of the vagina by effective contraction and retraction of the uterus. Thereafter, it is expelled out by either voluntary contraction of abdominal muscles (bearing down efforts) or by manipulative procedure.

Mechanism of control of bleeding: After placental separation, innumerable torn sinuses which have free circulation of blood from uterine and ovarian vessels have to be obliterated. **The occlusion is affected by complete retraction** whereby the arterioles, as they pass tortuously through the interlacing intermediate layer of the myometrium, are literally clamped (Fig. 6.15). It is the principal mechanism to prevent bleeding.

However, there is no stretching of the urethra as was previously thought. Rather, the urethra is pushed anteriorly, with the neck of the bladder still lying in the vulnerable position behind the symphysis pubis. The changes in the posterior structures due to downward and backward displacement are marked when the head is sufficiently low down and in the stage of "crowning". The perineum which is a triangular area of about 4 cm thickness, becomes a thinned out, membranous structure of less than 1 cm thickness. The anus, from being a closed opening, becomes dilated to the extent of 2–3 cm. The anococcygeal raphe is also thinned and stretched. Thus, the posterior wall of the birth canal becomes about 23 cm (9") in length; 11.5 cm (4½") for the depth, of the sacrum and 11.5 cm (4½") for the stretched soft tissue, while its anterior wall remains the same 4 cm (1½"), in length. The canal becomes almost a semicircle.

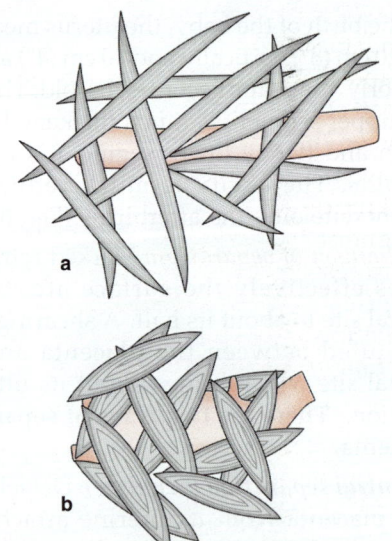

Fig. 6.15: Blood vessels. **a.** running through the interlacing muscle fibres, **b.** literally clamped due to effective retraction of the uterine muscles

MANAGEMENT OF NORMAL LABOUR

General considerations: Labour events have got great psychological/emotional and social impact on the woman and her family. She experiences stress, physical pain and fear of dangers. The care given should be tactful/sensitive and respectful to her. Privacy must be maintained. She is explained about the events from time to time. Comfortable environment, skill and confidence of the care giver and the emotional support are all essential so that a woman can give birth with dignity.

Management of normal labour aims at maximal observation with minimal active intervention. **The idea** is to maintain the normalcy and to detect any deviation from the normal at the earliest possible moment.

ANTISEPTICS AND ASEPSIS

Scrupulous surgical cleanliness and asepsis on the part of the patients and the attendants involved in the delivery process are to be maintained.

Patient care: Shaving of the vulva need not be mandatory. In the West they don't do. The vulva and the perineum are washed liberally with soap and water and then with 10% Dettol solution or Hibitane (chlorhexidine) 1 in 2000.

The woman should take a shower or bath, wear laundered gown and stay mobile. Throughout labour she is given continued encouragement and emotional support. *Antiseptic and aseptic precautions are to be taken during vaginal examination and during conduction of delivery.*

VAGINAL EXAMINATION IN LABOUR

First vaginal examination should be done by a senior doctor to be more reliable and informative. The examination is done with the patient lying in dorsal position.

PRELIMINARIES

1. *Toileting:* The hands and forearms should be washed with soap and running water, a scrubbing brush should be used for the finger nails. The procedure should take at least 3 minutes.
2. *Sterile pair of gloves* is to be put on.
3. Vulval toileting has previously been performed. Vulva should once more be swabbed from before backwards with antiseptic lotion like 10% Dettol or Hibitane 1 in 2000. The same solution is poured over the vulva by separating the labia minora by the fingers of left hand.
4. *Gloved middle and index fingers of the right hand* smeared liberally with antiseptic cream like Cetavlon are introduced into the vagina after separating the labia by two fingers of the left hand.
5. Complete examination should be done before fingers are withdrawn.
6. Vaginal examination should be kept as minimum as possible to avoid risks of infection.

The following pieces of information are to be noted and recorded carefully
- Degree of cervical dilatation in centimeters.
- Degree of effacement of cervix.
- Status of membranes and, if ruptured, colour of the liquor.
- Presenting part and its position by noting the fontanelles and sagittal suture in relation to the quadrants of the pelvis.
- Caput or moulding of the head and, if present, to note its degree.
- Station of the head in relation to ischial spines (Fig. 6.16).

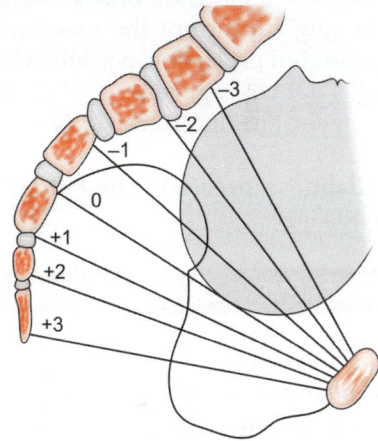

Fig. 6.16: Station of the head in relation to ischial spines

Spines are the most prominent bony projections felt on internal examination and the bispinous diameter is the shortest diameter of the pelvis in transverse plane being 10.5 cm. The station is said to be '0' if the presenting part is at the level of the spines. The station is stated in minus figures, if it is above the spines (– 1 cm, – 2 cm, – 3 cm, – 4 cm and – 5 cm) and in plus figures if it is below the spines (+ 1 cm, + 2 cm, + 3 cm, + 4 cm and + 5 cm).

INDICATIONS OF VAGINAL EXAMINATION

Whatever aseptic technique is employed, there is always some chance of introducing infection

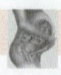

especially after rupture of the membranes. **Hence, vaginal examination should be restricted to a minimum.**

- At the onset of labour—to confirm the onset of labour and to detect precisely the presenting part and its position. Pelvic assessment especially in primigravidae, should be done during the initial examination.
- The progress of labour can be judged on periodic examinations noting the dilatation of the cervix and descent of the head in relation to the spines (station). Generally, it is done at an interval of 3–4 hours.
- Following rupture of the membranes to exclude cord prolapse especially where the head is not yet engaged.
- Whenever any interference is contemplated.
- To diagnose precisely the beginning of second stage.

MANAGEMENT OF THE FIRST STAGE

PRINCIPLES

1. *Non-interference with watchful expectancy* so as to prepare the patient for natural birth.
2. *To monitor carefully* the progress of labour, maternal conditions and fetal behaviour so as to detect any intrapartum complication early.

PRELIMINARIES

This consists of basic evaluation of the current clinical condition.

- Enquiry is to be made about the onset of labour pains or leakage of liquor, if any.
- Thorough general and obstetrical examinations, including vaginal examination, are to be carried out and recorded.
- Records of antenatal visits, investigation reports and any specific treatment given, if available, are to be reviewed.

ACTUAL MANAGEMENT

- **General**
  - *Antiseptic dressing*
  - *Encouragement and assurance* are given to keep up the morale.
  - *Constant supervision* is ensured.
- *Bowel:* An educated woman may be instructed to come to the hospital after evacuating the bowel by taking a suppository earlier. An enema with soap and water or glycerine suppository is traditionally given in early stage. This may be given if the rectum feels loaded on vaginal examination.
- *Rest and ambulation:* If the membranes are intact, the patient is allowed to walk about. This attitude prevents venacaval compression and encourages descent of the head. Ambulation can reduce the duration of labour, need of analgesia and improves maternal comfort. If, however, labour is monitored electronically or analgesic drug is given, she should be in bed.
- *Diet:* There is delayed emptying of the stomach in labour. **Food is withheld during active labour.** Fluids in the form of plain water, ice chips or fruit juice may be given in early labour. Intravenous fluid with ringer solution is started where any intervention is anticipated.
- *Bladder care:* Patient is encouraged to pass urine by herself as full bladder often inhibits uterine contraction and may lead to infection. If the woman cannot go to the toilet, she is given a bed pan. Privacy must be maintained and comfort must be ensured. If the patient fails to pass urine, especially in late first stage, catheterization is to be done with strict aseptic precautions.
- **Promoting physical comfort**
  - General body wash
  - Mouth washing

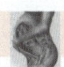

– Combing of hair
– Changing of soiled gowns
– Back rub

- *Relief of pain:* The common analgesic drug used is pethidine 50–100 mg intramuscularly when the pains are well established in the active phase of labour. If necessary, it is repeated after 4 hours. Pethidine is an effective analgesic as well as a sedative. Metoclopramide 10 mg. IM is commonly given to combat vomiting due to pethidine. Pethidine crosses the placenta and is a respiratory depressant to the neonate. ***The drug should not be given if delivery is anticipated within two hours.***

- **Assessment of progress of labour and partograph recording.**

Abdominal findings

1. *Uterine contractions:* The nature of uterine contractions, as regards to its intensity, frequency and duration, is assessed. The number of contractions in 10 minutes and duration of each contraction in seconds are recorded in the partograph.
2. *Pelvic grip:* Gradual disappearance of poles of the head (sinciput and occiput) which were felt previously.
3. Shifting of the maximal impulse of the fetal heart beat downwards and medially.

- **To note the fetal well-being**
  Fetal heart rate (FHR) along with its rhythm and intensity should be noted every half hour in the first stage and every 15 minutes in second stage or following rupture of the membranes. To be of value, the observation should be made immediately following uterine contraction. The count should be made for 60 seconds. To avoid confusion of maternal and fetal heart rates, maternal pulse should be counted. Otherwise maternal tachycardia may be wrongly treated as fetal heart rate. Normal fetal heart rate ranges from 110–150 per minute.

- **Vaginal examination**
  – Dilatation of the cervix in centimetres in relation to hours of labour is a reliable index to note the progress of labour.
  – To note the position of the head and degree of flexion.
  – To note the station of the head in relation to the ischial spines.
  – *Colour of the liquor* (clear or meconium stained) if the membranes are ruptured.
  – *Degree of moulding of the head:* Moulding occurs first at the junction of occipitoparietal bones and then between the parietal bones
  – *Caput formation:* Progressive increase is more important than its mere presence.

EVIDENCES OF FOETAL DISTRESS

To watch the maternal condition

Routine check up includes
- To record two hourly pulse, blood pressure and temperature
- To observe the tongue periodically for hydration
- To note the urine output/urine for acetone/glucose and IV fluids/drugs.

Evidence of maternal distress

- Anxious look with sunken eyes
- Dehydration/dry tongue
- Acetone smell in breath
- Rising pulse rate of 100 per minute or more
- Hot/dry vagina often with offensive discharge
- Scanty high coloured urine with presence of acetone.

MANAGEMENT OF THE SECOND STAGE

The transition from the first stage to the second stage is evidenced by the following features.

 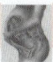

- Increasing intensity of uterine contractions.
- Appearance of bearing down efforts.
- Urge to defecate with descent of the presenting part.
- Complete dilatation of the cervix as evidenced on vaginal examination.

Principles

1. To assist in the natural expulsion of the fetus slowly and steadily.
2. To prevent perineal injuries.

General measures

- The patient should be in bed.
- Constant supervision is mandatory and the FHR is recorded at every five minutes.
- Vaginal examination is done at the beginning of the second stage not only to confirm its onset but also to detect any accidental cord prolapse. The position and the station of the head are once more to be reviewed and the progressive descent of the head is ensured.

Preparation for delivery

- Position: Dorsal position with 15° left lateral tilt is commonly favoured as it avoids aortocaval compression and facilitates pushing effort.
- The accoucheur scrubs up and puts on sterile gown, mask and gloves and stands on the right side of the table.
- Toileting the external genitalia and inner side of the thighs is done with cotton swabs soaked in Savlon or Dettol solution. One sterile sheet is placed beneath the buttocks of the patient and one over the abdomen. Sterilized leggings are to be used. Essential aseptic procedures are remembered as 3 'C's:
  1. Clean hands
  2. Clean surface
  3. Clean cutting and ligaturing of the cord.
- To catheterize the bladder, if it is full.

Conduction of delivery

The assistance required in spontaneous delivery is divided into three phases:

- Delivery of the head
- Delivery of the shoulders
- Delivery of the trunk

Delivery of the head: The principles to be followed are to maintain flexion of the head, to prevent its early extension and to regulate its slow escape out of the vulval outlet.

- The patient is encouraged for the bearing down efforts during uterine contractions.
- When the scalp is visible for about 5 cm in diameter, flexion of the head is maintained during contractions. This is achieved by pushing the occiput downwards and backwards by using thumb and index fingers of the left hand while pressing the perineum by the right palm with a sterile vulval pad.
- The process is repeated during subsequent contractions until the subocciput is placed under the symphysis pubis. At this stage, the maximum diameter of the head (biparietal diameter) stretches the vulval outlet without any recession of the head even after the contraction is over and it is called "crowning of the head". The purpose of increasing the flexion of the head is to ensure that the small suboccipitofrontal diameter 10 cm (4") distends the vulval outlet instead of larger occipitofrontal diameter 11.5 cm (4½") (Fig. 6.17).
- When the perineum is fully stretched episiotomy is done at this stage after prior infiltration with 10 ml of 1% lignocaine. Bulging thinned out perineum is a better criterion than the visibility of 4–5 cm of scalp to decide the time of performing episiotomy.
- Slow delivery of the head in between the contractions is to be regulated. This is accomplished by pushing the chin with a sterile towel gauze covered fingers of the

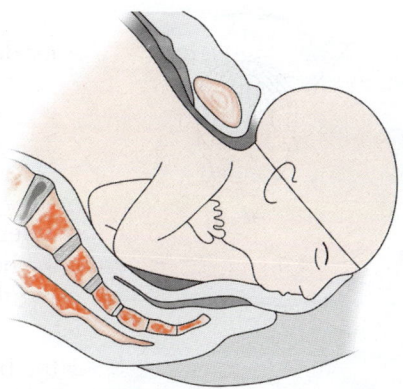

Fig. 6.17: Suboccipitofrontal diameter distending the vulval outlet

right hand placed over the anococcygeal region while the left hand exerts pressure on the occiput. The forehead, nose, mouth and the chin are thus born successively over the stretched perineum by extension (Fig. 6.18).

- **Care following delivery of the head**
  - Immediately following delivery of the head, **the mucus and blood in the mouth and pharynx are to be wiped**

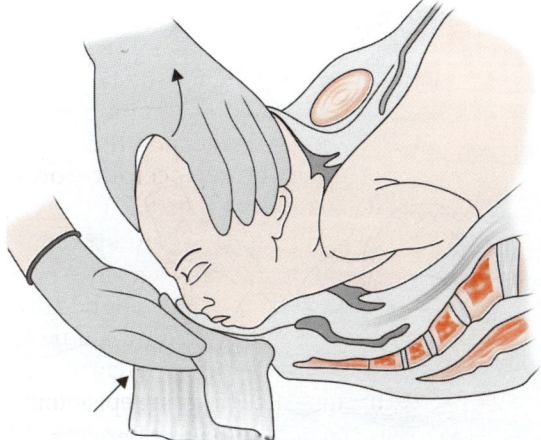

Fig. 6.18: Assisted delivery of the head by extension, exerting an upward pressure to the chin by the right hand placed over the anococcygeal raphe

with sterile gauze piece on a little finger. Alternatively, mechanical or electrical sucker may be used.

- **The eyelids are then wiped with sterile dry cotton swabs** using one for each eye starting from the medial to the lateral canthus to minimize contamination of the conjunctival sac.
- **The neck is then palpated to exclude the presence of any loop of cord (20–25%).** If it is found and if loose enough, it should be slipped over the head or over the shoulders as the baby is being born. But if it is sufficiently tight enough, it is cut in between two pairs of Kocher's forceps placed 1 inch apart.

- **Prevention of perineal laceration:** More attention should be paid not to the perineum but to the controlled delivery of the head.
  - **Delivery by early extension is to be avoided.** Flexion of the subocciput comes under the symphysis pubis so that lesser suboccipitofrontal 10 cm (4") diameter emerges out of the introitus.
  - **Spontaneous forcible delivery of the head is to be avoided** by assuring the patient not to bear down during contractions.
  - **To deliver the head in between contractions**
  - **To perform timely episiotomy** (when indicated)
  - **To take care during delivery of the shoulders** as the wider bisacromial diameter (12 cm) emerges out of the introitus.

*Delivery of the shoulders: **Do not be hasty in delivery of the shoulders.*** Wait for the uterine contractions to come and for the movements of restitution and external rotation of the head to occur (Fig. 6.19). During the next contraction, the anterior shoulder is born behind the symphysis. If there is delay, the head is grasped

 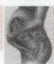

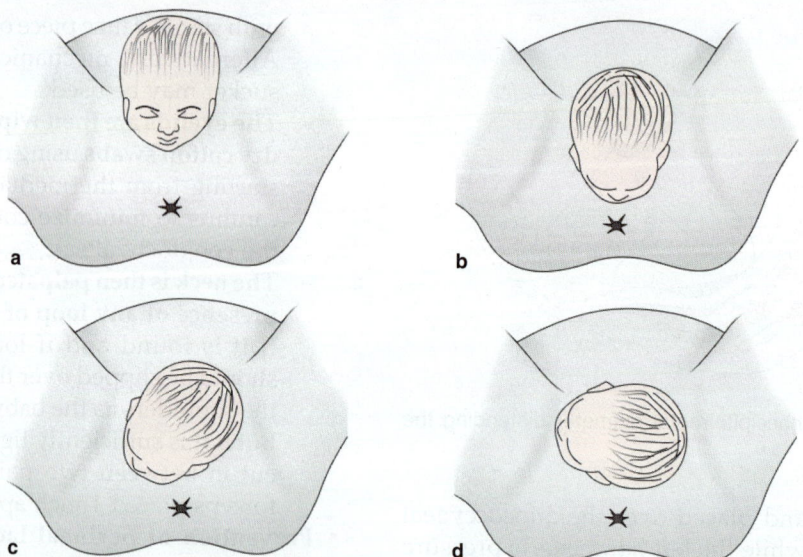

Fig. 6.19: **a.** Head is born by extension, **b.** Head drops down with the face close to the anus, **c.** Restitution, **d.** External rotation

by both hands and is gently drawn posteriorly until the anterior shoulder is released from under the pubis. By drawing the head in upward direction, the posterior shoulder is delivered out of the perineum (Fig. 6.20). *Traction on the head should be gentle* to avoid excessive stretching of the neck causing injury to the brachial plexus, haematoma of the neck or fracture of the clavicle.

Delivery of the trunk: After the delivery of the shoulders, the forefinger of each hand are inserted under the axillae and the trunk is delivered gently by lateral flexion.

IMMEDIATE CARE OF THE NEWBORN

- Soon after the delivery of the baby, it should be placed on a tray covered with clean dry linen with the head slightly downwards (15°). It facilitates drainage of the mucus accumulated in the tracheobronchial tree by gravity. The tray is placed between the legs of the mother and should be at a lower level than

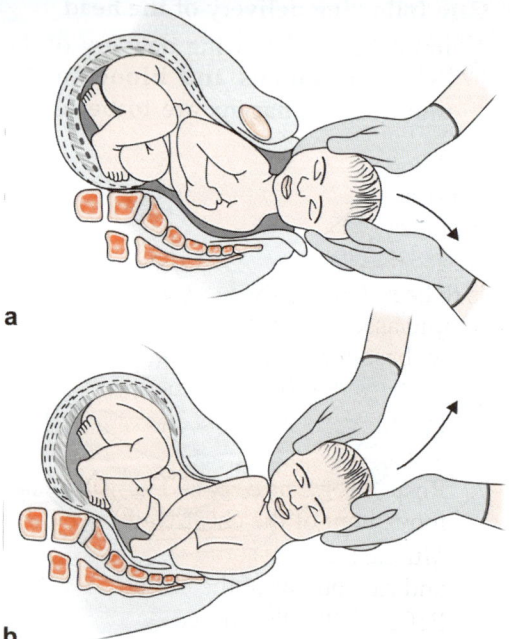

Fig. 6.20: Assisted delivery of the shoulders. **a.** Anterior shoulder, **b.** Posterior shoulder

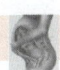

- Anxiety related to uncertain outcome of labour and birth.
- Pain, related to uterine contractions
- Fluid volume deficit related to lack of fluid intake.
- Communication, impaired verbal, related to inability to understand medical terminology or English.
- Knowledge deficit related to the labour process.
- Urinary elimination, altered related to pressure of uterus on bladder.
- Nutrition: less than body requirements, related to lack of nutrient intake, medical limitation of oral intake.
- Self-esteem disturbance related to body exposure.
- Risk for ascending genital tract infection related to multiple vaginal examinations.
- Anxiety related to unknown surroundings and hospital procedures
- Risk for fetal injury related to uteroplacental insufficiency
- Risk for maternal injury and infection related to the second stage of labour.
- Risk for altered parenting related to delayed bonding.

the uterus to facilitate gravitation of blood from the placenta to the infant.

- Air passage should be cleared of mucus and liquor by gentle suction.
- **Apgar rating** at 1 minute and at 5 minutes is to be recorded. The Apgar score permits a rapid assessment of the need for resuscitation based on five signs that indicate the physiologic state of the neonate.
  1. Heart rate, based on auscultation with a stethoscope
  2. Respiratory rate, based on observed movement of the chest wall
  3. Muscle tone, based on degree of flexion and movement of the extremities
  4. Reflex irritability, based on response to gentle slaps on the soles of the feet
  5. Colour, described as pallid, cyanotic or pink.

Each item is scored as a 0,1 or 2. Evaluations are made 1 and 5 minutes afterbirth. Scores of 0 to 3 indicate severe distress, scores of 4 to 6 indicate moderate difficulty and scores of 10 indicate that the infant should have no difficulty adjusting to extrauterine life. Apgar scores do not predict future neurologic outcome, but the 5 minute score does correlate with the degree of risk for neonatal morbidity and mortality.

- **Clamping and ligature of the cord:** The cord is clamped by two Kocher's forceps, the near one is placed 5 cm away from the umbilicus and is cut in between. Two separate cord ligatures are applied with sterile cotton threads 1 cm apart using reef-knot, the proximal one being placed 2.5 cm away from the navel. Squeezing the cord with fingers prior to applying ligatures prevents accidental inclusion of embryonic remnants. Leaving behind a length of the cord attached to the navel not only prevents inclusion of the embryonic structure, if present, but also facilitates control of primary haemorrhage due to a slipped ligature. The cord is divided with scissors about 1 cm beyond the ligatures taking aseptic precautions so as to prevent cord sepsis. Presence of any abnormality in cord vessels (single umbilical artery) is to be noted. The cut end is then covered with sterile gauze piece after making sure that there is no bleeding.

Delay in clamping for 2–3 minutes or till cessation of the cord pulsation facilitates transfer of 80–100 ml blood from the compressed placenta to a baby when placed below the level of uterus. This is beneficial to a mature baby but may be deleterious to a preterm or a low birth weight baby due to hypervolaemia. But early clamping should be done in cases of Rh incompatibility (to

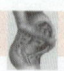

prevent antibody transfer from the mother to the baby) or babies born asphyxiated or one of a diabetic mother.

- **Quick check is made to** detect any gross abnormality and the baby is wrapped with a warm towel. The identification tape is tied on the wrist of both the baby and the mother. Once the management of the third stage is over (usually 10–20 minutes), baby is given to the mother or to the nurse.

The initial physical assessment includes a brief review of systems (Box 6.2)

1. **External:** Note skin color, staining or wasting (dysmaturity), note any birthmarks, note length of nails and creases on soles of feet, check for presence of breast tissue, assess nasal patency by covering one nostril at a time while observing respirations and color, amniotic fluid (staining may indicate fetal hypoxia, offensive odor may indicate intrauterine infection).

2. **Chest:** Palpate for point of maximal impulse (PMI) and auscultate for rate and quality of heart tones and murmurs, note character of respirations and presence of crackles or rhonchi, note equality of breath sounds on each side of chest by holding stethoscope in each axilla.

3. **Abdomen:** Verify presence of a rounded abdomen and absence of anomalies, note number of vessels in cord.

4. **Neurologic:** Check muscle tone and reflex reaction, assess Moro reflex, palpate anterior fontanelle for fullness or bulge, note by palpation the presence and size of the fontanelles and sutures.

5. **Other observations:** Note gross structural malformations obvious at birth.

The initial examination of the newborn can occur while the nurse is drying and wrapping the infant, or observations can be made while the infant is lying on the mother's abdomen or in her arms immediately after birth.

MANAGEMENT OF THE THIRD STAGE

The third stage is the most critical stage of labour: Previously uneventful first and second stages can become abnormal within a minute with disastrous consequences.

Third stage includes separation, descent and expulsion of the placenta with its membranes.

SIGNS

Pains

For a short time, the patient experiences no pain. However, intermittent discomfort in the lower abdomen reappears, corresponding with the uterine contractions.

Before separation

- *Per abdomen*: Uterus becomes discoid in shape, firm in feel and non-ballottable. Fundal height reaches slightly below the umbilicus.

Box 6.2 Initial physical assessments by body system

CNS	Moves extremities, muscle tone good symmetric features, movement, suck, rooting, Moro response, grasp reflexes good anterior fontanelle soft and flat.
CV	Heart rate strong and regular, no murmurs heard, pulses strong/equal bilaterally.
RESP	Lungs clear to auscultation bilaterally, no retractions or nasal flaring, respiratory rate, 30–60 breaths/min, chest expansion symmetric, no upper airway congestion.
GU	*Male:* urethral opening at tip of penis, testes descended bilaterally. *Female:* vaginal opening apparent
GI	Abdomen soft, no distention, cord attached and clamped, anus appears patent.
ENT	Eyes clear, palates intact, nares patent
Skin	Colour [ ] pink, acrocyanotic, no lesions or abrasions, no peeling, birthmarks, caput/molding, vacuum "cap", forceps marks, other.

- *Per vaginam*: There may be slight trickling of blood. Length of the umbilical cord, as visible from outside, remains static.

After separation

- *Per abdomen*: Uterus becomes globular, firm and ballottable. The fundal height is slightly raised as the separated placenta comes down in the lower segment and the contracted uterus rests on top of it. There may be slight bulging in the suprapubic region due to distension of the lower segment by the separated placenta.
- *Per vaginam*: There may be slight gush of vaginal bleeding. Permanent lengthening of the cord is established. This can be elicited by pushing down the fundus when a length of cord comes outside the vulva which remains permanent, even after the pressure is released.

Expulsion of placenta and membranes

The expulsion is achieved either by voluntary bearing down efforts or more commonly aided by manipulative procedure. The "afterbirth" delivery is soon followed by slight to moderate bleeding amounting to 100–250 ml.

Maternal signs

There may be chills and occasional shivering.

The principles underlying the management of third stage are to ensure strict vigilance and to follow the management guidelines strictly in practice so as to prevent the complications, the important one being postpartum haemorrhage.

Steps of management: Two methods of management are currently in practice.

1. Expectant management
2. Active management

Expectant management (traditional)

In this management, *the placental separation and its descent into the vagina are allowed to occur spontaneously.* Minimal assistance may be given for the placental expulsion if it needed.

- *Constant watch* is mandatory and the patient should not be left alone.
- *A hand is placed over the fundus*
  - *To recognize* the signs of separation of placenta
  - *To note* the state of uterine activity–contraction and relaxation
  - *To detect*, though rare, cupping of the fundus which is an early evidence of inversion of the uterus.

  Desire to fiddle with fundus or massage the uterus strongly to be condemned. The patient is expected to expel the placenta within 20 minutes with the aid of gravity.

- **Expulsion of the placenta:** *Only when the features of lower placental separation and its descent into the lower segment are confirmed,* the patient is asked to bear down simultaneously with the hardening of the uterus. The raised intra-abdominal pressure is often adequate to expel the placenta. If the patient fails to expel, one can wait safely up to 10 minutes if there is no bleeding. As soon as the placenta passes through the introitus, it is grasped by the hands and twisted round and round with gentle traction so that the membranes are stripped intact. If the membranes threaten to tear, they are caught hold of by sponge holding forceps and in similar twisting movements, the rest of the membranes are delivered. *Gentleness, patience and care are prerequisites for* complete delivery of the membranes.

Assisted expulsion

1. **Controlled cord traction (modified Brandt-Andrews method):** The palmar surface of the fingers of the left hand is placed above the symphysis pubis approximately at the junction of upper and lower uterine segment (Fig. 6.21). The body of the uterus is pushed upwards and backwards,

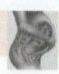

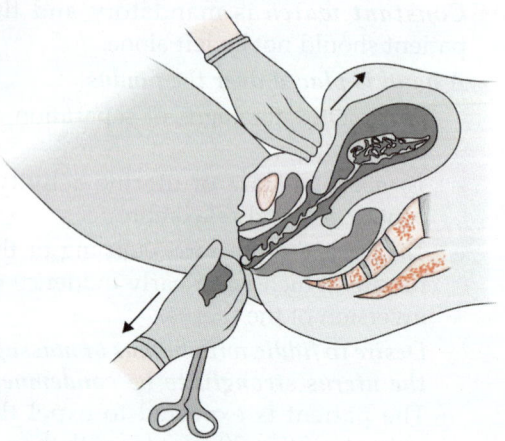

Fig. 6.21: Expulsion of the placenta by controlled cord traction

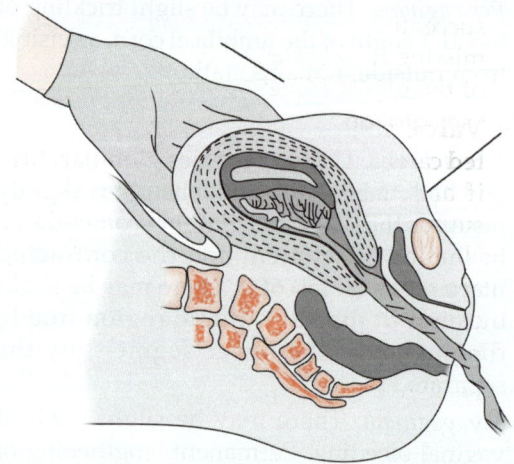

Fig. 6.22: Expression of the placenta by fundal pressure

towards the umbilicus while by the right hand, steady tension (but not too strong traction) is given in downward and backward direction holding the clamp until the placenta comes outside the introitus. The procedure is to be adopted only when the uterus is hard and contracted.

2. **Fundal pressure:** *The fundus is pushed downwards and backwards* after placing four fingers behind the fundus and the thumb in front using the uterus as a sort of piston. *The pressure must be given only when the uterus becomes hard.* If it is not, then make it hard by gentle rubbing. The pressure is to be withdrawn as soon as the placenta passes through the introitus. *If the baby is macerated or premature, this method is preferable to cord traction* as the tensile strength of the cord is much reduced in both the instances (Fig. 6.22).

The cord may be accidentally torn which is not likely to cause any problem. The sterile gloved hand should be introduced and the placenta is to be grasped and extracted.

- **The uterus is massaged** to make it hard, which facilitates expulsion of retained clots if any. Injection of oxytocin (5–10 units) IV

or methergin 0.2 mg is given intramuscularly. Oxytocin is more stable and has lesser side effects (nausea, vomiting, rise of BP) compared to ergometrine.

- **Examination of the placental membranes and cord:** The placenta is placed on a tray and is washed out in running tap water to remove the blood and clots. The maternal surface is first inspected for its completeness and anomalies. *The maternal surface* is covered with greyish decidua (spongy layer of the decidua basalis). Normally, the cotyledons are placed in close approximation and any gap indicates a missing cotyledon. *The membranes,* chorion and amnion, are to be examined carefully for completeness and presence of abnormal vessels indicative of succenturiate lobe. *The amnion is shiny but the chorion is shaggy.* The cut end of the cord is inspected for number of blood vessels. *Normally, there are two umbilical arteries and one umbilical vein. An oval gap in the chorion with torn ends of blood vessels running up to the margin of the gap indicates a missing succenturiate lobe.* The absence of a cotyledon or evidence of a missing

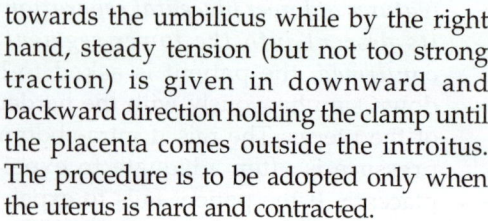

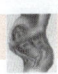

succenturiate lobe or evidence of significant missing membranes demands exploration of the uterus urgently.

- **Vulva, vagina and perineum are inspected** carefully for injuries and to be repaired, if any. The episiotomy wound is now sutured. The vulva and adjoining part are cleaned with cotton swabs soaked in antiseptic solution. A sterile pad is placed over the vulva.

- **Fourth stage,** pulse, blood pressure, behaviour of the uterus and any abnormal vaginal bleedings, is to be watched at least for 1 hour after delivery. When fully satisfied that the general condition is good, pulse and blood pressure are steady, the uterus is well contracted and there is no abnormal vaginal bleeding, the patient is sent to the ward.

Active management of third stage (Fig. 6.23)

The underlying principle in active management is to excite powerful uterine contractions following birth of the anterior shoulder by parenteral oxytocin which facilitates not only early separation of the placenta but also produces effective uterine contractions following its separation.

The advantages are

1. To minimize blood loss in third stage approximately to 1/5th and

2. To shorten the duration of third stage to half.

The only disadvantage is slight increased incidence of retained placenta (1–2%) and consequent increased incidence of manual removal. Of course, accidental administration during delivery of the first baby in undiagnosed twins produces grave danger to the unborn second baby caused by asphyxia due to tetanic contraction of the uterus. *Thus, it is imperative to limit its use in twins only during delivery of the second baby.*

Limitation: To be effective, it should be administered in proper time followed by slow delivery of the baby and followed by rapid delivery of the placenta. Thus, it may be an ideal procedure while conducting delivery.

PARTOGRAPH

Friedman first devised it: It is a composite graphical record of cervical dilatation and descent of head against duration of labour in hours OR

Partogram is a graphical record of cervical dilation in centimeters against duration of labour in hours. It also gives information about fetal and maternal conditions that are all recorded on a single sheet of paper.

The components of a partograph are:

a. Patient identification .

b Time–recorded at hourly interval. Zero time for spontaneous labour is the time of admission in the labour ward and for induced labour is the time of induction.

c. Fetal heart rate

d. State of membranes and colour of liquor: to mark 'I' for intact membranes, 'C' for clear and 'M' for meconium stained liquor

e. Cervical dilation and decent of the head

f. Uterine contractions

g. Drugs and fluids

h. Blood pressure

i. Oxytocin

j. Urine analysis

k. Vital signs record

Partogram: It is a sigmoid curve and the first stage of labour has got two phases a **latent phase** and an **active phase**. The active phase has got three components.

- Acceleration phase with cervical dilation of 2.5–4 cm

- Phase of maximum slope of 4–9 cm dilation

- Phase of deceleration of 9–10 cm dilation

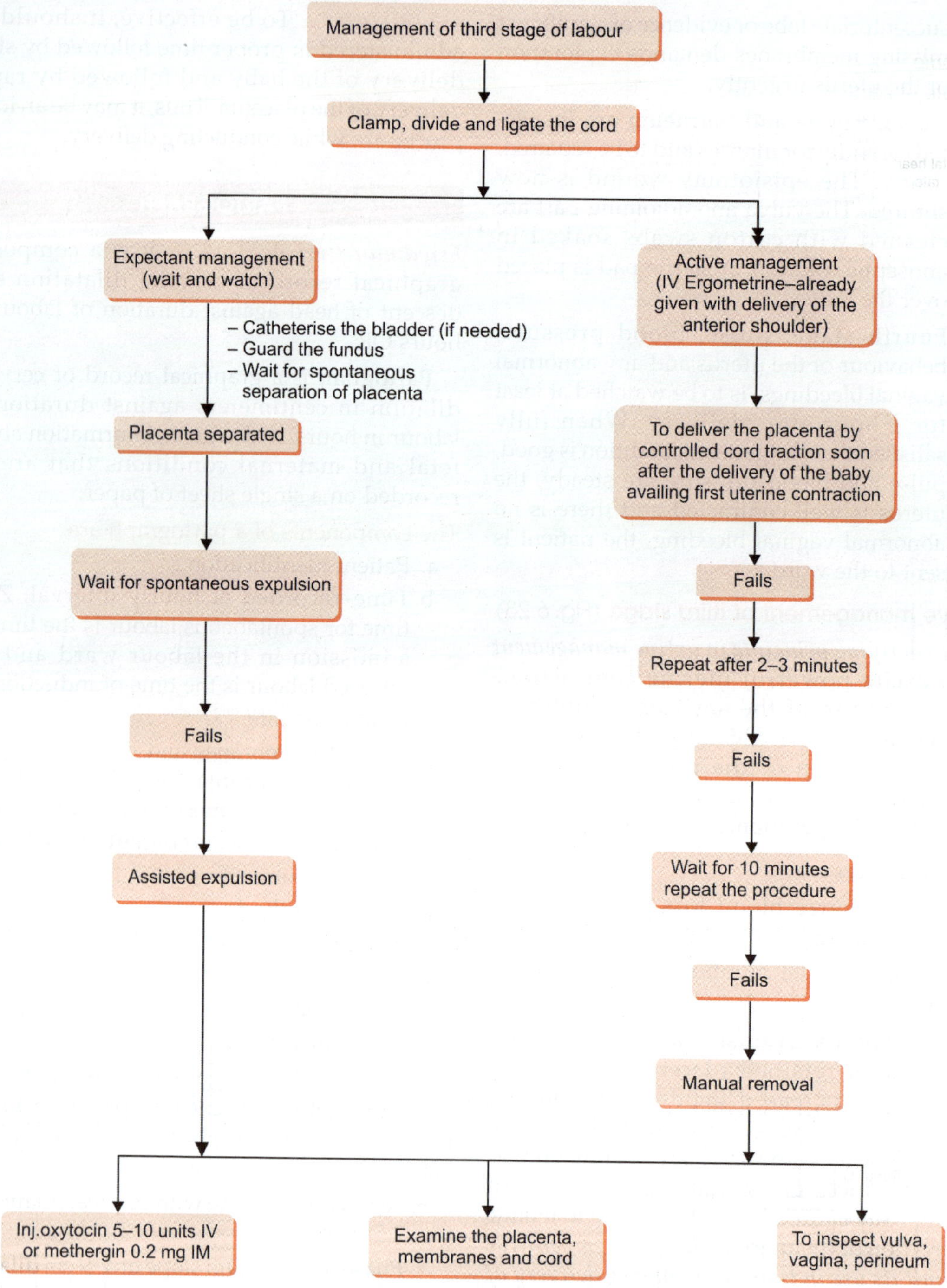

Management of third stage of labour

↓

Clamp, divide and ligate the cord

Expectant management (wait and watch)

Active management (IV Ergometrine–already given with delivery of the anterior shoulder)

– Catheterise the bladder (if needed)
– Guard the fundus
– Wait for spontaneous separation of placenta

Placenta separated

To deliver the placenta by controlled cord traction soon after the delivery of the baby availing first uterine contraction

Wait for spontaneous expulsion

Fails

Fails

Repeat after 2–3 minutes

Fails

Assisted expulsion

Wait for 10 minutes repeat the procedure

Fails

Manual removal

Inj.oxytocin 5–10 units IV or methergin 0.2 mg IM

Examine the placenta, membranes and cord

To inspect vulva, vagina, perineum

Fig. 6.23: Scheme of management of third stage

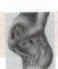

PARTOGRAPH

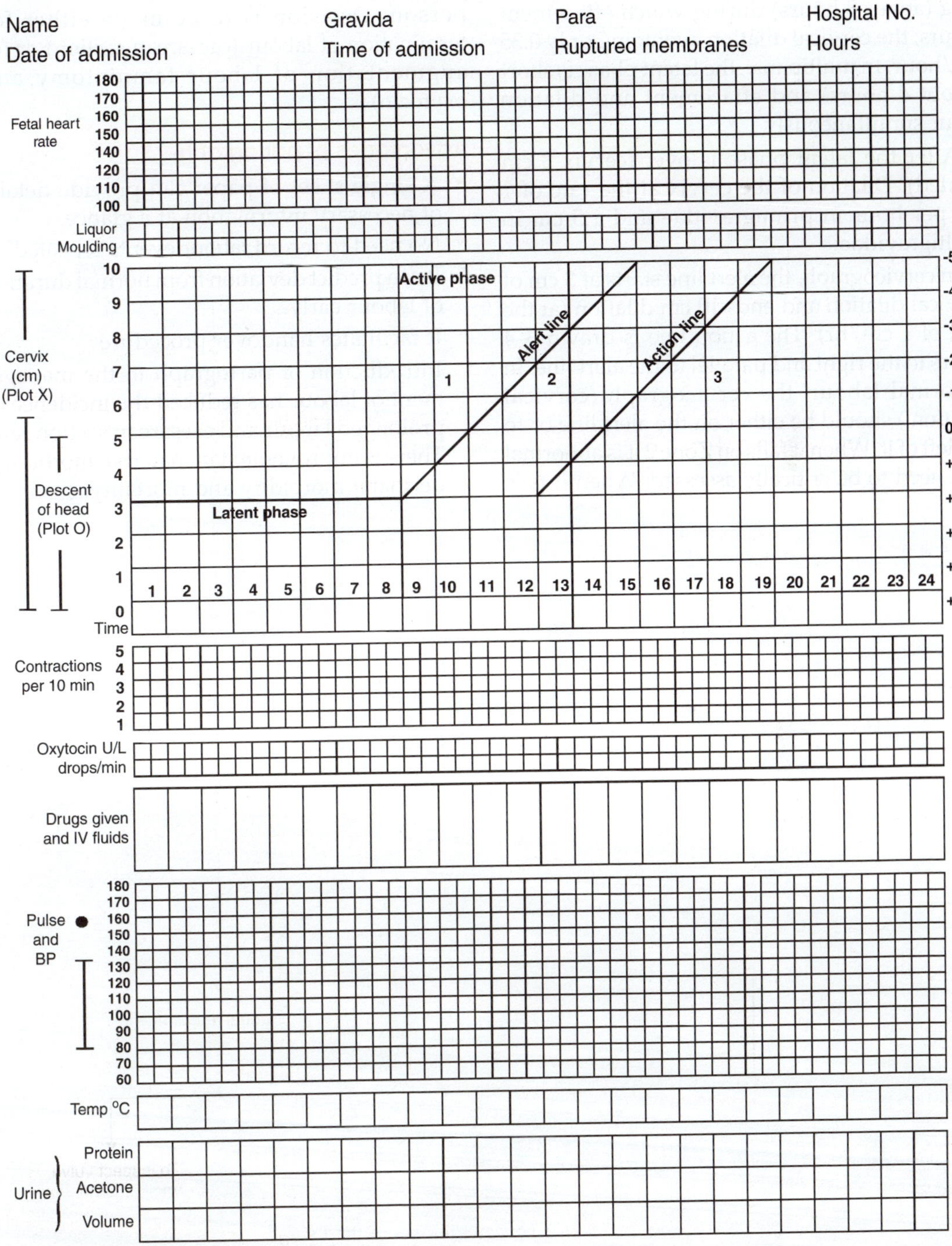

Name   Gravida   Para   Hospital No.

Date of admission   Time of admission   Ruptured membranes   Hours

Fetal heart rate: 180 170 160 150 140 120 110 100

Liquor / Moulding

Cervix (cm) (Plot X) 10 9 8 7 6 5 4 3 2 1 0

Active phase

Alert line

Action line

1   2   3

Latent phase

-5 -4 -3 -2 -1 0 +1 +2 +3 +4 +5

Descent of head (Plot O)

Time: 1 2 3 4 5 6 7 8 9 10 11 12 13 14 15 16 17 18 19 20 21 22 23 24

Contractions per 10 min 5 4 3 2 1

Oxytocin U/L drops/min

Drugs given and IV fluids

Pulse ● and BP 180 170 160 150 140 130 120 110 100 90 80 70 60

Temp °C

Urine { Protein / Acetone / Volume

(Adopted from WHO publication)

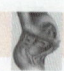

In primigravidae, the latent phase is often long (about 8 hours) during which effacement occurs; the cervical dilation averaging only 0.35 cm/hour. In multiparae, the latent phase is short (about 4 hours) and effacement and dilation occur simultaneously .

After the latent phase is over (cervix 3 cm dilated). Dilation of the cervix at the rate of 1 cm per hour in primigravidae and 1.5 cm in multigravidae.

In cervicograph, the alert line starts at 3 cm of cervical dilation and ends 10 cm dilation (at the rate of 1 cm/hr). The action line is drawn 3–4 hours to the right and parallel to the alert line. In a normal labour, the cervicograph (cervical dilation) should be either on the alert line or to the left of it. When it falls on Zone 2 it is abnormal and need to be critically assessed. When it falls on Zone 3 case should be reassessed by a senior person. Decision is to be made either for termination of labour (caesarean section) or for augmentation of labour (amniotomy and oxytocin).

Advantages of partograph

- A single sheet of paper can provide details of necessary information at a glance
- No need to record labour events repeatedly.
- It can predict deviation from normal duration of labour early.
- It facilitates handover procedure
- Introduction of partograph in the management of labour has reduced the incidence of prolonged labour and caesarean section rate. There is improvement in maternal morbidity, perinatal morbidity and mortality.

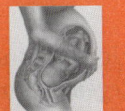

7

Normal Puerperium

OUTLINE

- Involution of the uterus
- Involution of other pelvic structures
- Lochia
- General physiological changes
- Lactation
- Management of normal puerperium
- Postpartum exercise

The puerperium is the period during which the maternal organs, particularly the reproductive organs return to the non-pregnant or near normal state with the exception of the lactating breast which remain active throughout this period.

Definition

Puerperium is the period following childbirth during which the body tissues, especially the pelvic organs revert back approximately to the pre-pregnant state both anatomically and physiologically. Involution is the process whereby the genital organs revert back approximately to the state as they were before pregnancy.

Duration

Puerperium begins as soon as the placenta is expelled and *lasts for approximately 6 weeks.* The period is arbitrarily divided into:
1. Immediate—within 24 hours
2. Early—up to 7 days
3. Remote—up to 6 weeks

INVOLUTION OF THE UTERUS

ANATOMICAL CONSIDERATION

Uterus

Immediately following delivery, the uterus becomes firm and retracted with alternate hardening and softening. The uterus measures about 20 × 12 × 7.5 cm (length, breadth and thickness) and weighs about 1000 gm. At the end of 6 weeks, its measurement is almost similar to that of the non-pregnant state and weighs about 60 gm (Fig. 7.1).

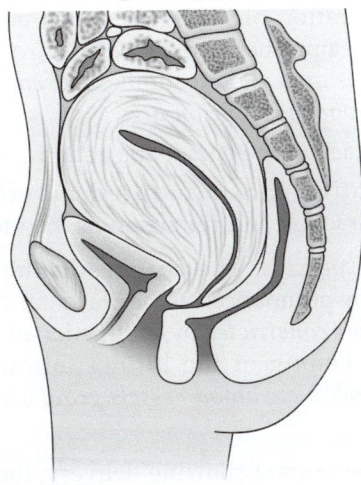

Fig. 7.1: Sagittal section showing uterus five days after delivery

Lower uterine segment

Immediately following delivery, the lower segment becomes a thin, flabby, collapsed structure.

Cervix

The cervix contracts slowly; the external os admits two fingers for a few days but by the end of first week, narrows down to admit the tip of a finger only. The external os never reverts back to the nulliparous state.

Physiological consideration

Changes occur in the following components:

1. Muscles
2. Blood vessels
3. Endometrium

Muscles

During puerperium, the number of muscle fibres is not decreased but there is substantial reduction of the myometrial cell size. Withdrawal of the steroid hormones, oestrogen and progesterone, may lead to increase in the activity of the uterine collagenase and the release of proteolytic enzyme. Autolysis of the protoplasm occurs by the proteolytic enzyme with liberation of peptones which enter the blood stream. These are excreted through the kidneys as urea and creatinine. *The conditions which favour involution are:*

1. Efficacy of the enzymatic action
2. Relative anoxia induced by effective contraction and retraction of the uterus.

Blood vessels: The changes of the blood vessels are pronounced at the placental site. *The arteries are constricted* by contraction of its wall and thickening of the intima followed by thrombosis. *New blood vessels grow* inside the thrombi.

Endometrium: Following delivery, the major part of the decidua is cast off with the expulsion of the placenta and the membranes, more at the placental site. The endometrium left behind varies in thickness from 2–5 mm. *Regeneration occurs from the epithelium of the uterine gland mouths and interglandular stromal cells.* Regeneration of the epithelium is completed by 10th day and the entire endometrium is restored during the 3rd week except at the placental site where it takes about 6 weeks.

Clinical assessment of involution

The rate of involution of the uterus can be *assessed clinically by noting the height of the fundus of the uterus in relation to the symphysis pubis.* The measurement should be taken carefully at a fixed time everyday, preferably by the same observer. *Bladder must be emptied beforehand* and preferably the bowel too, as the full bladder and the loaded bowel may raise the level of the fundus of the uterus. *The uterus is to be centralised* and with a measuring tape, the fundal height is measured above the symphysis pubis. Following delivery, the fundus lies about 13.5 cm (5 ½") above the symphysis pubis. During the first 24 hours, the level remains constant; thereafter there is a steady decrease in height by 1.25 cm (½") in 24 hours, *so that by the end of second week, the uterus becomes a pelvic organ.* The rate of involution thereafter slows down until 6 weeks, the uterus becomes almost normal in size.

The involution may be affected adversely and is called subinvolution. Sometimes, the involution may be prolonged in women who are lactating so that the uterus may be smaller in size, superinvolution. The uterus, however, returns to normal size if the lactation is withheld.

INVOLUTION OF OTHER PELVIC STRUCTURES

VAGINA

The distensible vagina, noticed soon afterbirth, takes a long time (4–8 weeks) to involute. It

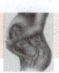

regains its tone but never to the virginal state. The mucosa remains delicate for the first few weeks and submucous venous congestion persists even longer. It is the reason to withhold surgery on puerperal vagina. Rugae partially reappear at third week but never to the same degree as in pre-pregnant state. The introitus remains permanently larger than the virginal state. Hymen is lacerated and is represented by nodular tags, the carunculae myrtiformes.

Broad ligaments and round ligaments require considerable time to recover from the stretching and laxation.

Pelvic floor and pelvic fascia take a long time to involute from the stretching effect during parturition.

LOCHIA

It is the vaginal discharge for the first fortnight during puerperium. The discharge originates from the uterine body, cervix and vagina.

Odour and reaction

It has got a peculiar offensive fishy smell. Its reaction is alkaline tending to become acid towards the end.

Colour

Depending upon the variation of the colour of the discharge, it is named as:

1. **Lochia rubra** (red) 1–4 days.
2. **Lochia serosa** yellowish or pink or pale brownish 5–9 days.
3. **Lochia alba** (pale white) 10–15 days.

Composition

Lochia rubra consists of blood, sheds of fetal membranes and decidua, vernix caseosa, lanugo and meconium.

Lochia serosa consists of less RBC but more leukocytes, wound exudate, mucus from the cervix and microorganisms (anaerobic Streptococci and Staphylococci). *The presence of bacteria is not pathognomonic unless associated with clinical signs of sepsis.*

Lochia alba contains plenty of decidual cells, leucocytes, mucus, cholestrin crystals, fatty and granular epithelial cells and microorganisms.

Amount

The average amount of discharge, for the first 5–6 days, is estimated to be 250 ml.

If a mother has excessive lochia, a clean pad should be applied and checked within 15 minutes. The number of perineal pads applied during a given period should be counted, or the pads weighed to help determine the amount of vaginal discharge. One gram of weight equals 1 ml of blood. In addition, the woman's fundus should be checked for firmness. Nurses often estimate the amount of lochia in the following terms, which are commonly described with the approximate size of the area soiled in 1 hour.

- **Scant:** Less than a 1-inch stain on a perineal pad
- **Small (slight):** Smaller than a 4-inch stain
- Moderate: Smaller than a 6-inch stain
- **Heavy (large):** Larger than a 6-inch stain
- **Excessive:** Pad saturation within 15 minutes.

Normal duration

The normal duration may extend upto 3 weeks. The red lochia may persist for longer duration specially in women who get up from the bed for the first time in later period. The discharge may be scanty, specially following premature labour and cesarean birth or may be excessive in twin delivery or hydramnios.

Clinical importance

The character of the lochial discharge gives useful information about the abnormal puerperal state. *The vulval pads are to be inspected daily to get information.*

- **Odour:** If offensive, indicates infection. *Retained plug or cotton piece inside the vagina should be kept in mind.*
- **Amount:** Scanty or absent, signifies infection or lochiometra. If excessive, indicates infection.

 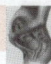

- **Colour:** Persistence of red colour beyond the normal limit signifies subinvolution or retained bits of conceptus.
- **Duration:** Duration of the lochia alba beyond 3 weeks suggests local genital lesion.

GENERAL PHYSIOLOGICAL CHANGES

Pulse

For a few hours after normal delivery, the pulse rate is likely to be raised, which settles down to normal during the second day. In some, it may be abnormally slowed down and persists for 1–2 days may be due to rest, diminished food intake and excessive fluid excretion.

Temperature

The temperature should not be above 37.2°C (99°F) within the first 24 hours. There may be slight reactionary rise following delivery by 0.5°F but comes down to normal within 12 hours. On the 3rd day, there may be slight rise of temperature due to breast engorgement which should not last for more than 24 hours. *However, genitourinary tract infection should be excluded if there is rise of temperature.*

Urinary tract

The bladder wall becomes oedematous and hyperaemic and often shows evidences of submucous extravasation of blood. Intravesical pressure due to trauma the bladder may be over distended without any desire to pass urine. *Stagnation of the urine along with a devitalised bladder wall contribute to the urinary tract infection in puerperium.* Dilated ureters and renal pelvis return to normal size within 8 weeks.

Gastrointestinal tract

Increased thirst in early puerperium is due to loss of fluid during labour, in the lochia, diuresis and perspiration. *Slight intestinal paresis* leads to constipation. Lack of tone of the perineal and abdominal muscles and reflex pain in the perineal region are also contributing factors for constipation.

Weight loss

In addition to the weight loss as a consequence of the expulsion of the uterine contents, a further loss of about 2 kg (5 lb) occurs during puerperium chiefly caused by diuresis.

Fluid loss

There is a net fluid loss of at least 2 litres during the first week and an additional 1.5 litres during the next 5 weeks.

Blood values

Immediately following delivery, there is slight *decrease of blood volume* due to dehydration and blood loss. The blood volume returns to the non-pregnant level by the second week. *Cardiac output* rises soon after delivery.

RBC volume and haematocrit values return to normal by the end of first week. *Leuco-cytosis* to the extent of 30,000 per cu.mm occurs following delivery probably in response to stress of labour. *Platelet count* decreases soon after the separation of the placenta but secondary elevation occurs, with increase in platelet adhesiveness between 4–10 days. *Fibrinogen level* remains high up to the second week of puerperium, resulting in persistent high level of ESR in puerperium as during pregnancy. A hypercoagulable state persists and fibrinolytic activity is enhanced.

Menstruation and ovulation (Fig. 7.2)

The onset of the first menstrual period following delivery is very variable and depends more than anything on lactation. *If the patient does not breastfeed her baby,* the menstruation returns by 6th week following delivery in about 40% and by 12th week in 80% of cases. *If the patient breastfeeds her baby,* the menstruation may be suspended in about 70% until the baby stops breastfeeding. However, menses may start even

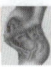

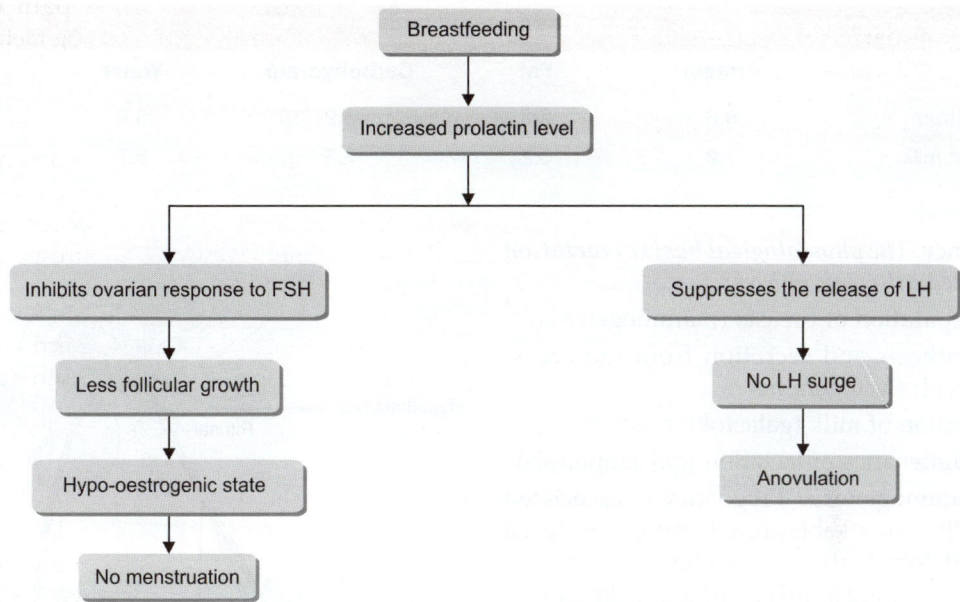

Increased frequency and duration of suckling is associated with high prolactin level, prolonged ovarian suppression and lactational amenorrhoea

Fig. 7.2: Scheme of mechanism of amenorrhoea and anovulation in lactating mothers

before cessation of breastfeeding in the remaining 30%.

In non-lactating mothers, ovulation may occur as early as 4 weeks and in lactating mothers, about 10 weeks after delivery. Thus, lactation provides a natural method of contraception and contributes to spacing of pregnancies. *However, ovulation may precede the first menstrual period in about one-third and it is possible for the patient to become pregnant before she menstruates following her confinement.*

LACTATION

For the first two days following delivery, no further anatomic changes in the breasts occur. The secretion from the breasts, called colostrum which starts during pregnancy, becomes more abundant during the period.

Composition of the colostrum

It is deep yellow serous fluid, alkaline in reaction. It has got a higher specific gravity; a high protein, vitamin A, sodium and chloride content but has got lower carbohydrate, fat and potassium than the breast milk. It contains antibody (IgA) produced locally (Table 7.1).

Microscopically: It contains fat globules, colostrum corpuscles and acinar epithelial cells.

Advantages

1. The antibodies (IgA, IgG, IgM) and humoral factors (lactoferrin) provides immunological defence to the new born.
2. It has laxative action on the baby because of *large fat* globules.

PHYSIOLOGY OF LACTATION

Although lactation starts following delivery, the preparation for effective lactation starts during

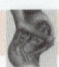

Table 7.1: Percentage composition of colostrum and breast milk

	Protein	Fat	Carbohydrate	Water
Colostrum	8.6	2.3	3.2	8.6
Breast milk	1.2	3.2	7.5	8.7

pregnancy. *The physiological basis of lactation is divided into four phases:*

1. Preparation of breasts (mammogenesis)
2. Synthesis and secretion from the breast alveoli (lactogenesis)
3. Ejection of milk (galactokinesis)
4. Maintenance of lactation (galactopoiesis)

- **Mammogenesis:** Pregnancy is associated with a remarkable growth of both the ductal and lobuloalveolar systems. *An intact nerve supply is not essential for the growth of the mammary glands during pregnancy.*

- **Lactogenesis:** Though some secretory activity is evident (colostrum) during pregnancy and accelerated following delivery, *milk secretion actually starts on 3rd or 4th postpartum day.* Around this time, the breasts become engorged, tense, tender and feel warm. Inspite of a high prolactin level during pregnancy, milk secretion is kept in abeyance. Probably, the steroids, oestrogen and progesterone circulating during pregnancy, make the breast tissues unresponsive to prolactin. The secretory activity is enhanced directly or indirectly by growth hormone, thyroxine, glucocorticoids and insulin.

- **Galactokinesis:** Discharge of milk from the mammary glands depends not only on the suction exerted by the baby during suckling but also on the contractile mechanism which expresses the milk from the alveoli into the ducts.

During suckling, a conditioned reflex is set up (Fig.7.3). The ascending impulses from the nipple pass to the supraoptic nucleus and

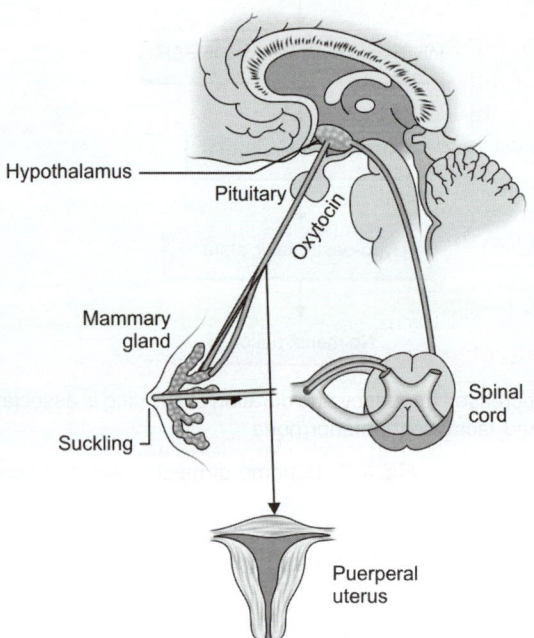

Fig. 7.3: Lactation reflex

then along the hypothalamo-pituitary axis to the posterior pituitary. Oxytocin is liberated from the posterior pituitary which, in addition to its oxytocic effect, produces contraction of the myoepithelial cells of the alveoli and the ducts containing the milk. This is the **milk ejection** or **milk let down** reflex whereby the milk is forced down into the ampulla of the lactiferous ducts, wherefrom it can be expressed by the mother or sucked out by the baby.

The milk ejection reflex is inhibited by factors such as pain, breast engorgement or adverse psychic condition.

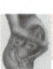

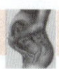

- **Galactopoiesis:** Prolactin appears to be the single most important galactopoietic hormone. *For maintenance of effective and continuous lactation, suckling is essential.* It is not only essential for the removal of milk from the glands, but it also causes the release of prolactin.

Milk production

In the first postpartum week, the total amount of milk yield in 24 hours is calculated to be 60 multiplied by the number of postpartum days and is expressed in terms of millilitres. Thus, the milk yield on 4th day is about $60 \times 4 = 240$ ml. A milk yield of 120–180 ml per feeding is usual by the end of second week.

Stimulation of lactation

The following are the methods that can be adopted with advantages to improve adequate milk yield:

- **During pregnancy**
  - To improve the maternal instinct to nurse the baby mentioning the advantages of breastfeeding.
  - Care and preparation of the nipple including teaching the patient as to how to express out the colostrum and to take care of the crust formed on the nipples.
- **Following delivery**
  - To put the baby to the breast immediately interval for 3 minutes from the first day, if the condition permits/demands feeding.
  - Plenty of fluids to drink.
  - To avoid engorgement and trapping of milk, manual expression prior to nursing is done.

Suppression of lactation

This becomes necessary if the baby is born dead or dies in the neonatal period or when the patient does not like to breastfeed her baby or if breastfeeding is contraindicated. This can be effective, either by using hormones or by mechanical means.

- **Drugs:** Combination of testosterone and oestrogen preparation (Mixogen)—2 ampoules intramuscularly. *The risk of using oestrogenic preparations* in puerperium includes thromboembolic manifestation or late postpartum blood loss.
- **Mechanical:** This is an effective procedure in cases *where the lactation is—to be suppressed after the establishment of milk secretion.*
  - The patient should stop breastfeeding.
  - She should not express or pump out the milk from the breast.
  - A tight compression bandage is applied for about 2–3 days.
  - Analgesic tablet containing aspirin and codeine preparation may be given to relieve pain.

MANAGEMENT OF NORMAL PUERPERIUM

The underlying principles in management are

1. *To give all out attention* to restore the health status of the mother
2. *To prevent infection*
3. *To take care of the breasts,* including promotion of lactation and nursing of the child
4. *To motivate the mother* for contraceptive acceptance.

Immediate attention

Immediately following delivery, the patient should be closely observed. She may be given a drink to her likings or something to eat, if she is hungry. If the patient is exhausted and tired, a sedative like diazepam 10 mg intramuscularly may be given to ensure good sleep.

Rest and ambulance

Reasonable period of 8–12 hours rest is enough for most of the patients. After a good resting period, the patient becomes fresh and can breastfeed the baby or moves out of bed to go to the toilet. **Now-a-days, early ambulation is favoured.**

Advantages of early ambulation

1. Provides a sense of well-being; bladder complications and constipation are reduced.
2. Facilitates uterine drainage and hastens involution of the uterus.
3. Lessens puerperal venous thrombosis and embolic phenomenon. *However, early ambulation does not mean return to normal activities which should be restricted for at least 6 weeks.* During this period, she should take as much rest as possible and avoid strenuous work especially, lifting, straining and pushing. The patient is to spend some of the resting time in prone position to promote anteversion of the uterus. The patient is advised to take at least 2 hours of rest after her midday meal.

Hospital stay

Early discharge from the hospital is an almost universal procedure. If adequate coverage of supervision by the health visitors is provided, there is no harm in early discharge.

Diet

The patient should be on a light diet on the first day and normal diet may be resumed from the 2nd day. *If the patient is lactating,* high calories, adequate protein, fat, plenty of fluids, minerals and vitamins are to be given. However, in non-lactating mothers, a non-pregnant diet is enough.

Care of the bladder

The patient is encouraged to pass urine 6–8 hours following delivery and thereafter at 4–6 hours interval. At times, *the patient fails to pass urine and the causes are*

1. Lack of privacy
2. Unaccustomed position
3. Reflex from the perineal injuries

Table 7.2: Nursing diagnosis applicable to post-partum period

- Pain related to afterpains of the contracting uterus and episiotomy repair.
- Risk for fluid volume deficit, related to fluid loss secondary to uterine atony.
- Risk for Infection, related to childbirth trauma to tissues
- Urinary retention related to urinary meatus edema and trauma.
- Sleep pattern disturbance related to discomforts of childbirth.
- Knowledge deficit related to insufficient understanding about postpartum changes.
- Anxiety related to assuming parental role.
- Breastfeeding, ineffective, related to inexperience and lack of knowledge.
- Knowledge deficit related to lack of experience in infant care.

Maintaining privacy or alteration in the position or allowing the patient to use the toilet, if not contraindicated, usually serves the purpose. *If the patient still fails to pass urine, catheterisation should be done and kept for 24 hours.*

Care of the bowel

The problem of constipation is much less because of early ambulant and liberalisation of the dietary intake. A diet containing sufficient roughage and fluids is enough to move the bowel. If necessary, mild laxative such as milk of magnesia 4–6 teaspoons may be given at bed time.

Sleep

The patient is in need of rest, both physical and mental. So she should be protected against worries and undue fatigue. This is because of hypersensitive state of the nervous system. Sleep may be ensured by giving diazepam, orally at bed time. If there is some discomfort, such as after pains or painful piles or engorged breasts, they should be dealt with adequate

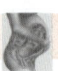

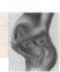

analgesics, e.g. aspirin (0.6 gm) with codeine (30–60 mg) orally 4–6 hourly as necessary.

Care of the vulva and episiotomy wound

Shortly after delivery, the vulva and buttocks are washed with soap water down over the anus and a sterile pad is applied. The perineal wound should be dressed with antiseptic powder after each act of micturition and defaecation or at least twice a day.

The state of healing is assessed by observing for redness, edema, ecchymosis (bruising), discharge and approximation of the wound (REEDA scale). Foul odour accompanied by drainage indicates infection; therefore further examination of the incision and area of warmth and tenderness should be made.

Care of the breasts

The nipples should be washed with sterile water before each feeding. It should be cleaned, dried and kept covered by clean linen after the feeding is over. A nursing brassiere provides comfortable support. They should be softened by a compress of sterile olive oil for 24 hours and then washed with soap and water.

Rooming-in or bedding-in

There is no need for a mother and her baby to lie separately after a normal delivery. The baby should be kept in her bed or in a cot besides her bed. This not only establishes the mother-child relationship but also the mother is conversant with the art of baby care so that she can take full care of the baby while at home.

Asepsis and antiseptics

Asepsis must be maintained especially during the first week of puerperium. The uterus provides an ideal environment for the growth of the organisms. The gaping vaginal introitus

---

Table 7.3: Self perineal care

- Explain procedure to woman
- Gather supplies needed
- Assist the woman to bathroom
- Wash hands before and after each perineal care.
- Remove soiled pad from front to back: discard in waste container
- Squeeze peri bottle or pour warm water or cleansing solution over perineum without opening labia.
- Pat dry. Use each cotton one time, pat from front to back then discard cotton.
- Apply medicated ointment, or pad, as directed. Do not apply perineal pad for 1 to 2 minutes. (otherwise, medication will be absorbed in pad)
- Apply clean perineal pad from front to back, touching only sides and outside of pad.
- Do not flush toilet until she is standing upright; otherwise the flushing water can spray perineum.
- Always do perineal care after each voiding, stool or atleast every 4 hours during puerperium.
- Report clots, increase in flow, or excessive cramping.

Box 7.1: Conditions that make women at high-risk for postpartal infection

1. Rupture of the membranes over 24 hours before delivery (bacteria may have started to invade the uterus while the fetus was still in utero)
2. Placental fragments that have been retained within the uterus (the tissue necroses and serves as an excellent bed for bacterial growth)
3. Postpartal haemorrhage (the woman's general condition is weakened)
4. Pre-existing anaemia (the body's defense against infection is lowered)
5. Prolonged and difficult labour, particularly instrument deliveries (trauma to the tissue may leave lacerations of fissures or easy portals of entry for infection)
6. Internal fetal heart monitoring (contamination may have been introduced with the placement of the scalp electrode)
7. Local vaginal infection was present at the time of delivery (direct spread of infection occurred)
8. The uterus was explored following delivery for a retained placenta or abnormal bleeding site (infection was introduced with exploration).

facilitates entry of organisms. The general resistance is also lowered following childbirth process. Liberal use of local antiseptics, aseptic measures during perineal wound dressing, use of clean bed linen and clothing are positive steps. To keep the room dust free and restriction of visitors to a minimum, especially those who have got septic foci, could be of help in reducing exogenous infection.

Immunisation

1. Administration of anti-D-gamma globulin to unimmunised Rh-negative mother bearing Rh-positive baby.
2. Women who are susceptible to rubella can be vaccinated safely with live attenuated rubella virus.
3. The booster dose of tetanus toxoid should be given at the time of discharge/if it is not given during pregnancy.

Table 7.4: Postpartal discharge instructions	
Implementation	**Rationale**
Work	All woman should avoid heavy work (lifting or straining) for at least the first 3 weeks following birth. It is usually advised that she doesn't return to an outside job for at least 3 weeks (better 6 weeks) not only for her own health but also for enjoyment of the early weeks with her newborn.
Rest	The woman should plan at least one rest period a day and try to get a good night's sleep. She can rest during the day when her newborn is sleeping unless she has other children or an aged parent to care for.
Exercise	The woman should limit the number of stairs she climbs to 1 flight/day for the 1st week at home. Beginning the 2nd week, if her lochial discharge is normal, she may start to expand this activity. She should continue with muscle strengthening exercises such as sit ups and leg raising.
Hygiene	The woman may take either tub baths or showers. She should continue to apply any cream or ointment ordered for the perineal area and remember to continue to cleanse her perineum from front to back. Any perineal stitches will be absorbed within 10 days.
Coitus	Coitus is safe as soon as the woman's lochia has turned to alba and if she has an episiotomy, it is healed (about the 3rd week after delivery). Vaginal cells may not be as thick as formerly because prepregnancy hormone balance has not yet completely returned. Use of a contraceptive foam of lubricating jelly will aid comfort.
Contraception	The woman should begin a contraception measure with the initiation of coitus (if she desires contraception). If she wishes an IUD, this may be fitted immediately following delivery or at her 1st postpartal check-up. Oral contraceptives are begun about 2–3 weeks after delivery. Until she returns for this check-up, she can use an over-the-counter spermicidal jelly and her sexual partner, a condom to provide a high level of protection.
Follow-up	The woman should notify her physician or nurse-midwife if she notices an increase, not a decrease, in lochial discharge or if lochia serosa or lochia alba becomes lochia rubra. Delayed postpartal haemorrhage can occur in women who become extremely fatigued. Getting adequate rest during her first week at home will do much to prevent the possibility of this complication. Four to six weeks after birth the woman should return to her physician or nurse-midwife for an examination.

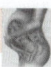

MANAGEMENT OF AILMENTS

- **After pain:** *It is the infrequent, spasmodic pain felt in the lower abdomen after delivery* for a variable period of 2–4 days. Presence of blood clots or bits of the after births lead to spasmodic hypertonic contractions of the uterus in an attempt to expel them out. This is commonly met in primiparae. The pain may also be due to ischaemia caused by vigorous uterine contraction especially in multiparae. The treatment includes massaging the uterus with expulsion of the clot followed by administration of tablet ergometrine 1 mg or intramuscular injection of 0.5 mg in the atonic variety. In the ischaemic type, analgesics and antispasmodics are helpful.
- **Pain on the perineum:** *Never, forget to examine the perineum when analgesic is to be administered to relieve pain.* Early detection of vulvovaginal haematoma can thus be made.
- **Correction of anaemia:** Majority of the women in the tropics remain in an anaemic state following delivery. Supplementary iron therapy (ferrous sulphate 200 mg), is to be given daily for a minimum period of 4–6 weeks.

POSTPARTUM EXERCISE

Abdominal breathing: Lie on back with knees bent. Inhale deeply through nose. Keep ribs stationary and allow abdomen to expand upward. Exhale slowly but forcefully while contracting the abdominal muscles; hold for 3–5 seconds while exhaling and relax.

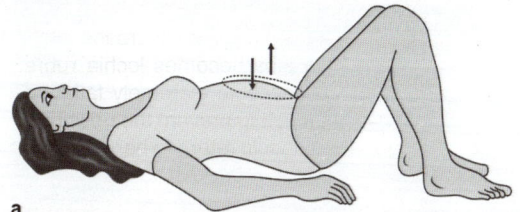

a

Reach for the knees: Lie on back with knees bent. While inhaling, deeply lower chin onto chest. While exhaling, raise head and shoulders slowly and smoothly and reach for knees with arms outstretched. The body should only rise as far as the back will naturally bend while waist remains on floor or bed. Slowly and smoothly lower head and shoulders back to starting position and relax.

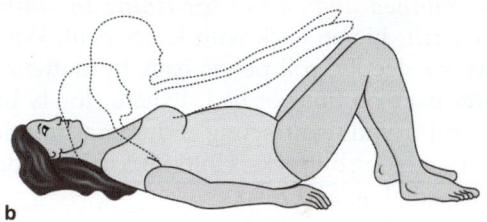

b

Double knee roll: Lie on back with knees bent. Keeping shoulders flat and feet stationary, slowly and smoothly roll knees over to the left to touch floor or bed. Maintaining a smooth motion, roll knees back over to the right until they touch floor or bed. Return to starting position and relax.

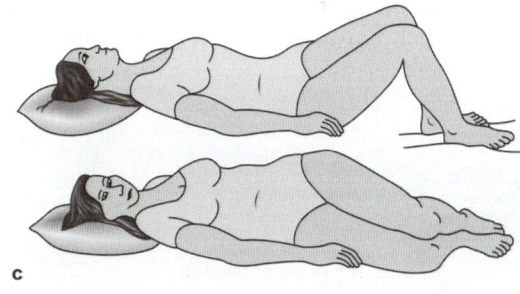

c

Leg roll: Lie on back with legs straight. Keeping shoulders flat and legs straight, slowly and smoothly lift left leg and roll it over to touch the right side of floor or bed and return to starting position. Repeat, rolling right leg over to touch left side of floor or bed and relax.

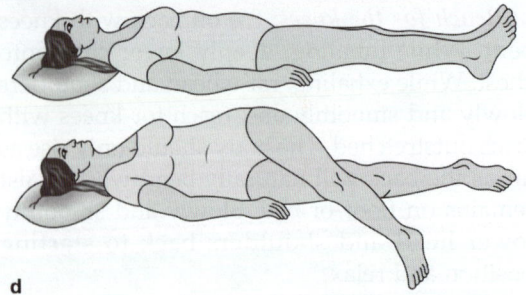

d

Combined abdominal breathing in supine pelvic tilt: Lie on back with knees bent. While inhaling deeply, roll pelvis back by flattening lower back on floor or bed. Exhale slowly but forcefully while contracting abdominal muscles and tightening buttocks. Hold for 3 to 5 seconds while exhaling and relax.

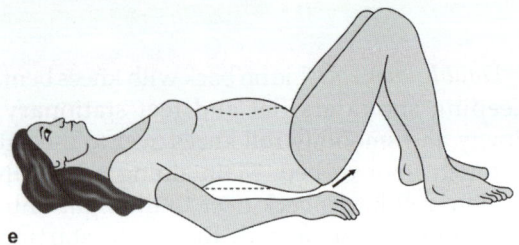

e

Buttocks lift: Lie on back with arms at sides, knees bent and feet flat. Slowly raise buttocks and arch back. Return slowly to starting position.

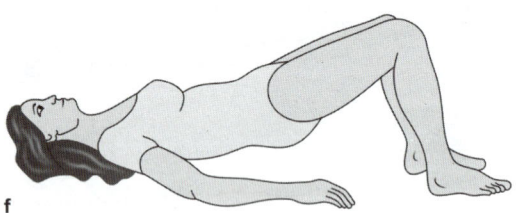

f

Single knee roll: Lie on back with right leg straight and left leg bent at the knee. Keeping shoulders flat, slowly and smoothly roll left knee over to the right to touch floor or bed and then back to starting position. Reverse position of legs. Roll right knee over to the left to touch or floor or bed and return to starting position. Relax.

Arm raises: Lie on back with arms extended at 90° angle from body. Raise arms so they are perpendicular and hands touch lower slowly.

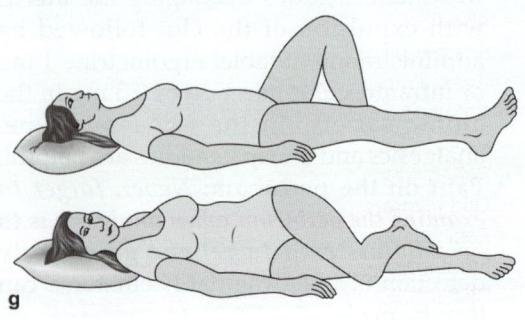

g

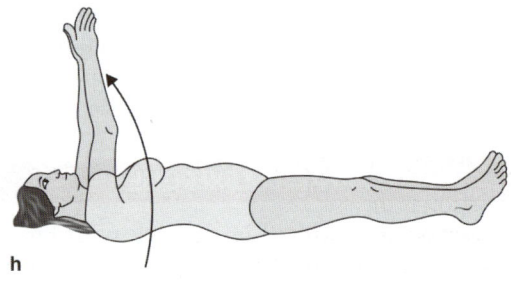

h

Figs 7.4a to h: Postpartum exercise should begin as soon as possible. Woman should start with simple exercises and gradually progress to more strenuous ones

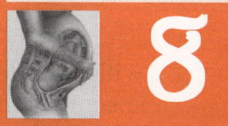

8

Obstetric Disorders in Pregnancy

OUTLINE

- Abortion
- Ectopic pregnancy
- Gestational trophoblastic diseases
- Antepartum haemorrhage
- Multiple pregnancy
- Polyhydramnios
- Oligohydramnios
- Post maturity
- Intrauterine fetal death
- Stillbirth
- Abnormalities of placenta and cord

ABORTION

SPONTANEOUS ABORTION (MISCARRIAGE)

Definition

Abortion is the termination of pregnancy before the period of viability which is considered to occur at 20th week.

CLASSIFICATION OF VARIETIES (Fig. 8.1)

Etiology

The etiology of abortion is often complex and obscure. The causes of abortion are usually divided into:

- Ovular or fetal
- Maternal environment
- Paternal factor
- Unknown

OVO-FETAL FACTORS

1. The ovo-fetal factors usually operate in fetal wastage. Meticulous histological and cytogenic study of the abortus reveals gross defects in the ovum or the fetus. The defects include chromosomal abnormality (commonest one being autosomal trisomy, monosomy), gross congenital malformation, blighted ovum (ovum without embryo) and hydropic degeneration of the villi. In early weeks, death or disease of the fetus often proceeds the expulsive action of the uterus.

2. Interference with the circulation in the umbilical cord by knots, twists or entanglements may cause death of the fetus and its expulsion.

3. Low attachment of the placenta or faulty placental formation (circumvallate) may interfere with placental circulation.

4. Twins or hydramnios (acute) by rapidly stretching the myometrium may cause abortion.

MATERNAL FACTORS (15%)

Maternal factors usually operate in late abortion leading sometimes to expulsion of a living foetus which, of course, is too small to survive.

a. *Maternal illness*
   1. *Infection:* Viral infection specially of rubella and cytomegalic inclusion disease produces congenital malformation and abortion if contracted in

139

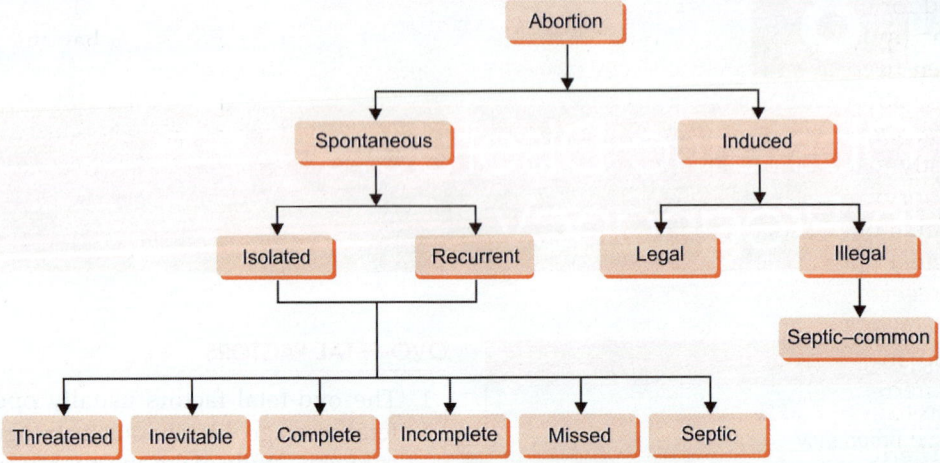

Fig. 8.1: Classification of varieties

early weeks of pregnancy. The viruses of hepatitis, parvovirus, influenza have got lethal action on the fetus causing its death and expulsion. Parasitic (malaria) and protozoal infection (toxoplasmosis) may produce abortion if contracted in early pregnancy. Spriochaetes hardly produce abortion before 20th week because of effective thickness of the placental barrier. Hyperpyrexia may precipitate abortion by increasing uterine irritability.

2. *Maternal hypoxia and shock:* Acute or chronic respiratory disease, heart failure, severe anaemia or anaesthetic complications may produce anoxic state which may precipitate abortion. Severe gastroenteritis or cholera which is prevalent in, the tropics is often an important cause.

3. *Chronic illness:* Hypertension, chronic nephritis and chronic wasting diseases are responsible for late abortion by producing placental infarction resulting in fetal anoxia.

4. *Endocrine factors:* An increased association of abortion is found in conditions of hypothyroidism, hyper-thyroidism and diabetes mellitus. Inadequate corpus luteal state is considered to be related with unsatisfactory ovular growth and development and hence its expulsion.

b. *Trauma*
  1. Direct trauma on the abdominal wall by blow or fall may be related to abortion. But fortunately except in abortion prone women, pregnancy remains undisturbed.
  2. *Psychic:* Emotional upset or change in environment may lead to abortion by affecting the uterine activity.
  3. In susceptible individual, even a minor trauma in the form of a journey along rough road, internal examination in early months or eliciting Hegar's sign or sexual intercourse in early months is enough to excite abortion.
  4. Amniocentesis, chorion villus sampling or abdominal surgery in early months may cause abortion.

c. *Toxic agents:* Environmental toxins like lead, arsenic, anaesthetic gases, tobacco, caffeine, alcohol, radiation in excess amount increase the risk of abortion. Drugs used for epilepsy or antimalarial preparations (quinine) are not so much harmful when used in therapeutic doses so as to cause abortion.

d. *Cervicouterine factors:* These are related mostly to the second trimester abortions.

   1. Cervical incompetence, either congenital or acquired is one of the commonest causes of midtrimester and recurrent abortions.

   2. Congenital malformation of the uterus in the form of bicornuate or septate uterus may be responsible for midtrimester or recurrent abortion.

   3. Uterine tumour (fibroid) specially of the submucous variety might be responsible not only for infertility but also for abortion due to distortion of the uterine cavity and increased uterine irritability.

   4. Retroverted uterus, is not responsible for abortion but its association might be due to its failure to rectify between 12 and 14 weeks due to adhesions or due to trauma during sexual intercourse or it could be due to disturbance in uterine vascularity.

e. *Immunological:* Presence of autoimmune factors like lupus anticoagulant and antiphospholipid antibodies increase the risk of abortion. Alloimmune factors have been observed in cases with recurrent pregnancy loss.

f. *Blood group incompatibility:* Incompatible ABO group matings may be responsible for early pregnancy wastage and often recurrent but Rh incompatibility is a rare cause of death of the fetus before 28th week. Couple with group 'A' husband and group 'O' wife have got higher incidence of abortion.

g. *Premature rupture of the membranes* inevitably leads to abortion.

h. *Dietetic factors:* Deficiency of folic acid or vitamin E is often held responsible.

Paternal factors

Defective sperm, contributing half the number of the chromosomes to the ovum, may result in abortion, but it is difficult to prove. However, some women who abort habitually may have normal pregnancies following marriage with a different man.

Unknown (25%)

Inspite of the numerous factors mentioned, it is indeed difficult, in a majority, to pinpoint the cause or abortion in clinical practice. Too often, more than one factor is present. Immunological causes of abortion have recently gained attention.

Mechanism of abortion

In the early weeks, death of the ovum occurs first, followed by its expulsion. In the later weeks, maternal environmental factors are involved leading to expulsion of the foetus which may have signs of life but is too small to survive.

- *Before 8 weeks:* The ovum, surrounded by the villi with the decidual coverings, is expelled out intact. Sometimes, the external os fails to dilate so that the entire mass is accommodated in the dilated cervical canal and is called cervical abortion (Fig. 8.2).

- *8–14 weeks:* Expulsion of the fetus commonly occurs leaving behind the placenta and the membranes. A part of it may be partially separated with brisk haemorrhage or remains totally attached to the uterine wall.

- *Beyond 14th week:* The process of expulsion is similar to that of a "mini labour". The fetus is expelled first followed by expulsion of the placenta after a varying interval.

THREATENED ABORTION

Definition

It is a clinical entity where the process of abortion has started but has not progressed to a state from which recovery is impossible.

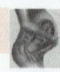

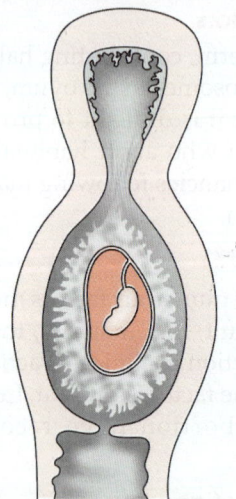

Fig. 8.2: Cervical abortion

Clinical features

Symptoms
1. Period of amenorrhoea
2. Scanty bright red bleeding of blood stained discharge
3. No abdominal pain, at times lower abdominal period-like discomfort.
4. No history of expulsion of any fleshy lump.

Signs
1. Per abdomen and bimanual examination, gravid uterus is felt soft, enlarged corresponding to period of amenorrhoea.
2. On speculum and vaginal palpation cervical os is closed. Stained discharge is present.

Investigations

Routine investigations include
1. **Blood** for haemoglobin estimation, ABO and Rh grouping. Blood transfusion may be required urgently if abortion becomes inevitable and anti-D gamma globulin has to be given in Rh negative non-immunized women.
2. **Urine** for immunological test of pregnancy. This is done to confirm the fetal death in

cases of continued bleeding. However, the test remains positive for a variable period even after the fetal death.

Special investigation

The ultrasonographic (transvaginal) findings may be:
1. A well formed gestation ring with central echoes from the embryo indicating healthy fetus.
2. Observation of fetal cardiac motion. With this there is 98% chance of continuation of pregnancy.
3. A blighted ovum is evidenced by loss of definition of the gestation sac, smaller mean gestational sac diameter, absent fetal echoes and absent fetal cardiac movements.

Treatment

- **Bed rest:** The patient should be in bed for few days until bleeding stops. Prolonged restriction of activity has got no therapeutic value. However, with history of previous early pregnancy wastage, the period of rest should be extended to about two weeks beyond the period at which the previous wastage occurred.
- **Drugs:** Sedation and relief of pain may be ensured by phenobarbitone 30 mg or diazepam 5 mg tablet twice daily. Bowel should be left alone for 48 hours. Mild laxative (milk of magnesia) 4 teaspoons at bed time may be prescribed later on, if required. Enema should not be given (Fig. 8.3).

General measures

1. The patient is advised to preserve the vulval pads and anything expelled out per vaginam, for inspection.
2. To report if bleeding and/or pain becomes aggravated.
3. Routine note of pulse, temperature and vaginal bleeding.

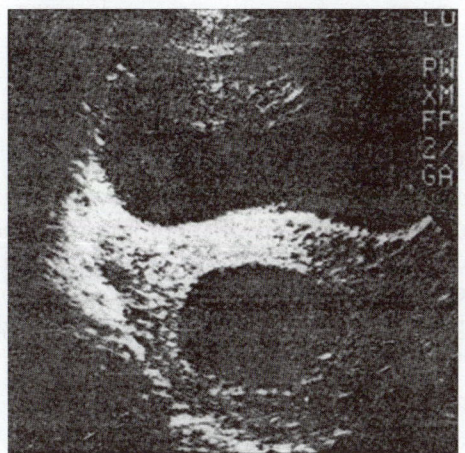

Fig. 8.3: Ultrasonographic picture of blighted ovum

Advice on discharge

The patient should limit her activities for at least two weeks and avoid heavy work, strenuous exercise and excitement. Coitus is contraindicated during this period. She should be re-examined after one month to note the growth of the uterus and advised to consult the physician if bleeding recurs.

INEVITABLE ABORTION (Fig. 8.4)

Definition

It is the clinical type of abortion where the changes have progressed to a state from where continuation of pregnancy is impossible.

Clinical features

Symptoms
1. History of amenorrhoea for months
2. Frank vaginal bleeding at times with clots
3. Severe colicky lower abdominal pain
4. No tissue is expelled
5. She may faint due to heavy blood loss

Signs
1. Maternal vital signs may remain normal in majority. In few signs of shock due to blood loss—tachycardia, hypotension (below 100 mm Hg systolic), cold clammy skin.
2. *Uterine size*: Uterus is felt firm (contracted)
3. *Pelvic exam*: Internal cervical os dilates admitting index finger; conceptus is felt by finger. Frank blood and clots in vagina.

Complications
1. *Blood loss*—Shock and death
2. Infection of conceptus and uterus

Management

The principles in the management are:
1. To take appropriate measures to look after the general condition.
2. To accelerate the process of expulsion.
3. To maintain strict asepsis as outlined in conduction of labour.

General measures

Morphine 15 mg is given intramuscularly. Excessive bleeding should be promptly controlled

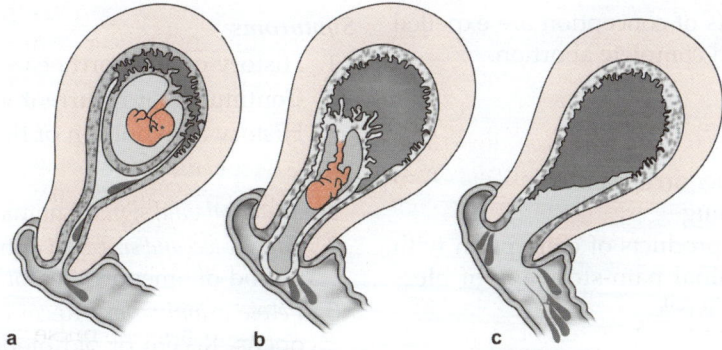

Fig. 8.4: a. Threatened abortion, **b.** Inevitable abortion, **c.** Incomplete abortion

by administering methergin 0.2 mg if the cervix is dilated and the size of the uterus is less than 12 weeks. The shock is corrected by intravenous fluid therapy and blood transfusion.

Active treatment

a. *Before 12 weeks*
1. Dilatation and evacuation followed by curettage of the uterine cavity by blunt curette under general anaesthesia is quite effective and a safe procedure.
2. Alternatively, suction evacuation followed by curettage may be employed.

b. *After 12 weeks*
1. The uterine contraction is accelerated by oxytocin drip (10 units in 500 ml of 5% dextrose) 40–60 drops per minute. If the fetus is expelled and the placenta is retained, it is removed by ovum forceps, if lying separated. If the placenta is not separated, digital separation followed by its evacuation is to be done under general anaesthesia.
2. If bleeding is profuse with the cervix closed (suggestive of low implantation of placenta) evacuation of the uterus may have to be done by abdominal hysterotomy.

COMPLETE ABORTION

Definition

When the products of conception are expelled in mass, it is called complete abortion.

Clinical features

Symptoms
1. History of amenorrhoea
2. Vaginal bleeding
3. Expulsion of products of conception with lower abdominal pain-stoppage of bleeding within a week.

Signs
1. Maternal vital signs normal

2. *Pelvic examination*—Os closed, uterus remains firm. Red discharge comes trace in recent case. Fleshy mass expelled is found to be intact conceptus.

Management

The effect of blood loss, if any, should be assessed and treated. If there is doubt about complete expulsion of the products, uterine curettage should be done. Transvaginal sonography is useful to prevent unnecessary surgical procedure.

Rh negative women

A Rh negative patient without antibody in her system should be protected by Anti-D gamma globulin—50 microgram or 100 microgram intramuscularly in cases of early abortion or late abortion respectively within 72 hours. However, Anti-D may not be required in a case with complete miscarriage before 12 weeks gestation where no instrumentation has been done.

INCOMPLETE ABORTION

Definition

When the entire products of conception are not expelled, instead a part of it is left inside the uterine cavity, it is called incomplete abortion. This is the commonest type met amongst women, hospitalized for abortion complications.

Clinical features

Symptoms
1. History of amenorrhoea
2. Continuous or recurrent vaginal bleeding
3. History of expulsion of fleshy tissue

Signs
1. *Maternal vital signs:* Anemia may be present
2. *Uterine feel and size:* Soft or firm, smaller than period of amenorrhoea or corresponding.
3. *Pelvic examination:* Recent one-internal os opens. Recent or old blood clot; os closes but becomes patulous.

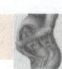

Termination

The products left behind may lead to:

1. Profuse bleeding
2. Sepsis
3. Placental polyp
4. Rarely choriocarcinoma

Management

- *In recent cases*—the same principles are to be followed like that of the inevitable abortion. It is emphasized, that the patient may be in a state of shock due to blood loss. She should be resuscitated before any active treatment is undertaken.
  - *Early abortion*: Dilatation and evacuation under general anaesthesia is to be done.
  - *Late abortion*: The uterus is explored under general anaesthesia and the products left behind is either removed by ovum forceps or by blunt curette.
- *In late cases,* dilatation and curettage operation is to be done to remove the bits of tissues left behind. The removed materials are subjected to a histological examination.

MISSED ABORTION (SILENT MISCARRIAGE)

Definition

When the fetus is dead and retained inside the uterus for a variable period, it is called missed abortion or silent miscarriage or early fetal demise.

Pathology

The causes of prolonged retention of the dead fetus in the uterus is not clear. Beyond 12 weeks, the retained fetus becomes macerated or mummified. The liquor amnii gets absorbed and the placenta becomes pale, thin and may be adherent. Before 12 weeks, the pathological process differs when the ovum is more or less completely surrounded by the chorionic villi.

CARNEOUS MOLE (SYN: BLOOD MOLE, FLESHY MOLE OR TUBEROUS MOLE)

It is the pathological variant of missed abortion affecting the foetus before 12 weeks. Small repeated haemorrhages in the chorio-decidual space distrupt the villi from its attachments. The bleeding is slight so it does not cause rupture of the decidua as a blood mole. By this time, the ovum becomes dead and is either completely absorbed or remains as a rudimentary structure. Gradually, the fluid portion of the blood surrounding the ovum gets absorbed and the wall becomes fleshy, hence the term fleshy or carneous mole (Fig. 8.5).

Clinical features (early pregnancy)

Symptoms

1. History of amenorrhoea
2. An episode of vaginal bleeding followed by continuous dark discharge.
3. Pain is absent
4. No expulsion of fleshy tissue

Signs

1. Maternal vital signs are normal
2. Uterine size (per abdomen and pelvic exam) is definately smaller than period of amenorrhoea.
3. Feel of uterus—firm.

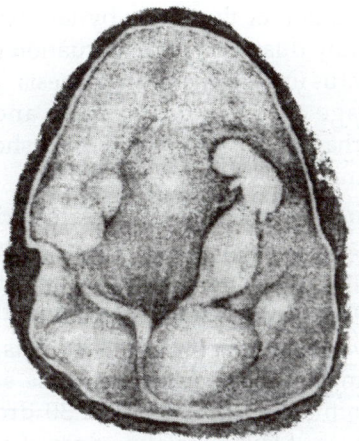

Fig. 8.5: A carneous mole

4. Vaginal exam—cervical os is closed.
5. Dark tarry vaginal discharge
6. Urinary hCG is shows falling concentration till it comes negative by two weeks times. Clinical diagnosis of missed abortion can be made by 4 weeks time when all above signs could be ascertained.
7. *Ultrasonography:* Abdominal or transvaginal
8. *Early pregnancy:* Ultrasonography shows absent foetal heart motion, blighted ovum, distorted gestation sac. Serum progesterone level fall < 10 ng/ml.
9. *Midpregnancy:* Absent foetal cardiac motion and overlapping of skull bone.

Complications

Haemorrhage from uterus, gum, urinary tract, infection site rarely develops in missed abortion over 6 weeks duration and in mid pregnancy. Thromboplastin gets absorbed from gestation sac →lowering of plasma fibrinogen, platelet, factor VIII →disseminated intravascular coagulation (DIC) →coagulation defect → bleeding.

Management

Uterus is less than 12 weeks: Vaginal evacuation can be carried out without delay. This can be effectively done by suction evacuation or slow dilatation of the cervix by laminaria tent followed by dilatation and evacuation (D & E) of the uterus under general anaesthesia. The risk of damage to the uterine walls and brisk haemorrhage during the operation should be kept in mind.

Uterus more than 12 weeks: The same principles of the management protocol as advocated in the intrauterine fetal death are to be followed. Induction is done by the following methods:

- *Oxytocin:* To start with 10–20 units of oxytocin in 500 ml of 5% dextrose saline is administered in drip with 30 drops per minute. If fails, escalating dose of oxytocin to the maximum of 100 units, in a pint of

5% dextrose saline at a drip rate of 30 drops per minute, may be used with precaution.

- *Prostaglandins:* Prostaglandin is more effective than oxytocin in such cases. The following procedures may be employed :
  - Intramuscular administration of 15 methyl $PGF_{2\alpha}$ (carboprost tromethamine) 250 ng at three hourly intervals for a maximum of 10 such.
  - Prostaglandin E_1 analogue (misoprost) 250 mg tablet is inserted into the posterior vaginal fornix every 4 hours for a maximum 5 such.

SEPTIC ABORTION

Definition

Any abortion associated with clinical evidences of infection of the uterus and its contents, is called septic abortion. Although clinical criteria vary, abortion is usually considered septic when there are:

1. Rise of temperature of at least 100.4°F (38°C) for 24 hours or more
2. Offensive or purulent vaginal discharge
3. Other evidences of pelvic infection such as lower abdominal pain and tenderness.

Incidence

It is difficult to work out the overall incidence of septic abortion. About 10% of abortions requiring admission to hospital are septic. The majority of septic abortion are associated with incomplete abortion. While in the majority of cases the infection occurs following illegal induced abortion but infection can occur even after spontaneous abortion.

Mode of infection

The micro-organisms involved in the sepsis are usually those normally present in the vagina (endogenous). Thus, their growth in culture media has to be interpreted in relation to clinical manifestation. The micro-organisms are:

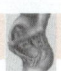
1. *Anaerobic:* Bacteroides group (fragilis), anaerobic *Streptococci*, *Cl. welchii*, and tetanus bacillus.
2. *Aerobic:* Escherichia coli (*E. coli*), *Klebsiella*, *Staphylococcus*, *Pseudomonas* and haemolytic *Streptococcus* (usually exogenous). Mixed infection is more common.

Pathology

Infection colonises in necrotic product of conception → endometritis → spread of infection; to uterine wall and beyond → peritonitis, septicaemia.

Clinical features

1. History of amenorrhoea
2. Vaginal bleeding followed by foul smelling vaginal discharge
3. Pain lower abdomen
4. Product may or may not be expelled.
5. Fever with chill

Signs

Maternal vital signs: High temperature, tachycardia, septic shock, jaundice, oliguria, anuria, per abdomen-tender lower abdomen, tender and rigid abdomen in generalised peritonitis.

Pelvic examination

1. Gravid uterus is felt same or smaller sized, firm, tender on movement, closed or open os.
2. Foul purulent discharge from uterus.

Investigations

Routine investigations include

1. Cervical or high vaginal swab is taken prior to internal examination for
   * Culture in aerobic and anaerobic media to find out the dominant micro-organisms
   * Sensitivity of the micro-organisms to antibiotics
   * Smear for gram stain. Gram negative organisms are—*E. coli*, *Pseudomonas*, Bacteroides, etc. Gram-positive organisms are—*Staphylococci*, anaerobic *Streptococci*, *Cl. welchii*, *Cl. tetani*, etc.
2. Blood for haemoglobin estimation, total and differential count of white cells, ABO and Rh grouping.
3. Urine analysis including culture.

Special investigations

1. Ultrasonography pelvis and abdomen to detect intrauterine retained products of conception, pyometra, foreign body—intrauterine or intra-abdominal, free fluid in the peritoneal cavity or in the pouch of Douglas.
2. X-ray abdomen and pelvis—not commonly done these days.
3. Blood
   * *Culture:* If associated with spell of chills and rigors
   * *Serum electrolytes:* As an adjunct to the management protocol of endotoxic shock.
   * Coagulation profile

Complications

Immediate: The major complications of septic abortion are dependent more on the nature of the abortion in which the sepsis occurs. Practically all the fatal complications are associated with illegally induced abortions confined to the Grade III types.

* Haemorrhage related due to abortion process and also due to the injury inflicted during the interference.
* Injury may occur to the uterus and also to the adjacent structures particularly gut.
* Spread of infection leads to
1. *Generalized peritonitis:* The infection reaches through:
   * The uterine tubes
   * Perforation of the uterus
   * Bursting of the microabscess in the uterine wall and
   * Injury to the gut.

2. *Endotoxic shock:* Mostly due to *E. coli* or *Cl. welchii* infection.
3. *Acute renal failure:* Multiple factors are involved producing patchy cortical necrosis or acute tubular necrosis. It is common in infection with *Cl. welchii*.
4. Thrombophlebitis

All these lead to increased maternal deaths, the magnitude of which is to the extent of about 20–25% as per hospital statistics. The risk is about 50 times more in illegal induced abortion than in legal abortion.

Remote: The remote complications include:

1. Chronic debility
2. Chronic pelvic pain and backache
3. Dyspareunia
4. Ectopic pregnancy
5. Secondary infertility due to tubal blockage
6. Emotional depression

Prevention

1. To take meticulous antiseptic and aseptic precautions either during internal examination or during operation in spontaneous abortion, as outlined in conduction of labour.
2. An inevitable or incomplete abortion should be made complete as early as possible.
3. To boost up family planning acceptance in order to curb the unwanted pregnancies.
4. Rigid enforcement of legalized abortion in practice and to curb the prevalence of illegal abortions. Education, motivation and extension of the facilities are sine-qua-non to get the real benefit out of it.

MANAGEMENT

General management

- Hospitalization even with a case of mild infection is preferable. The patient should be kept in isolation, if possible.
- To take high vaginal or cervical swab for culture, drug sensitivity test and Gram stain.

- Vaginal examination is then made to note the state of the abortion process and extension of the infection. If the products are found loosely lying in the cervix, they should be removed by sponge holding forceps.
- Overall assessment of the case is to be done and the patient is put in accordance with the clinical grading.
- Investigation protocols as outlined before are done, as required and where available.
- To formulate the line of treatment which aims at
  - To control sepsis
  - To remove the source of infection
  - To give supportive therapy to bring back the normal homeostatic and cellular metabolism.
  - To remain vigilant in order to assess the response of treatment.

Grade I

Drugs

1. Antibiotics (*see* below)
2. Prophylactic antigas-gangrene serum (AGS) of 8000 units and 3000 units of antitetanus serum (ATS) intramuscularly are given if there is a history of interference.
3. Analgesics and sedatives, as required, are to be prescribed.

Blood transfusion: Early and adequate blood transfusion is not only helpful to improve the body resistance and anaemia but is also effective to prevent or minimize shock and oliguria.

Evacuation of the uterus: As abortion is often incomplete, evacuation should be performed at a convenient time within 24 hours following antibiotic therapy. Excessive bleeding is, of course, an urgent indication for evacuation. Early emptying not only minimizes the risk of haemorrhage but also removes the nidus of infection. Gentleness and avoidance of vigorous curettage are to be followed to minimize the risk

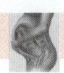
of injury to the soft uterus and spread of infection into the deeper tissues.

Grade II

Drugs: Antibiotics—mixed infections including gram positive, gram negative and anaerobic organisms are common. Ideal antibiotic regimens should cover all of them.

1. *For gram positive aerobes*
   - Aqueous penicillin G 5 million units IV every 6 hours
   - Ampicillin 0.5–1 gm IV every 6 hours.
2. *Gram negative aerobes*
   - Gentamicin 1.5 mg/kg IV every 8 hours (serum level to be monitored in a case with renal failure and dose to be adjusted accordingly).
   - Cefuroxime 1.5 gm, IV every 8 hours.
3. *For anaerobes:* Metronidazole 500 mg IV every 8 hours, or Clindamycin 600 mg IV every 6 hours.

Antibiotic regimens have to be modified according to the culture and sensitivity report as obtained later on. Analgesic, A.G.S. and A.T.S. are given as in Grade I. Blood transfusion, in adequate amount, is more often needed than in Grade I cases.

Clinical monitoring: To note pulse, respiration, temperature, urinary output and progress of the pain, tenderness and mass in lower abdomen.

Surgery

1. *Evacuation of the uterus:* Evacuation should be withheld for at least 48 hours after the infection is controlled and becomes localized, the only exception being excessive bleeding.
2. *Posterior colpotomy:* When the infection is legalized in the pouch of Douglas, pelvic abscess is formed. It is evidenced by spiky rise of temperature, rectal tenesmus (frequent loose stool mixed with mucus) and boggy mass felt through the posterior fornix. Posterior colpotomy and drainage of the pus relieve the symptoms and improve the general outlook of the patient.

Grade III

Antibiotics are discussed above. Clinical monitoring is to be conducted as outlined in grade II. Supportive therapy is directed to treat generalized peritonitis by gastric suction and intravenous saline infusion.

Active surgery

Along with the antibiotic therapy and the resuscitation of the patient with the fluid and electrolyte, the patient should be assessed as to whether active surgery is needed. The indications of active surgery are:

1. Injury to the uterus
2. Suspected injury to the gut
3. Presence of foreign body in the abdomen as evidenced by the sonography or X-ray or felt through the fornix on bimanual examination
4. Unresponsive peritonitis suggestive of collection of pus
5. Septic shock or oliguria not responding to the conservative treatment
6. Uterus too big to be safely evacuated per vagina.

The laparotomy should be done by experienced surgeon with a skilled anaesthetist. Removal of the uterus should be done by its own merit irrespective of parity. Adnexa is to be removed or preserved according to the pathology found. Thorough inspection of the gut and omentum for evidence of any injury is mandatory. Even when nothing is found on laparotomy, simple drainage of the pus is effective.

Unsafe Abortion

It is defined to the procedure of termination of unwanted pregnancy either by persons lacking the necessary skills or in an environment lacking the minimal standards or both

Table 8.1: Comparison and management of spontaneous abortion (miscarriage)

Type	Cramps	Bleeding	Tissue passed	Cervical opening	Uterine size	Nursing management
Threatened	Slight (with or without cramps)	Slight to moderate (bleeding ceases)	None	Closed	Commensurate with date	Bed rest, sedation, avoidance of coitus, ultrasound. Observe amount of bleeding (save pads). Woman to gradually increase activity. Do pregnancy tests. Give Rh(D) immunoglobulin within 72 hours if indicated.
Inevitable	Moderate	Moderate to severe	None	Open with membranes or tissues bulging the ruptured membranes	Commensurate with date	Bed rest, sedation. Transfusion may be indicated. Observe amount of bleeding, color (save pads). Give RhoGAM if indicated.
Incomplete	Severe	Severe and continuous	Placental or fetal tissue	Open with tissue in cervical canal or passage of tissue	Smaller than date	Bed rest, sedation. Observe to determine how much tissue is passed; save all available tissues. Carefully record vital signs. D and C as necessary. Give RhoGAM if indicated.
Complete	None	Minimal	Complete placenta and fetus	Closed with no tissue in cervical canal	Smaller than date	Observe to determine if the all tissue is passed (save pads). Give RhoGAM if indicated.
Missed	None; no life felt	Brownish discharge	None; prolonged retention of tissue	Closed	Smaller than expected	No specific treatment available. Oxytocics may be used to induce labour and delivery. Check for coagulation defect (DIC).
Recurrent (habitual)						Comprehensive and conservative care essential in early months. Shirodkar surgery done if necessary for incompetent cervix.

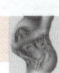

(WHO 1992). 90% of unsafe abortions are in the developing countries comprising 13% of all maternal deaths (WHO 1998). All most all the complications are preventable if it is performed in a safe manner with proper post abortion care services.

Case history: The patient had three consecutive midtrimester abortions. Hysterography reveals bicornuate uterus. Uteroculoplasty was done. Pregnancy occurred one year later, which was delivered by caesarean section at 39 weeks.

MEDICAL TERMINATION OF PREGNANCY (MTP)

Since legalisation of abortion in India, deliberate induction of abortion by a registered medical practitioner in the interest of mother's health and life is protected under the MTP act. The following provisions are laid down.

- The continuation of pregnancy would involve serious risk of life or grave injury to the physical and mental health of the pregnant woman.
- There is a substantial risk of the child being born with serious physical and mental abnormalities so as to be handicapped in life.
- When the pregnancy is caused by rape, both in cases of major and minor girl and in mentally imbalanced women.
- Pregnancy caused as a result of failure of a contraceptive

In practice, the following are the indications for termination under the MTP Act

- *To save the life of the mother* (Therapeutic or Medical termination) : The indications are limited and scarcely justifiable now a days except in the following cases:
  - Pulmonary tuberculosis, when superimposed pregnancy deteriorates the condition,
  - Cardiac diseases (Grade III & IV) with history of decompensation in the previous pregnancy or in between the

pregnancies are justifiable indications for termination in the first trimester,
  - Chronic glomerulonephritis
  - Malignant hypertension
  - Intractable hyperemesis gravidarum
  - Cervical or breast malignancy
  - Diabetes mellitus with retinopathy
  - Epilepsy or psychiatric illness with the advice of a psychiatrist.
- *Social indications:* This is almost the sole indication and is covered under the provision "to prevent grave injury to the physical and mental health of the pregnant woman". In about 80%, it is limited to parous women having unplanned pregnancy with low socioeconomic status. Pregnancy caused by rape or unwanted pregnancy caused due to failure of any contraceptive device also falls in this category (20%).
- *Eugenic:* This is done under the provision of "substantial risk of the child being born with serious physical and mental abnormalities so as to be handicapped in life". The indication is rare.
  - Chromosomal and enzymatic abnormalities of the fetus which are identified as factors responsible for transmission of certain inherited disorders.
  - When the fetus is likely to be deformed due to action of teratogenic drugs or radiation exposure in early pregnancy. Taking hormones either in the form of tablets or injections for diagnosis of pregnancy or accidental pelvic X-ray (having less than 10 rad) is not a justifiable indication specially in first pregnancy, for termination.
  - Rubella, a viral infection affecting in the first trimester, is an indication for termination.
  - History of one or both parents being mentally defective or previous children being malformed, can be a reason for termination in consultation with a geneticist.

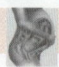

ECTOPIC PREGNANCY

Ectopic pregnancy still contributes significantly to the cause of maternal mortality and morbidity. While there has been about four fold increase in incidence over the couple of decades, but the mortality has been slashed down to about 80 percent. Advance in ultrasound particularly transvaginal imaging and sensitive β hCG assay have considerably improved the diagnostic capability at the early stage even prior to its termination.

Definition

An ectopic pregnancy is one in which the fertilized ovum is implanted and develops outside the normal uterine cavity.

Sites of implantation (Fig. 8.6)

TUBAL PREGNANCY

Frequency

The incidence has increased. The reasons are increased prevalence of chronic pelvic inflammatory disease, tubal plastic operations,

Table 8.2: Nursing Diagnosis related to Abortions

- Fear related to potential loss of pregnancy
- Knowledge deficit related to the cause of abortion.
- Pain related to abdominal cramping with contractions of uterine muscles.
- Self-esteem, situational low, related to feelings of guilt and blame for abortion.
- Risk for fluid volume deficit related to hemorrhage, related to retention of tissue and surgery required to empty uterus.
- Spiritual distress related to couple's preference in religious rites is not carried out.
- Risk for Injury, related to pregnancy termination.
- Risk for infection related to incomplete abortion.
- Anxiety related to pregnancy outcome and uncertainity of future pregnancies.
- Risk for maternal injury related to fetal autolysis or Rh Iso immunization

ovulation induction and IUD use. Early diagnosis and therapy has helped to reduce maternal deaths due to ectopic pregnancy. The incidence varies from 1 in 300 to 1 in 150 deliveries.

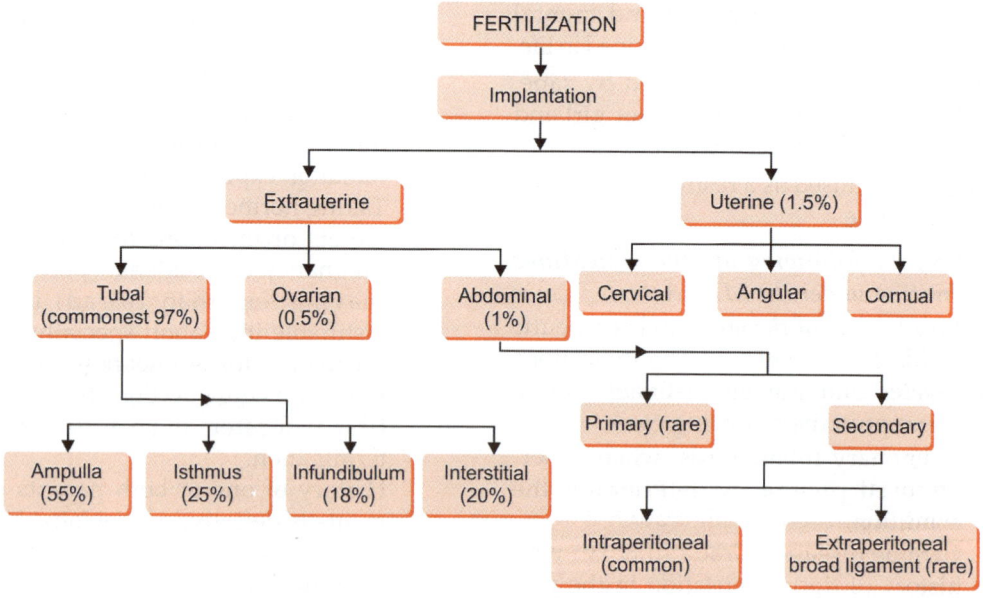

Fig. 8.6: Sites of implantation

Etiology

Factors which are responsible for the fertilized ovum to remain in the tube are

- Factors preventing or delaying the migration of the fertilized ovum to the uterine cavity
- Factors facilitating nidation of the fertilized ovum in the tubal mucosa.

Factors delaying or preventing migration

Pelvic inflammatory disease (PID) increases the risk of ectopic pregnancy by 6–10 fold.

a. Loss of cilia of the lining epithelium and impairment of muscular peristalsis
b. Narrowing of the tubal lumen
c. Formation of pockets due to adhesions between mucosal folds
d. Peritubal adhesions resulting in kinking and angulation of the tube.

Iatrogenic

1. *Contraception failure:* The absolute number of ectopic pregnancy is infact diminished with use of any contraceptive because pregnancy occurs less often. But in selected contraception failure, there is increased incidence of ectopic pregnancy.
   a. *IUCD:* It prevents intrauterine pregnancy effectively, tubal implantation to a lesser extent and the ovarian pregnancy not at all. There is thus relative increase in tubal pregnancy (7 times more) should pregnancy occur with IUCD in situ.
   b. *Sterilization operation:* There is 15–50 percent chance of being ectopic if pregnancy occurs following tubal sterilization. The risk is highest following laparoscopic fulguration without tubal resection.
   c. *Use of progestin only pill* or postcoital oestrogen preparations increases the

> **Box 8.1:** Risk factors of ectopic pregnancy
>
> - History of PID
> - History of tubal ligation
> - Contraception failure
> - Previous ectopic pregnancy
> - Tubal reconstructive surgery
> - History of infertility
> - ART particularly if the tubes are patent but damaged
> - IUD use
> - Previous induced abortion

chance of tubal pregnancy probably by impaired tubal motility.

2. *Tubal surgery:* Tubal reconstructive surgery to improve the fertility increases the risk of tubal pregnancy significantly.
3. *Intrapelvic adhesions* following pelvic surgery.
4. *ART:* Tubal pregnancy is increased following ovulation induction and IVF-ET arid GIFT procedures.
5. *Others*
   a. *Previous ectopic pregnancy:* There is 10–15% chances of repeat ectopic pregnancy.
   b. *Prior induced abortion* significantly increases the risk.
   c. *Developmental defects of the tube*
      - Elongation
      - Diverticulum
   d. Transperitoneal migration of the ovum—contralateral presence of corpus luteum is noticed in tubal pregnancy in about 10% cases.

Factors facilitating nidation in the tube

1. Early resumption of the trophoblastic activity is probably due to premature degeneration of the zona pellucida.
2. Increased decidual reaction
3. Tubal endometriosis

 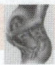

MORBID ANATOMY

Changes in the tube

1. Implantation in the tube occurs more commonly in intercolumnar fashion i.e. in between two mucosal folds
2. Decidual change at the site of implantation is minimal. The muscles undergo limited hyperplasia and hypertrophy but more stretching. Blood vessels are engorged
3. The ovum burrows through the mucous membrane and lies deep in the muscle layers—so called intramuscular implantation.
4. A pseudocapsularis is formed consisting of fibrin, lining epithelium and few muscle fibers
5. Blood vessels are eroded by the chorionic villi and the blood accumulates in between the ovum and the pseudocapsularis
6. The tube on the implantation site is distended and the wall is thinned out. The thinness is due to distension by the growing ovum/accumulation of blood and erosion by the chorionic villi.
7. Further changes in the tube specially at the site of implantation depend on the mode of termination of the pregnancy which invariably occurs within 6–8 weeks.

Changes in the uterus

Under the influence of oestrogen, progesterone and chorionic gonadotrophin, there is varying amount of enlargement of the uterus with increased vascularity. The decidua develops all the characteristics of intrauterine pregnancy except that it contains no evidence of chorionic villi. When the ovum is dead, it is either disintegrated and comes out piecemeal or comes in a single piece (decidual cast).

MODE OF TERMINATION (Fig. 8.7)

Because of the unfavourable environment, early interruption of pregnancy is inevitable within 6–8 weeks. The modes of termination are as follows:

Tubal mole: The formation of the tubal mole is similar to that formed in uterine pregnancy. The fate of the mole is either (Fig. 8.8).

- Complete absorption
- Expulsion through the abdominal ostium as tubal abortion with a variable amount of internal haemorrhage.

The encysted blood so collected in the pouch of Douglas, is called pelvic haematocele.

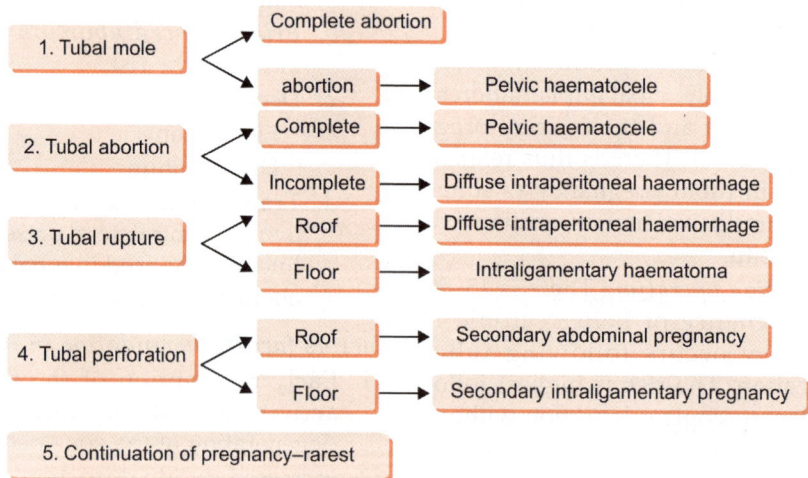

Fig. 8.7: Mode of termination

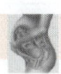

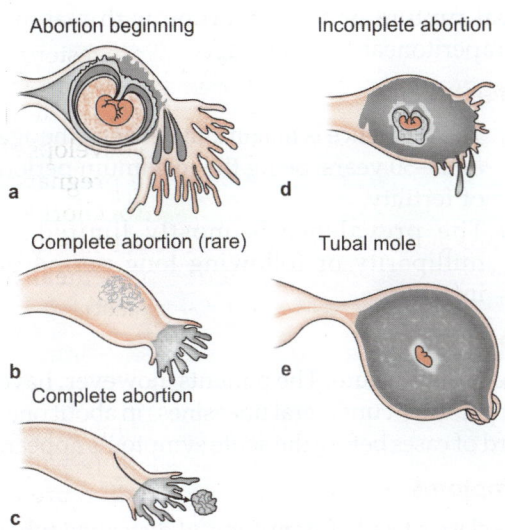

Fig. 8.8: Mode of termination of tubal abortion

Tubal abortion: This is the common mode of termination, if implantation occurs in the ampulla or infundibulum. Prior to abortion, the ovum may be converted into mole or else, a living ovum is aborted.

Tubal rupture: Tubal rupture is predominantly common in isthmic and interstitial implantation. Isthmic rupture usually occurs at 6–8 weeks, the ampullary one at 8–12 weeks and the interstitial one at about 4 months.

Depending upon the site of rupture

- *Intraperitoneal rupture:* This type of rupture is common. The rent is situated on the roof or sides of the tube. The bleeding is intraperitoneal.
- *Extraperitoneal rupture (intra-ligamentary):* This type of rupture is rare and occurs when the rent lies on the floor of the tube where the broad ligament is attached. It is commonly met in isthmic implantation.

Secondary abdominal pregnancy: the prerequisites for the continuation of fetal growth outside the tube (Fig. 8.9)

1. Perforation of the tubal wall should be a slow process
2. Amnion must be intact
3. Placental chorion should escape injury from the rupture
4. Herniation of the amniotic sac with the living ovum and the placenta should occur through the rent.
5. Placenta gets attached to the neighbouring structures and new vascular connection should be re-established. The fibrin is

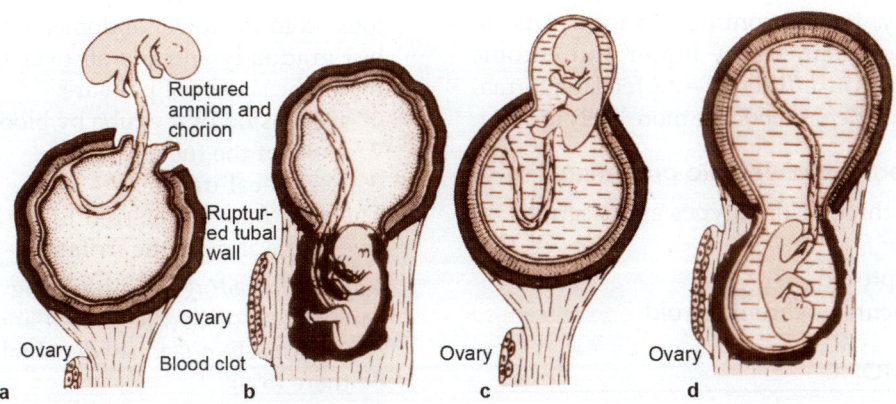

Fig. 8.9: Fate of tubal rupture. **a.** Intraperitoneal, **b.** Extraperitoneal with broad ligament haematoma, **c.** Secondary abdominal, **d.** Secondary broad ligament

 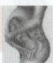

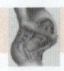

deposited over the exposed amnion to constitute a secondary amniotic sac.

6. Intestine, omentum and adjacent structures get adherent to the secondary sac.

Secondary broad ligament pregnancy

Pregnancy may continue in the same process as in abdominal pregnancy. The growth of the pregnancy is limited—between the two layers of the peritoneum which may be stripped off the pelvic floor. Occasionally, the sac may rupture secondarily at a later period and the fetus is extruded into the peritoneal cavity, with—the placenta attached in its original position, forming a secondary abdominal pregnancy.

Fate of secondary abdominal pregnancy

- Death of the ovum with complete absorption
- Catastrophe may occur due to separation of the placenta leading to the death of the ovum with massive intraperitoneal haemorrhage.
- The gestation sac may be infected and a fistulous communication with the intestine, bladder, vagina or through the umbilicus may occur.
- The fetus dies (majority) and undergoes mummification or adipocere formation or becomes calcified to form lithopaedion.
- Rarely, it may continue to term. Due to environment, scanty liquor and chronic placental insufficiency—the fetal malformation and deformation are more likely to occur.

Clinical features of ectopic pregnancy

Clinically three distinct types are described:
- Acute
- Unruptured
- Sub-acute or chronic or old

ACUTE ECTOPIC

An acute ectopic is fortunately less common (about 30%) and it is associated with cases of tubal rupture or tubal abortion with massive intraperitoneal haemorrhage.

Patient profile

1. The incidence is maximum between the age of 20–30 years, being the maximum period of fertility.
2. The prevalence is mostly limited to nulliparity or following long period of infertility.

Mode of onset

The onset is acute. The patients, however, have got persistent unilateral uneasiness in about one-third of cases before the acute symptoms appear.

Symptoms

The classic triad of symptoms of disturbed tubal pregnancy are amenorrhoea (75%) followed by abdominal pain (100%) and lastly, appearance of vaginal bleeding (70%).

- *A short period of amenorrhoea* of 6–8 weeks or a delayed period or slight spotting on the expected date of the period is usually present.
- *Abdominal pain* is the most constant feature of the triad. The pain is acute, agonizing or colicky in nature. In between the colicky pains, the patient remains in agony, a feature which differentiates it from intestinal colic. Initially, the pain is located in the lower abdomen on one side but gradually spreads all over the abdomen. The causes of pain are:
  1. Distension of the tube by blood
  2. Colic of the tubal muscles
  3. Peritoneal irritation

  The pain may be referred to the shoulder due to diaphragmatic irritation.
- *Vaginal bleeding:* The bleeding is slight, sanguinous or dark coloured and usually continuous. Expulsion of decidual cast may be there (5%).
- *Feeling of nausea, vomiting, fainting attacks even to the extent of syncope may*

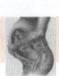

be present. The syncopal attack (10%) is peculiar to ectopic and is probably due to reflex vasomotor disturbance caused by irritation of the peritoneum by the blood.

On examination

- General look is diagnostic of acute ectopic. The patient lies quiet and conscious, perspires and looks blanched.
- Pallor is usually severe and depends on the amount of internal haemorrhage and is significantly out of proportion to the visible vaginal bleeding, if any.
- Features of shock are evidenced by the rapid and feeble pulse, fall of the blood pressure and cold and clammy extremities.
- Abdominal examination reveals the abdomen is tense, timid and tender. The tenderness is mostly limited to the lower abdomen. No mass is usually felt. Shifting dullness may be elicited. Gut may be distended.
- Bimanual examination may precipitate more intraperitoneal bleeding due to manipulation. The findings are:
  – Vaginal mucosa—blanched white.
  – Uterus seems normal in size or slightly bulky
  – Extreme tenderness on fornix palpation or on movement of the cervix (75%).
  – No mass is usually felt through the fornix.
  – The uterus floats as if in water

UNRUPTURED TUBAL ECTOPIC

High degree of suspicion and an ectopic conscious clinician can only diagnose the entity at its prerupture state. It is most often diagnosed accidentally during laparoscopy or laparotomy. The physician should include ectopic pregnancy in the differential diagnosis when a sexually active female has abnormal bleeding and/or abdominal pain.

Symptoms

- Presence of delayed period or spotting with features suggestive of pregnancy.
- Uneasiness on one side of the flank which is continuous or at times colicky in nature.

Signs

Bimanual examination

1. Uterus is slightly smaller than the period of amenorrhoea showing evidence of early pregnancy
2. A pulsatile small, well circumscribed tender mass may be felt through one fornix separated from the uterus.

Investigations

With the advent of transvaginal sonography (TVS), highly sensitive radioimmunoassay of β hCG and laparoscopy, more and more ectopics are now diagnosed in unruptured state.

CHRONIC OR OLD ECTOPIC

Onset

The onset is insidious. The patient had previous attacks of acute pain from which she had recovered or she has chronic features from the beginning.

Symptoms

- Amenorrhoea of short period of 6–8 weeks is usually present.
- Lower abdominal pain is present with varying degrees. It starts as an acute one and gradually becomes dull or colicky in nature.
- Vaginal bleeding appears sooner or later following the pain. It is scanty sanguinous or dark coloured and continuous in nature.
- *Other symptoms:* There may be features of bladder irritation—dysuria, frequency or even retention of urine. Rectal tenesmus may appear specially following infected haematocele. Rise of temperature may be due to infection or due to absorption of the

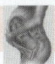

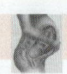

products of degenerated blood accumulated in the abdomen.

On examination

- The patient looks ill
- Varying degree of pallor is present which is not proportionate to the continued vaginal bleeding.
- Persistent high pulse rate
- Features of shock are absent
- Temperature may be slightly elevated to 38°C.
- Abdominal examination
  1. Tenderness and muscle guard on the lower abdomen specially on the affected side is a striking feature.
  2. A mass in the lower abdomen may be felt which is irregular and tender.
  3. Cullen's sign: Dark bluish discolouration surrounding the umbilicus, if found, suggests intraperitoneal haemorrhage.
- Bimanual examination is painful and reveals
  1. Vaginal mucosa—pale
  2. Uterus seems to be normal in size or bulky
  3. Extreme tenderness on movement of the cervix.
  4. An ill defined, boggy and extremely tender mass is felt through the-posterolateral fornix extending to the pouch of Douglas. The mass may push the uterus to the opposite side.
- Rectal examination corroborates the pelvic findings.
- Examination under anaesthesia (EUA) is helpful to evaluate the pelvic findings but accidental tubal rupture may be provoked during manipulation.

DIAGNOSIS OF ECTOPIC PREGNANCY

Acute ectopic

The classic history of acute abdominal catastrophe with fainting attack and collapse associated with features of intra-abdominal haemorrhage in a woman of child bearing age points to a certain diagnosis of acute ectopic.

No time should be wasted for investigation other than estimation of haemoglobin and blood grouping (ABO and Rh).

EUA: Extreme tenderness on vaginal examination, which is of significance, cannot be elicited by EUA. Moreover, at times, it proves risky as the manipulation may provoke further bleeding.

Differential diagnosis: The conditions which simulate acute ectopic are:

1. Acute appendicitis
2. Perforated peptic ulcer
3. Twisted ovarian tumour
4. Ruptured endometrial cyst
5. Ruptured corpus luteal cyst

SUBACUTE (CHRONIC) ECTOPIC

It is indeed difficult at times to diagnose old ectopics. The confusing features are:

1. Absence of amenorrhoea
2. Absence of vaginal bleeding
3. Vaginal bleeding followed by pain
4. Apparently normal general condition
5. Presence of bilateral mass on internal examination.
6. Previous history of tubectomy operation or IUD insertion

Investigations for the diagnosis of tubal ectopic pregnancy

a. *Blood examination* should be done as a routine for:
   1. Haemoglobin
   2. ABO and Rh grouping
   3. Total white cell count and differential count
   4. ESR

There may be varying degrees of leucocytosis and ESR.

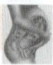

b. *Culdocentesis* is simple and safe. Where sensitive TVS or laparoscopy is not readily available, culdocentesis is still a diagnostic alternative. Through a 18 gauze lumbar puncture needle fitted with a syringe, the posterior fornix is punctured to gain access to the pouch of Douglas. Aspiration of nonclotting blood signifies collection of intraperitoneal blood.

c. *Estimation of β hCG:* The suspicious findings are:

1. Lower concentration of β hCG compared to normal intrauterine pregnancy.
2. Doubling time in plasma fails to occur in 2 days.

d. *Sonography:* Transvaginal sonography (TVS) is more informative. The diagnostic features are:

1. Absence of intrauterine pregnancy with a positive pregnancy test.
2. Fluid in the pouch of Douglas
3. Adnexal mass clearly separated from the ovary.

Colour Doppler sonography: (TV-CDS)—can identify the placental shape (ring-of-fire pattern) and blood flow pattern outside the uterine cavity.

e. *Combination of quantitative β hCG values and sonography*

1. When the β hCG value is greater than 1500 IU/L and there is an empty uterine cavity, ectopic pregnancy is more likely.
2. Failure to double the value of β hCG by 48 hours along with an empty uterus is very much suggestive

f. *Laparoscopy* offers benefit in cases of confusion with other pelvic lesions. It should be employed only when the patient is haemodynamically stable.

Advantages are

1. Confirmation of diagnosis
2. Removal of the ectopic mass using operative procedures at the same time.

3. Direct injection of chemotherapeutic agents in to the ectopic mass—when medical management is decided.

g. *Dilatation and curettage:* Identification of decidua without villi structure is very much suggestive. Chorionic villi that float in normal saline as lacy fronds, is diagnostic of intrauterine pregnancy.

h. *Serum progesterone:* Level greater than 25 ng/ml is suggestive of viable intrauterine pregnancy whereas level less than 5 ng/ml suggests an ectopic or abnormal intrauterine pregnancy.

i. *Laparotomy* offers benefit when in doubt and the old axion, *open and see* holds good.

Differential diagnosis

1. Incomplete abortion in retroverted uterus
2. Salphingitis
3. Appendicitis
4. Twisted ovarian tumour
5. Ruptured chocolate cyst

INTERSTITIAL PREGNANCY (Fig. 8.10)

It is the rarest variety of tubal pregnancy. Because of the thick and vascular musculature of the uterine wall with greater distensibility,

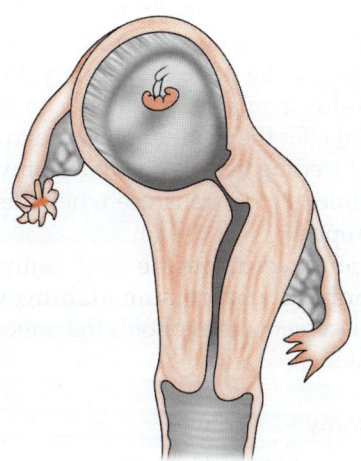

Fig. 8.10: Interstitial pregnancy

the fetus grows dissecting the muscle fibres for a longer period (12–14 weeks) before termination occurs. The usual termination is rupture associated with massive intraperitoneal haemorrhage due to its combined vasculari-sation by the uterine and ovarian arteries. On rare occasion, abortion occurs through the uterine cavity.

The diagnosis before rupture is very difficult. However, the diagnosis is revealed on laparotomy following termination as rupture. Hysterectomy is commonly done.

MANAGEMENT OF ECTOPIC PREGNANCY

ACUTE

Principle

The principle in the management of acute ectopic is resuscitation and laparotomy and not resuscitation followed by laparotomy.

Anti-shock treatment

Anti-shock measures are to be taken energetically with simultaneous preparation for urgent laparotomy.

- Ringer's solution (crystalloid) is started, if necessary with venesection.
- Arrangement is made for blood transfusion. Even if blood is not available laparotomy is to be done desperately. When the blood is available, it is better to be transfused after the clamps are placed to occlude the bleeding vessels on laparotomy, as it is of little help to transfuse when the vessels are open.
- After drawing the blood samples for grouping and cross matching volume replacement with colloids (haemocele) is to be done.

Laparotomy

Indications of laparotomy are:
1. Patient haemodynamically unstable

2. Laparoscopy contraindicated.
3. Evidence of rupture: The principle in laparotomy is "quick in quick out."
   - *Salpingectomy* is the definitive surgery. The excised tube should be sent for histological examination (Fig. 8.11).
   - The ipsilateral ovary and its vascular supply is preserved. Oophorectomy is done only if the ovary is damaged beyond salvage or is pathological
   - Place of subtotal hysterectomy: In interstitial pregnancy, the rupture rent is so big and the general condition is so low that, most often, a quick subtotal hysterectomy is done. However, if the condition permits and the uterine conservation is desirable, resection of the uterus may be attempted.

Place of autotransfusion: Its routine use is not advocated because of its adverse reaction. In case, where donated blood is not available, the fresh blood from the peritoneal cavity may be collected for auto transfusion. The collection is done through strainer consisting of 4–5 layers of sterile gauze pieces into a bottle containing citrate solution (3.8%) in the proportion of five parts of blood to one part of citrate solution.

CHRONIC ECTOPIC

All cases of chronic or suspected ectopic are to be admitted as an emergency. The patient is

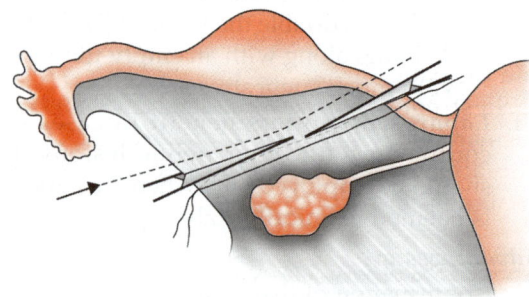

Fig. 8.11: Salpingectomy. Note the placement of the clamps

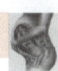

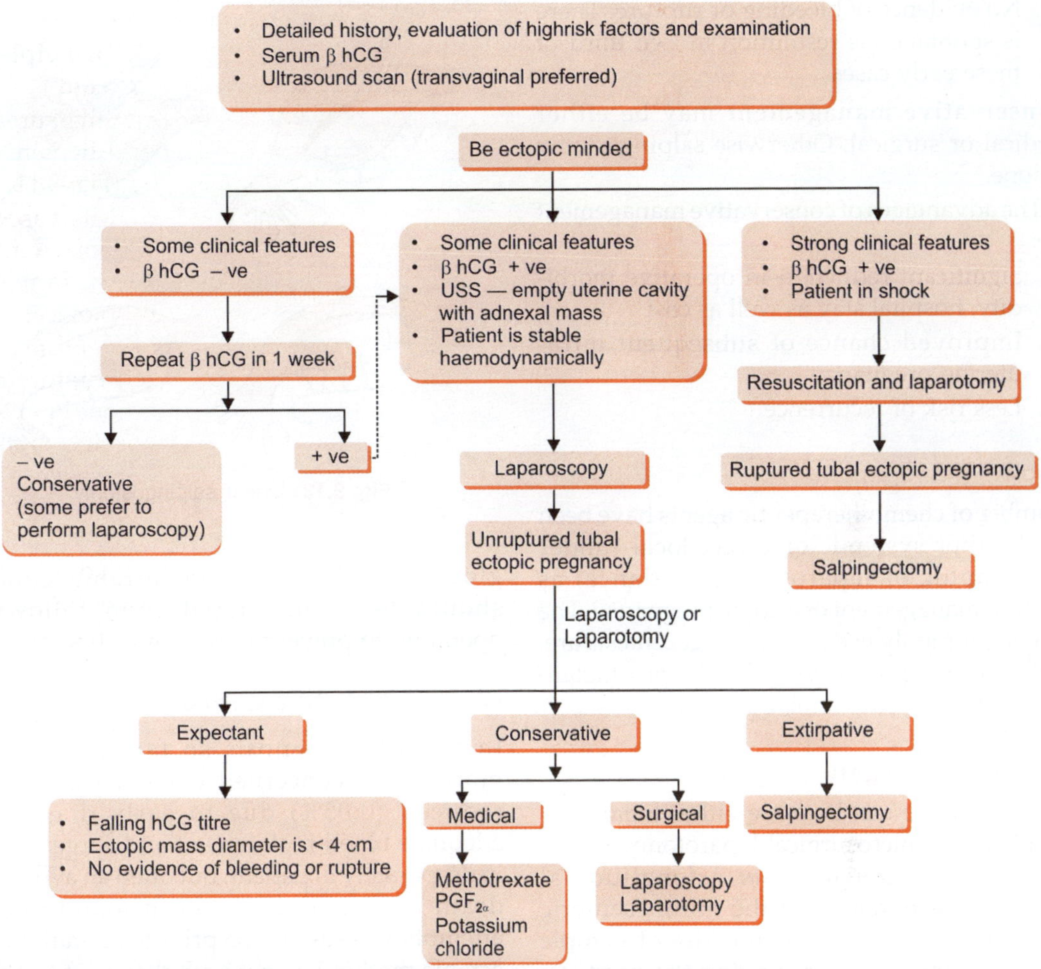

- Detailed history, evaluation of highrisk factors and examination
- Serum β hCG
- Ultrasound scan (transvaginal preferred)

Be ectopic minded

- Some clinical features
- β hCG – ve

- Some clinical features
- β hCG + ve
- USS — empty uterine cavity with adnexal mass
- Patient is stable haemodynamically

- Strong clinical features
- β hCG + ve
- Patient in shock

Repeat β hCG in 1 week

Resuscitation and laparotomy

– ve
Conservative
(some prefer to perform laparoscopy)

+ ve

Laparoscopy

Ruptured tubal ectopic pregnancy

Unruptured tubal ectopic pregnancy

Salpingectomy

Laparoscopy or Laparotomy

Expectant

Conservative

Extirpative

- Falling hCG titre
- Ectopic mass diameter is < 4 cm
- No evidence of bleeding or rupture

Medical

Surgical

Salpingectomy

Methotrexate
PGF$_{2\alpha}$
Potassium chloride

Laparoscopy
Laparotomy

Fig. 8.12: Scheme of management of tubal ectopic pregnancy

kept under observation, investigations are done and the patient is put up for laparotomy at the earliest convenient time. Usually a pelvic haematocele is found. Blood clots are removed. The affected tube is identified and salpingectomy is commonly done.

Resumption of ovulation and contraception: About 15% of women ovulate by 19 days and about 25% ovulate by the 30th postoperative day. Contraception should ideally be commenced at the time of hospital discharge.

UNRUPTURED TUBAL PREGNANCY

Management

- Expectant
- Conservative
- Salpingectomy

Expectant management: Where only observation is done hoping spontaneous resolution. Indications are:
1. Falling hCG titre
2. Ectopic mass < 4 cm

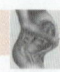

3. No evidence of bleeding or rupture. There is spontaneous resolution in two third of these early cases.

Conservative management may be either medical or surgical. Otherwise salpingectomy is done.

The advantages of conservative management are:

1. Significant reduction in operative morbidity, hospital stay as well as cost
2. Improved chance of subsequent intrauterine pregnancy
3. Less risk of recurrence

Medical management

Number of chemotherapeutic agents have been used either systemic or direct local (under sonographic or laparoscopic guidance) as medical management of ectopic pregnancy. The drugs commonly used for salpingocentesis are: methotrexate, potassium chloride, prostaglandin ($PGF_{2\alpha}$), hyperosmolar glucose.

Conservative surgery

The procedure can be done either laparoscopically or by microsurgical laparotomy.

1. *Linear salpingostomy:* A longitudinal incision is made on the antimesenteric border directly over the site of ectopic pregnancy. After removing the products (by fingers, scalpel handle or by suction), the incision line is kept open to be healed later on by secondary intention. Haemostasis is achieved by electrocautery or laser (Fig. 8.13).
2. *Segmental resection:* This is of choice in isthmic pregnancy. End to end anastomosis can be done immediately or at a later date after appropriate counselling of the patient.
3. *Salpingectomy* is done when whole of the tube damaged

Rh negative women: In Rh negative women not yet sensitized to Rh antigen, anti-D gamma

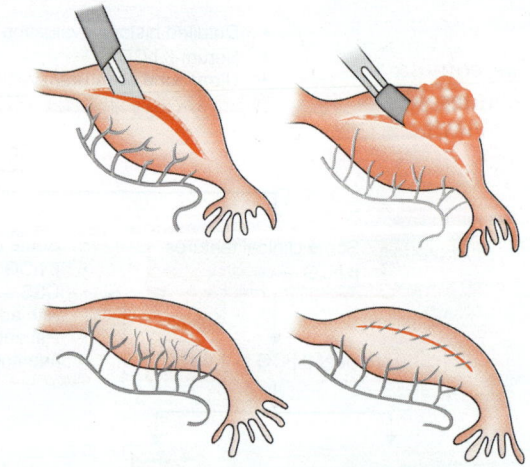

Fig. 8.13: Linear salpingostomy

globulin—50 microgram intramuscularly should be administered soon following operation to prevent isoimmunization.

PROGNOSIS OF TUBAL PREGNANCY

Immediate prognosis so far as maternal mortality is concerned has been markedly reduced (0.05%) due to early diagnosis, adequate blood replacement and surgery even in desperately ill patient. But often an avoidable death from ectopic has been found due to attempts at resuscitation prior to operation. An ectopic mother has got ever chance of a viable birth in 1 in 3 and a chance of recurrence of ectopic in 1 in 10.

GESTATIONAL TROPHOBLASTIC DISEASES (GTDs)

Definition

The GTDs refers to the spectrum of proliferative abnormalities of the trophoblast associated with pregnancy. Contrary to normal pregnancy, in GTDs abnormal growth and development of the trophoblast continues even beyond the end of pregnancy.

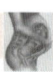

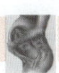

Classification (Box 8.2)

The conventional histological classification, includes—hydatidiform mole, invasive mole and choriocarcinoma.

Box 8.2: Classification of GTDs

- Hydatidiform mole
  - Complete or classic mole
  - Incomplete or partial mole
- Gestational trophoblastic neoplasia (GTN)
  - Persistent trophoblastic disease
  - Placental site trophoblastic tumour
  - Invasive mole
  - Choriocarcinoma
- Nonmetastatic   • Metastatic
  - Low-risk—good prognosis
  - High-risk—poor prognosis

HYDATIDIFORM MOLE (SYN: VESICULAR MOLE)

Types

- Complete
- Incomplete

Definition (Figs 8.14 and 8.15)

It is an abnormal condition of the ovum where there are partly degeneration and partly hyperplastic changes in the young chorionic villi. These result in the formation of clusters of small cysts of varying sizes. Because of its superficial resemblance to hydatid cyst, it is named as hydatidiform mole. It is best regarded as a benign neoplasia of the chorion with malignant potential.

Incidence

The molar pregnancy is common in Oriental Countries—Philippines, China, Indonesia, Japan, India, Central and Latin America and Africa. *The highest incidence is in Philippines being 1 in 80 pregnancies* and lowest in European countries and USA being about 1 in 2000. The incidence, in India, is about *1 in 400.*

Etiology

The cause is not definitely known, but it appears to be related to the *ovular defect* as it sometimes affects one ovum of a twin pregnancy. However, the following factors and hypotheses have been forwarded:

- Its prevalence is highest in teenage pregnancies and in those women over 35 years of age.
- The prevalence appears to vary with race and ethnic origin.
- Faulty nutrition caused by inadequate intake of high class protein could partly explain its prevalence in the Oriental Countries. Low dietary intake of carotene is associated with increased risk.

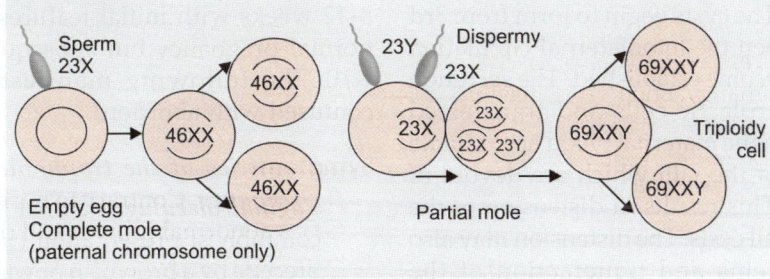

Fig. 8.14: Chromosome of hydatidiform mole

 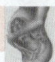

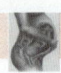

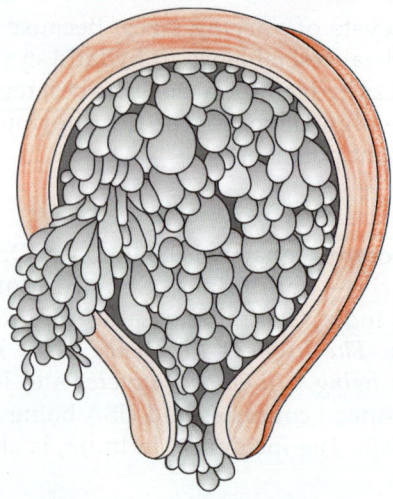

Fig. 8.15: Hydatidiform mole

- Disturbed maternal immune mechanisms suggested by:
  - Rise in gammaglobulin level in absence of hepatic disease
  - Increased association of AB blood group which possesses no ABO antibody.
- Cytogenetic abnormality: *In general, complete moles have a 46, XX karyotype, the molar chromosomes are derived entirely from the father.*
- History of prior hydatidiform mole increases the chance of recurrence.

Pathology

It is principally a disease of the chorion. Death of the ovum or failure of the embryo to grow is essential to develop complete (classic) hydatidiform mole. The cysts begin to form from 3rd to 5th week when the fetomaternal circulation normally has become established. The secretion from the hyperplastic cells and transferred substances from the maternal blood accumulate in the stroma of the villi which are devoid of blood vessels. This results in distension of the villi to form small cysts. The distension may also be due to oedema and liquefaction of the stroma. *Vesicle fluid is interstitial fluid and is almost similar to ascitic or oedema fluid, but rich in hCG.*

NAKED EYE APPEARANCE

The mass filling the uterus is made of multiple chains and clusters of cysts of varying sizes. *There is no trace of embryo or the amniotic sac.* Hemorrhage, if occurs, takes place in the decidual space.

MICROSCOPIC APPEARANCE

The basic findings are
1. There is marked proliferation of the syncytial and cytotrophoblastic epithelium.
2. Marked thinning of the stromal tissue due to accumulation of fluid.
3. There is absence of blood vessels which seems primary rather than due to pressure atrophy.
4. The villus pattern is distinctly maintained.

OVARIAN CHANGES

Bilateral lutein cysts are present in about 50 percent. These are due to excessive production of chorionic gonadotrophin. These regress spontaneously within two months after expulsion of mole. The contained fluid is rich in chorionic gonadotrophin. *It also contains oestrogen and progesterone.*

Clinical features

Age and parity: It is prevalent amongst teenaged and elderly patients with high parity. The patient gives history of amenorrhoea of 8–12 weeks with initial features suggestive of normal pregnancy but subsequently presents with the following manifestations (often confused with abortion).

Symptoms

- *Vaginal bleeding:* Vaginal bleeding is the commonest presentation (90%). It may be precede by a brownish or watery discharge. The blood may be mixed with fluid from

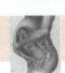

ruptured cyst giving the appearance of discharge "white currant in red currant juice".

- *Varying degree of lower abdominal pain may be due to*
  - Over distension of the uterus
  - Concealed hemorrhage
  - Rarely perforation of the uterus by the invasive mole
  - Infection
  - Uterine contractions to expel out the contents.
- **Constitutional symptoms**
  - *The patient becomes sick* without any apparent reason.
  - *Vomiting of pregnancy becomes excessive* to the stage of hyperemesis in 15% cases. It is probably related to excess chorionic gonadotrophin.
  - *Breathlessness* due to pulmonary embolisation of the trophoblastic cells (2%).
  - *Thyrotoxic features* of tremors or tachycardia are present on occasion (10%). It is probably due to increased chorionic thyrotrophin.
- *Expulsion of grape-like vesicles per vaginam is diagnostic of vesicular mole.* Actually, in approximately 50% of cases the mole is not suspected until it is expelled in part or whole.
- History of quickening is absent.

Signs

- Features suggestive of early months of pregnancy are evident.
- *The patient looks more ill* than can be accounted for.
- *Pallor* is unusually prominent, out of proportion to the visible blood loss and may be due to concealed hemorrhage.
- *Features of pre-eclampsia* (hypertension, oedema and/or proteinuria) are present in about 50%. On rare occasion, convulsion may occur. The pre-eclamptic process may be due to over distension of the uterus or

more probably, due to hyperactivity of the trophoblastic cells.

Per abdomen

- *The size of the uterus* is more than that expected for the period of amenorrhoea in 70%, corresponds with the period of amenorrhoea in 20% and smaller than the period of amenorrhoea in 10%. The frequent findings of undue enlargement of the uterus is due to exuberant growth of the vesicles and the concealed hemorrhage.
- *The feel of the uterus* is firm elastic (doughy). This is due to the absence of the amniotic fluid sac.
- *Fetal parts* are not felt, nor any fetal movements. External ballottement cannot be elicited.
- *Absence of fetal heart sound* which cannot be detected even by the Doppler effect cardioscope.

Vaginal examination

- *Internal ballottement* can not be elicited.
- *Unilateral or bilateral enlargement (theca lutein cyst) of the ovary* may be palpable in 25–50% of cases. The enlarged ovary may not be palpable due to the enlarged uterus.
- *Finding of vesicles* in the vaginal discharge is pathognomonic of hydatidiform mole.
- If the cervical os is open, instead of the membranes, blood clot or the vesicles may be felt.

Investigations

- Full blood count, ABO and Rh grouping.
- Hepatic, renal and thyroid function tests are carried out.
- *Sonography:* Characteristic echogram of molar pregnancy is 'snow storm' appearance (Fig. 8.16).
- *Quantitative estimation of chorionic gonadotrophin:* High hCG titre in urine diluted up to 1 in 200 to 1 in 500 beyond 100 days of gestation is very much suggestive.

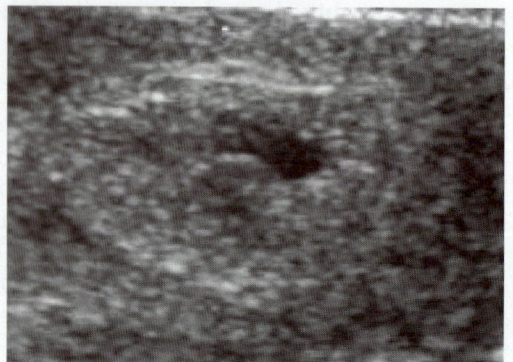

Fig. 8.16: 'Snow storm' appearance of hydatidiform mole

- *Straight X-ray abdomen:* If the uterine size is more than 16 weeks, a negative fetal shadow may be of help.

COMPLICATIONS

Immediate

1. *Hemorrhage and shock*: The causes of hemorrhage are:
   a. Separation of the vesicles from its attachment to the decidua. The hemorrhage may be concealed or revealed.
   b. Massive intraperitoneal hemorrhage which may be the first feature of a perforating mole.
   c. During evacuation of the mole due to
      - Atonic uterus
      - Uterine injury

2. **Sepsis:** The increased risk of sepsis is due to:
   a. As there are no protective membranes, the vaginal organisms can creep up into the uterine cavity.
   b. Presence of degenerated vesicles, sloughing decidua and old blood favours nidation of bacterial growth.
   c. Lowered body resistance due to chronic blood loss and associated pre-eclampsia.
   d. Increased operative interference.

3. **Perforation of the uterus:** The uterus may be injured due to
   a. Perforating mole—which may produce massive intraperitoneal hemorrhage,
   b. During vaginal evacuation specially by conventional (D & E) method or during curettage following suction evacuation.

4. **Pre-eclampsia** with convulsion on rare occasion.

5. **Acute pulmonary insufficiency due to** pulmonary embolisation of the trophoblastic cells with or without villi stroma. Symptoms usually begins within 4–6 hours following evacuation.

6. **Coagulation failure** due to pulmonary embolisation of trophoblastic cells as they cause fibrin and platelet deposition within the vascular tree.

Late: **The development of choriocarcinoma** following hydatidiform mole ranges between **2–10%. The following are the known risk factors** which are more likely to be associated with the malignant changes.

- Patients above the age of 35 irrespective of parity
- Patients having previous 3 or more births irrespective of age. Age is probably more important than the parity.
- Initial hCG levels in urine of over 100,000 I.U./24 hours.
- Histologically proven infiltrative mole
- Previous history of molar pregnancy
- A women with group A or AB with husband group O.

Prognosis

Immediate risk from hemorrhage and sepsis are markedly diminished due to blood transfusion and antibiotics.

Management

The principles in the management are:
- To give adequate supportive therapy to restore the blood loss.

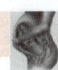

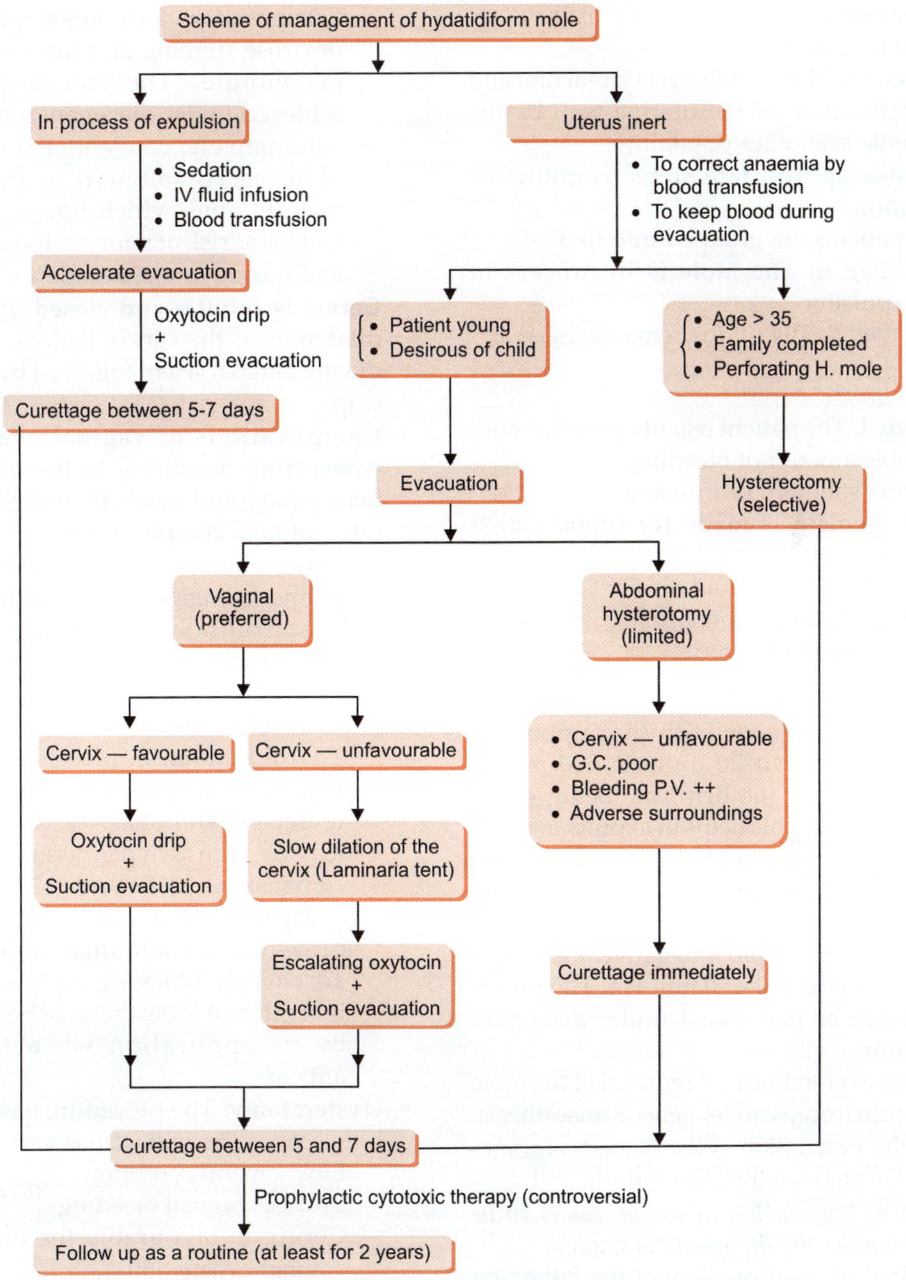

Scheme of management of hydatidiform mole

In process of expulsion
- Sedation
- IV fluid infusion
- Blood transfusion

Accelerate evacuation

Oxytocin drip
+
Suction evacuation

Curettage between 5-7 days

Uterus inert
- To correct anaemia by blood transfusion
- To keep blood during evacuation

- Patient young
- Desirous of child

- Age > 35
- Family completed
- Perforating H. mole

Evacuation

Hysterectomy (selective)

Vaginal (preferred)

Abdominal hysterotomy (limited)

Cervix — favourable

Cervix — unfavourable

- Cervix — unfavourable
- G.C. poor
- Bleeding P.V. ++
- Adverse surroundings

Oxytocin drip + Suction evacuation

Slow dilation of the cervix (Laminaria tent)

Escalating oxytocin + Suction evacuation

Curettage immediately

Curettage between 5 and 7 days

Prophylactic cytotoxic therapy (controversial)

Follow up as a routine (at least for 2 years)

Fig. 8.17: Scheme of management of hydatidiform mole

- To evacuate the uterus as soon as the diagnosis is made:
  - As risk of hemorrhage is a real one and
  - Perforation of the uterine wall by the mole is another possibility.
- To take appropriate steps to minimise infection.
- The patients are grouped into two
  - *Group A:* The mole is in process of expulsion.
  - *Group B:* The uterus remains inert.

SUPPORTIVE THERAPY

- *Group A:* The patient usually presents with variable amount of bleeding.
- Ringers solution, IV infusion
- Arrangement is made for blood transfusion.
- *Group B:* Blood should also be kept ready prior to elective termination.
- Evacuation of the uterus

Definitive management

Group A: Simultaneous with the supportive therapy, oxytocin 10–20 units in 500 ml 5% dextrose is set up, the drip rate being 40–60 drops per minute. This helps in expulsion of the mole with minimal blood loss. The expulsion process is enhanced by any of the following methods.

- *Suction evacuation:* A negative pressure is applied up to 200–250 mm Hg. The procedure can be performed under diazepam sedation.
- Digital exploration and removal of the mole by ovum forceps under general anaesthesia.

After the evacuation is completed, ergometrine 0.2 mg is given intramuscularly.

Group B: *Evacuation of the uterus is to be done as soon as the diagnosis is made.*

- **Vaginal evacuation:** Any of the following methods of termination may be followed
- **Cervix is favourable**
  - *The preferred method is suction evacuation supplemented by oxytocin drip*

(20 units of oxytocin in 500 ml 5 percent dextrose running at a rate of 30 drops per minute). The procedure can be achieved under diazepam sedation,
  - Alternatively, conventional dilatation of the cervix followed by evacuation may be done which however carries increased risk of injury to the soft cervix and incomplete evacuation.
- **Cervix is tubular and closed:** Prior slow dilatation of the cervix is done by introducing laminaria tent followed by oxytocin drip.
- **Complications of vaginal evacuation:** Apart from the injury to the uterus and hemorrhage and shock, there are two more rare but fatal complications
  - Acute pulmonary insufficiency due to pulmonary embolisation of the trophoblastic cells. Symptoms of acute chest pain, tachycardia, tachypnoea and dyspnoea develop about 4–6 hours following evacuation.
  - **Thyroid storm:** In presence of hyperthyroid state when evacuation is done under general anaesthesia, the acute features such as hyperthermia, delirium, convulsions, coma and cardiovascular collapse develop. The condition can be prevented by administration of beta adrenergic blocking agents prior to induction of anaesthesia or be corrected by its application when the state appears.
- **Hysterotomy:** The procedure has got very little scope. *The indications are*
  - Low general condition
  - Profuse vaginal bleeding
  - Cervix unfavourable for immediate vaginal evacuation
  - Unfavourable surroundings.

The advantages are
- Less blood loss in the evacuation procedure
- Complete evacuation ensured

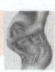

- Better control of post evacuation atonic uterus, if occurs
- Curettage can be done effectively in the same sitting.
- **Hysterectomy:** This is indicated in
- Patients with age over 35
- Patients completed the family irrespective of age. These are definitely high risk patients as far as the development of future malignancy is concerned. The operation is applicable to the same patient profile with spontaneous expulsion of mole and the surgery is to be done within 5 days.

Following evacuation anti-D immuno-globulin should be given to the Rh negative nonimmunised patient.

Follow-up

Routine follow up is mandatory to all cases for at least 1 year. The prime objective is to diag-nose persistent trophoblastic proliferation that is considered malignant. The occurrence of choriocarcinoma is mostly confined to this period.

Follow-up protocols

The follow-up protocols include
1. History and clinical examination
2. hCG assay
3. Chest X-ray

Methods employed in each visit

1. *Enquire* about relevant symptoms like irregular vaginal bleeding, persistent cough, breathlessness or hemoptysis.
2. *Abdominovaginal examination to note*
   - Involution of the uterus
   - Ovarian size and
   - Malignant deposit if any, in the anterior vaginal wall. The lutein cysts usually regress within two months.

3. *Investigations*
   - *Detection of hCG in urine or serum:* Urine or serum assays are carried out at every visit.
   - *Chest X-ray:* Atleast monthly till the hCG level becomes normal. Thereafter, it should be done at 3, 6 and 12 months following evacuation of mole.
   - *To repeat uterine curettage*
     - Sub-involution of the uterus without any evidence of fall in hCG titre.
     - Continued or reappearance of irre-gular bleeding.
     - hCG titre remains positive even after 6 weeks following evacuation.

Nursing diagnosis

1. **Risk for fluid volume deficit related to evacuation of hydatidiform mole.**
   Interventions
   1. Monitor vital signs and blood pressure.
   2. Monitor amount of bleeding by menstrual pad count and/on weight.
   3. Obtain preoperative laboratory work ordered.
      a. CBC
      b. Quantitative beta-hCG
      c. Clotting studies; platelets, fibrinogen.
      d. Urinalysis.
      e. Chest X-ray
   4. Begin or maintain IV line with 18 gauge or larger intracatheter.
   5. Administer ordered IV fluids for volu-me expansion without overloading.
   6. Careful intake and output.

2. **Grief related to loss of pregnancy.**
   Interventions
   1. Encourage verbalization of client's feelings.
   2. Assist client/family in identifying coping mechanisms.
   3. Be realistic with information given.
   4. Allow client/family to participate in plan of care whenever possible.

3. **Risk for altered health maintenance related to insufficient knowledge of trophoblastic disease.**

Interventions

1. Encourage compliance with a close follow-up regimen.
   a. Ultrasound test often are repeated, especially of bleeding recurs.
   b. Maternal status
      1. Hypovolemia
      2. Anemia
      3. Coagulopathy
      4. Fatigue
      5. Signs of labour
      6. Avoidance of coitus.
2. Discuss contraceptive options to prevent pregnancy for 1 year

4. **Anxiety related to fear of carcinoma secondary to trophoblastic disease.**

Interventions

1. Encourage client to verbalize concerns
2. Clarify the relatively low risk of conversion to carcinoma.

ANTEPARTUM HAEMORRHAGE

Definition

It is defined as bleeding from or into the genital tract after the 28th week of pregnancy but before the birth of the baby. The incidence is about 3% amongst hospital deliveries.

Causes (Fig. 8.18)

The causes of antepartum haemorrhage fall into the following categories.

PLACENTA PRAEVIA

Definition

When the placenta is implanted partially or completely over the lower uterine segment it is called placenta praevia.

Incidence

About one-third cases of antepartum haemorrhage belong to placenta praevia. The incidence of placenta praevia ranges from 0.5–1% amongst hospital deliveries. In 80% cases, it is found to multiparous women. The incidence is increased beyond the age of 35, with high birth order pregnancies and in multiple pregnancy.

Etiology

The exact cause of implantation of the placenta in the lower segment is not known. *The following theories are postulated.*

- *Dropping down theory:* The fertilized ovum drops down and is implanted in the lower segment. Poor decidual reaction in the upper uterine segment may be the cause. Failure of zona pellucida to disappear in time can be hypothetical possibility.

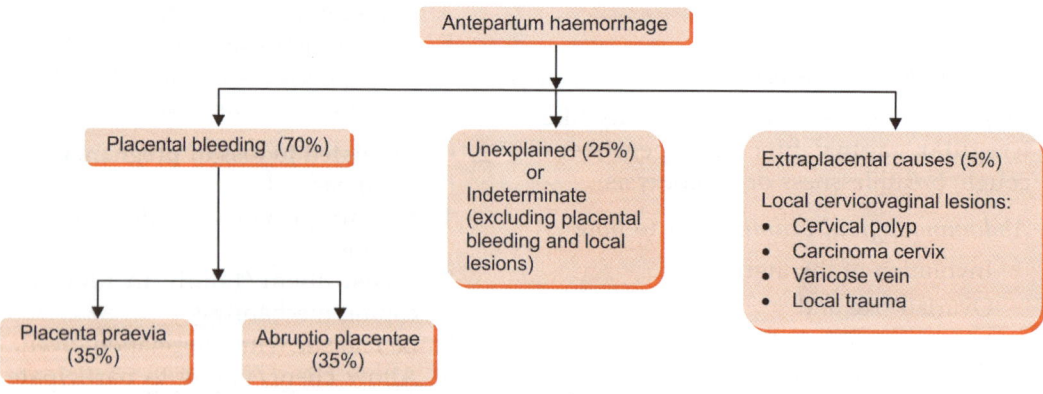

Fig. 8.18: Causes of antepartum haemorrhage

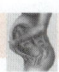

- *Persistence of chronic activity* in the decidua capsularis.
- *Defective decidua,* results in spreading of the chronic villi over a wide area in the uterine wall to get nourishment.
- *Big surface area of the placenta* as in twins may encroach onto lower segment.

The predisposing factors for placenta praevia are

1. Multiparity
2. Increased maternal age
3. History of previous caesarean section or any other scar in the uterus (myomectomy)
4. Placental size and abnormality (succenturiate lobes).

Types of degrees (Fig. 8.19)

Four degrees are presently recognised.

Degree I; Lam (incomplete or partial placenta praevia): The placenta covers the internal os when it is closed, but partially covers it when fully dilated.

Degree IV (central or total placenta praevia): The placenta completely covers the internal os even after it is fully dilated.

For clinical purpose, the types are graded into mild degree (type-I and II anterior) and major degree (type-II posterior, III and IV).

Dangerous placenta praevia is the name given to the type II posterior placenta praevia.

1. Because of the curved birth canal major thickness of the placenta (about 2.5 cm) overlies the sacral, promontory, thereby diminishing the anteroposterior diameter of the inlet and prevents engagement of the presenting part. This hinders effective compression of the separated placenta to stop bleeding.
2. Placenta is more likely to be compressed, if vaginal delivery is allowed.
3. More chance of cord compression or cord prolapse. The last two may produce fetal anoxia or even death.

Clinical features

Symptoms

1. Bleeding per vagina is painless apparently causeless and recurrent. Bleeding starts spontaneously often during sleep. The first attack of bleeding starts any time from 28th week, till delivery with highest incidence at 36–38 weeks of pregnancy and may cease spontaneously within a few hours.
2. Pain in abdomen is absent unless spontaneous labour ensures.

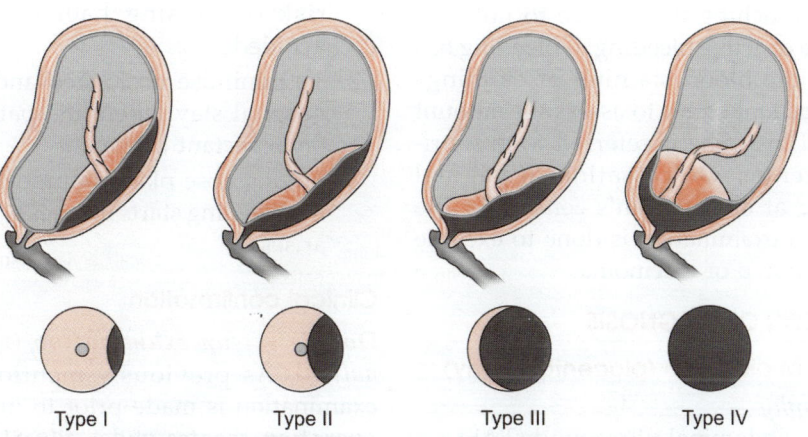

Fig. 8.19: Degrees of placenta praevia with findings on vaginal examination

Type I   Type II   Type III   Type IV

 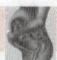

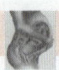

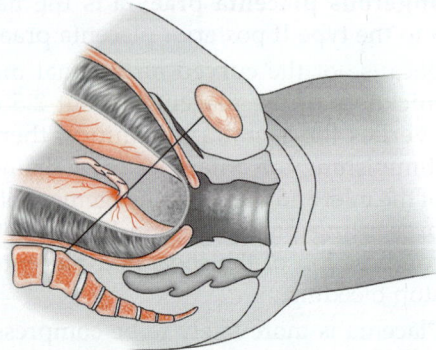

Fig. 8.20: Type II posterior placenta praevia. Note the effective reduction of the anteroposterior diameter of the inlet in contrast to type II anterior

Signs
1. Patient shows evidence of late pregnancy
2. Evidences of blood loss, e.g. shock and/or anemia may be present depending on the degree of haemorrhage.
3. Per abdomen: Obstetric findings—the abdomen is soft and the uterus is of normal consistency. The foetus is felt normally; the presenting part remains usually non engaged. Malpresentations or unstable lie are more commonly encountered. F.H.S. is audible except in cases of marked separation of the placenta where it is absent.
4. Vulval inspection (only looking at vulva but not touching it) is made to note the presence of active bleeding; if bleeding has ceased, the blood staining of clothings should be looked for to assess the amount of blood loss. She is referred to obstetrician's center. On cessation of vaginal bleeding at obstetrician's centre, gentile speculum examination is done to exclude cervical polyp or carcinoma.

CONFIRMATION OF DIAGNOSIS

Localisation of placenta (placentography)

1. *Sonography*
   - Trans abdominal ultrasound (TAS)
   - Transvaginal ultrasound (TVS)
   - Transperineal ultrasound
   - Colour Doppler flow study
2. *Magnetic resonance imaging* (MRI)
3. *Radiography* (rarely done)
   - Soft tissue radiography
   - Displacement radiography
4. *Radioactive isotopes*
   Iodine 132 or 131 or Technetium 99 (*obsolete*)

Clinical

- By internal examination (double set up examination)
- Direct visualization during caesarean section
- Examination of the placenta following vaginal delivery.

PLACENTOGRAPHY

Sonography: Sonography provides the simplest, most precise and safest method of placental localisation.

In addition, it is helpful for assessing the fetal size and status.

Advantages

The advantages of such investigations are:
1. Diagnostic vaginal examination with the risk of causing haemorrhage can be avoided.
2. To minimise prolonged and unnecessary hospital stay where the patient is placed on expectant treatment.
3. To diagnose placenta praevia even before the bleeding starts in cases where suspicion arises.

Clinical confirmation

Double set-up examination (*vaginal examination*): As previously mentioned, vaginal examination is made prior to inference *in the operation theatre under anaesthesia keeping everything ready for caesarean section.*

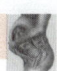

Palpation of the placenta on the lower segment not only conclusively confirms the clinical diagnosis but also identifies its degree.

Visualization of the placenta implantation on the lower segment can be confirmed during caesarean section.

Examination of the placenta following vaginal delivery reveals

1. A tongue shaped comparatively thin segment of placental tissue projecting beyond the main placental mass with evidences of degeneration.
2. Rent on the membranes is situated on the margin of the placenta.
3. Abnormal attachment of the cord (marginal or membranous) is more common.

COMPLICATIONS

Maternal

During pregnancy

1. *Antepartum haemorrhage with varying degrees of shock* is an available complication of placenta praevia.
2. *Malpresentation* is common.
3. *Premature labour* either spontaneous or induced is common.

During labour: The following complications occur:

1. *Early rupture of the membranes*
2. *Cord prolapse* is due to abnormal attachment of the cord.
3. *Slow dilatation* of the cervix
4. *Intrapartum haemorrhage* may occur due to further separation of placenta with dilatation of the cervix.
5. *Increased incidence of operative interference*
6. *Postpartum haemorrhage is due to*
   - *Imperfect retraction* of the lower uterine segment on which the placenta is implanted.
   - *Large surface area of placenta* with atonic uterus due to pre-existing anaemia.

- Occasional association of *morbidly adherent placenta on the lower segment.*
- *Trauma to the cervix and lower segment* because of extreme softness and vascularity.

7. *Retained placenta is due to*
   - Increased surface area
   - Morbid adhesion

Puerperium

1. *Sepsis is increased due to*
   - Increased operative interference
   - Placental site near to the vagina
   - Anaemia and devitalised state of the patient
2. *Subinvolution*
3. *Embolism*

Fetal

1. *Low birth weight* babies are quite common which may be the effect of preterm labour either spontaneous or induced.
2. *Asphyxia* is common and it may be the effect of
   - Early separation of placenta.
   - Compression of the placenta.
   - Compression of the cord.
3. *Intrauterine death*
4. Birth injuries are more common due to increased operative interference.
5. *Congenital malformation* is three times more common in placenta praevia.

PROGNOSIS

Maternal

There has been a substantial *reduction of maternal deaths* in placenta praevia throughout the globe but more appreciably noticed in the developed countries. *But in the developing countries,* because of wide gaps in the extension of the medical facilities and also the difference in patients profile between the urban and the vast rural population (70% of the population). Inadequate antenatal care, delay in referral,

 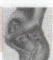

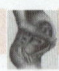

road and transport difficulties contribute to the poor outcome. *The ultimate causes of death are haemorrhage and shock.*

The **morbidity** is somewhat raised due to operative delivery.

Fetal

The reduction of the perinatal mortality is not so gratifying as compared to that of maternal mortality. *The reduction of deaths is principally due to* judicious extension of expectant treatment thereby reducing the loss from prematurity, liberal use of caesarean section which greatly lessens the loss from anoxia and improvement in the neonatal care unit. But still the perinatal mortality ranges from 10 to 25%. *The causes of death are*

1. Prematurity
2. Asphyxia
3. Congenital malformation.

MANAGEMENT

Prevention

Placenta praevia is one of the inherent obstetric hazards. *Thus to minimise the risks, the following guidelines are useful.*

- *Adequate antenatal care* to improve the health status of women, specially correction of anaemia, so that the patient can withstand blood loss.
- *Antenatal diagnosis* of low lying placenta at 20 weeks with routine ultra sound needs repeat ultra sound examination at 34 weeks to confirm the diagnosis.
- *Significance of warning haemorrhage* should not be ignored or underestimated.
- *Family planning and limitation of births* have been proved to lower the incidence of placenta praevia in the hospital statistics.

At home

1. The patient is immediately *put to bed rest.*
2. Injection *morphine* 15 mg is given intramuscularly.

3. *To assess the blood loss*
   - Inspection of the clothings soaked with blood.
   - To note the pulse, blood pressure and degree of anaemia.

4. *Quick but gentle abdominal examination* to mark the height of the uterus, to auscultate the fetal heart sound and to note any tenderness on the uterus.

5. *Vaginal examination must not be done.* Only inspection is done to see whether the bleeding continues or ceases and to put a sterile vulval pad.

Transfer to hospital

Arrangement is made to shift the patient to an equipped hospital (having facilities of blood transfusion, emergency caesarean section and neonatal care unit). If the patient is transferred to a peripheral health centre she should be shifted to a specialised centre at the earliest opportunity. An intravenous dextrose-saline drip should be started in the health centre if the patient had significant amount of haemorrhage and kept running during transport. Patient should be accompanied by two or three persons fit for donation of blood, if necessary.

ABRUPTIO PLACENTAE

Definition

It is one form of antepartum haemorrhage where the bleeding occurs due to premature separation of normally situated placenta. Out of the various nomenclatures, abruptio placentae seems to be appropriate one.

Incidence

Hospital records show incidence of 1 in 250 deliveries. Multigravida shows higher incidence. It is prone to recur. In two-thirds abruption occurs before 36 weeks.

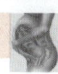

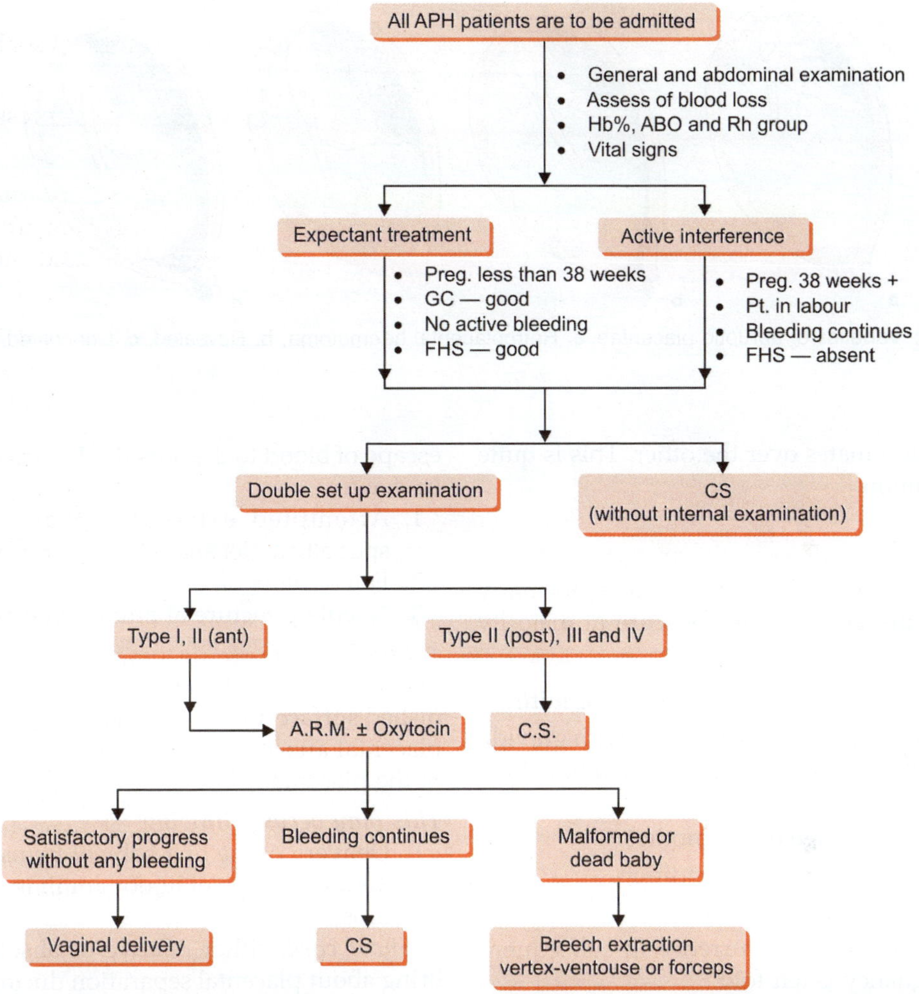

All APH patients are to be admitted

- General and abdominal examination
- Assess of blood loss
- Hb%, ABO and Rh group
- Vital signs

Expectant treatment

- Preg. less than 38 weeks
- GC — good
- No active bleeding
- FHS — good

Active interference

- Preg. 38 weeks +
- Pt. in labour
- Bleeding continues
- FHS — absent

Double set up examination

CS
(without internal examination)

Type I, II (ant)

Type II (post), III and IV

A.R.M. ± Oxytocin

C.S.

Satisfactory progress
without any bleeding

Bleeding continues

Malformed or
dead baby

Vaginal delivery

CS

Breech extraction
vertex-ventouse or forceps

Fig. 8.21: Scheme of management of placenta praevia in hospital

Varieties (Fig. 8.22)

1. *Revealed:* Following separation of the placenta, the blood insinuates downwards between the membranes and the decidua. Ultimately, the blood comes out of the cervical canal to be visible externally. This is the commonest type.
2. *Concealed:* The blood collects behind the separated placenta or collected in between the membranes and decidua. The collected blood is prevented from coming out of the cervix by the presenting part which presses on the lower segment. At times, the blood may percolate into the amniotic sac after rupturing the membranes. In any of the circumstances blood is not visible outside. This type is rare.
3. *Mixed:* In this type, some part of the blood collects inside (concealed) and a part is expelled out (revealed). Usually one variety

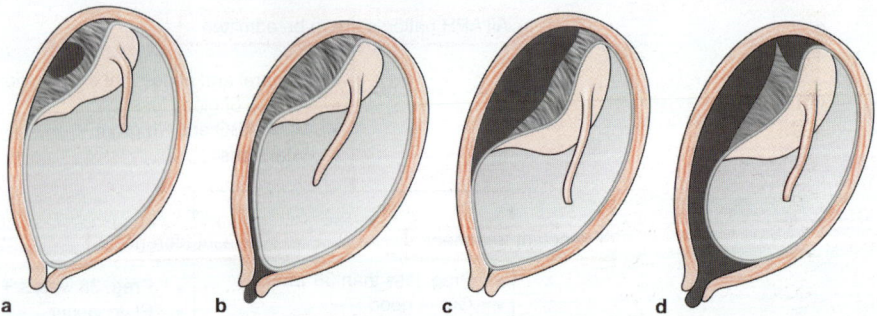

Fig. 8.22: Varieties of abruptio placentae. **a.** Retroplacental haematoma, **b.** Revealed, **c.** Concealed, **d.** Mixed

predominates over the other. This is quite common.

Etiology

The exact cause of separation of a normally situated placenta remains obscure in majority of cases.

The prevalence is more in association with

1. High birth order pregnancies with gravida 5 and above three times more common than in first birth
2. Advancing age of the mother
3. Poor socioeconomic condition
4. Malnutrition, smoking
5. A tendency of recurrence in subsequent pregnancy is ten-fold.

Relation with pre-eclampsia: The mechanism of the placental separation in pre-eclampsia is as follows. Spasm of the uterine vessels supplying the placental surface leads to capillary anoxia. This results in damage of the endothelium distal to the spasm. When the spasm disappears, the capillaries cannot cope with the blood flow which follows—resulting in extravasation of blood and subplacental haematoma. The initial separation may be central or marginal.

Trauma: Traumatic separation of the placenta usually leads to its marginal separation with escape of blood to the outside. *The trauma may be due to:*

1. Attempted external cephalic version specially under anaesthesia using great force
2. Fall or blow on the abdomen
3. Needle puncture at amniocentesis.

Sudden uterine decompression: Sudden decompression of the uterus leads to diminished surface area of the uterus adjacent to the placental attachment and results in separation of the placenta.

This may occur following

1. Delivery of the first baby of twins
2. Sudden escape of liquor amnii in hydramnios.

Short cord, either relative or absolute, can bring about placental separation during labour by mechanical pull.

Supine hypotension syndrome: In this condition which occurs in pregnancy there is passive engorgement of the uterine and placental vessels resulting in rupture and extravasation of the blood.

Folic acid deficiency: Deficiency of folic acid without evidence of overt megaloblastic erythropoiesis has been blamed to be the cause of separation of placenta.

Torsion of the uterine leads to increased venous pressure and rupture of the veins with separation of the placenta.

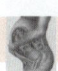

Clinical classification

Depending upon the degree of placental abruption and its clinical effects, the cases are graded as follows:

- **Grade 0:** Clinical feature suggestive of placental separation may be absent. The diagnosis is made after inspection of placenta following delivery.
- **Grade 1**
  - External bleeding is present.
  - Tenderness on the uterus may or may not be present.
  - **Shock is absent**
  - **FHS** is good
- **Grade 2**
  - External bleeding may or may not be present.
  - *Uterine tenderness is always present.*
  - Shock is absent.
  - *Fetal distress or even fetal death occurs.*
- **Grade 3**
  - External bleeding may or may not be present.
  - *Uterine tenderness is marked.*
  - Shock is pronounced
  - *Fetal death is the rule*
  - Associated coagulation defect or anuria may complicate.

Pathology

In mild cases (revealed type), a small blood clot can be adherent to the maternal surface of the placenta and on separation of the clot, the area is found to be depressed in placental maternal surface.

In severe concealed type (Couvelaire uterus) the retroplacental clot is large one; over and above, there are muscular and vascular injuries in the uterine wall especially at the site of the placental attachment. There are haemorrhagic infiltration from capillaries in the uterine musculature, oedema on the serous surface sometimes, free blood can be found in the peritoneal covering of the uterus, and necrosis in the muscles and also ecchymoses.

Changes in the liver and kidney: In severe type of abruptio placentae Fibrin knots, a thrombotic lesion in the hepatic sinusoids have been described specific of abruptio placentae.

Renal changes: oliguria and anuria may develop. These changes are those of acute tubular necrosis in mild form and renal cortical necrosis in severe form.

Coagulation failure: Defibrination and excess fibrinolysis: Certain unusual haemorrhages occur at needle puncture site, haematuria cutaneous ecchymoses, postpartum haemorrhage etc. About 5% abruptio placentae develops coagulation failure, excess fibrinolysis and haemorrhagic state. Coagulation failure is detected by prolonged coagulation time, lowered platelet, fibrinogen count and excess fibrinolysis by elevated fibrinogen-fibrin degradation products in serum. The latter is anticoagulant.

Clinical features

The clinical features depend on

1. Degree of separation of placenta
2. Speed at which separation occurs
3. Amount of blood concealed inside the uterine cavity. The clinical features of the revealed and mixed variety are given in tabulated form (Table 8.3).

Complications

Maternal

1. Shock due to haemorrhage and injury to the uterus.
2. Sepsis
3. Haemorrhage—antepartum, intrapartum and postpartum
4. Uterine rupture in Couvelaire uetrus
5. Coagulation defect
6. Anuria

Fetal risk

The fetal mortality in revealed type goes upto 25% but in concealed type it is 100%. The chief

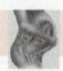

Table 8.3: Distinguishing features of placenta praevia and abruptio placentae

	Placenta praevia	Abruptio placentae
1. Clinical features		
• Nature of bleeding	• Painless, apparently causeless and recurrent • Bleeding is always revealed	• Painful, often attributed to pre-eclampsia or trauma and continuous • Revealed, concealed or usually mixed
• Character of blood	Bright red	Dark coloured
• General condition and anaemia	Proportionate to visible blood loss	Out of proportion to the visible blood loss in concealed or mixed variety.
• Features of pre-eclampsia	Not relevant	Present in one-third cases.
2. Abdominal examination		
• Height of uterus	Proportionate height	may be disproportionately enlarged in concealed type
• Feel of uterus	Soft and relaxed	May be tense, tender and rigid
• Malpresentation	Malpresentation is common. The head is high floating.	Unrelated, the head may be engaged
• FHS	Usually present	Usually absent specially in concealed type
3. Placentography	Placenta in lower segment	Placenta in upper segment.
4. Vaginal examination	Placenta is felt on the lower segment.	Placenta is not felt on lower segment Blood clots should not be confused with placenta.

factors for fetal mortality are prematurity and anoxia due to separation of the placenta.

Definitive treatment

- *Sedation* is ensured by giving Inj. morphine 15 mg intramuscularly.
- *Blood sample is taken* (as mentioned in revealed type).
- *To correct hypovolaemic shock*—normal saline or haemocele infusion with a wide bore cannula is started and arrangement is made for urgent massive fresh blood transfusion. Blood pressure is not a reliable guide to assess the shock, as it may be maintained at a deceptively high level due to severe degree of vasospasm or capillary bed blockage. *Blood transfusion prevents* ischaemic renal damage by maintaining blood pressure, prevents the blood coagulation disorders and ensures the patient to be in a better position to withstand postpartum haemorrhage.

- *Artificial rupture of the membranes* is to be done at the earliest moment if the membranes are found intact. Oxytocin drip should be started, if not contraindicated.

The advantages of amniotomy are

1. To expedite delivery
2. To minimise two other grave complications—renal cortical necrosis and blood coagulation disorders.

Vaginal delivery: Following rupture of the membranes with or without adding oxytocin,

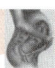

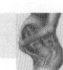

Table 8.4: Clinical features of revealed and mixed variety

	Revealed	Mixed (concealed features predominate)
Symptoms	Abdominal discomfort or pain followed by vaginal bleeding (usually slight)	The patient is seized with acute intense pain abdomen followed by slight vaginal bleeding. The pain becomes continuous.
• Character of bleeding	Continuous dark colour (slight to moderate)	Continuous, dark colour (usually slight) or blood stained serous discharge.
• General condition	Proportionate to the visible blood loss, shock is usually absent	* Shock is pronounced which is out of proportion to the visible blood loss.
• Pallor	Related with the visible blood loss	Pallor is usually severe and out of proportion to the visible bleeding.
• Features of pre-eclampsia	May be absent	Frequent association either pre-existing or appear.
• Uterine height	Proportionate to the period of gestation.	may be disproportionately enlarged and globular.
• Uterine feel	Normal feel with localised tenderness.	Uterus is tense, tender and rigid.
• Fetal parts	Can be identified easily	Difficult to make out.
• F.H.S.	Usually present	Usually absent
• Urine output	Normal	Usually diminished.

Investigations: Ultrasonography is less reliable for diagnosis, though retroplacental mass could be seen in some cases.

Laboratory

• Blood : Hb%	Low value proportionate to the blood loss	Markedly lower, out of proportion to the visible blood loss.
• Coagulation profile	Usually undisturbed	Variable disturbance • Clotting time increased • Fibrinogen level—low • Platelet count—low
• Urine for protein	May be absent	* * Usually present
• Confusion in diagnosis	With placenta praevia. As such vaginal examination is withheld unless certain in the diagnosis.	With acute obstetrical-gynaecological-surgical complication

*   **Shock:** While shock may be due to blood loss and hypovolaemia but disproportionate shock may appear in the same mechanism similar to that found in crush syndrome.

**   **Shock proteinuria:** It may be due to absorption of some autolytic substances from the separated placental tissue or may be the effect of intrarenal vasospasm.

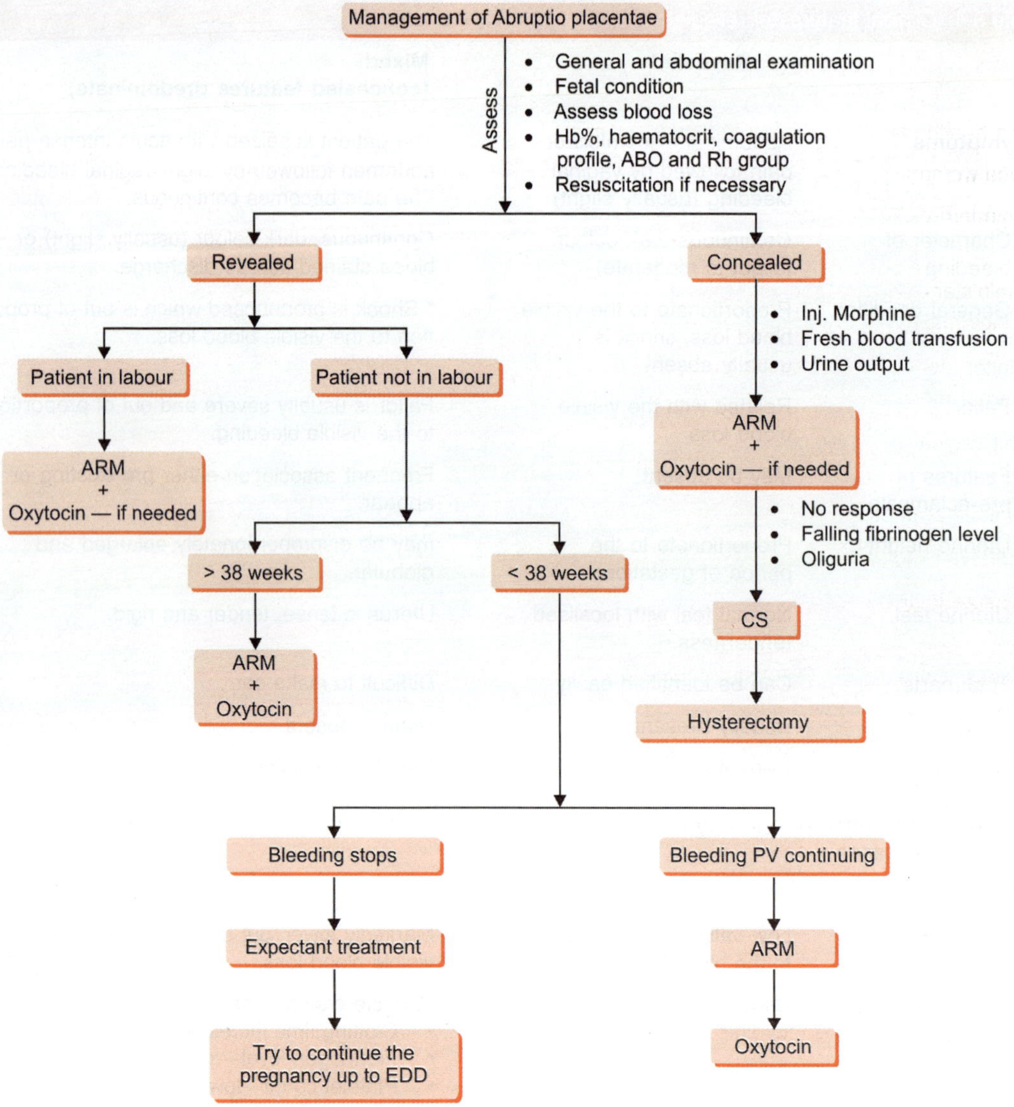

```
                    ┌─────────────────────────────────────┐
                    │   Management of Abruptio placentae   │
                    └─────────────────────────────────────┘
```

Assess
- General and abdominal examination
- Fetal condition
- Assess blood loss
- Hb%, haematocrit, coagulation profile, ABO and Rh group
- Resuscitation if necessary

Revealed → Concealed

Concealed:
- Inj. Morphine
- Fresh blood transfusion
- Urine output

Revealed:
- Patient in labour
- Patient not in labour

Patient in labour → ARM + Oxytocin — if needed

Patient not in labour → > 38 weeks / < 38 weeks

> 38 weeks → ARM + Oxytocin

Concealed → ARM + Oxytocin — if needed
- No response
- Falling fibrinogen level
- Oliguria
→ CS → Hysterectomy

Bleeding stops → Expectant treatment → Try to continue the pregnancy up to EDD

Bleeding PV continuing → ARM → Oxytocin

Fig. 8.23: Scheme of management of abruptio placentae

labour is usually completed quickly (usually within 6 hrs.).

MULTIPLE PREGNANCY

When more than one fetus simultaneously develops in the uterus, it is called multiple pregnancy. Simultaneous development of two fetus (twins) is the commonest, although rare, development of three fetuses (triplets), four fetuses (quadruplets) or six fetuses (sextuplets) may also occur.

TWINS

Simultaneous development of two fetuses is the commonest variety of multiple pregnancy.

180

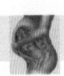
Table 8.5: Emergency implementations for bleeding in pregnancy

Implementation	Rationale
Alert health care team of emergency situation	Provides maximum coordination of care
Place woman flat in bed on her side	Maintains optimal placental and renal function
Begin intravenous fluid such as lactated Ringer's	Replaces intravascular fluid volume, intravenous line is established if blood replacement will be needed
Administer oxygen as necessary at 6–10 liters/min by face mask	Provides adequate fetal oxygenation despite lowered maternal circulating blood volume
Monitor uterine contractions and fetal heart rate by external monitor	Assess whether labor is present and fetal status, external system avoids cervical trauma
Omit vaginal examination	Prevents tearing of placenta if placenta previa is cause of bleeding
Withhold oral fluid	Anticipates need for emergency surgery
Order type and cross match of two units whole blood	Preparation for restoring circulating maternal blood volume
Measure intake and output	Enables assessment of renal function (will decrease to under 30 ml/h with massive circulating volume loss.
Assess vital signs (pulse, respirations and blood pressure every 15 min) apply pulse oximeter and automatic BP cuff as necessary	Provides baseline data on maternal response to blood loss
Assist with placement of CVP and blood determinations	Provides more accurate data on maternal hemodynamic state
Measure maternal blood loss by weighing perineal pads, save any tissue passed	Saturating a sanitary pad in less than 1 hour is heavy blood loss, tissue may be abnormal trophoblast tissue
Set aside 5 ml of blood drawn intravenously in a clean test tube, observe in 5 min for clot formation	Tests for possible blood coagulation problem (disseminated intravascular coagulation; suspect this if no clot forms within time limit)
Assist with ultrasound examination	Supplies information on placental and fetal well-being
Maintain a positive attitude toward fetal outcome	Supports mother-child bonding
Support woman's self-esteem	Supports problem solving as this is lessened by poor self-esteem

Varieties

1. *Binovular twins:* It is the commonest (two-thirds) and results from the fertilization of two ova.
2. *Uniovular twins* (one-third) results from the fertilization of the single ovum.

Genesis of twins

Binovular twins (Syn: fraternal, dizygotic) result from fertilization of two ova, most likely ruptures from two distinct Graafian follicles usually of the same or one from each ovary, by two sperms during a single ovarian cycle. Their subsequent implantation and development differ little from those of a single fertilized ovum. *The babies bear only fraternal resemblance to each other* (that of brothers and sisters from different births) and hence called fraternal twins.

In uniovular twins (Syn: identical, monozygotic), the twinning may occur at different periods after fertilization and this markedly influences the process of implantation and the formation of the fetal membranes. The exact stage at which *the separation occurs, is probably after the formation of inner cell mass (between 4th to 8th day).* Thus, two embryos will develop enclosed by a single chorion and having a single placenta and two separate amniotic sacs *(diamniotic-monochorionic).*

On extremely rare occasions, *division occurs after the development of embryonic disc* resulting in the formation of *conjoined twins* called - Siamese twins. *Four types of fusion may occur*

1. Thoracopagus (commonest)
2. Pyopagus
3. Craniopagus
4. Ischiopagus

Determination of zygosity

With the advent of organ transplantation, the identification of the zygosity of the multiple foetuses has assumed much importance.

Examination of placenta and membranes

- *Binovular twins* (Fig. 8.24)
  1. There are two placentae, either completely separated or more commonly fused at the margin appearing to be one (9 out of 10).
  2. Each foetus is surrounded by a separate amnion and chorion.
  3. *As such, the intervening membranes consist of 4 layers*—amnion, chorion, and amnion, chorion.
- *Uniovular twins*
  1. The placenta is single.
  2. Each fetus is surrounded by a separate amniotic sac with the chorionic layer common to both (diamniotic-monochorionic).

SEX

While twins having opposite sex are always binovular and twins of the same sex are not always uniovular but the *uniovular twins are always of the same sex.*

Incidence

In India the incidence is about 1 in 80. While the incidence of monozygotic twins remains fairly constant throughout the globe being 1 in 250.

According to Hellin's (1895) rules, the mathematical frequency of multiple birth is twins 1 in 80 pregnancies, triplets 1 in 80^2 and quadruplets 1 in 80^3 and so on.

Table 8.6: Summary of determination of zygosity

	Placenta	Communicating vessels	Intervening membranes	Sex	Genetic features (dominant blood group)	Skin grafting (reciprocal)	Follow-up
Uniovular	One	Present	2 amnions	Always identical	Same	Acceptance	Usually identical
Binovular	Two (most often fused)	Absent	4 (2 amnions) and (2 chorions)	May differ	Differ	Rejection	Not identical

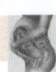

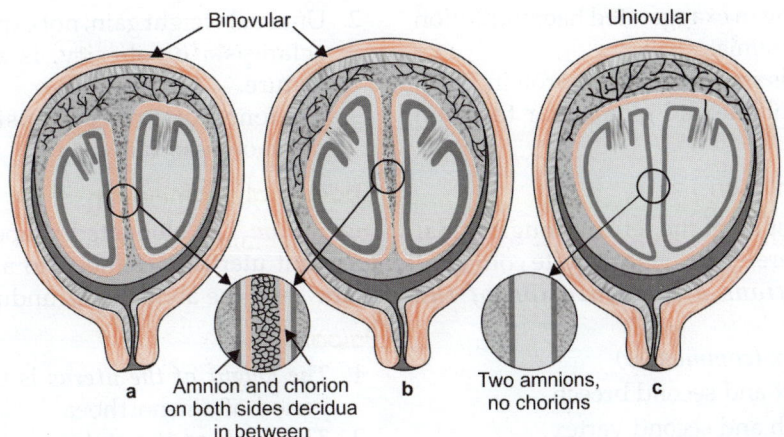

Binovular

Uniovular

a   Amnion and chorion   b   Two amnions,   c
     on both sides decidua   no chorions
     in between

Fig. 8.24: Twin placenta. Binovular twins have two placentae, may be separated or fused without any vascular communications, intervening membranes consist of 4 layers. Uniovular twins have got one placenta with free internal vascular anastomosis, the intervening membranes consist of 2 layers

Etiology

The cause of twinning is not known. *The frequency of uniovular twins remain constant throughout the globe* and is probably related to maternal environmental factors.

Prevalence of binovular twins is related to

- *Race:* The frequency is highest amongst Negroes, lowest amongst Mongols and intermediate amongst Caucasians.
- *Hereditary:* There is hereditary predisposition likely to be *more transmitted through the female (maternal side).*
- *Advancing age of the mother:* The *maximum being between the age of 30–35 years.*
- *Influence of parity:* The incidence is increased with increasing parity specially *from 5th gravida onwards.*
- *Iatrogenic:* Drugs used for induction of ovulation may produce multiple fetuses following gonadotrophin therapy.
- *Fetus papyraceous or compressus* (Fig. 8.25) is a state which occurs if one of the fetuses dies early. The dead fetus is flattened and compressed between the membranes of the living fetus and the uterine wall. It may

occur in both varieties of twins, but *is more common in uniovular twins* and is discovered at delivery or earlier by sonar.

- *Maternal physiological changes:* Multiple pregnancy imposes physical changes on the mother in excess of those seen in singleton pregnancy.
  1. There is increase in weight gain and cardiac output.
  2. Plasma volume is increased by an addition of 500 ml. There is no corresponding increase in red cell volume

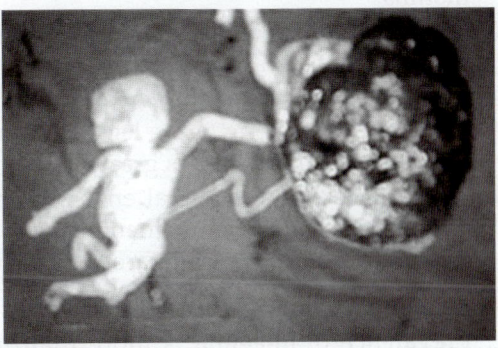

Fig. 8.25: Fetus papyraceous or compressus

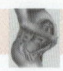

resulting in exaggerated haemodilution and anaemia.

3. There is increased a fetoprotein level, tidal volume and glomerular filtration rate.

Lie and presentation

The commonest lie of the fetus is longitudinal (90%) but malpresentations are quite common. *The combinations of presentation of the fetuses are*

1. Both vertex *(commonest)*
2. First vertex and second breech
3. First breech and second vertex
4. Both breech
5. First vertex and second transverse and so on, *but rarest one, being both transverse when the possibility of conjoined twins should be ruled out.*

DIAGNOSIS

History

1. History of *ovulation inducing drugs* specially gonadotropins, for infertility
2. Family history of twinning

Symptoms

Minor ailments of normal pregnancy are often exaggerated. Some of the symptoms are related to the undue enlargement of the uterus:

1. Increased nausea and vomiting in early months.
2. Cardiorespiratory embarrassment which is evident in the later months—such as palpitation or shortness of breath.
3. Tendency of swelling of the legs, varicose veins and haemorrhoids is greater.
4. Unusual rate of abdominal enlargement and excessive fetal movements may be noticed by an experienced parous mother.

General examination

1. Prevalence of anaemia is more than in singleton pregnancy.

2. Unusual weight gain, not explained by pre-eclampsia or obesity, is an important feature.
3. Evidence of pre-eclampsia (25%) is a common association.

Abdominal examination

Inspection: The elongated shape of a normal pregnant uterus is changed to a more "barrel shape" and the abdomen is unduly enlarged.

Palpation

1. *The height of the uterus* is more than the period of amenorrhoea.
2. *The girth of the abdomen* at the level of umbilicus is more than the normal average at term (100 cm).
3. *Palpation of too many fetal parts.*
4. *Finding of two fetal heads or three fetal poles* make the clinical diagnosis almost certain.

Auscultation

Simultaneous hearing of *two distinct fetal heart sounds located at separate spots with a silent area in between* the difference in heart rates is at least 10 beats per minute.

Internal examination

In some cases, one head is felt deep in the pelvis, while the other one is located by abdominal examination.

Investigations

- **Sonography**
  - Two gestational sacs can be detected as early as 10th week of pregnancy.
  - Detection of two fetal heads and their accurate measurement of biparietal diameters can be made by the 14th week.
  - For assessment of placentation, sonar is done between 16 and 24 weeks
  - For assessment of IUGR, it should be repeatedly (2–3 weeks interval) employed in second half of pregnancy.

- *Radiography* is done less often these days. Two fetal heads and spines could be seen.
- *Biochemical tests:* Maternal serum chorionic gonadotrophin, a fetoprotein and unconjugated oestriol are approximately double than those of singleton pregnancies.

Differential diagnosis

1. Hydramnios
2. Big baby
3. Fibroid or ovarian tumour with pregnancy
4. Ascites with pregnancy

Complications

1. Maternal
   - Pregnancy
   - Labour
   - Puerperium
2. Fetal

Maternal

During pregnancy

- *Nausea and vomiting* with increased frequency and severity.
- *Anaemia* is more common in twin pregnancy. This is because of increased iron and folate requirements by the two fetuses. Deficiency of folic acid leads to increased incidence of megaloblastic anaemia.
- *Pre-eclampsia (25%)* is increased three times over singleton pregnancy.
- *Hydramnios (10%) is more common in uniovular twins and usually involves the second sac.*
- *Antepartum haemorrhage* may occur with slight increased frequency. *The increased incidence of placenta praevia* is due to bigger size of the placenta encroaching on to the lower segment. *The separation of normally situated placenta may be due to*
  1. Increased incidence of P.I.H.
  2. Sudden escape of liquor following rupture of the membranes of the hydramniotic sac.
  3. Deficiency of folic acid.

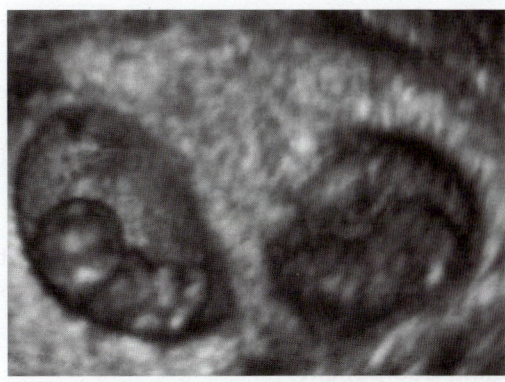

Fig. 8.26: Sonogram X-ray showing two fetal heads

4. Following delivery of the first baby due to sudden shrinkage of the uterine wall.
- *Malpresentation* is quite common in twins compared to singleton pregnancies and is *more common in the second baby.*
- *Preterm labour (30%)* frequently occurs and the mean gestational period for twins is 37 weeks. Over distension of the uterus, hydramnios and premature rupture of the membranes are responsible for preterm labour.
- *Mechanical distress* such as palpitation, dyspnoea, varicosities and haemorrhoids may be increased compared to a singleton pregnancy.

During labour

- *Early rupture of the membranes and cord prolapse.* Cord prolapse is five times more common than in singleton pregnancy and is more common in relation to the second baby.
- *Increased operative interference* is due to high prevalence of malpresentation with its associated complications.
- *Bleeding* following the birth of the first baby, may at times, be alarming and is due to separation of the placenta following reduction of placental site.

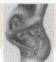

- *Postpartum haemorrhage* is the real danger in twins. *It is due to*
  1. Atony of the uterine muscle due to over distension of the uterus.
  2. A longer time taken by the big placenta to separate.
  3. Bigger surface area of the placenta.
  4. Implantation of a part of the placenta in the lower segment which is less retractile.

During puerperium

There is increased incidence of
- Subinvolution—because of bigger size of the uterus.
- Infection—because of increased operative interference, pre-existing anaemia and blood loss during delivery.
- Failing lactation

FETAL

- *Miscarriage rate* is increased.
- *Premature rate (80%)* is very much increased
- *Intrauterine death of one fetus*—Intrauterine death is increased more in uniovular one. The deaths are due to cord compression, completion for nourishment or congenital malformation.
- *Fetal anomalies* are increased two folds over the singleton pregnancy, more in uniovular twins. They are in the form of an encephaly, hydrocephalus, cardiac anomalies or Down's syndrome.
- *Asphyxia and stillbirth* are more common due to increased prevalence of pre-eclampsia, malpresentation, placental abruption and increased operative interferences. The second baby is more at risk.

Prognosis

Maternal mortality is increased in twins than in a singleton pregnancy. *Death is mostly due to haemorrhage (before, during and after delivery), pre-eclampsia and anaemia.*

Perinatal mortality is markedly *increased mainly due to prematurity* and is 4–5 times higher than in a singleton pregnancy. *The second baby is more at risk (50%) than the first one due to*
1. Retraction of uterus leading to placental insufficiency.
2. Increased operative interference.
3. Increased incidence of cord prolapse.

TWIN TRANSFUSION SYNDROME

It is a clinicopathological state, *exclusively met with in uniovular twins*, where one twin appears to bleed into the other through some kind of placental vascular anastomosis. Clinical manifestations of twin transfusion syndrome occur when there is anastomosis between artery and vein.

As a result the receptor twin becomes larger, polycythemic, hypertensive and hypervolaemic, at the expense of the donor twin which becomes smaller, anaemic, hypotensive and hypovolaemic. Difference of haemoglobin concentration between the two, usually exceeds 5 gm% and estimated fetal weight discrepancy is 25% or more.

ANTENATAL MANAGEMENT

The essence of successful outcome of a twin pregnancy is to diagnose it at the earliest period of gestation. This will help the mother to take additional care not only for her own benefit but also for the foetuses.

Advice

- *Diet:* Increased dietary supplement is needed for increased energy supply to the extent of 300 kcal. per day, over and above that needed in a singleton pregnancy.

- *Increased rest* at home and early cessation of work is advised to prevent preterm labour and other complications.

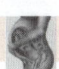

- *Supplement therapy*
  - Iron therapy is to be increased to the extent of 60–80 mg per day.
  - Additional vitamins, calcium and folic acid (1 mg) are to be given, over and above those prescribed for a singleton pregnancy.
- *Interval of antenatal visit* should be more frequent to detect at the earliest, the evidences of anaemia, preterm labour or pre-eclampsia.
- *Fetal growth assessment* should be done by ultrasound.

Hospitalisation

Elective: The patient may be *admitted around 32th week if she requests it for* **rest.** Bed rest not only ensures physical and mental rest but improves utero placental circulation.

This results in
1. Increased birth weight of the babies
2. Decreased frequency of pre-eclampsia
3. Decreased frequency of preterm labour
4. Lowered perinatal mortality

Emergency: Development of complicating factors necessitates urgent admission irrespective of the period of gestation.

MANAGEMENT DURING LABOUR

Place of delivery: As the twin pregnancy is considered a 'high-risk', the patient should be confined in an equipped hospital preferably having an intensive neonatal care unit.

First stage

Usual conduction of the first stage as outlined for a singleton fetus, is to be followed with additional precautions.
- *The patient should be kept in bed* and the enema withheld. These are to prevent early rupture of the membranes.
- *Use of analgesic drugs* is to be limited as the babies are small and rapid delivery may

occur. *Epidural analgesia* is preferred as it facilitates manipulation of second fetus should it prove necessary.
- *Careful fetal monitoring* is to be done.
- *Internal examination should be done* soon after the rupture of the membranes to exclude cord prolapse.
- *An intravenous line with ringer's solution should be set up.*
- *One unit of compatible and cross matched blood* should be made readily available.
- *Neonatologist* should be present at the time of delivery.

Delivery of the first baby

The delivery should be conducted in the same guidelines as mentioned in normal labour.
1. *Liberal episiotomy* under local filtration with 1% lignocaine saves both the forecoming or the aftercoming head of the premature baby from the intracranial damages.
2. *Forceps delivery,* if needed, should be done *preferably under pudendal block anaesthesia.*
3. *Do not give intravenous ergometrine with the delivery of the anterior shoulder of the first baby.*
4. *Clamp the cord at two places and cut in between,* to prevent exsanguination of the second baby through communicating placental circulation in uniovular twins.
5. *At least, 8–10 cm of cord is left behind* if administration of any drug or transfusion is required.
6. *The baby is labelled as No. 1*

Conduction of labour after the delivery of the first baby

Principles

The principles is to expedite the delivery of the second baby. The second baby is put under strain due to placental insufficiency caused by uterine retraction following the birth of the first baby.

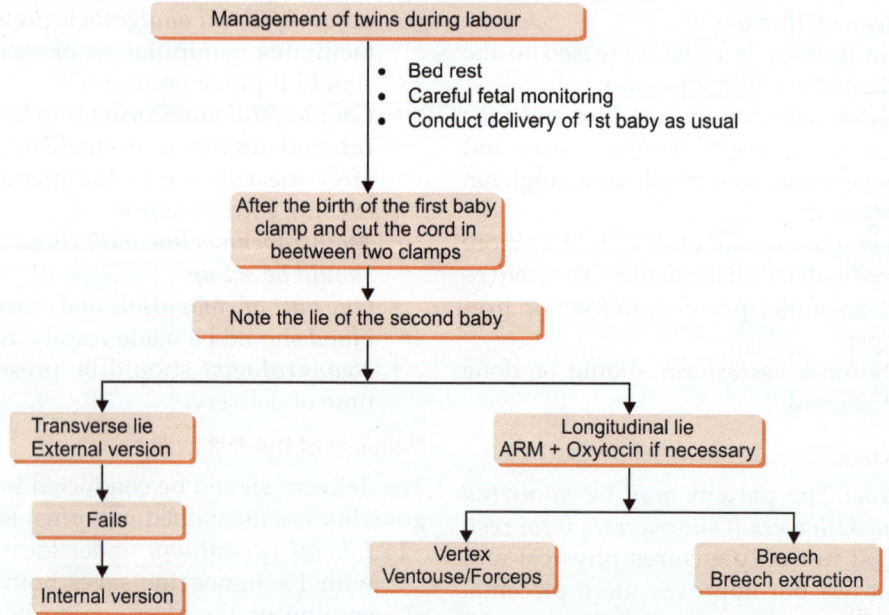

Fig. 8.27: Scheme of management of twins during labour

Management of third stage

The risk of postpartum haemorrhage can be minimized by routine administration of 0.2 mg. methergin intravenously with the delivery of the anterior shoulder of the second baby. The placenta is to be delivered by controlled cord traction. It is a sound practice to continue the oxytocin drip for at least one hour, following delivery of the second baby. A blood loss of more than average should be immediately replaced by blood transfusion, already kept at hand.

Indications of caesarean section

The indications are broadly divided into:
- Obstetric causes
- For twins

Obstetric indication

1. Placenta praevia
2. Severe pre-eclampsia
3. Previous caesarean section
4. Cord prolapse of the first baby

5. Abnormal uterine contraction
6. Contracted pelvis

For twins

1. Both the fetuses or even the first fetus with noncephalic (breech or transverse) presentation
2. Twins with complications: IUGR, conjoined twins
3. Monoamniotic twins
4. Collision of both the heads at brim preventing engagement of either head.

There is no valid reason to perform caesarean section in all cases of second twins of noncephalic presentation.

POLYHYDRAMNIOS (SYN : HYDRAMNIOS)

Definition

Anatomically the polyhydramnios is defined as a state where liquor amnii exceeds 2000 ml.

Incidence

Because of different criteria used in the definition of polyhydramnios, the incident varies from 0.5–1% of cases. It is more common in multiparae than primigravidae.

Etiology

It may be the result of deficient absorption as well as excessive production of liquor amnii/ which may be temporary or permanent. While certain maternal or fetal factors are found to be associated with hydramnios/yet the cause remains unknown in about 50%. The composition of the liquor amnii/however, remains normal.

1. Fetal anomalies

Congenital fetal malformations is associated with polyhydramnios in about 20% cases

- Anencephaly—hydramnios is found in association with anencephaly in about 50% cases. The causes of excessive production of liquor amnii may be due to:
  - Transudation from the exposed meninges
  - Absence of fetal swallowing reflex
  - Possible suppression of fetal anti-diuretic hormone leading to excessive urination.
- Open spina bifida—increased transudation from the meninges.
- Oesophageal or duodenal atresia - preventing swallowing of the liquor. However, hydramnios is associated only in about 15% cases of oesophageal atresia.
- Facial clefts and neck masses—by interfering normal swallowing.
- Hydrops fetalis due to rhesus isoimmunization, cardiothoracic anomalies and fetal cirrhosis are often associated with hydramnios.

2. Placenta

Chorioangioma of the placenta: Tumour growing from a single villus consisting of hyperplasia of blood vessels and connective tissue results in increased transudation.

3. Multiple pregnancy

Multiple pregnancy is about 10 times more common than its overall incidence. Hydramnios is more common in uniovular twins, usually affecting the second sac.

4. Maternal

- *Diabetes:* It is more common in hydramnios. Hydramnios is associated with diabetes in about 30% cases. However, with adequate supervision, the incidence of hydramnios can be lowered. It is presumed that a raised maternal blood sugar→raised fetal blood sugar → fetal diuresis→ hydramnios.
- *Cardiac or renal disease:* May lead to oedema of the placenta leading to increase in transudation.

Clinical types

Depending on the rapidity of onset, hydramnios may be:

- Chronic (commonest)—onset is insidious taking few weeks.
- Acute (extremely rare)—onset is sudden, within few days or may appear acutely on pre-existing chronic variety.

CHRONIC POLYHYDRAMNIOS

In the majority of cases, the accumulation of liquor is gradual and as such, the patient is not very much inconvenienced.

Symptoms

The symptoms are mainly from mechanical causes.

- Respiratory—the patient may suffer from dyspnoea or even remain in the sitting position for easier breathing.
- Palpitation

Table 8.7: Complications of multifetal pregnancy

Maternal	Fetal
Nausea, Vomiting	Abortion
Anaemia	Vanishing twin/ Fetus papyraceous
PIH and pre-eclampsia	Preterm birth
Polyhydramnios/ Oligohydramnios	Fetal anomalies
Preterm labour	Discordant growth
Malpresentation	Intrauterine death of one fetus
Antepartum heamorrhage	Twin transfusion syndrome
Mechanical distress (dyspnoea, palpitation)	Cord prolapse, locked twins
Prolonged labour	(↑) Perinatal mortality
Operative haemorrhage Postpartum haemorrhage (↑) Postnatal support	

- Oedema of the legs, varicosities in the legs or vulva and haemorrhoids.

Signs

- The patient may be in a dyspnoeic state in the lying down position.
- Evidences of pre-eclampsia (oedema, hypertension and proteinuria) may be present.

ABDOMINAL EXAMINATION

Inspection

- Abdomen is markedly enlarged, looks globular with fullness at the flanks.
- The skin is tense/shiny with large striae.

Palpation

- Height of the uterus is more than the period of amenorrhoea.
- Girth of the abdomen round the umbilicus is more than normal.
- Fluid thrill can be elicited in all directions over the uterus.

- Fetal parts cannot be well denned; so also the presentation or the position. External ballottement can be elicited more easily.

Auscultation

Fetal heart sound is not heard distinctly, although its presence can be picked up by Doppler.

Internal examination

The cervix is pulled up/may be partially taken up or at times, dilated, to admit a finger tip through which tense bulged membranes can be felt.

Investigations

- *Sonography:* Sonography is helpful
  - To detect abnormally large echo-free space between the fetus and the uterine wall (single pool > 8 cm). Amniotic fluid index (AFI) is more than 20 cm
  - To exclude multiple fetuses
  - To note the lie and presentation of the fetus
  - To diagnose any fetal congenital malformation.
- *Radiography:* Not commonly performed these days. The X-ray plate may be hazy and at times, it may not be possible to exclude with certainty multiple pregnancy or bony congenital malformation of the fetus.
- *Blood*
  - ABO and Rh grouping—rhesus iso-immunization may cause hydrops fetalis and fetal ascites.
  - Post prandial sugar and if necessary glucose tolerance test.
- *Amniotic fluid:* Estimation of alpha feto-protein which is markedly elevated in the presence of a fetus with an open neural tube defect.

Differential diagnosis

- Twins

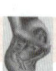

- Pregnancy with huge ovarian cyst
- Maternal ascites

Complications

The complications of hydramnios are grouped into
- Maternal
- Fetal

Maternal

During pregnancy
1. Pre-eclampsia (25%)
2. Malpresentation and persistence of floating head
3. Premature rupture of the membranes
4. Preterm labour either spontaneous or induced
5. Accidental haemorrhage due to decrease in the surface area of the emptying uterus beneath the placenta, following sudden escape of liquor amnii.

During labour
1. Early rupture of the membranes
2. Cord prolapse
3. Uterine inertia
4. Increased operative delivery due to malpresentation
5. Retained placenta, postpartum haemorrhage and shock.

Puerperium
1. Subinvolution
2. Increased puerperal morbidity due to infection resulting from increased operative interference and blood loss.

Fetal

There is increased perinatal mortality to the extent of about 50%. The deaths are mostly due to prematurity and congenital abnormality (20%).

MANAGEMENT

Recently there has been a falling trend in the incidence of hydramnios of severe magnitude.

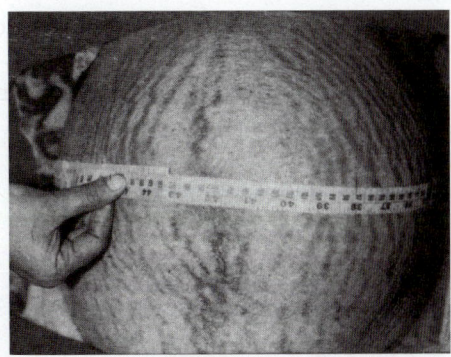

Fig. 8.28: Abdominal girth round the umbilicus is more than normal

The reasons are:
- Early detection and control of diabetes.
- Rhesus isoimmunization is now preventable.
- Genetic counselling in early months and detection of fetal congenital abnormalities with ultrasound and their termination, reduce their number in late pregnancy.

Minor degree hydramnios

It is commonly found in midtrimester and usually requires no treatment/ except extra bed rest for a few days. The excess liquor is expected to be diminished as pregnancy advances.

Severe degree hydramnios

In view of the risks involved and the high perinatal mortality rate, the patient should be shifted in a hospital equipped to deal with "high-risk" patients.

Principles

1. To relieve the symptoms
2. To find out the cause
3. To avoid and to deal with the complication.
- *Supportive therapy* includes bed rest, if necessary, with a back rest; analgesics and sedatives as and when required and treatment of the associated conditions like pre-eclampsia or diabetes on the usual line. The use of diuretic is of little value. Indomethacin given orally to the mother

 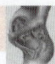

(25 mg every 6 hours) has been found to decrease amniotic fluid.

- Investigations are done to exclude congenital fetal malformations

Further management depends on

1. Response to treatment
2. Period of gestation
3. Presence of fetal malformation
4. Associated complicating factors.

Uncomplicated cases (no demonstrable fetal malformation)

1. Response to treatment is good: The pregnancy is to be continued awaiting spontaneous delivery at term.
2. Unresponsive (with maternal distress)
   a. *Pregnancy less than 37 weeks:* An attempt is made to relieve the distress with a hope of continuation of pregnancy by amniocentesis. Slow decompression is done at the rate of about 500 ml per hour and the amount of fluid to be removed should be sufficient enough to relieve the mechanical distress. Ordinarily, it should not exceed 1–1.5 litrer. Because of slow decompression., chance of accidental haemorrhage is less but liquor amnii may again accumulate soon or later for which the procedure may have to be repeated.
   b. *Pregnancy more than 37 weeks:* Induction of labour should be done. The following procedures may be helpful. Amniocentesis →drainage of good amount of liquor amnii →to check the favourable lie and presentation of the fetus →a stabilising oxytocin infusion is started → low rupture of the membranes is done when the lie becomes stable and the presenting part gets fixed to the pelvis. This will minimise sudden decompression with

separation of the placenta, change in lie of the fetus-and cord prolapse. High rupture of the membranes with Drew-Smythe catheter may lead to accidental low rupture of the membranes and escape of gush of liquor amnii with its incidental hazards.

With congenital fetal abnormality

Termination of pregnancy is to be done irrespective of the duration of pregnancy. The patient is relieved of symptoms and unnecessary development of pregnancy complications are also avoided. Amniocentesis is done to drain good amount of liquor amnii. Thereafter induction by vaginal PGE$_2$ gel insertion followed by low rupture of membranes is done. If, accidentally, low rupture of the membranes occurs, escape of gush of liquor should be immediately controlled by placing the palm over the introitus to avoid accidental haemorrhage. The lie should be checked and if found longitudinal, oxytocin infusion may be started.

During labour: Usual management is followed as outlined in twin pregnancy. Internal examination should be done soon after the rupture of the membranes to exclude cord prolapse. If the uterine contraction becomes sluggish, oxytocin infusion may be started, if not contraindicated. To prevent postpartum haemorrhage, intravenous methergin 0.2 mg should be given with the delivery of the anterior shoulder. One must remain vigilant following the birth of the baby for retained placenta, postpartum haemorrhage and shock. Oesophageal atresia of the baby should be excluded by passing a rubber catheter down to the stomach.

ACUTE POLYHYDRAMNIOS

The onset is acute and the fluid accumulates within a few days. It usually occurs before 20 weeks of pregnancy. It is usually associated

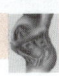

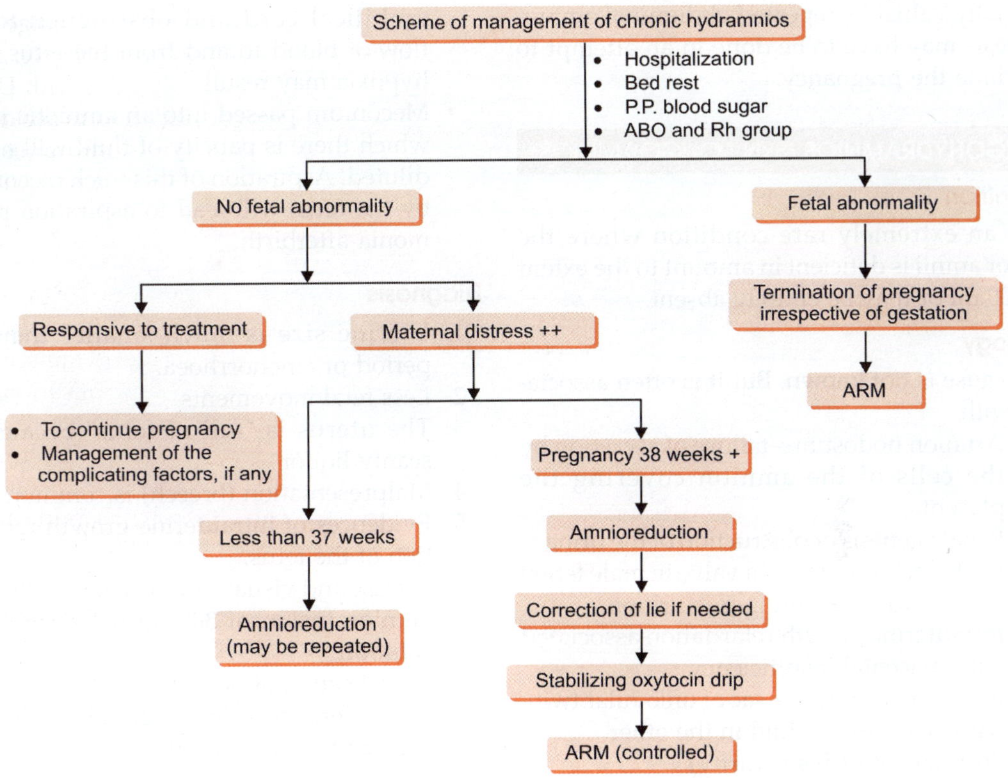

Scheme of management of chronic hydramnios

- Hospitalization
- Bed rest
- P.P. blood sugar
- ABO and Rh group

No fetal abnormality

Fetal abnormality

Termination of pregnancy irrespective of gestation

ARM

Responsive to treatment

Maternal distress ++

- To continue pregnancy
- Management of the complicating factors, if any

Pregnancy 38 weeks +

Less than 37 weeks

Amnioreduction

Amnioreduction (may be repeated)

Correction of lie if needed

Stabilizing oxytocin drip

ARM (controlled)

Fig. 8.29: Scheme of management of chronic hydramnios

with uniovular twins or chorioangioma of the placenta.

Symptoms

Features of acute abdomen predominate—such as abdominal pain, nausea and vomiting.

Signs

1. The patient looks ill
2. Absence of features of shock
3. Oedema of the legs or presence of other associated features of pre-eclampsia.
4. Abdomen is hugely enlarged more than the period of amenorrhoea.
5. Fluid thrill is present
6. Fetal part cannot be felt nor is the fetal heart sound audible

7. Internal examination reveals—taking up of the cervix or even dilatation of the os through which the bulged membranes are felt.
8. Sonograph shows multiple fetuses or at times fetal abnormalities, with radiography often the plates become too hazy to interpret.

Differential diagnosis includes

1. Accidental haemorrhage
2. Retroverted gravid uterus
3. Hydatidiform mole

Treatment

Most often, spontaneous abortion occurs. To relieve the distress, decompression has to be done. On rare occasions where the baby is specially valuable, repeated abdominal amnio-centesis may have to be done in an attempt to continue the pregnancy.

OLIGOHYDRAMNIOS (SYN.: OLIGOAMNIOS)

Definition

It is an extremely rare condition where the liquor amnii is deficient in amount to the extent of 100 ml or may be entirely absent.

Etiology

The cause is not known. But it is often associated with

1. Arnnion nodosum—failure of secretion by the cells of the amnion covering the placenta
2. Renal agenesis or obstruction of the urinary tract (posterior urethral valve in male fetus) of the fetus preventing micturition.
3. Intrauterine growth retardation associated with placental insufficiency
4. It may affect only one sac of uniovular twin, with an excess of fluid in the other
5. Postmaturity (dysmaturity)

Effects of oligohydramnios

Early pregnancy: When oligohydramnios occurs in early pregnancy there may be fetal deformities

- Amniotic adhesions or bands may cause deformities like amputation of fetal limbs, or constriction and obstruction of the umbilical cord.
- Pressure deformities such as club feet
- Pulmonary hypoplasia has been reported
- The skin becomes dry, leathery and wrinkled.

Late pregnancy: The markedly reduced volume of amniotic fluid can cause several problems.

- It is a sign of fetal jeopardy as in cases of IUGR.
- Close adaptation between the fetus and the uterine wall can lead to pressure on the

umbilical cord and obstruction to the flow of blood to and from the fetus, fetal hypoxia may result.

- Meconium passed into an amniotic sac in which there is paucity of fluid will not be diluted. Aspiration of this thick meconium by the fetus will lead to aspiration pneumonia afterbirth.

Diagnosis

1. Uterine size is much smaller than the period of amenorrhoea.
2. Less fetal movements
3. The uterus is "full of fetus" because of scanty liquor
4. Malpresentation (breech) is common
5. Evidences of intrauterine growth retardation of the fetus.
6. Ultrasound visualisation is done following amnioinfusion of 300 ml of warm saline solution.
7. Visualisation of normal filling and emptying of fetal bladder essentially rules out urinary tract abnormality

Complications

Fetal

1. Abortion
2. Deformity due to intra-amniotic adhesions or due to compression. The deformities include alteration in shape of the skull, wryneck, club foot, or even amputation of the limb.
3. Fetal pulmonary hypoplasia (may be the cause or effect).
4. Cord compression
5. Fetal mortality is high
6. Fetal distress in labour and common complications

Maternal

1. Prolonged labour due to inertia
2. Increased operative interference due to malpresentation. The sum effect may lead to increased maternal morbidity.

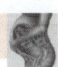

Treatment

Premature rupture of the membranes is common. Labour may be protracted and the contractions are more painful. Fetal distress occurs frequently. Because of frequent association of fetal malformation, vaginal delivery is favoured.

POSTMATURITY (SYN : POST-TERM PREGNANCY)

The expected date of confinement is calculated by the Naegele's rule. Term is reached 40 weeks (280 days) after the first day of the last normal menstrual period. It is based on the belief that conception takes place on about the 14th day of her cycle.

Definition

Any pregnancy which has passed beyond the expected date of delivery, is called a prolonged or postdated pregnancy. But for clinical purposes, a pregnancy continuing beyond two weeks of the expected date of delivery is called postmaturity or post-term pregnancy.

Incidence

About 6 to 8% pregnancies go beyond 42 weeks. But in many instances of suspected post-term pregnancy the gestational period may not have been correctly calculated.

Limitations of diagnosis

It is difficult to arrive at the true incidence of post-dated (post-term) pregnancies because of several shortcomings such as:

- Women whose cycle is longer than 28 days or whose ovulation occurred late.
- Mistakes dates. The patient often cannot recall the exact date of her LMP.
- History of previous irregular cycles
- Pregnancy following immediately after stopping or oral contraceptive pills.
- Women have been known to falsify the menstrual history for social reasons.

Etiology

Certain factors related with post-maturity are: **Hereditary factor** might play some role as it often runs in the family and often manifests in consecutive pregnancies in the same individual. **High standard of living with sedentary habits** often tends to prolong the pregnancy. Of interest, there is prolongation of pregnancy in anencephaly without polyhydramnios. The theory of initiation of labour operating through fetal hypothalamopituitaryadrenal axis is not applicable in **anencephaly** and hence prolongation of pregnancy occurs. Placental sulphatase deficiency, fetal adrenal hypoplasia, though rare conditions, are associated with prolonged pregnancy. **Elderly primigravidae or elderly multiparae** are more likely to have prolonged pregnancy. Previous history of a post-term pregnancy has a 50% chance of recurrence.

Diagnosis

It is indeed difficult to diagnose postmaturity when the case is first seen beyond the expected date. Every possible effort should be made with available resources to diagnose at least the maturity of the fetus, if not the postmaturity. The following are the useful clinical guides

1. *Menstrual history:* If the patient is sure about her date with previous history of regular cycles, it is a fairly reliable diagnostic aid in the calculation of the period of gestation. But in cases of mistaken maturity or pregnancy occurring during lactational amenorrhoea or soon following withdrawal of the 'pill', confusion arises. In such cases, the previous well documented antenatal records of first visit in first trimester as mentioned, if available, are useful guides.

2. The suspected clinical findings those are evident when an otherwise uncomplicated case overrun the expected date by two weeks are:

 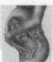

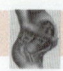

- **Weight:** Regular periodic weight checking reveals stationary or even falling weight.
- **Girth of the abdomen:** Normally, the girth of the abdomen at the level of umbilicus increases steadily upto the completion of 38 weeks and then remains steady upto term. Thereafter, the girth gradually diminishes because of diminishing liquor.
- **History of false pain:** Appearance of false pain followed by its subsidence with continuation of pregnancy is suggestive- The false pain is presumed to coincide with the expected date.
- **Obstetric palpation:** The following findings, taken together, help in the diagnosis of the maturity of the fetus'. These are height of the uterus, size of the fetus and hardness of the skull bones. As the liquor amnii diminishes, the uterus feels "full of fetus"—a feature usually associated with postmaturity.
- **Internal examination:** While a ripe cervix is usually suggestive of fetal maturity, to find an unripe cervix does not exclude maturity. Feeling of hard skull bones either through the cervix or through the fornix usually suggests maturity.

Investigations

The investigations are directed:
- To confirm the fetal maturity
- To detect evidences of placental insufficiency

Assessment of fetal maturity

- **Sonography:** Accurate assessment of gestational age is the most useful contribution of ultrasound. But it is essential that correct parameters are used at a particular gestational age.
- **Amniocentesis:** The biochemical and cytological parameters help in the assessment of maturity.

- **Straight X-ray abdomen:** Overall fetal shadow, thickness and density of the skull bone shadow, appearance and density of the ossification centres in the upper end of the tibia (38–40 weeks) and lower end of the femur (36–37 weeks) are taken together to assess the maturity.

Evidences of placental insufficiency

Assessment of placental dysfunction and fetal jeopardy have to be inferred with the available gadgets. Absence of umbilical artery end diastolic frequency indicates fetal jeopardy.

Clinical concept

In addition to the increased length of gestation at which the baby is delivered, the following criteria have been used to establish the diagnosis of postmaturity retrospectively, i.e. after the birth of the baby.

- **Baby**
  1. Weight and length are of 4 kg and 54 cm respectively. Both are variable and even an underweight baby may be born.
  2. *General appearance:* Baby looks thin and old. There is absence of vernix caseosa. Body and the cord are stained with greenish yellow colour. Head is hard without much evidence of moulding. Nails are protruding beyond the nail beds.
- **Liquor amnii:** Scanty and may be saffron coloured with meconium.
- **Placenta:** There is evidence of ageing of the placenta manifested by excessive infarction and calcification.
- **Cord:** There is diminished quantity of Wharton's jelly which may precipitate cord compression.

DANGERS

Fetal

During pregnancy: There is chance of fetal hypoxia, due to placental insufficiency.

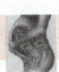

During labour: There is increased incidence of asphyxia and intracranial damage due to

1. Aggravation of pre-existing hypoxia leads to increased fetal distress.
2. Increased incidence of difficult labour due to big size baby, non-moulding of the head due to hardening of the skull bones and occasional shoulder dystocia.
3. Increased incidence of operative delivery.
4. Scanty liquor amnii and less Wharton's jelly in the cord favour cord compression.

Following birth

1. Meconium aspiration syndrome and atelectasis are the result of premature attempt at respiratory efforts due to intrauterine anoxia with consequent inhalation of meconium containing liquor amnii.
2. Low Apgar scores.
3. Hypoglycaemia and polycythemia specially occur in growth retarded post-term babies.

Maternal

There is increased morbidity, incidental to hazards of induction, instrumental and operative delivery. Postmaturity per se does not put the mother at risk.

MANAGEMENT

Before formulating the management, one should be certain about the maturity of the fetus with the available parameters as previously described. Increased fetal surveillance is maintained. For the formulation of management, the cases are grouped into:

- Uncomplicated
- Complicated

Uncomplicated

- *Selective induction:* In this regime, the pregnancy may be allowed to continue till spontaneous onset of labour. However, periodic assessment of fetal well being is to

be done so that early evidences of fetal compromise can be dealt with by induction.

- *Routine induction:* The expectant attitude is extended for 10–14 days past the expected date hoping spontaneous onset of labour during the period without undue risk. During this period careful fetal monitoring should be performed at regular intervals.

Induction

It is preferable to induce between 10 and 14 days, a little earlier in primigravidae.

If the cervix is favourable (ripe), induction is to be done by stripping of the membranes or by low rupture of the membranes. If the liquor is found clear, oxytocin infusion is added to be more effective. Careful fetal monitoring is mandatory. If the liquor amnii is thickly meconium stained, suggestive of chronic placental insufficiency, caesarean section is justified.

If the cervix is unripe, it is made favourable by vaginal administration of PGE_2 gel. This is followed by low rupture of the membranes. Oxytocin infusion is added when required.

Complicated group: (associated with complicating factors)

- *Elective caesarean section:* It is advisable when postmaturity is associated with complicating factors like contracted pelvis, post caesarean pregnancy, malpresentation, elderly primigravidae, etc.
- Associated complications likely to produce placental insufficiency preeclampsia, history of bleeding during pregnancy, diabetes and Rh negative pregnancy should not be allowed to go post expected date and termination is to be done by the safest method—induction or caesarean section.

Care during labour

Whether spontaneous or induced, the labour is expected to be prolonged because of a big and

 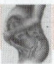

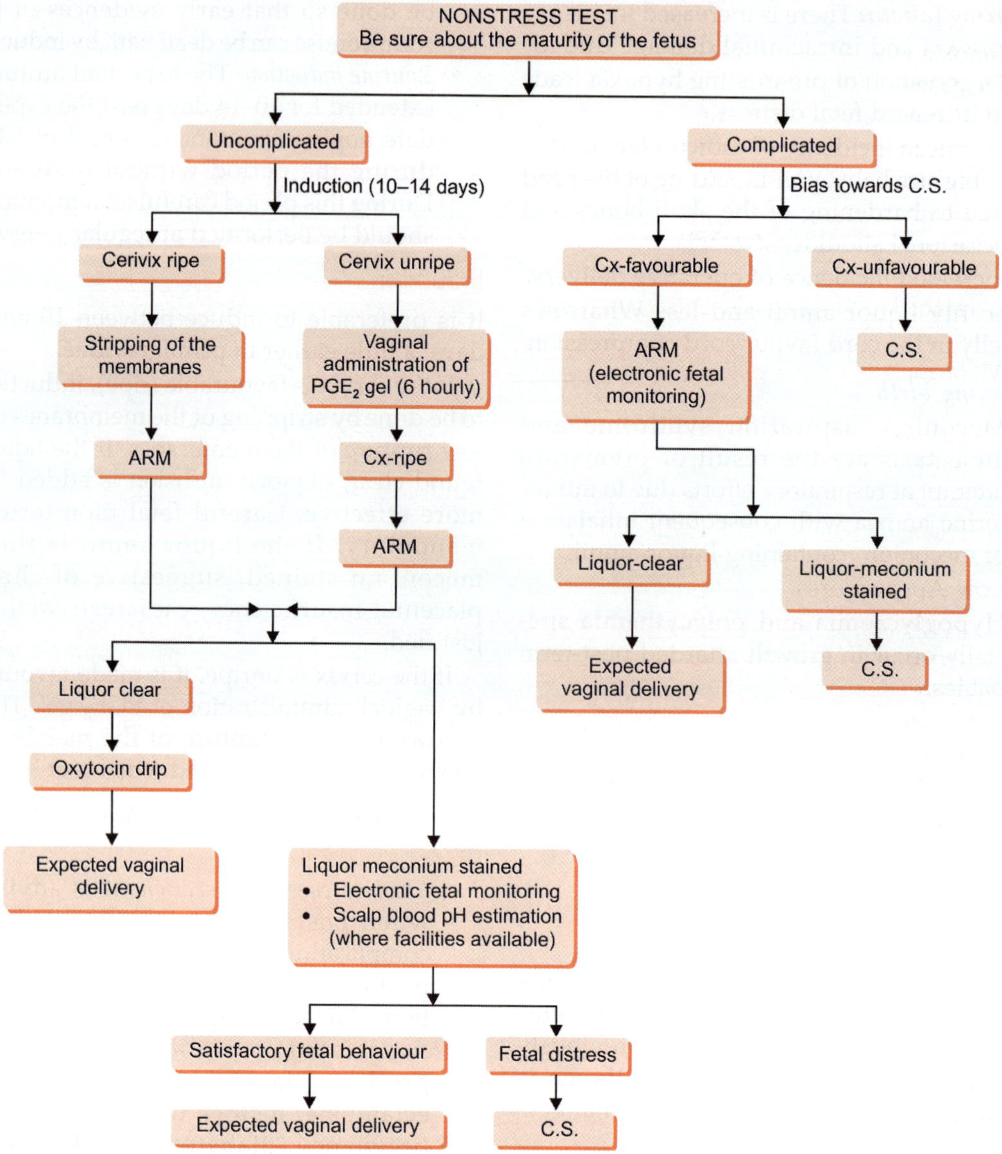

```
                    NONSTRESS TEST
              Be sure about the maturity of the fetus
```

Uncomplicated — Induction (10–14 days)

- **Cerivix ripe**
  - Stripping of the membranes
    - ARM

- **Cervix unripe**
  - Vaginal administration of PGE₂ gel (6 hourly)
    - Cx-ripe
      - ARM

- **Liquor clear**
  - Oxytocin drip
    - Expected vaginal delivery

- **Liquor meconium stained**
  - Electronic fetal monitoring
  - Scalp blood pH estimation (where facilities available)
    - Satisfactory fetal behaviour
      - Expected vaginal delivery
    - Fetal distress
      - C.S.

Complicated — Bias towards C.S.

- **Cx-favourable**
  - ARM (electronic fetal monitoring)
    - Liquor-clear
      - Expected vaginal delivery
    - Liquor-meconium stained
      - C.S.

- **Cx-unfavourable**
  - C.S.

Fig. 8.30: Scheme of management of postmaturity

poor moulding of the head. More analgesics is required for pain relief. Possibility of shoulder is to be kept in mind. Careful fetal monitoring with available gadgets is to be done. If fetal distress appears, prompt delivery either by caesarean section or by forceps is to be done.

INTRAUTERINE FETAL DEATH

Antepartum death occurring beyond 28 weeks is termed as intrauterine death and it usually results in the delivery of a macerated fetus.

Causes

Fetal anoxia is a cause in most cases.

1. **Diseases of pregnancy**
   - Pre-eclampsia: Placental insufficiency due to maternal hypotension is the most common cause of intrauterine fetal death.
   - *Antepartum haemorrhage:* Accidental haemorrhage and placenta praevia; if placental separation occurs for more than one third area of the placenta.
2. **Maternal diseases in pregnancy**
   - Chronic hypotension
   - Chronic renal disease
   - Syphilis
   - Severe anemia
   - Diabetes mellitus
   - Acute maternal illness: Maternal hyperpyrexia as in malaria, enteric fever, acute pyelonephritis, maternal hypotension as in severe diarrhoea.
   - *Drug effect:* Prolonged frusemide therapy
3. **Fetal reasons**
   - Postmaturity
   - Genetic defective and congenital malformation
   - Erythroblastosis
   - Idiopathic

Diagnosis

Repeated examinations are often required to confirm the diagnosis.

Symptoms

Absence of fetal movements which were previously experienced by the patient.

Signs

Retrogression of the positive breast changes that occur during pregnancy is evident after variable period following death of the fetus.

Per abdomen

- Gradual retrogression of the height of the uterus so that it becomes smaller than the period of amenorrhoea.
- Uterine tone is diminished and the uterus feels flaccid. Braxton-Hicks contraction is not easily felt.
- Fetal movements are not felt during palpation.
- Fetal heart sound which was audible before is absent and is very much suggestive. Doppler effect of ultrasound is a better alternative to the ordinary stethoscope.
- Egg-shell crackling feel of the fetal head.

Investigations

- *Sonography:* The evidences are:
  - Lack of all fetal motions (including cardiac) during a 10 minute period of careful observation with a real-time sonar is a strong presumptive evidence of fetal death.
  - Gradually, oligohydramnios and collapsed cranial bones are evident.
- *Straight X-ray abdomen:* The following features may be found in varying degree, or in combination.

  Spalding sign: The irregular overlapping of the cranial bones on one another is due liquefaction of the brain matter and softening of the ligamentous structures supporting the vault. It usually appears 7 days after death.
  - Hyperflexion of the spine is more common. In some cases hyperextension of the neck is seen.
  - Crowding of the ribs shadow with loss of normal parallelism.
  - Appearance of gas shadow (Robert's sign) in the chambers of the heart and great vessels may appear as early as 12 hours but difficult to interpret.

Investigations protocol in IUD

Investigation protocols are directed

- To confirm the diagnosis by sonography or radiology.
- To estimate the blood fibrinogen level and partial thromboplastin time periodically,

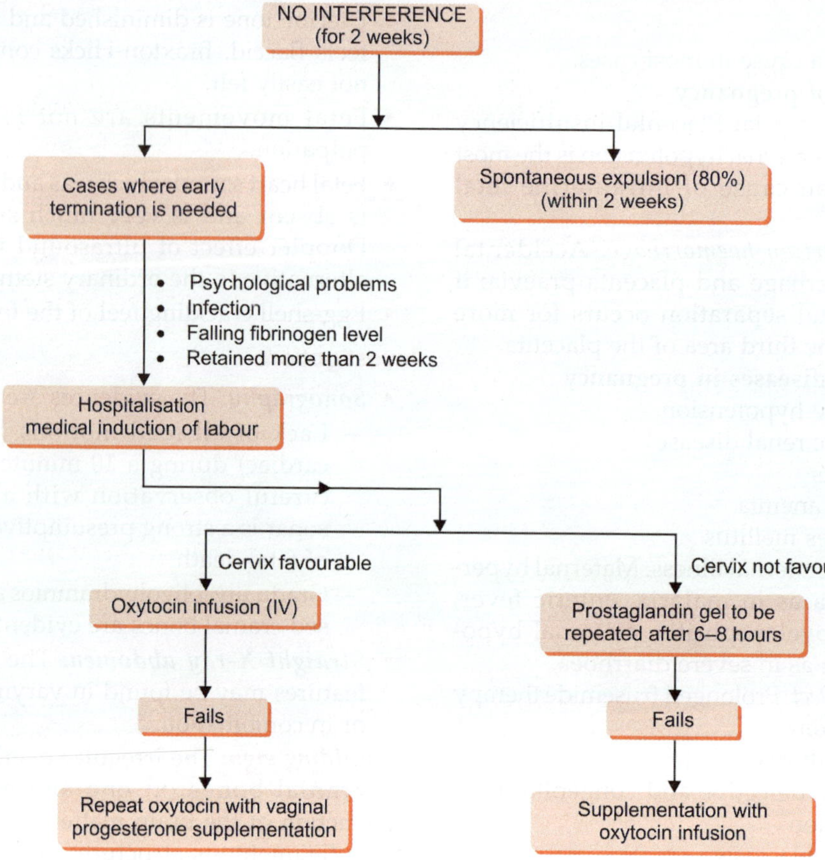

```
                          ┌─────────────────────┐
                          │   NO INTERFERENCE   │
                          │     (for 2 weeks)   │
                          └──────────┬──────────┘
              ┌──────────────────────┴──────────────────────┐
              ▼                                              ▼
  ┌───────────────────────┐                    ┌───────────────────────────┐
  │   Cases where early   │                    │ Spontaneous expulsion (80%)│
  │  termination is needed│                    │    (within 2 weeks)        │
  └───────────┬───────────┘                    └───────────────────────────┘

        • Psychological problems
        • Infection
        • Falling fibrinogen level
        • Retained more than 2 weeks

  ┌───────────────────────┐
  │    Hospitalisation     │
  │ medical induction of labour│
  └───────────┬───────────┘
       ┌───────┴────────────────────────────────┐
       ▼                                         ▼
  Cervix favourable                       Cervix not favourable
  ┌───────────────────────┐              ┌───────────────────────────┐
  │  Oxytocin infusion (IV)│              │  Prostaglandin gel to be   │
  │                       │              │ repeated after 6–8 hours   │
  └───────────┬───────────┘              └──────────┬────────────────┘
              ▼                                     ▼
        ┌──────────┐                          ┌──────────┐
        │  Fails   │                          │  Fails   │
        └────┬─────┘                          └────┬─────┘
             ▼                                     ▼
  ┌───────────────────────┐              ┌───────────────────────────┐
  │ Repeat oxytocin with vaginal│        │  Supplementation with      │
  │ progesterone supplementation│        │   oxytocin infusion         │
  └───────────────────────┘              └───────────────────────────┘
```

Fig. 8.31: Scheme of management of intrauterine fetal death

specially if the fetus is retained for more than 2 weeks.

• To find out the cause of death.

Haematological examination consists of ABO and Rh grouping, VDRL, post prandial blood sugar, HbAIC, urea, creatinine estimations, thyroid profile, TORCH screening, lupus anticoagulant and anticardiolipin antibodies. Urine examination for casts and pus cells. Naked eye examination of the placenta and the cord including histology and examination of the baby including autopsy may give some clue as to the cause of death.

Post-mortem studies may not be informative, except in cases of congenital malformations as the tissues are softened and necrotic, precluding proper examination.

Complications

1. Psychological upset often becomes a problem.
2. Infection—so long as the membranes are intact, infection is unlikely but once the membranes rupture, infection, especially by gas forming organisms like *Cl. welchii* may occur.
3. Blood coagulation disorders—if the fetus is retained for more than 4 weeks (as occur in 10–20% cases), there is a possibility of defibrination from 'silent' disseminated intravascular coagulopathy (DIC).

4. During labour—Uterine inertia, retained placenta and postpartum haemorrhage.

Prevention

While IUD cannot be totally prevented, the following guidelines can help to reduce its incidence

- Regular antenatal care—to prevent, detect at the earliest and institute effective therapy likely to cause fetal death.
- To screen out the "at-risk mothers", to monitor carefully for the assessment of fetal well being and to terminate the pregnancy at the earliest evidences of fetal compromise.

MANAGEMENT

Expectant attitude (non-interference)

The patient and her relatives are likely to be upset psychologically but they should be assured of safety of non-interference. In about 80% of cases spontaneous expulsion occurs within 2 weeks of death. The patient may remain at home for the first 2 weeks with the advice to come to the hospital for delivery. If spontaneous expulsion fails to occur within 2 weeks, the patient is to be admitted. Fibrinogen estimation should be done every week, if not twice a week. A falling blood fibrinogen level approaching 150 mg% should be arrested by controlled infusion of heparin.

Interference

The indications of interference are:

- Psychological upset of the patient—common
- Manifestations of uterine infection
- Falling fibrinogen level—the fibrinogen level should be elevated well above the critical level before interference.
- Tendency of prolongation of pregnancy beyond 2 weeks.

Early termination is now favoured as

1. Reliable diagnosis could be made with real time ultra sonography quickly

2. Prostaglandins are available for effective induction
3. Complications could be avoided.

Methods of termination

The termination should always be done by medical induction

- *Oxytocin infusion:* This is widely practised and effective in cases where the cervix is favourable. To begin with, 5–10 units of oxytocin in 500 ml of Ringer's solution is administered through intravenous infusion drip. Consecutive two bottles may be administered at a time. In case of failure, an escalating dose of oxytocin is used on the next day. To start with, a drip is set up with 20 units of oxytocin in 500 ml of Ringer's solution and run 30 drops per minute (80 mU/minute). The strength of the drip may be increased to 40 units after the first bottle, if the contraction fails to start. The risk of antidiuretic effect with such a high dose of oxytocin should be kept in mind and hence not more than two bottles should be infused at a time. If the uterus still remains refractory, the same procedure is repeated after vaginal administration of prostaglandin gel.
- *Prostaglandins:* Vaginal administration of prostaglandin (PGE$_2$) gel or lipid pessary high in the posterior fornix is very effective for induction where the cervix is unfavourable. This may have to be repeated after 6–8 hours. Misoprostol (PGE$_1$) 50 mg vaginal is also effective. The procedure may be supplemented with oxytocin infusion.

Place of caesarean section in a case with IUD is limited. Major degree placenta praevia/previous caesarean section (two or more) and transverse lie are the common ones.

STILLBIRTH

A stillbirth is a birth of newborn after 28th completed week (weighing 1000 gm or more) when

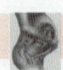

the baby does not breathe or show any sign of life after delivery.

Such deaths include antepartum deaths (macerated) and intrapartum deaths (fresh stillbirths). Stillbirths rate is the number of such deaths per 1000 total births (live and still).

Etiology

Fetal hypoxia is the most important cause.

Maternal: Maternal anemia and hypertension in labour cause placental insufficiency and fetal death.

Placental: Uterine action in labour enhances fetal hypoxia due to placental insufficiency already existing during pregnancy. Placental separation, hypertonic uterine inertia, uterine retraction after premature rupture of membranes, retraction ring in obstructed labour or tetanic spasm of uterus following injudicious oxytocic administration are important causes to interfere placental function and fetal death in labour. Prolonged and obstructed labour in late admissions is an important cause.

Umbilical cord accidents: Prolapse of cord in labour, cord compression by after coming head of breech, multiple turns around fetal neck or body or very rarely true knot are causes of fetal death.

Fetal causes: Low birth weight baby is delivered stillborn. Fetal hypoxia in labour and birth trauma are important causes. This results from delivery breech, difficult forceps deliveries, prolonged labour, precipitate labour, excessive moulding of fetal head due to cephalopelvic disproportion, rigid cervix or perineum. Fetal hypoxia may also cause intracranial haemorrhage especially in prematures. Babies with congenital malformation may die during labour or be delivered by destructive operations.

Analgesics and anaesthetics administered to mother during labour may depress the fetal respiratory centre especially in prematures.

Prevention

1. *Attending all pre-natal appointments:* It is important to attend regular pre-natal appointments throughout pregnancy to make sure baby is developing properly and also that placenta is healthy or of normal size.

2. *Monitoring fetal movements:* After 26 weeks of pregnancy, it is recommended that all pregnant women monitor the fetal movements and number of kicks that fetus makes every day. If baby is kicking less than ten times a day or seems to be abnormally quiet, to consult health care provider.

3. *Avoid infection:* Many infection responsible for still birth are preventible during pregnancy. Antenatal mother must get tested for STD's, including chlamydia, gonorrhoea and syphilis early in pregnancy.

4. *To report pain or bleeding:* Antenatal mother must monitor for any abnormal bleeding or pains during pregnancy.

ABNORMALITIES OF PLACENTA AND CORD

There is a marked variation in the morphology including size, shape and weight of the placenta. Variation of the cord is also quite common. Only those of clinical importance are described.

LARGE PLACENTA (MORE THAN 500 GM)

Occurs in syphilis, diabetes mellitus, largest in erythroblastosis foetalis.

PLACENTA SUCCENTURIATA (Fig. 8.32)

Morphology: One (usual) or more small lobes of placenta, size of a cotyledon, may be placed at varying distances from the main placental margin. A leash of vessels connecting the main to the small lobe traverse through the membranes. The accessory lobe is developed from

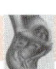

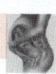

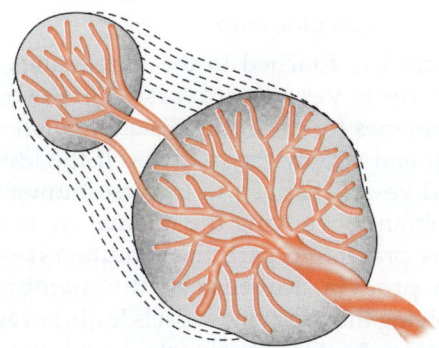

Fig. 8.32: Succenturiata placenta

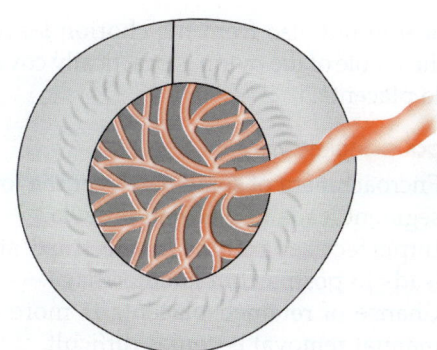

Fig. 8.33: Circumvallate placenta

the activated villi on the chorionic laeve. In case of absence of communicating blood vessels, it is called placenta spuria. The incidence of placenta succenturiata is about 3%.

Diagnosis: Diagnosis is made following inspection of the placenta after its expulsion.

1. With intact lobe the features have already been described.
2. With missing lobe
   a. There is a gap in the chorion
   b. Torn ends of blood vessels are found on the margin of the gap.

Clinical significance: If the succenturiate lobe is retained, following birth of the placenta, it may lead to

1. Postpartum haemorrhage which may be primary or secondary
2. Subinvolution
3. Uterine sepsis
4. Polyp formation

Treatment: Whenever the diagnosis of missing lobe is made, exploration of the uterus and removal of the lobe under general anaesthesia is to be done.

PLACENTA EXTRACHORIALIS

Two types are described

1. Circumvallate placenta (Fig. 8.33)
2. Placenta marginata

Morphology

Circumvallate placenta

1. The fetal surface is divided into a central depressed zone surrounded by a thickened white ring which is usually complete. The ring is situated at varying distances from the margin of the placenta. The ring is composed of a double fold of amnion and chorion with degenerated decidua and fibrin in between.
2. Vessels radiate from the cord insertion as far as the ring and then disappear from view.
3. The peripheral zone outside the ring is thicker and the edge is elevated and rounded.

Placenta marginata: A thin fibrous ring is present at the margin of the chorionic plate where the fetal vessels appear to terminate.

Clinical significance: There is increased chance of

1. Abortion
2. Hydrorrhoea gravidarum (excessive watery vaginal discharge)
3. Antepartum haemorrhage
4. Growth retardation of the baby
5. Preterm delivery
6. Retained placenta or membranes

PLACENTA MEMBRANECAE

The placenta is undually large and thin. The placenta not only develops from the chorion frondosum but also from the chorion leave so that the whole of the ovum is practically covered by the placenta.

Clinical significance

1. Encroachment of some part over the lower segment leads to placenta praevia.
2. Imperfect separation in the third stage leads to postpartum haemorrhage.
3. Chance of retained placenta is more and manual removal becomes difficult.

PLACENTA ACCRETA AND INCRETA

In placenta accreta the decidua is entirely absent; in increta the muscles have been invaded by the villi. Fortunately such morbid adhesion is usually partial, rarely complete. As an extreme rarity, placenta percreta—villi perforating the uterine wall can occur, The endometrial scarring due to vigorous curettage, severe infection is a predisposing factor of morbid additions of placenta.

CORD ABNORMALITIES

Battledore placenta (Fig. 8.34)

The cord is attached to the margin of the placenta. If associated with low implantation of the placenta, there is chance of cord compression in vaginal delivery leading to fetal anoxia or even death; otherwise, it has got little clinical significance.

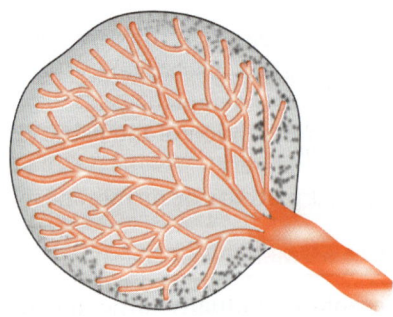

Fig. 8.34: Battledore placenta

Velamentous placenta

The cord is attached to the membranes. The branching vessels traverse between the membranes for a varying distance before they reach and supply the placenta. If the leash of blood vessels happen to traverse through the membranes overlying the internal os, in front of the presenting part, the condition is called vasa praevia. Rupture of the membranes involving the overlying vessels leads to vaginal bleeding. As it is entirely fetal blood, this may result in fetal exsanguination and even death (Fig. 8.35).

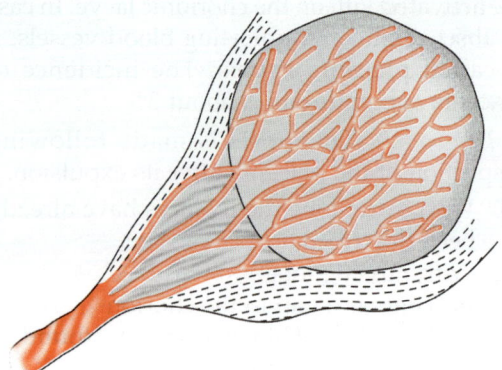

Fig. 8.35: Velamentous placenta

Bipartite placenta

Two complete and separate parts are present, each with a cord leaving it. The bipartite cord joins a short distance from the two parts of the placenta. This is different from the two placenta in a twin pregnancy, where there are also two umbilical cords, but these do not join at any point. Where there is a succenturate lobe, the vessels are attached to the placenta directly and never join the cord.

Tripartite placenta

A *tripartite placenta* is similar but with three distinct parts.

Except for the dangers noted above these varieties of conformation have no clinical significance.

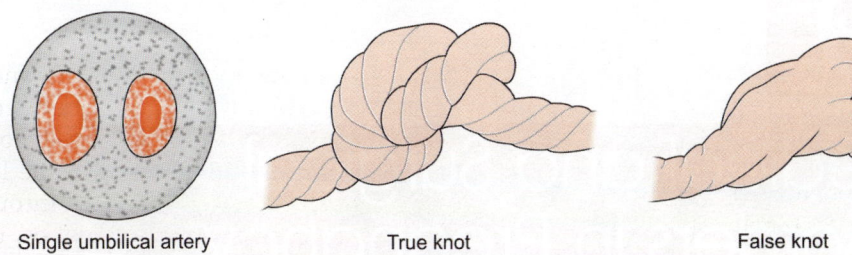

| Single umbilical artery | True knot | False knot |

Fig. 8.36: Abnormalities in the umbilical cord

Management

In the presence of fetal bleeding, urgent delivery is essential either vaginally or by caesarean section. The infant's haemoglobin should be estimated and if necessary, blood transfusion be carried out. If the baby is dead, vaginal delivery is awaited.

Abnormal length

The cord may be unduly long or short.

Short cord: The short cord may be true (less than 20 cm or 8") or commonly relative due to entanglement of the cord round any fetal part. In exceptional circumstances, the cord may be absent and the placenta may be attached to the liver as in examples.

Clinical significance

In either variety, it may cause
1. Failure of external version
2. Prevent descent of the presenting part specially during labour
3. Separation of a normally situated placenta
4. Favour malpresentation

Long cord: The clinical significance due to the presence of a long cord is that there is an increased chance of
1. Cord prolapse

2. Cord entanglement round the neck or the body. The condition may produce sufficient compression on the cord vessels so as to produce fetal distress or rarely death.
3. True knot is rare. Even with true knot the fetal vessels are protected from compression, by the Wharton's jelly. False knots are the result of accumulation of Wharton's jelly or due to varices.

Single umbilical artery

Single umbilical artery is present in about 1–2 per cent of cases. It may be due to failure of development of one artery or due to its atrophy in later months. It is more common in twins and in babies, born of diabetic mothers or in polyhydramnios. It is frequently associated with congenital malformation of the fetus (10–20 per cent). There is increased chances of miscarriage, prematurity, IUGR and increased perinatal mortality.

Knots in the cord

- *True knot:* It occurs in 1% deliveries when cord is long and fetus actively moves. It is common in monoamniotic twins. Perinatal loss increases threefold.
- *False knot:* It occurs from kinking of vessels and a developmental variation. It has no clinical importance.

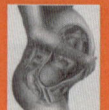

9

Medical and Surgical Disorders in Pregnancy

OUTLINE

- Hypertensive disorders in pregnancy
- Anaemia in pregnancy
- Heart disease
- Asthma
- Diabetes
- Thyroid disorders
- Epilepsy
- Hyperemesis gravidarum
- Rh incompatibility
- Jaundice
- Infections in pregnancy

HYPERTENSIVE DISORDERS IN PREGNANCY

Hypertension is one of the common complication with in pregnancy and contributes significantly to maternal and perinatal morbidity and mortality.

PREGNANCY INDUCED HYPERTENSION (PIH)

Pregnancy induced hypertension (PIH) is divided into three clinical types
- Pre-eclampsia
- Eclampsia
- Gestational hypertension

PRE-ECLAMPSIA

Definition

Pre-eclampsia is a multi system disorder of unknown etiology characterised by develop-ment of hypertension to the extent of 140/90 mm Hg or more with proteinuria and edema or both induced by pregnancy after the 20th week in a previously normotensive and non-proteinuria patient. The pre-eclamptic features may appear, even before the 20th week as in cases of hydatidiform mole and acute poly-hydramnios.

Classification

Pre-eclampsia may appear as a primary disorder or it may complicate pre-existing pathology like chronic hypertension or chronic nephritis. The classification of hypertension in pregnancy, the two conditions are often incorporated.

1. **Primary:** 70%
   - Pre-eclampsia
   - Eclampsia (with convulsion)
2. **Secondary:** 30%
   - Pre-eclampsia—eclampsia superimposed on chronic hypertension (25%)
   - Pre-eclampsia—eclampsia superimposed on chronic nephritis (5%)

Diagnostic criteria of pregnancy induced hypertension

Hypertension: *An absolute rise of blood pressure at least 140/90 mm Hg,* if the previous blood pressure is not known or a rise in systolic pressure of at least 30 mm Hg or a rise in diastolic pressure of at least 15 mm Hg over the previously known pressure is called pregnancy induced hypertension.

Calculation based on mean arterial pressure (MAP) as advocated by page

$$\frac{\text{Systolic pressure} + (\text{diastolic pressure} \times 2)}{3} = \text{MAP}$$

A rise of 20 mm Hg over the previous reading, or when the MAP is 105 mm Hg or more should be considered as significant.

Oedema: Demonstration of *pitting oedema over the ankles* after 12 hours bed rest or rapid gain in weight of more than 1 lb a week or more than 5 lb a month in the later months of pregnancy may be the earliest evidence of pre-eclampsia.

Proteinuria: Presence of protein in 24 hours urine of more than 0.3 gm or more than 1 gm per litre in 2 or more midstream specimens obtained 6 hours apart in the absence of urinary tract infection is considered significant.

Incidence

The incidence in primigravidae is about 10% and multigravidae 5%.

Predisposing factors

There is increased association of pre-eclampsia with the following :

1. Elderly and young primigravidae
2. Family history of pre-eclampsia, eclampsia or hypertension
3. Poor and underprivileged sector—more due to neglect in antenatal care rather than nutritional cause.
4. Pregnancy complications such as hydatidiform mole, multiple pregnancy, polyhydramnios, Rh incompatibility
5. Medical disorders—hypertension, nephritis, diabetes
6. New paternity
7. Hereditary—thought to be single recessive gene disorder. Cigarette smoking reduces the risk.

Etiology of pregnancy induced hypertension (Fig. 9.1)

Hypertension

The underlying basic pathology is intense *vasospasm,* affecting almost all the vessels, particularly those of uterus, kidney and brain. The responsible agent for vasospasm, still has not been isolated precisely, but it seems certain to be humoral in origin.

The following are the possibilities

- Increased normal circulating pressor substances or appearance of a new pressor agent.
- Vascular system is sensitised, so that the normal circulating pressor substances act adversely.
- Diminished vascular refractoriness to the normal circulating pressor substances.

There is, as yet, no proof of appearance of any new pressor substance nor any increase of normal circulating pressor substances like renin-angiotensin complex or vasopressin or epinephrine in pre-eclampsia.

In normal pregnancy

1. Angiotensin-II (part of ex; globulin) is destroyed by angiotensinase which is liberated from the placenta. Thus, the blood pressure is stabilized.
2. The vascular system becomes refractory, selectively to pressor agent angiotensin-II. This is probably brought out by *vascular synthesis of prostaglandin I_2 and nitric oxide (NO)* which have got vasodilator effect. The interaction between the two systems stabilizes the blood pressure in normal pregnancy.

In pre-eclampsia

1. There is an *imbalance of different components of prostaglandins*—relative or absolute deficiency of vasodilator prostaglandin (PGI_2), synthesized in vascular

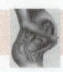

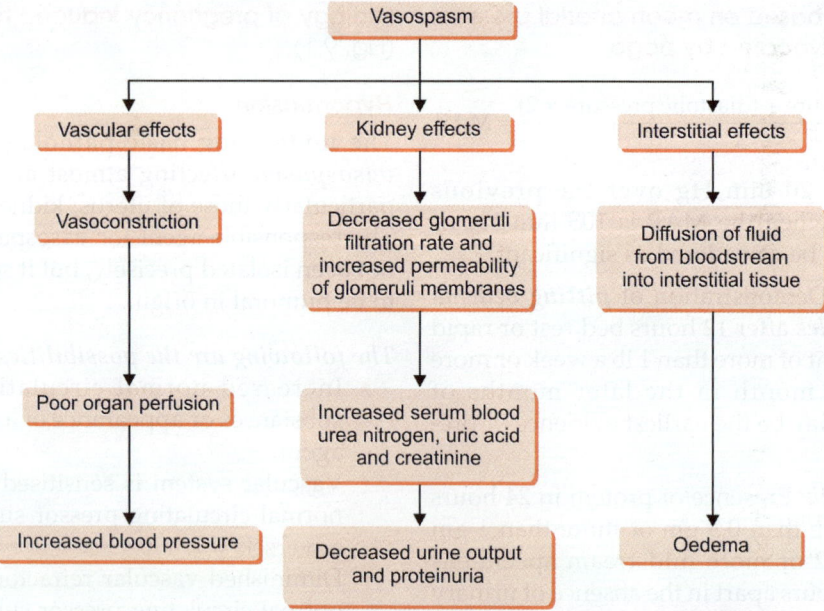

Fig. 9.1: Physiologic changes with pregnancy induced hypertension

endothelium and increased synthesis of thromboxane (TXA_2), a potent vasocons-trictor in platelets.

2. *There is increased vascular sensitivity to the pressor agent angiotensin-II.* The sensitizing substances are yet to be explored. The role of steroid sex hormones oestrogen, progesterone or other metabolites still remain speculative. Increased vasocons-trictor effect on the sensitised blood vessels is due to the elevated concentration of sodium in the extracellular mucopoly-saccharides on the arterial wall.

3. **Nitric oxide (NO):** It is synthesized in the vascular endothelium and syncytiotropho-blast from L-arginine. It significantly relaxes vascular smooth muscle, inhibits platelet aggregation and prevents inter-villous thrombosis. Deficiency of nitric oxide contributes to the development of hypertension.

4. **Endothelin-1** is synthesized by endothelial cells and it is a potent vasoconstrictor compared to angiotensin II. Endothelin-1 also contributes to the cause of hyper-tension. Hence pre-eclampsia is charac-terised by complex *endothelial cell dysfunction* resulting in imbalance of vasodilators such as PGI_2 and NO on one hand and vasoconstrictors such as angiotensin II, TXA_2 and endothelin-I on the other.

5. It has been suggested that abnormality is due to a *single recessive immune response gene* of homozygous in nature. *Lupus anti-coagulant (LA) and Anticardiolipin anti-bodies (ACAs)* also have been associated with pre-eclampsia.

6. *Angiotensinase activity is depressed,* more so following proteinuria with elimination of α_2 globulin.

Oedema

The cause of excessive accumulation of fluids in the extracellular tissue spaces is not clear. Excessive retention of sodium in the oedematous state is *probably due to increased aldosterone out of activation of corticosterone by angiotensin-II.* But paradoxically in severe pre-eclampsia, aldosterone level falls. Diminished renal blood flow, decreased glomerular filtration rate and increased tubular reabsorption are also responsible for retention of sodium.

Proteinuria

The probable chain of events is as follows. Spasm of the afferent glomerular arterioles→ anoxic damage to the endothelium of the glomerular tuft → increased capillary permeability→increased leakage of proteins. Tubular reabsorption is simultaneously depressed. *Albumin constitutes 50–60% and alpha globulin constitutes 10–15% of the total proteins excreted in the urine.*

PATHOPHYSIOLOGY

It becomes evident in severe pre-eclampsia and eclampsia. Pathological changes are vascular injury as fibrinoid atheros, capillary—arteriolar thrombosis, haemorrhage surrounding area.

- *Brain* becomes oedematous with capillary haemorrhage, thrombosis, patchy areas of necrosis.
- *Venticular haemorrhage:* Clinically irritability of CNS, hyperactive reflexes.
- *Liver:* Enlarges subcapsular haemorrhage, microscopic
  - Periportal haemorrhagic necrosis at periphery of lobule.
  - Fatty change 3 thrombi in portal capillaries.

Complications

- *Liver* may rupture. Hepatic dysfunctions— jaundice, enzymes raised.
- *Kidney:* Normal size or slightly enlarged, microscopic. Avascular glomeruli with endothelial and epithelial cellular swelling.

- *Glomerural endotheliosis,* mesangial cells increase. Tubular epithelial degeneration and desquamation.

Effect

- *Renal blood flow* is reduced, protenuria, oliguria, anuria. Kidneys fully recover following delivery.
- *Heart:* Cloudy swelling to fatty change, lungs become congested.
- *Adrenal haemorrhage (eclampsia)*
- *Stamach haemorrhage*
- *Placenta:* Progressive reduction in maternal placental blood flow to one third (placental insufficiency) causes intrauterine growth retardation.

Hypoxia leads to hyperplasia of structures - increased syncytial sprouting, proliferation of cytotophoblast and thickening of basement membranes. White infarcts could not be correlated.

Acute red infarcts may be present due to maternal blood sinus thrombosis.

Placental blood vessel show acute fibrinoid necrosis, fibrin deposit and medial necrosis (acute atherosis).

Water and electrolyte

Two stages

- *Early stage* of sodium and water retention increases plasma volume and interstitial water retention →generalized edema. Capillary permeability increases.
  Salt (sodium chloride) content of interstitial fluid rises. Sodium shifts into arterial wall. Raised plasma prolactin causes vascular sensitivity or salt retaining in arteriole. Ascites may develop.
- *Late stage* of sodium retention and generalized vasoconstriction characterized by decreased plasma volume. Plasma bicarbonate falls.

Haemodynamic changes

1. Cardiac contractility is rarely impaired.

 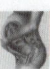

2. Cardiac afterload (ventricular wall tension during systole) is elevated.

3. Cardiac period (endodiastolic filling pressure) is usually normal or low.

4. Cardiac output falls with increases hypertension. Peripheral vasodilators improve cardiac output.

5. Blood volume is reduced due to haemoconcentration

6. Haematocrit value rises.

Hormonal changes

- In severe preeclampsia plasma oestrogen—progesterone are reduced.
- Plasma hCG is constantly elevated.
- Plasma prolactin level is elevated.
- Amniotic fluid prolactin rises.
- Aldosterone is lower in mild pre-eclampsia, further reduced in severe pre-eclampsia.

Coagulation

Disseminated intravascular coagulation: Thromboplastin absorption from throphoplast into maternal circulation →varying degree of intravascular coagulation (disseminated intravascular coagulation D.I.C.) can develop in the form of platelet—fibrin thrombi in microcirculation of brain, pituitary, kidney, heart, lungs, placenta →reduced circulating platelet →increase in fibrin degradation products →plasma fibrinogen falls. Soluble fibrin monomer complexes rise. Plasma antithrombin III falls. DIC is the effect rather than cause of PIH.

CLINICAL TYPES

- *Mild:* This includes cases of sustained rise of blood pressure of more than 140/90 mm Hg but less than 160 systolic or 110 diastolic without significant proteinuria.
- *Severe:* Severe pre-eclampsia is diagnosed when one or more of the following manifestations exists.

1. A persistent diastolic pressure of > 110 mm Hg.
2. Persistent severe epigastric pain
3. Cerebral or visual disturbances
4. Oliguria.
5. Protein excretion of > 5 gm/day.
6. Platelet count < 1,00,000/Ul.
7. Elevated liver enzymes.
8. Retinal haemorrhages, exudates or papilledema.
9. Intrauterine growth restriction of the fetus.
10. Pulmonary oedema.

From the prognostic point of view, a diastolic rise of blood pressure is more important than the systolic rise.

CLINICAL FEATURES

Pre-eclampsia frequently occurs in primigravidae (70%). It is more often associated with obstetrical medical complications such as multiple pregnancy, polyhydramnios, pre-existing hypertension, diabetes, etc. The clinical manifestations appear usually after the 20th week.

Onset

The onset is usually insidious and the syndrome runs a slow course. On rare occasion, however, the onset becomes acute and follows a rapid course.

Symptoms

Pre-eclampsia is principally a syndrome of signs and when symptoms appear, it is usually late.

Mild symptoms: Slight swelling over the ankles which persists on rising from the bed in the morning or tightness of the ring on the finger is the early manifestation of pre-eclampsia oedema. Gradually, the swelling may extend to the face, abdominal wall, vulva and even the whole body.

Alarming symptoms: The following are the ominous symptoms which may be evident either singly or in combination. *These are usually associated with acute onset of the syndrome.*

1. *Headache*—either located over the occipital or frontal region,
2. *Disturbed sleep*
3. *Diminished urinary output*—urinary output of less than 500 ml in 24 hours is very ominous.
4. *Epigastric pain*—acute pain in the epigastric region associated with vomiting, at times coffee colour, is due to haemorrhagic gastritis or due to subcapsular haemorrhage in the liver.
5. *Eye symptoms*—there may be blurring or dimness of vision or at times complete blindness. Vision is usually regained within 4–6 weeks following delivery. The eye symptoms are due to spasm of retinal vessels, oedema and retinal detachment.

Signs

1. *Abnormal weight gain:* Abnormal weight gain within a short span of time probably appears even before the visible oedema. *A rapid gain in weight of more than 5 lb a month or more than 1 lb a week in later months of pregnancy is significant.*
2. *Rise of blood pressure:* The rise of blood pressure is usually insidious but may be abrupt. The diastolic pressure usually tends to rise first followed by the systolic pressure.
3. *Oedema:* Visible oedema over the ankles on rising from the bed in the morning is pathological. The oedema may spread to other parts of the body in uncared cases. Sudden and generalised oedema may indicate imminent eclampsia. Observation of edema in addition to hypertension warrants additional investigation. Edema is assessed for distribution, degree and pitting.

Dependent edema is edema of the lowest or most dependent parts of the body, where hydrostatic pressure is greatest. If a pregnant woman is ambulatory, this edema may first be evident in the feet and ankles. If the pregnant woman is confined to bed, the edema is more likely to occur in the sacral region.

Pitting edema is edema that leaves a small depression or pit after finger pressure is applied to the swollen area. The pit, which caused by movement of fluid to adjacent tissue away from the point of pressure, normally disappears within 10 to 30 seconds. Although the amount of edema is difficult to quantitate. The method described may be used to record relative degree of edema formation.

4. *There is no manifestation* of chronic cardiovascular or renal pathology.
5. *Abdominal examination* may reveal evidences of chronic placental insufficiency such as scanty liquor or growth retardation of the fetus.

Thus, the manifestations of pre-eclampsia usually appear in the following order—rapid gain in weight →visible oedema and/or hypertension →proteinuria.

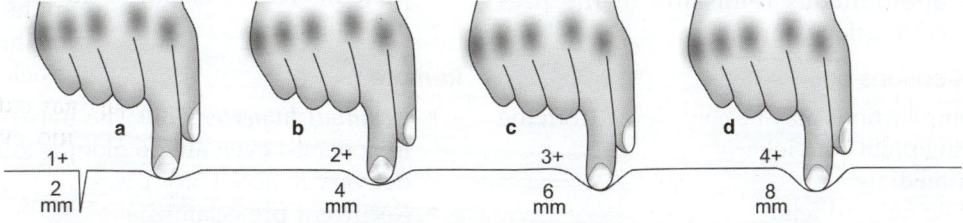

Fig 9.2: Assessment of pitting edema: a +1, b +2, c +3, d +4

 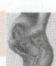

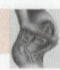

Investigations

- *Urine:* Proteinuria is the last feature of pre-eclampsia to appear. It may be trace or at times copious. There may be few hyaline casts, epithelial cells or even few red cells.
- *Ophthalmoscopic examination:* In severe cases there may be retinal oedema, constriction of the arterioles, alteration of normal ratio of vein.
- *Blood values:* A serum uric acid level *(biochemical marker of pre-eclampsia)* of more than 4.5 mg% indicates the presence of pre-eclampsia. Blood urea level remains normal or slightly raised. Serum creatinine level may be more than 1 mg/dl. There may be thrombocytopenia of varying degrees. Hepatic enzyme levels may be increased.
- **Antenatal fetal monitoring:** *Antenatal fetal* well being assessment is done by clinical examination, daily fetal kick count, ultrasonography for fetal growth and liquor pockets, cardiotocography.

Course of the disease

Pre-eclampsia is usually insidious in onset and runs a slow course. The following course of events may occur:

- *If detected early:* With prompt and effective treatment the pre-eclampsia features may subside completely.
- *If left untreated and uncared for*
  - The pre-eclampsia features remain stationary.
  - Aggravation of the pre-eclamptic features.
  - Eclampsia
  - Spontaneous remission of the pre-eclamptic features.

Complications

The complications may be considered from the following points of view:

1. **Immediate**
   Maternal and fetal
2. **Remote**

Immediate

Maternal
- *During pregnancy*
  - Eclampsia (2%)
  - Accidental haemorrhage
  - Oliguria and anuria
  - Dimness of vision and even blindness
  - Preterm labour
  - **HELLP** syndrome (haemolytic anaemia, elevated liver enzymes, low platelet count).
- *During labour*
  - Eclampsia
  - Postpartum haemorrhage—may be related with coagulation failure.
- *Puerperium*
  - *Eclampsia:* Usually occurs within 48 hours
  - *Shock:* Puerperal vasomotor collapse is associated with reduced concentration of sodium and chloride.
  - *Sepsis:* Due to increased incidence of induction, operative interference and low vitality.

Fetal

The fetal risk is related to the severity of pre-eclampsia, duration of the disease and degree of proteinuria.

1. Intrauterine death—due to spasm of utero-placental circulation leading to accidental haemorrhage or acute red infarction.
2. Intra-uterine growth restriction—due to chronic placental insufficiency
3. Asphyxia
4. Prematurity—either due to spontaneous preterm onset of labour or due to preterm induction.

Remote

- *Residual hypertension:* The hypertension may persist even after 6 months following delivery in about 50% cases.
- Recurrent pre-eclampsia
- Chronic nephritis

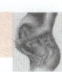

PROGNOSIS

The prognosis of pre-eclampsia depends on the period of gestation, severity of disease and response to treatment.

Immediate

If the pre-eclampsia is detected early, with prompt and effective treatment the pre-eclamptic features subside completely and the prognosis is not unfavourable, both for the mother and the baby. However, if the cases are left uncared for, as happens in the developing countries or with cases of acute onset, serious complications are likely to occur. In such conditions, both the mother and the baby are in danger.

Maternal mortality: Increased maternal deaths are mainly related to eclampsia, accidental haemorrhage, acute renal failure, pulmonary oedema, disseminated intravascular coagulopathy and HELLP syndrome.

Perinatal mortality: Although the maternal mortality has been reduced significantly, the perinatal mortality still remains very high even in the developed countries (7–10%). In the developing countries, the perinatal mortality remains to the extent of about 20%, about 50% of which being stillborn.

Remote

There is no evidence to suggest that severity of pre-eclampsia or its duration has got an effect on the development of residual hypertension (50%) or recurrent pre-eclampsia (25%) in subsequent pregnancies.

PREDICTION AND PREVENTION

Pre-eclampsia is not a totally preventable disease. Somewhat, it is found more related to chains of social ills such as poor maternal nutrition, limited or no antenatal care and poor reproductive education. However, some specific "high risk" factors leading to pre-eclampsia may be identified in an individual. These are:

1. Primigravida specially with young and elderly
2. Poor nutrition
3. Low level of education
4. Presence of complicating factors like pre-existing hypertension, twins, polyhydramnios, clinical or latent diabetes, nephritis, etc.
5. History of pre-eclampsia or hypertension in the family or in previous pregnancy
6. Abnormal weight gain
7. Rising serum uric acid level.

The following regime should be enforced in such a group of patients in an attempt to prevent or to detect early manifestations of pre-eclampsia.

- Regular antenatal check up at frequent interval from the beginning of pregnancy to detect at the earliest, the rapid gain in weight or a tendency of rising blood pressure specially the diastolic one.
- The patient is advised to take adequate rest in bed on her left side at least extra 2 hours at noon from the 20th week of pregnancy onwards.
- Low dose aspirin 60 mg daily beginning early in pregnancy in potentially high risk patients seems promising. It selectively reduces platelet thromboxane production. Aspirin in low doses is known to inhibit cyclo-oxygenase in platelets thereby preventing the formation of thromboxane A_2 without interfering with prostacyclin generation.
- Calcium supplementation (2 gm per day) reduces the risk of pre-eclampsia.
- Antioxidants, vitamins E & C, taking from 16 to 22 weeks onwards reduce the risk of pre-eclampsia. She should be on a well balanced diet rich in protein.

MANAGEMENT

So long as the etiology of pre-eclampsia remains obscure, the treatment is mostly empirical and symptomatic. While measures are directed to relieve oedema and hypertension, there is no specific therapy to proteinuria which automatically subsides with the control of hypertension.

Objectives are

1. To correct/stabilize the altered physiology.
2. Prevention of complications.
3. Prevention of eclampsia.
4. Delivery of a healthy baby, in optimal time with minimum maternal morbidity.

Hospital or home treatment: Ideally all patients of pre-eclampsia are to be admitted in the hospital for effective treatment. Rest, high protein diet and mild sedative at bed time are prescribed and the patient is investigated and checked after or week or even earlier. If treatment fails, the patient is to be admitted. It is essential that she should be warned against the ominous symptoms such as headache, visual disturbances, vomiting, epigastric pain or scanty urine.

Treatment modalities

Rest: The patient should be in bed preferably in left lateral position as much as possible to lessen the effects of venacaval compression. Rest

is to be continued till all the pre-eclamptic manifestations subside.

1. **Rest** increases the renal blood flow → diuresis
2. Increases the uterine blood flow → improves the placental perfusion
3. Reduces the blood pressure.

Diet: The diet should contain adequate amount of protein (about 100 gm). Salt is neither restricted nor forced. Fluids need not be restricted. Total calorie approximate 1600 cal/day.

Sedative: To cut down emotional factor, mild sedative may be given orally as phenobarbitone 60 mg or diazepam 5 mg at bed time or more frequently.

Laxative: If the patient is constipated, a mild laxative like milk of magnesia 4 teaspoons at bed time may be given.

Diuretics: The diuretics should not be used injudiciously as they cause harm to the baby by diminishing placental perfusion and by electrolyte imbalance. **The compelling reasons for its use are:**

1. Cardiac failure
2. Pulmonary oedema
3. Along with selective antihypertensive drug therapy (diazoxide group) where blood-pressure reduction is associated with fluid retention.
4. Massive oedema, not relieved by rest and producing discomfort to the patient. The most potent diuretic commonly used is frusemide (lasix) 40 mg—given orally after breakfast for 5 days in a week.

Antihypertensive: The compelling indications of its use are:

1. Persistent rise of blood pressure specially where the diastolic pressure is over 110 mm Hg. The use is more urgent if associated with proteinuria.
2. In severe pre-eclampsia to bring down the blood pressure during continued preg-

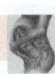

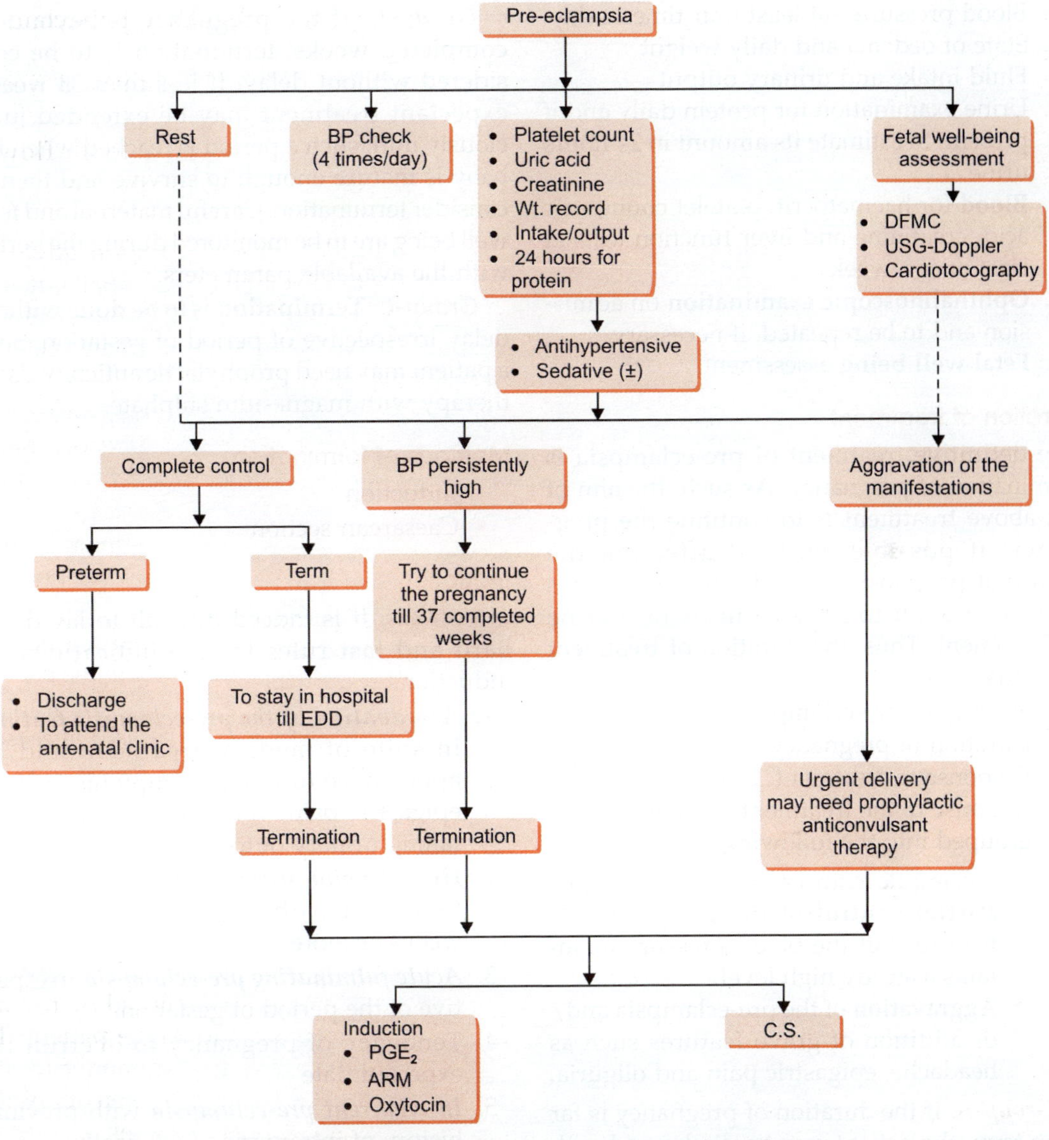

Pre-eclampsia

Rest

BP check
(4 times/day)

- Platelet count
- Uric acid
- Creatinine
- Wt. record
- Intake/output
- 24 hours for
  protein

Fetal well-being
assessment

- DFMC
- USG-Doppler
- Cardiotocography

- Antihypertensive
- Sedative (±)

Complete control

BP persistently
high

Aggravation of the
manifestations

Preterm

Term

Try to continue
the pregnancy
till 37 completed
weeks

- Discharge
- To attend the
  antenatal clinic

To stay in hospital
till EDD

Urgent delivery
may need prophylactic
anticonvulsant
therapy

Termination

Termination

Induction
- PGE$_2$
- ARM
- Oxytocin

C.S.

Fig 9.2: Scheme of management of pre-eclampsia

nancy and during the period of induction of labour. The common oral drugs used are either methyl dopa (Aldomet) 0.5–2 g/day or adrenoreceptor antagonist (both alpha and beta blocker)–labetalol 200 mg 6–8 hrly. If the blood pressure is not under control, nifedipine, a calcium channel blocker at a dose of 10–20 mg retard twice a day or hydralazine 25 mg twice daily is added.

Progress chart

The effect of treatment should be evaluated by maintaining a chart which records the following:

1. Blood pressure—at least four times a day
2. State of oedema and daily weight
3. Fluid intake and urinary output
4. Urine examination for protein daily and if present, to estimate its amount in 24 hours urine
5. **Blood** for haematocrit, platelet count, uric acid, creatinine and liver function tests at least once a week
6. **Ophthalmoscopic examination** on admission and to be repeated, if necessary
7. **Fetal well being** assessment.

Duration of treatment

The definitive treatment of pre-eclampsia is termination of pregnancy. As such, the aim of the above treatment is to continue the pregnancy, if possible, without affecting the maternal prognosis until the fetus becomes mature enough to survive in extra-uterine environment. Thus, the duration of treatment depends on

1. Severity of pre-eclampsia
2. Duration of pregnancy
3. Response to treatment. Depending on the response to the treatment, the patients are grouped into the following:

    Pre-eclamptic features completely subside.
    - **Partial control** of the pre-eclamptic features but the blood pressure maintains a steady high level.
    - **Aggravation** of the pre-eclampsia and/or addition of grave features such as headache, epigastric pain and oliguria.

Group-A: If the duration of pregnancy is far from term, the patient may be discharged with advice to attend the antenatal clinic after one week. If the patient is near term, she should be kept for a few days till completion of 37th week. Thereafter, decision is to be taken either to terminate the pregnancy or to wait for spontaneous onset of labour by the due date. It is not wise to allow the pregnancy to continue beyond the expected date.

Group-B: If the pregnancy is beyond 37 completed weeks, termination is to be considered without delay. If less than 38 weeks, expectant treatment may be extended judiciously until such a period is reached when the baby is mature enough to survive and then to consider termination. Careful maternal and fetal well being are to be monitored during the period with the available parameters.

Group-C: **Termination is to be done** without delay irrespective of period of gestation. Such a patient may need prophylactic anticonvulsant therapy with magnesium sulphate.

Methods of termination

- Induction
- Caesarean section

Induction

Indications: It is indeed difficult to lay down hard and fast rules for the indications for induction.

1. *Aggravation of the pre-eclamptic features* in spite of medical treatment and/or appearance of newer symptoms such as epigastric pain, vomiting, eye symptoms, falling urinary output.
2. *Hypertension persists* in spite of medical treatment with pregnancy reaching 38 weeks or more.
3. *Acute fulminating pre-eclampsia* irrespective of the period of gestation.
4. Tendency of pregnancy to overrun the expected date
5. *In recurrent pre-eclampsia* with previous history of intrauterine fetal death.

Methods: **If the cervix is ripe,** surgical induction by low rupture of the membranes is the method of choice. Oxytocin infusion may be added to accelerate the process in selected cases. **If the cervix is unripe** and the termination is not an urgent one, prostaglandin (PGE_2) gel 500 ug intracervical or 1–2 mg in the posterior fornix is inserted to make the cervix

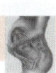

ripe when low rupture of the membranes can be performed.

CAESAREAN SECTION

Indications

1. *When an urgent termination is indicated but the cervix is unfavourable* (unripe and closed) for surgical induction.
2. *Severe pre-eclampsia* with a tendency to prolong the induction—delivery interval.
3. *Associated complicating factors* such as elderly primigravidae, contracted pelvis, malpresentation etc.

Management during labour

Blood pressure tends to rise during labour and convulsions may occur (intra-partum eclampsia). The patient *should be in bed. Liberal sedatives* should be given in the form of pethidine 75–100 mg intramuscularly and to be repeated at intervals. *Antihypertensive drugs* may be given if the blood pressure becomes high. *Blood pressure and urinary output are to be noted* regularly so as to detect imminent eclampsia. Careful monitoring of the fetal well being is mandatory.

Labour duration is curtailed by low rupture of the membranes in the first stage; and forceps or ventouse in second stage. *Intravenous ergometrine following the delivery of the anterior shoulder is withheld* as it may cause further rise of blood pressure. However, there is no contraindication of intramuscular ergometrine. *The patient should be sedated immediately following delivery* of the baby with intramuscular morphine 15 mg to prevent postpartum eclampsia and to keep the patient under close observation for several hours.

Puerperium

The patient is to be watched closely for at least 48 hours, the period during which convulsions usually occur. Tab phenobarbitone 60 mg in repeated doses can produce effective sedation.

Hypertensive drug is to continue if the diastolic pressure is raised beyond 100 mm Hg. *The patient is to be kept in the hospital,* till the blood pressure is brought down to a safe level and proteinuria disappears.

ECLAMPSIA

The term eclampsia is derived from a Greek word, meaning *like a flash of lightening*. It may occur quite abruptly, without any warning manifestations.

Pre-eclampsia when complicated with convulsion and/or coma is called eclampsia.

Incidence

The hospital incidence in India ranges from 1 in 500 to 1 in 30. It is more common in primigravidae (75%), five times more common in twins than in singleton pregnancies and occurs between the 36th week and term in more than 50%.

Cause of convulsion

The cause of cerebral irritation leading to convulsion is not clear. The irritation may be provoked by:

1. *Anoxia:* Spasm of the cerebral vessels following hypertension → increased cerebral vascular resistance → fall in cerebral oxygen consumption → anoxia.
2. *Cerebral oedema:* May contribute to irritation.
3. *Cerebral dysrhythmia:* Increases following anoxia or oedema.

Onset of fits

Fits occur more commonly beyond the 36th week (more than 50%). On rare occasions, convulsion may occur in early months as in hydatidiform mole.

- *Antepartum (50%):* Fits occur before the onset of labour. More often, labour starts soon after and at times it is impossible to differentiate it from intrapartum mole.

 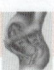

- **Intrapartum (30%):** Fits occur for the first time during labour.
- **Postpartum (20%):** Fits occur for the first time in puerperium, usually within 48 hours of delivery. Fits occurring beyond 7 days of delivery, reasonably rules out eclampsia.

CLINICAL FEATURES

Except on rare occasions, an eclamptic patient always shows previous manifestations of acute fulminating pre-eclampsia *called premonitory symptoms.*

Eclamptic convulsion or fit: The fits are epileptiform and consist of four stages.

- *Premonitory stage:* The patient becomes unconscious. There is twitching of the muscles of the face, tongue and limbs. Eye balls roll or are turned to one side and become fixed. This stage lasts for about 30 seconds.
- *Tonic stage:* The whole body goes into a tonic spasm—the trunk-opisthotonus, limbs are flexed and hands clenched. Respiration ceases and the tongue protrudes between the teeth. Cyanosis appears. Eyeballs become fixed. This stage lasts for about 30 seconds.
- *Clonic stage:* All the voluntary muscles undergo alternate contraction and relaxation. The twitchings start in the face then involve one side of the extremities and ultimately the whole body is involved in the convulsion. Biting of the tongue occurs. Breathing is stertorous and blood stained frothy secretions fill the mouth; cyanosis gradually disappears. This stage lasts for 1–4 minutes.
- *Stage of coma:* Following the fit, the patient passes on to the stage of coma. It may last for a brief period or in others deep coma persists till another convulsion. On occasion, the patient appears to be in a confused state following the fit and fails to remember the happenings. Rarely, the coma occurs without prior convulsion.

The fits are usually multiple, recurring at varying intervals. *When it occurs in quick succession it is called status eclampticus.* Following the convulsions, the temperature usually rises; pulse and respiration rates are increased and so also the blood pressure. The urinary output is markedly diminished, proteinuria is pronounced and the blood uric acid is raised.

- *Management during fit*
  1. In the premonitory stage, a mouth gag is placed in between the teeth to prevent tongue bite and should be removed after the clonic phase is over.
  2. The air passage is to be cleared off the mucus with a mucus sucker. The patient's head is to be turned to one side and the pillow is taken off. Raising the foot end of the bed, facilitates postural drainage of the upper respiratory tract.
  3. Oxygen is given until cyanosis disappears.

Status eclampticus: **Thiopentone sodium 0.5 gm** dissolved in 20 ml of 5% dextrose is given intravenously very slowly. The procedure should be supervised by an expert anaesthetist. *If the procedure fails,* use of complete anaesthesia, muscle relaxant and assisted

---

Box 9.2: After convulsion

- Observe for post convulsion coma, incontinence
- Use suction as needed
- Administer oxygen via face mask at 10 liters/min
- Start IV fluids
- Give magnesium sulfate or anticonvulsant drug as ordered
- Insert indwelling urinary catheter
- Monitor vital signs
- Monitor fetal and uterine status
- Provided hygeine and a quite enviornment
- Be prepared for delivery

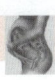

ventilation can be employed. *In unresponsive cases,* caesarean section in ideal surroundings may be a life saving attempt.

Complications

- Injuries—tongue bite, injuries due to falling out of bed, bed sore.
- Pulmonary oedema—due to leaky blood capillaries.
- Pneumonia—aspiration, hypostatic or infective.
- Acute left ventricular failure
- Hyperpyrexia
- Hepatic necrosis
- Postpartum shock
- Disturbed vision—due to retinal oedema or detachment—usually reversible.
- Puerperal sepsis
- Cerebral haemorrhage
- Renal failure
- DIC
- Pulmonary embolism, psychosis

PROGNOSIS

Maternal

Immediate: Once the convulsion occurs, the prognosis becomes uncertain. Prognosis depends on many factors and the ominous features are:

1. Long interval between the onset of fit and commencement of treatment.
2. Antepartum eclampsia specially with long delivery interval.
3. Number of fits more than 10.
4. Coma in between fits.
5. Temperature over 102°F with pulse rate above 120/minute.
6. Blood pressure over 200 mm Hg systolic.
7. Oliguria (< 400 ml/24 hours) with proteinuria > 5 gm/24 hours.
8. Non-response to treatment.
9. Jaundice

Mortality: Maternal mortality in eclampsia is very high in India and varies from 2 to 30%, much more in rural based hospital than in the urban counterpart. However, if treated early and adequately, the mortality should be even less than 2%.

Causes of maternal deaths

1. Cardiac failure
2. Pulmonary oedema
3. Aspiration and/or septic pneumonia
4. Cerebral haemorrhage
5. Anuria
6. Pulmonary embolism
7. Postpartum shock
8. Puerperal sepsis

Remote: If the patient recovers from acute illness, she is likely to recover rapidly within 2–3 weeks.

Fetal

The perinatal mortality is very high to the extent of about 30–50%. The causes are:

1. **Prematurity**—spontaneous or induced.
2. **Intrauterine asphyxia** due to placental insufficiency arising out of infarction, retro-placental haemorrhage and spasm of uteroplacental vasculature.
3. **Effects of the drugs** used to control convulsions
4. **Trauma** during operative delivery.

MANAGEMENT

First aid treatment outside the hospital: The patient, either at home or in the peripheral health centres should be shifted urgently to the referral hospitals. There is no place of continuing the treatment in such places. The patient must be heavily sedated before moving her to the hospital.

Hospital treatment: the principles

- Resuscitation—maintain airway
- Arrest convulsions
- Organise investigations
- Ventilatory support (if needed)

 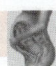

- Haemodynamic stabilisation (control BP)
- Delivery by 6–8 hours
- Postpartum care (intensive)

General management: (medical and nursing)
- *The patient should be placed in a railed cot in an isolated room,* protected from noxious stimuli which might provoke further fits. The patient is to lie on her side to minimise venacaval compression. Airway is maintained, oxygen is administered. If the patient is unconscious, the position should be changed at intervals to prevent hypostatic pneumonia and bedsore. The patient should have a doctor or at least, a trained nurse for constant supervision.
- *Detailed history is to be taken* from the relatives, relevant to the diagnosis of eclampsia, duration of pregnancy, number of fits and nature of medication administered outside.
- *Only when the patient is properly sedated,* a thorough but quick general, abdominal and vaginal examinations are made. If the patient is unconscious, a self retaining catheter is introduced and the urine is tested for protein. The continuous drainage facilitates measurement of the urinary output, periodic urine analysis and prevention of soiling of the bed due to incontinence, likely to occur during fits.
- *Half hourly pulse, respiration rates and blood pressure* to be recorded. Hourly urinary output is to be noted. If undelivered, the uterus should be palpated at regular intervals to detect the progress of labour and the fetal heart rate is to be monitored. Immediately after a convulsion, fetal bradycardia is common probably due to maternal acidosis and hypoxia induced by the fit.
- *Fluid balance:* Crystalloid solution (Ringer's solution) is started as a first choice. Total *fluids should not exceed the previous 24 hours urinary output plus 1000 ml.*

Normally, it should not exceed 2 liters in 24 hours. Infusion of balanced salt solution should be at the rate of 75–100 ml/hr.
- *Antibiotic:* To prevent infection, *ampicillin 500 mg IM or IV six hourly* is administered.

Specific management
1. **Anticonvulsant and sedative regime:** The various anticonvulsant regimes that are in use, maintain the fundamental principles as laid down by Stroganoff (1930).
   - **Magnesium sulphate** is the drug of choice. It reduces motor endplate sensitivity to acetylcholine and thereby reduces neuromuscular irritability. It induces cerebral vasodilatation, dilates uterine arteries, increases production of endothelial prostacyclin and inhibits platelet activation. It has no detrimental effects on the neonate within therapeutic level. It has got excellent result with maternal mortality of 0.4%.

Regimens of $MgSO_4$ for the management of severe pre-eclampsia and eclampsia
Loading Dose: 4 gm IV over 3–5 min followed by 10 gm deep IM (5 gm in each buttock)

Maintenance Dose: 5 gm IM 4 hourly in alternate buttock.

Repeat injections are given only if the knee jerks are present, urine output exceeds 30 ml/hour and the respiration rate is more than 12 per minute. *The therapeutic level of serum magnesium is 4–7 mEq/L.* Magnesium sulphate is continued for 24 hours after the last seizure.
- *Lytic cocktail regime:* Menon (1961) in India employed the regime using chlorpromazine, phenergan and pethidine and has got satisfactory result with reduction of **maternal mortality to 2.2%.**
- *Protocol:* On admission
  1. 25 mg chlorpromazine and 100 mg pethidine in 20 ml of 5% dextrose are given intravenously along with 50 mg chlorpromazine and 25 mg promethazine given intramuscularly.

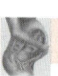

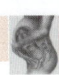

2. Subsequently, promethazine 25 mg and chlorpromazine 50 mg are given intramuscularly, alternatively at 4 hourly intervals, for a period up to 24 hours following the last fit. The dosage and time schedule are not rigid and can be modified according to the need of the case.

3. Intravenous 500 ml of 10% dextrose drip is started at the beginning with 100 mg pethidine; the drip rate is adjusted to 20–30 drops per minute. The drip rate should be so adjusted as to make the patient quiet. Not more than 2 liters of dextrose and in all 300 mg pethidine are to be given in 24 hours. *The pethidine drip should be continued up to 24 hours following the last fit.*

- *Diazepam therapy (Lean):* Diazepam is used in initial doses of 40 mg intravenously. A further 40 mg in 500 ml of 5% dextrose is infused at 30 drops per minute or adjusted as per need. *Maternal mortality rate using this regimen is 5.0%.*

- **Antihypertensives and diuretics:** Inspite of anticonvulsant and, sedative regime, if the blood pressure remains more than 160/110 mm Hg, antihypertensive drugs should be administered. Hydralazine is quite effective in such acute condition. A dose of 5 mg is given intravenously slowly and to be repeated after 20 minutes with 10 mg, if there is no response. The blood pressure should be monitored every 5 minutes. Hydralazine is next given whenever the diastolic pressure rises to 110 mm Hg. Alternatively Labetalol (combined a and p receptor blocker) is given by slow intravenous route 20 mg per hour, for smooth control of blood pressure. Dose may be doubled by every 30 min. Unlike hydralazine, labetalol does not precipitate headache and palpitation.

Presence of pulmonary oedema requires diuretics. In such cases, the potent one (frusemide) should be administered in doses of 20–40 mg intravenously and to be repeated at intervals.

Treatment of complications: Prophylactic use of antibiotics markedly reduces the complications like pulmonary and puerperal infection.

- *Pulmonary oedema:* Frusemide 40 mg IV followed by 20 → of mannitol IV reduces pulmonary oedema and also prevents adult respiratory distress syndrome. **Pulse oximeter** is very useful to monitor such a patient. Aspiration of the mucus from the tracheobronchial tree by a suction apparatus is done.
- *Heart failure:* Oxygen inhalation, parenteral lasix and digitalis are used.
- *Anuria:* It is often surprising that urine output returns to normal following termination of pregnancy.
- *Hyperpyrexia:* It is difficult to bring down the temperature as it is central in origin. However, cold sponging and antipyretics may be tried.
- *Psychosis:* Chlorpromazine or Eskazine (trifluoperazine) is quite effective.

Intensive care monitoring: Patient with multiple medical problems needs to be admitted in an intensive care unit where she is looked after by a team consisting of an obstetrician, a physician and an expert anaesthetist. Cardiac, renal or pulmonary complications are managed effectively. Use of blood gas analyser, pulse oximeter and central venous pressure monitor should be done depending on individual case.

ANEMIA IN PREGNANCY

Definition: (WHO)

Anemia in pregnancy is defined as the haemoglobin concentration in the peripheral blood is

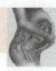

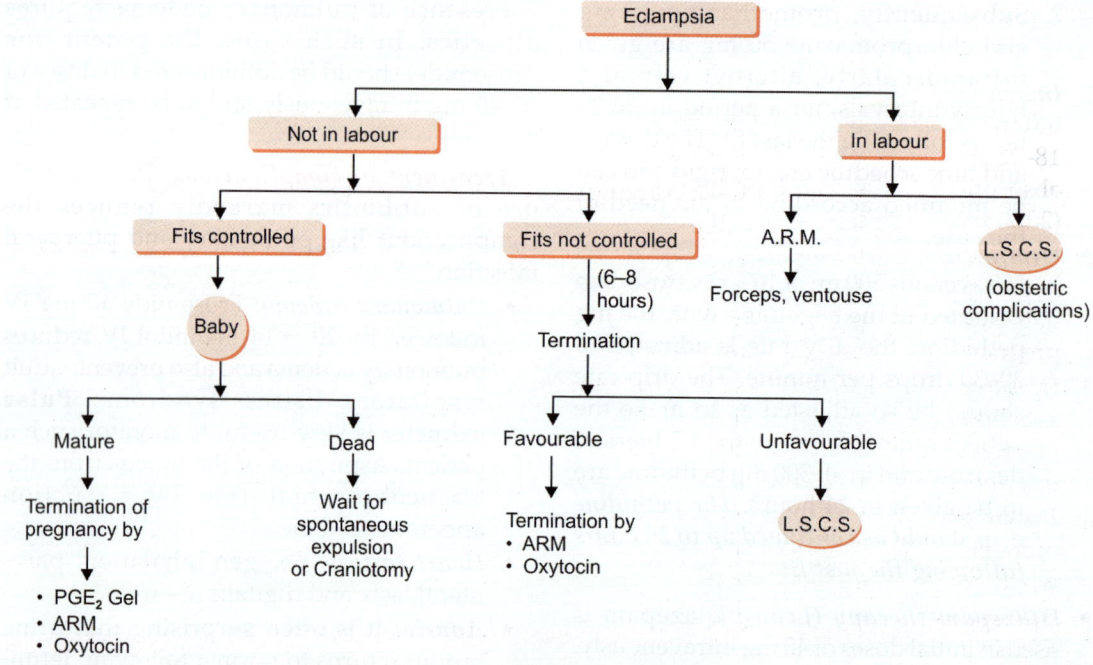

Fig. 9.3: Scheme of management of eclampsia

11 gm/100 ml or less. During pregnancy plasma volume expands resulting in haemoglobin dilution.

Classification

- Physiological anaemia of pregnancy
- Pathological anaemia

Pathological anaemia

1. Deficiency anaemia
   - Iron deficiency
   - Folic acid deficiency
   - Vitamin B_{12} deficiency
   - Protein deficiency
2. Haemorrhagic
   - Acute, e.g.: APH
   - Chronic, e.g.: Hookworm infestations, bleeding piles.
3. Hereditary
   - Thalassemias
   - Sickle cell anemia

- Haemoglobinopathies
4. Bone marrow insufficiency—aplasia due to radiation, drugs—aspirin
5. Anaemia of infection (malaria, tuberculosis)
6. Chronic disease or neoplasm

Physiological anaemia

There is disproportionate increase of plasma volume during pregnancy leads to apparent reduction of RBC, haemoglobin and haematocrit level.

The woman who has got sufficient iron reserve and is on balanced diet, is unlikely to develop anaemia during pregnancy inspite of an increased demand of iron. But inadequate food intake, repeated unplanned pregnancies, prepregnancy diminished store of iron, folic acid, gastric hyposecretion, diarrhoea, dysentery, infections, haemorrhage cause anaemia in pregnancy.

Factors which lead to the development of anemia during pregnancy

1. *Increased demands of iron:* An adequate balanced diet contains not more than 18–20 mg of iron and assuming that the absorption rate is increased by two-folds (20%) the demand is hardly fulfilled.
2. *Diminished intake of iron:* Apart from socioeconomic factors, faulty dietetic habits, loss of appetite and vomiting in pregnancy are responsible factors.
3. *Disturbed metabolism:* Pregnancy depresses the erythropoietic function of the bone marrow. Presence of infection markedly interferes with the erythropoiesis.
4. *Pre-pregnant health status:* It is the state of the stored iron which largely determines whether or not and how soon a pregnant woman will become anaemic.
5. *Excess demand*
   - Multiple pregnancy
   - Women with rapidly recurring pregnancy
   - Teenage pregnancies
   - Polymorphism

IRON DEFICIENCY ANAEMIA

Symptoms

- Lassitude, feeling of exhaustion, weakness
- Anorexia, indigestion
- Palpitation caused by ectopic beats
- Dyspnoea
- Giddiness
- Swelling of the legs

On examination

- Pallor—stomatitis, glossitis
- Oedema of the legs may be due to hypoproteinemia
- Soft systolic murmur
- Crepitations may be heard at the base of the lungs due to congestion.

Investigations

To note degree of anaemia

- Mild: 8–10 gm%
- Moderate: 8.7 gm%
- Severe: 7 gm%

To ascertain the type of anaemia

1. Peripheral blood smear (PBS): with leishman stain to study the morphology of the red cells
2. Hematological indices (lower limits)
   - Haemoglobin—10 gm%
   - Red blood cells—4 million/mm^3
   - PCV—30%
   - MCHC—30%
   - MCV—75 mm^3
   - MCH—25 pg
   - Serum iron—30 mg/100 ml.

To find out the cause of anaemia

1. *Examination of stool:* To detect helminthic infestations
2. *Urine:* Presence of protein, sugar and pus cells, culture and colony count
3. X-ray chest—pulmonary TB
4. Fractional test meal analysis of gastric juice to find out achlorhydria in pernicious anaemia.

Complications of severe anaemia

During pregnancy

1. Pre-eclampsia related to malnutrition and hypoproteinaemia
2. Inter current infection
3. Heart failure at 30–32 weeks of pregnancy
4. Preterm labour

During labour

1. Uterine inertia
2. Postpartum haemorrhage
3. Cardiac failure may be due to accelerated cardiac output (during labour or following delivery)
4. Shock

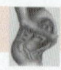

During puerperium

1. Puerperal sepsis
2. Subinvolution
3. Failing lactation
4. Puerperal venous thrombosis
5. Pulmonary embolism

Effects on baby

1. Low birth weight babies
2. IUD due to severe maternal anoxaemia
3. Increased neonatal death
4. Anaemia in baby

Treatment

Prophylactic

1. Avoidance of frequent child births
2. *Supplementary iron therapy:* 200 mg of $FeSO_4$ (60 mg of element Fe) along with 1mg folic acid. (Tea should be avoided within one hour of taking iron tablet.)
3. *Dietary prescription:* A realistic balanced diet, rich in iron and protien should be prescribed which should be within the reach of the patient and should be easily digestable. The foods rich in iron are liver, meat, egg, green vegetables, green peas, figs, beans, whole wheat and green plantains, onion stalks, jaggery. Iron utensils should preferably be used for cooking and the water used in rice and vegatable cooking should not be discarded.
4. *Adequate treatment:* To eradicate hookworm infestation, dysentery, malaria, bleeding piles and UTI.
5. Early detection of decreasing haemoglobin is to be made. Haemoglobin level should be estimated at the first antenatal visit, 30th week, finally at 36th week.

Curative

1. *Hospitalization:* Ideally all patients having haemoglobin level 9 gm per 100 ml or less should be admitted for investigation and treatment. But due to high prevalence of anaemia and inadequate hospital beds an arbitrary haemoglobin level of 7.5 gm% may be considered, when the patient should be hospitalized.
2. *Associated obstetrical—medical complication* even with moderate degree of anaemia.

General treatment include

- Diet rich in proteins, iron and vitamins is prescribed
- To improve appetite and facilitate digestion, preparation containing acid pepsin given after meals.
- To eradicate minimal septic focus—antibiotic therapy.
- Effective therapy to cure disease contributing to the cause of anaemia.

SPECIFIC THERAPY

Iron therapy

- Oral therapy
- Parenteral therapy

ORAL ROUTE

1. Fersolate tablet contian 200 mg of $FeSO_4$ thrice daily with or after meals. Treatment should be continued till blood picture becomes normal.
2. Maintenance dose—1 tablet daily to be continued for at least 100 days following delivery.

Contraindications of oral therapy

- Intolerance to oral iron
- *Severe anaemia in advanced pregnancy:* Considering the unpredictable absorption and utilization following oral therapy, parenteral therapy is the preferred choice.

PARENTERAL THERAPY

1. Intravenous route
   - Repeated injections
   - TDI—Total dose of infusion
2. Intramuscular route

Indications of parenteral therapy

- Intolerant to oral iron
- Does not respond to oral iron by one month excluding thalassaemia
- Irregular taking of oral iron.

The main advantage of parenteral therapy

The expected rise in haemoglobin concentration after parenteral therapy is 0.7–1 gm/100 ml/week.

Intravenous route

Total dose of infusion (TDI): The deficit of iron is first calculated and the total amount of iron required to correct the deficit is administered by a single sitting intrevenous infusion. The compound used is **iron dextran** compound, 1 ml of which contains 50 mg element iron and 1 ampoule contain 2 ml.

Advantages

- It eliminates repeated and painful intramuscular injections.
- The treatment is completed in a day and the patient may be discharged much earlier.
- It is less costly compared to repeated intramuscular therapy.

Estimation of the total requirements

0.3 × W (100 Hb%) mg of elemental iron. Where W = patient's weight in pounds. Hb% = observed haemoglobin concentration in percentage. Additional 50% is to be added for partial replenishment of the body store iron.

Example

The total elemental iron required in an anaemic patient weighing 100 lb with haemoglobin 50% is calculated as follows: 0.3 × 100 (100–50) = $^3/_{10}$ × 100 × 50 = 1500 mg. Add 50% = 750 mg. Total elemental iron required is 2250 mg.

Procedure

- The patient is admitted in the morning for infusion
- The required iron is mixed with 500 ml of 0.9% saline.
- Test dose of a few drops is given, wait for 5 minutes for reactions then procede.
- Precautions like those of blood transmission are to ba taken both prior and during the infusion process.
- The drip rate should be 10 drops per minute during the first 20 minutes and thereafter is increased to 40 drops per minute.
- Any adverse reaction like rigor, chest pain or hypotension calls for omission of the drip.

TDI reactions

Immediate vascular collapse, tachycardia, dyspnoea, cyanosis, vomiting, pyrexia. Painful arm in perivenous administration, late reactions, iron loading, hyperpigmentation of the skin.

Intramuscular therapy

- Iron dextran (inferon)
- Iron-sorbitol-citric acid complex in dextrin (jectofer)
- Total dose of iron-sorbitol complex is to be adjusted because of its 30% excretion in urine. Oral iron should be suspended atleast 24 hours prior to therapy to avoid reaction.

Procedure of injection

After an initial dose of 1 ml, the injections are given daily or on alternate days in doses of 2 ml intramuscularly. To prevent dark staining of the skin over the injection sites and to minimise pain the injections are given with a two inch needle deep into the upper outer quadrant of the buttock using a 'Z' technique. An additional precaution is to inject small quantity of air or saline down the needle before withdrawing it.

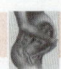

Risk of IM inferon

Staining of skin, abscess at injection site. Formation of sarcoma at IM injection site has been alleged on indiscriminate use of inferon. No such reactions could be seen with jectofer.

BLOOD TRANSFUSION

Indications

- To correct anaemia due to blood loss and to combat postpartum haemorrhage
- Patients with severe anaemia seen in late months of pregnancy
- Anaemia not responding to either oral or parenteral therapy
- Associated infection

The quality and quantity of blood: The blood to be transfused should be relatively fresh, properly typed, grouped and cross matched. Only packed cells are transfused. The quantity should be between 80 and 100 ml at a time. To allow time for readjustment, transfusion should not be repeated within 24 hours.

Risk of blood transfusion

- Premature labour may start which is more related to blood reaction.
- Cardiac failure with pulmonary edema because of overloading of the heart.
- Features of transfusion reaction

Management during labour

Ist stage

- Partography for labour is maintained
- Strict asepsis is maintained.
- Oxygen inhalation if necessary.
- Oral fluids is given, intravenous fluid is avoided.
- Injection pethidine can be given
- Packed cell blood transfusion is given in sever anaemia with heart failure.
- Close maternal and fetal monitoring is done

2nd stage

- Uterine inertia does not usually complicate.
- Prophylactic low forceps or vaccum delivery may be done to shorten the duration of second stage of labour. Strict asepsis is taken.
- Prophylactic IV ergometrine is given following the anterior shoulder delivery.

3rd stage

- One should be very vigilant during the third stage
- Fresh packed cell transfusion
- The danger of postpartum overloading of the heart should be avoided.

PUEPERIUM

- Prophylactic antibiotic
- Pre-delivery anti-anaemia therapy
- Warning about danger of recurrence of subsequent pregnancies.
- Contraceptive is provided since she is liable to have anaemia if repeat pregnancy comes early.
- Breastfeeding is encouraged

HAEMORRHAGIC ANAEMIA

Abortion, ectopic pregnancy, antepartum haemorrhage, postpartum haemorrhage make mother anaemic on recovery from hypo-volaemic shock. Bleeding piles, hook worm are additional common conditions. Anaemia becomes iron deficiency. Oral iron is the treatment.

Infections

Malaria, ankylostomiasis, dysenteries, kala azar, tuberculosis, pyelonephritis, bacterial and viral infections. Anaemia can be haemolytic iron deficiency (malaria), haemorrhagic (ankylostomiasis) or bone marrow depression (bacterial and viral); blood picture shows hypochromia microcytosis, normal or elevated serum iron.

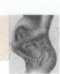

Aplastic or hypoplastic anaemia is rarely encountered during pregnancy. This may be (1) Primary congenital type, (2) secondary to drugs (cytotoxic), infection, irradiation, neoplastic infiltration, leukaemia. Severe anaemia and pancytopenia develop. Repeated blood transfusions are given, corticosteroid is continued. Therapeutic abortion is indicated.

SICKLE CELL HAEMOGLOBINOPATHIES

It is inherited disease caused by qualitative beta chain anomaly (glutamic radicle is replaced by valine) of Hb molecule characterized by formation of sickle shaped red cells in low oxygen tension.

Sickle cell disease in pregnancy (homozygous HbS, S)

1. Shortened red cell life span →haemolysis; persistent haemolytic anaemia from infancy
2. Painful repeated crisis—red cells in capillaries under low oxygen tension in chill or spontaneously become distorted to sickle cell, obstruct vessels and causes painful infarctive crisis in various organs (spleen, bone).
3. Folate deficiency is common

Effects on pregnancy

More frequent crisis, severe persistent anaemia, PIH like syndrome, bacteriuria, UTI. Pregnancy becomes hazardous.

Effect on mother

High maternal mortality (1.6%) and high perinatal mortality (30%). Infection, congestive heart failure; high incidence of abortion, preterm labour, IUGR.

Diagnosis

1. Refractory hypochromic anaemia (Hb7 gm%) or above and not responding to iron.
2. Screening test for sickle cell Hb by sickledex test.
3. Hb electrophoresis—HbF 2–20%, HbA, 2–4%, rest HbS (76%), no HbA.
4. Pain crisis in limb and abdomen.
5. Splenomegaly and hepatomegaly
6. Macrocytic anaemia may be associated. Sickling of some red cells can be seen on glass slide when mixed with 2% sodium metabisulphite.
7. Blood smear without crisis appears normal.

Treatment of sickle cell anaemia

- Partial exchange blood transfusion of HbA blood at second trimester and repeated every 2 weeks.
- For painful crisis pethidine is given.
- Folic acid 5 mg a day supplement is important. Labour is managed as in severe anaemia, oxygen therapy at times in extra need.
- Sterilization after one child is advisable.
- OC and IUCD are not recommended.

THALASSAEMIA IN PREGNANCY

Genetics

There is heredity single gene DNA mutation (deletion) in globin chain of haemoglobin resulting in red cell haemolysis. Disease is autosomal recessive following Mandelian law. If both parents are thalassaemia trait carrier, foetus has 1 in 4 chance of inheriting thalassaemia major. If one patient is thalassaemia carrier, foetus can be thalassaemia minor.

Types

1. Alpha thalassaemia—due to α chain DNA gene deletion defect in globin. This is common in South East Asia.

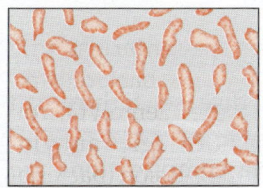
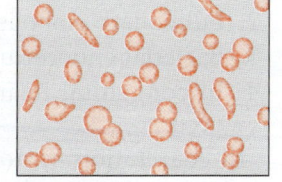

Fig. 9.4: Peripheral blood film with sickling of erythrocytes. Sickle test—RBC with 2% metabisulphite solution

2. Beta thalassaemia—β chain globin gene defect. β thalassaemia trait is commonest in India (80%) developing in late infancy and adult life. Type-1 β thalassaemia major usually does not survive to have pregnancy.

Antenatal foetal diagnosis of β thalassaemia

DNA mutation of foetal tissues is done from
- Chorion villus biopsy at 11–12th week
- Amniotic fluid foetal cells (16–18th week). On positive report for homogygous—β-thalassaemia major foetus. MTP is done by 20 weeks.

In case deleted DNA gene is not found in above foetal cells, pregnancy is permitted to continue with unaffected baby.

Obstetric features of β thalassaemic minor

1. Pregnancy is high-risk
2. Persistent chronic mild anaemia as Hb% is low. Peripheral blood smear—microcytic hypochronic (not iron deficient red cells) Serum iron is tested where high values may be present. Serum ferritin level comes low.
3. There can be associated iron deficiency anaemia where serum iron is low.
4. Splenomegaly
5. Placental hypertrophy, preterm labour, IUGR, stillbirth.

Treatment

1. Pregnancy with thalassaemia is referred to level II Care with haematologist .
2. No specific treatment
   - Only folic acid 5 mg a day if serum iron is more than 50 mg%.
   - Prophylactic and curative oral iron is given where there is combined nutritional iron deficiency anaemia (serum ferritin < 10 mg/L and serum iron is less than 50 mg%), but iron load is avoided.
3. Repeated blood transfusions are given. Under full care maternal mortality can be eliminated and also that of perinatal

mortality Birth of thalassaemia baby is prevented by current management.

HEART DISEASE IN PREGNANCY

Incidence of heart disease in pregnancy is 1% in India.

Types of heart disease in pregnancy

a. *Acquired Heart disease (90%):* Rheumatic valvular heart disease—mitral stenosis commonest (80%).
b. *Congenital heart disease (10%):* Atrial septal defect, patent ductus arteriosus, coarctation of aorta, etc.
c. *Cardiomyopathy* is a rare and highly fatal condition of myocardial failure of unknown aetiology occurring in puerperium and late pregnancy.

Cardiac physiology and haemodynamic changes with mitral valvular disease in pregnancy. Pregnancy puts on extra load on heart causing deterioration in cardiac functions because:

1. Heart in pregnancy is slightly enlarged and displaced outwards.
2. Heart has to work more due to extra blood volume of 25% during pregnancy.

Causes of death (complications) in heart disease in pregnancy, labour and puerperium.

1. Cardiac failure either in form of pulmonary oedema (less frequent) and congestive cardiac failure (more common). Cardiac failure may develop any time during pregnancy, labour, immediately after delivery (commonest).
2. Pulmonary embolism
3. Bacterial endocarditis
4. In congenital heart disease, failure can occur.

In coarctation of aorta complications are cerebral aneurysm, dissection of aorta, aortic rupture and cardiac failure.

Classification of heart disease in pregnancy

Grade I: Cardiac patient can carry normal active life without discomfort (breathless)—asymptomatic.

Grade II: Patient experiences breathless, exhaustion on ordinary physical activity. *Symptomatic on ordinary physical activity.*

Grade III: Patient experiences breathless, exhaustion even on light physical activity. *Symptomatic on light physical activity.*

Grade IV: Patient is unable to carry on any physical activity without being breathless. She is breathless even on rest (heart failure)—*symptomatic at rest.*

This functional assessment of cardiac lesion is made on her history of routine daily work. Grading is done at the time of examination of patient and may change during pregnancy.

Grading is based on subjective symptoms and does not relate to degree of cardiac lesion, it is of value when organic heart disease is diagnosed on objective signs.

Diagnosis of organic heart disease in pregnancy is made on

1. Aetiology
2. Structural lesion, e.g. mitral stenosis
3. Functional grading

MANAGEMENT

A. Antenatal care by obstetric specialist

For grade I and II

- *Clinic care:* Good antenatal care can prevent higher grade and cardiac failure.
- *Booking at first trimester:* Heart disease is clinically suspected or diagnosed by obstetrician. Referred to cardiologist for confirmation and cardiac treatment.
- *Home rest* throughout pregnancy is essential rest more hours in day time, 8 hours sleep at night.
- *All activities stopped:* Walking and light household work are permitted. Family members must support her, psychologically in particular.
- Health promotion by adequate food (without extra salt) and daily oral iron-folic acid.

She reports to clinic if breathless. She should avoid exposure to cold. Penicillin therapy is continued throughout pregnancy if she was on it as advised by cardiologist, to prevent recurrence of rheumatic fever. Inj. penidure LA 12 (benzathine penicillin) IM fortnightly is given throughout pregnancy.

- Hospital admission in high-risk pregnancy ward. For grade I she is admitted at end of 38 weeks.

For grade II

She is admitted at 28 weeks and kept in the hospital till delivery.

Grade III

Early pregnancy: Therapeutic abortion (MTP) is advised in a woman with a living baby. Hospitalisation throughout pregnancy if pregnancy is continued.

Grade IV

Immediate hospital admission and hospital care throughout pregnancy if she continues it.

Treatment of cardiac failure is promptly given on

1. Inj. morphine 5 mg IM
2. Propped up position
3. Oxygen inhalation
4. Monitoring of pulse rate, respiration rate
5. Urinary output
6. Diet: Milk, fruit juice, gradually on solid on improvement. No salty food or extra salt.
7. Fluid: Excess fluid is restricted
8. Drugs: Digitalisation, if tachycardia, cardiac failure, auricular fibrillation.

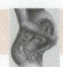

- Digoxin 0.5 mg IV followed by 0.25 mg orally every 6 hours till emergency passes off. Digitalis passes to foetus without having adverse effect in therapeutic doses.
- Diuretic: Frusemide—Inj. Lasix 20 mg IV in pulmonary oedema; oral lasix in congestive failure.
- Aminophylline 0.25–0.5 gm IV for bronchospasm followed by oral therapy.
- Anaemia is treated by hematinics, infection (respiratory) is treated by amoxycillin. Tab. Diazepam is given for sleep. Cardiologists care is given.

B. Cardiac surgery

Mitral valvotomy is now rarely performed during pregnancy. Prepregnancy mitral valvotomy is always preferred. Corrective surgery for congenital lesion is not undertaken during pregnancy

C. Obstetric treatment

Grade I and II: Patient wishing to have baby—pregnancy is left alone and continued with antenatal care as above. Vaginal delivery becomes easy and safer than caesarean section. Pregnancy usually goes to spontaneous labour. In overdated pregnancy when seldom occurs, induction of labour is done as a last measure.

Caesarean section is risky for cardiac woman since operation can precipitate heart failure (due to throwing of extra blood into circulation on uterine contraction following delivery). Other postoperative complications—pulmonary collapse, embolism are likely.

Caesarean section is rarely indicated on Obstetric reasons—cephalopelvic dispro-portion, abnormal presentation or APH.

Management in labour with heart disease

- She is prone to heart failure during labour.
- She is protected during

First stage

1. Semi recumbent position
2. Oxygen, inhalation if dyspnoea
3. Pethidine analgesia
4. Only oral fluid, intravenous fluid is avoided.
5. Monitoring of maternal pulse rate and cardiac failure. Partography is maintained.
6. Prophylactic antibiotic is given in labour—cephaxin (cephatoridine) 1 gm IV and genticyn 80 mg IM followed by second dose of both 8 hours later.

Second stage

This stage becomes usually quick in cardiac cases. For delay in progress in second stage low forceps or vacuum extraction is indicated. Perineal infiltration of xylocaine is suitable for this purpose.

Difficult forceps delivery is avoided. Anaesthesia for caesarean section is general or epidural by skilled anaesthesist.

Third stage is conducted conservatively

- *Prophylactic:* Intraveous methergin is avoided. Inj. methergin is given IM when active management is given.
- In case of postpartum haemorrhage inj. Methergin and oxytocin are given IM
- Oxytocin can be even given IV
- *Puerperium:* Delivered cardiac woman is carefully observed on her cardiac condition since she is prone to develop heart failure.
- *Breast feeding can be* given.
- She should move on the bed following delivery and go to toilet.
- She is discharged from hospital towards end of a week.
- *Contraception:* She should have one-two child by 30 years, Kohinoor is advised. CuT is feared to complicate bacterial endocarditis but can be given at 6th week. Oral contra-ceptive is not advisable. Tubectomy under general or local anaesthesia is performed after 3–4 days of delivery.

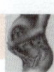
VARICOSE VEINS IN PREGNANCY

Sites are long or short saphenous veins on lower limbs and vulva. Varicosity progresses throughout pregnancy and is caused by predisposition, venous dilatation, pressure of gravid uterus on pelvic veins. Severe forms are rare in India.

Symptom: Asymptomatic or heaviness or pain at the site.

Signs: Prominent bluish tortuous veins at lower limb and vulva.

Complications: Oedema, varicose eczema ulcer, thrombophlebitis, sudden haemorrhage from vulval varices during delivery.

Treatment: To sit and lie with elevation of legs for some time in a day. To wear elastic stocking or bandage while up and about surgical treatment is not advocated during pregnancy.

DIABETES MELLITUS IN PREGNANCY

In the years before the discovery of insulin, foetal death was the rule and maternal morbidity (illness) was greatly increased when women with diabetes mellitus became pregnant. Today, technique such as multiple doses or constant infusion of insulin, home glucose testing, dietary counseling and advanced methods of foetal surveillance most often result in the birth of a healthy infant. Moreover, such measures permit the expectant mother to be an active participants in her own care that may reduce the risks of long-term complication from diabetes mellitus.

Diabetes mellitus is a chronic metabolic disorder due to either *insulin deficiency (relative or absolute)* or due to *peripheral tissue resistance* to the action of insulin. The ultimate effect is the *hyperglycaemia.* Two types are generally described.

PREGNANCY AND DIABETES

Pregnancy and diabetes are two distinct clinical entities; one is a normal physiological process that typically results in a positive outcome and other is a pathological disorder with inherent problems and complications. Gestational diabetes was first described by Heinrich Bennewitz, a graduate of Berlin University.

About 1–14 percent of all pregnancies are complicated by diabetes mellitus and 90 percent of them are gestational diabetes mellitus (GDM). Nearly 50 percent of women with GDM will become overt diabetes (type-2) over a period of 5 to 20 years.

Glycosuria in pregnancy

Repeat and random urine samples taken on one or more occasions throughout pregnancy reveal glycosuria in about 5–50 percent cases. During pregnancy, *renal threshold* is diminished due to the combined, effect of increased glomerular filtration and impaired tubular reabsorption of glucose. It is present most commonly in mid pregnancy. If glucose tolerance test is done, glucose leaks out in the urine even though the blood sugar level is well below 180 mg per 100 ml (normal renal threshold). No treatment is required and the condition disappears after delivery.

Significance

Glycosuria is specifically detected by testing a second fasting morning specimen of urine, collected a little later, after discarding the overnight urine. Fasting glycosuria if present, is ominous. Glycosuria on one occasion before 20th week and on two or more occasions, thereafter, is an indication for **glucose tolerance test.** Glycosuria occurring any time during pregnancy with a positive family history of diabetes or past history of having a baby weighing 4 kg or more should be similarly investigated.

Indications of glucose tolerance test

- Fasting glycosuria on one occasion before 20th week and on two or more occasions thereafter.

- Following a positive 'screening test'.
- If fasting blood sugar exceeds 95 mg/100 ml or if that after 2 hours of ingestion of 100 gm (WHO 75 gm) glucose is over 120 mg/100 ml.
- However, if the fasting plasma glucose value is ≥126 mg/dl and if confirmed on repeat test, there is no need to perform GTT as the woman is diabetic.

GESTATIONAL DIABETES MELLITUS

The term includes the cases with abnormal carbohydrate tolerance with onset or first detected during the present pregnancy.

Risk factors

1. Positive family history of diabetes should include uncles, aunts and grand parents.
2. Having a previous birth of an overweight baby of 4 kg or more.
3. Previous stillbirth with pancreatic islet hyperplasia revealed on autopsy.
4. Unexplained perinatal loss
5. Presence of polyhydramnios or recurrent vaginal candidiasis in present pregnancy.
6. Persistent glycosuria
7. Age over 30
8. Obesity

Screening

Screening strategy for detection of GDM are

1. *Low-risk:* Absence of any risk factors as mentioned above → blood glucose testing is not routinely required
2. *Average risk:* Some risk factors → perform screening set.
3. *High-risk:* Blood glucose test as soon as feasible.

   The method employed is by using 50 gm oral glucose tolerance test without regard to time of day or last meal, between 24–28 weeks of pregnancy.

   A plasma glucose value of 140 mg percent or that of whole blood of 130 mg percent at 1 hour is considered as cut off point *for consideration of a 100 gm (WHO 75 gm) glucose tolerance test.*

Hazards

1. Increased perinatal loss is associated with fasting hyperglycemia. Fetal anomalies are however not increased. This is due to the absence of metabolic disturbance during organogenesis.
2. Increased incidence of macrosomia.
3. Polyhydramnios.
4. Birth trauma.
5. Recurrence of GDM in subsequent pregnancies is about 50 percent.

MANAGEMENT

The patient needs more frequent antenatal supervision with periodic check up of **fasting blood glucose level which should be less than 95 mg percent.** The control of high blood glucose is done by restriction of **diet, exercise with or without insulin.** Human insulin should be started if fasting plasma glucose level exceeds 105 mg/dl and 2 hours post prandial value is greater than 130 mg/dl. even on diet control. **Diet** with 2000–2500 kcal/day for normal weight woman and restriction to 1200–1800 kcal/day for over weight woman is recommended. Exercise (aerobic, brisk walking) programmes are safe in pregnancy and may lessen the need of insulin therapy.

OBSTETRIC MANAGEMENT

Women with good glycemic control and who do not require insulin may wait for spontaneous onset of labour. However, elective delivery (induction or caesarean section) is considered in patients requiring insulin or with complications (macrosomia) at around 38 weeks.

Follow-up

Nearly 50 percent of women with GDM would develop overt diabetes over a follow-up period of 5–20 years. Women with fasting hyper-

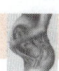
glycemia have got worse prognosis to develop type-2 diabetes and cardiovascular complications. Recurrence risk in subsequent pregnancy is more than 50 percent.

OVERT DIABETES

A patient with symptoms of diabetes mellitus and casual plasma glucose concentration 200 mg/dl or more is considered overt diabetic. The condition may be pre-existing or detected for the first time during present pregnancy. According to American Diabetic Association diagnosis is positive if

1. The fasting plasma glucose exceeds 126 mg/dl.
2. The 2 hour post glucose (75 gm) value exceeds 200 mg/dl.

Effects of pregnancy on diabetes mellitus

Diabetes mellitus in hyperglycemic state due to lack of insulin activity (dimensioned production and utilization).

Table 9.1: White's classification of pregnant diabetics	
Class A	Gestational diabetes
Class B	Overt diabetes—onset > age 20; duration < 10 years
Class C	Overt diabetes—onset < age 20; duration 10–19 years
Class D	Overt diabetes—onset < age 10; duration 20 years, benign retinopathy
Class E	Calcified pelvic vessels
Class F	Diabetic nephropathy with proteinuria
Class G	Malignant diabetic retinopathy

Table 9.2: Current classification of pregnant diabetics	
Group A	Gestational diabetes
Group B	Overt diabetes without vasculopathy
Group C	Diabetes with vasculopathy (retinopathy and/or nephropathy)

Effects

1. Hyperglycemia and glycosuria—thirst and polydipsia .
2. Increased fat catabolism conversion to free fatty acid, excess ketone bodies (acetone and β hydroxybutyric acid) ketosis acidosis, Na, K loss in urine.
3. Increased catabolism of amino acid leads to weight loss despite polyphagia.

First trimester: Insulin requirement falls to foetus and less carbohydrate intake (following sickness of pregnancy), hypoglycaemia on insulin therapy. Dose of insulin is controlled.

Early second trimester: Renal glycosuria due to lowering of renal threshold insulin requirements falls. Blood glucose is estimated for control of hyperglycaemia since glycosuria becomes misleading.

During second half of pregnancy: Insulin requirement increases due to contra insulin factors. Preexisting diabetes mellitus becomes unstable due to lack of insulin activity and effects of contra insulin factors. Ketosis develops in 10%. Risk to coma and foetal death increases.

Labour: Lack of carbohydrate intake and muscular exercise → hypoglcaemia unless she gets intravenous glucose and insulin.

Puerperium: Pregnancy contra insulin's are removed hyperglycaemia of pregnancy settles.

EFFECTS OF DIABETES ON PREGNANCY

During Pregnancy

- Spontaneous abortion increases with diabetes mellitus. The risk is related to poor glycaemic control.
- Infection increases in pregnant diabetic women. (Urinary and veginal infections increase resulting from glucose in the urine.) Infections are problematic in diabetic women because they encourage ketacidosis.
- Hydramnios increases causing over distention of the uterus, premature rupture

of membranes, preterm labour, and haemorrhage.

- Pregnancy—induced hypertension (PIH) increases with the preexisting vascular changes due to diabetes.
- Ketacidosis occurs most often in second and third trimesters when diabetogenic effect of the pregnancy is the greatest as insulin resistance increases. It is commonly a result of untreated hyperglycaemia, inappropriate dosage and maternal infections. Ketacidosis occurring during pregnancy can lead to fetal complications, even fetal death.
- Hypoglycaemia increases even with strict glycaemic control. Hypoglycaemia can be caused by overdose of insulin, skipped or late meals, or increased exercise. During the first trimester, serve hypoglycaemia can cause congenital fetal defects.

During labour

1. Prolongation of labour due to **big baby.**
2. Shoulder dystocia: Shoulder dystocia is due to disproportionate growth with increased shoulder/head ratio.
3. Perineal injuries
4. Postpartum haemorrhage
5. Operative interference

Puerperium

1. Puerperal sepsis
2. Lactation failure

Fetal risks

- **Fetal macrosomia (30–40%)** probably results from
  - **Maternal hyperglycaemia** →hypertrophy and hyperplasia of the fetal islets of Langerhans →increased secretion of fetal insulin →stimulates carbohydrate utilization and accumulation of fat. With good diabetic control, incidence of macrosomia is markedly reduced
  - **Elevation of maternal free fatty acid (FFA)** in diabetes leads to its increase

transfer to the fetus →acceleration of triglyceride synthesis →adiposity.
- **Congenital malformation** is related to the severity of diabetes affecting organogenesis in the first trimester.
- **Neonatal complications include**
  - Hypoglycaemia
  - Respiratory distress syndrome
  - Hyperbilirubinemia
  - Polycythaemia
  - Hypocalcaemia
  - Hypomagnesemia
  - Cardiomyopathy

Perinatal mortality: The overall perinatal mortality is increased 2–3 times. The neonatal deaths are principally due to hypoglycaemia, respiratory distress syndrome/polycythaemia and jaundice.

Management

Pre-conceptional counselling: Goal is to achieve tight control of diabetes before the onset of pregnancy. Ideally a diabetic woman should be seen jointly by the diabetologist, *obstetrician* and *dietician*. Fetal congenital malformations are significantly low (0.8–2%) in women who received pre-conceptional counselling. Women are taught for self glucose monitoring. Appropriate advice about diet and insulin is given. Chance of having a diabetic child is about 6% when father is only diabetic, rising to 20% if both the parents are diabetic.

Principles in the management

1. Careful antenatal supervision and control of the diabetes, so as to maintain the glucose level as near to physiological level as possible.
2. To find out the optimum time and method of delivery.
3. Arrangement for the care of the newborn.

Antenatal care: Antenatal supervision should be at monthly intervals up to 20 weeks and thereafter at 2 weeks intervals. At times patient needs admission for stabilization of

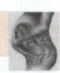

blood glucose and for monitoring the fetus. *The daily calorie requirement* is about 30–35 kcal per kg of body weight. Diet should contain carbohydrate 50%, protein 20% and fat 25–30%. Fat may be curtailed, if the patient is obese. Fibre containing diet is increased. Usually three meal regimen, with breakfast 25% of the total caloric intake/lunch 30%, dinner 30% and several snacks are quite suitable for most of the patients. *Frequent blood sugar estimation is required* as the urine examination for sugar is not informative. Monitoring of blood glucose by glucose meter can give an accurate idea about the control. In addition, glycosylated haemoglobin should be determined at the end of first trimester and three monthly thereafter. *Sonographic evaluation* in pregnancy (at 4–6 weeks interval) is extremely helpful, not only to diagnose varieties of congenital malformation of fetus but also to detect fetal macrosomia or growth restriction (rare). *Assessment of fetal well being is to be made from 28 weeks onwards. Biophysical profile* (twice weekly) should be performed when there is abnormal NST. *Doppler umbilical artery velocimetry* is useful in cases with vasculopathy.

Self-care in diabetes

- *Symptoms of hypoglycemia and ketoacidosis:* The pregnant diabetic woman must be able to recognize symptoms that indicate a change in glucose levels. She should be devised to check her capillary blood glucose level to see if it is above or below normal. In addition she should always carry a snack as a fast source of glucose. She should be devised to drink milk when possible to avoid a rebound of hyperglycemia.
- *Travel:* If insulin is required the woman should keep it refrigerated if necessary while she is travelling. A bracelet should be worn that identifies a woman as being diabetic.

- *Caesarean birth:* The woman should be advised that the possibility of a caesarean birth is increased.
- *Hospitalization:* The woman should be advised that she may be hospitalized two or three times during her pregnancy to evaluate glucose levels and adjust her insulin level.
- *Fetal monitoring:* The woman should be advised that fetal status will be assessed periodically during pregnancy.
- *Smoking:* The woman who smokes should be advised about the harmful effects of smoking on both the maternal vascular system and the development of the fetus.
- *Strict adherence to diet:* The woman should understand that during pregnancy, for the well being of the fetus, she must adhere to her diet.
- *Careful monitoring of glucose levels at home:* The woman should be advised that reliability in her daily record of glucose level is important in her care.
- *Careful monitoring of exercise.*

Insulin therapy

When diabetes is first detected during pregnancy and cannot be controlled by diet alone it should be treated with insulin. *A postprandial plasma glucose level of more than 140 mg% even on diet control is an indication of insulin therapy.* There is frequent change in insulin need during pregnancy and changes in the dosage are made in small increments at a time. Glycemic goals should be around 90 mg/dl before meals and not to exceed 120 mg/dl, 2 hours after meals. During the stabilization process of the insulin dose, frequent blood sugar estimation specially at night may be necessary using glucose meter (capillary whole blood, utilized for self monitoring, is equivalent to venous plasma). However, as pregnancy advances, "a double mixed regime" may be employed. The patient should receive three to four daily injections of a regular (human

 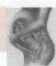

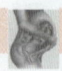

actrapid) and an intermediate acting insulin (isophane), the latter is to be given before dinner. The aim is to maintain the blood sugar level as near to normal as possible *without causing troublesome hypoglycaemia.* Use of subcutaneous insulin infusion by insulin pump is preferred as it is more physiological. *Oral antidiabetic drugs are avoided during pregnancy.* These drugs cross the placenta and may have teratogenic effect or produce neonatal hypoglycaemia.

Admission

In uncomplicated cases, the patient is admitted at 34–36 weeks. *Early hospitalization facilities:*
1. Stabilization of diabetes
2. Minimizes the incidence of pre-eclampsia, polyhydramnios and preterm labour.
3. To select out the appropriate time and method of delivery.

   Termination of pregnancy: An universal guideline cannot be formulated. But the fact that majority of intrauterine deaths of the fetus occur in the last two weeks of pregnancy, the termination should be done after 37 completed weeks. Facilities of an equipped *neonatal care unit* should be available. *Early delivery* may be considered when there is vascular complication (hypertension) or evidences of fetal compromise on antepartum monitoring.

Induction of labour

1. Multiparae with a good obstetric history.
2. Young primigravidae without any obstetric abnormality.
3. Presence of congenital malformation of the fetus

Methods

Prior to the day of induction of labour, the usual bed time dose of insulin is administered. No breakfast and no morning dose of insulin is given on the day of induction. Normal saline infusion is begun. Induction is done by low rupture of the membranes. Simultaneous oxytocin drip is started, if not contraindicated. An intravenous drip of one litre of 5% dextrose is set up with 10 units of soluble insulin. An infusion rate of 100–125 ml/hr (1–1.25 units/hr), will maintain a good glucose control to approximately 100 mg/dl. Insulin may also be infused from a syringe pump (0.25–2 units/hr). Blood glucose levels are estimated hourly with a glucose meter and the soluble insulin dose is adjusted accordingly. *Epidural analgesia is ideal* for pain relief. If the labour fails to start within 6–8 hours or if the labour progresses unsatisfactorily, caesarean section should be performed.

Caesarean section

1. Elderly primigravidae
2. Multigravidae with a bad obstetric history.
3. Diabetes with complications or difficult to control.
4. Obstetric complications like pre-eclampsia, polyhydramnios, malpresentation.
5. Fetal macrosomia (> 4 kg). As such 50% of diabetic mothers are delivered by caesarean section.

Procedure

Caesarean section is scheduled for early morning. On the day of operation, breakfast and the insulin dose are omitted. A 5% dextrose drip is started. The administration of dextrose drip and the insulin dose are to be maintained as mentioned in induction until the patient is able to take fluids by mouth. Continuous subcutaneous insulin infusion with insulin pump is preferred as it is more physiological. The insulin requirement suddenly falls following delivery and after the omission of the drip, prepregnant dose of insulin is to be administered or adjusted from the blood glucose level. *Epidural or spinal anaesthesia is better* than general anaesthesia as oral feeding could be started soon following the operation.

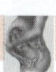

To control blood glucose

1. One litre of 5% dextrose drip is started with 10 units of soluble insulin.
2. A general guideline for insulin infusion rate is, 1 unit per hour for blood glucose of 70–130 mg/dl, 2 units per hour for blood glucose of 130–160 mg/dl and 3 units per hour for blood glucose of 160–200 mg/dl is followed. Use of motorized syringe pump for insulin infusion is convenient.
3. Hourly estimation of blood glucose levels is done with glucose meter and the insulin dose is adjusted accordingly. The blood glucose level should be maintained between 80–100 mg per 100 ml.

Place of awaiting spontaneous onset of labour at term

The following are the conditions where the pregnancy may be continued awaiting spontaneous onset of labour and vaginal delivery.

1. Young primigravidae or multiparae with good obstetric history.
2. Diabetes well controlled either by diet or insulin and without any obstetrical complication. However, in the absence of gadgets for assessment of fetal well being, it is risky to continue the pregnancy in such cases upto the EDD. *In any case, the pregnancy should not be allowed to overrun the expected date.*

Fetal monitoring: Constant watch to note the fetal condition is mandatory, preferably with continuous electronic fetal monitoring. CTG using a scalp electrode is maintained. Fetal scalp blood pH sampling is done whenever indicated. The combination of fetal hyperglycaemia and anoxia contribute not only to fetal distress but responsible for RDS. However, labour should not be allowed for more than an arbitrary 12 hours and should be augmented by low rupture of the membranes and oxytocin or delivered by caesarean section. Shoulder dystocia may be a problem. The cord should be clamped immediately after delivery to avoid hypervolaemia.

Examination of the placenta and cord: Placenta is large, the cord is thick and there is increased incidence of a single umbilical artery. Microscopically, villi show oedema and excessive syncitial knots, numerous cytotrophoblasts and thickened basement membrane. The term placentosis is given to such features.

Diabetic ketoacidosis pathology is insulin resistance →lipolysis →enhanced ketogenesis →fall in plasma HCO_3^- and pH (< 7.30).

Management is done in an acute care unit. *Parameters to assess are* degree of acidosis, alterations in the level of arterial blood gas, blood glucose, ketones and electrolytes.

- *IV insulin:* 0.2–0.4 units/kg (loading dose) →2.0–10.0 units/hour (maintenance with frequent capillary glucose measurement).
- *Fluids:* Isotonic NaCl 4–6 liters in first 12 hours. 5% Dextrose in normal saline when blood glucose is 200 mg/dl.
- *Potassium:* If reduced or normal—infusion 15–20 mEq/hour.
- *Bicarbonate:* If pH < 7.10 add 44 mEq to IL of 0.45 normal saline.

Puerperium: Antibiotics should be given prophylactically to minimize infection. *Insulin requirement falls* dramatically following delivery. She is to revert to the insulin regime as was prior to pregnancy. A fresh blood glucose level after 24 hours will help to adjust the dose of insulin. Women who breast feed should have additional 500 kcal daily in diet. In lactating women insulin dose is lower.

Care of the baby

A neonatologist should be present at the time of delivery. The baby should preferably be kept in an intensive neonatal care unit and to remain vigilant for at least 48 hours, to detect and to treat effectively any complication likely to arise.

- Asphyxia is anticipated and is treated effectively.
- To look for any congenital malformation.
- All babies should have blood glucose checked within 2 hours of birth.
- All babies should receive 1 mg vitamin K intramuscularly.
- Early breast feeding within ½-1 hour is advocated and to be repeated at three to four hourly intervals thereafter to minimize hypoglycaemia and hyperbilirubinaemia.

Improvement in the care of diabetes in pregnancy has reduced perinatal mortality significantly (< 5%).

Contraception

Barrier method of contraceptives is ideal for spacing of births. Low dose combined oral pills containing third generation progestins, are effective and have got minimal effect on carbohydrate metabolism. Main worry is their effect on vascular disease. Progestin only pill is a suitable alternative. The IUCD is avoided for fear of pelvic infection. Permanent sterilization is considered when family is completed.

HYPEREMESIS GRAVIDARUM

Hyperemesis Gravidarum is a disorder of early Pregnancy that is characterized by severe nausea and vomiting. Hyperemesis occurs in 0.5 to 10 cases per 1,000 pregnancies. The disorder most often appears between 8 and 12 weeks gestation and usually resolves by week 16.

Definition

It is a severe type of vomiting of pregnancy which has got deleterious effect on the health of the mother and/or incapacitates her in day to day activities.

Etiology

1. It is mostly limited to the first trimester.
2. It is more common in first pregnancy.

3. It has got a familial history.
4. It is more common in hydatidiform mole and multiple pregnancy.
5. It is common in unplanned pregnancies.

THEORIES

1. **Hormonal**
   - High levels of human chorionic gonadotrophin, also the increased association with hydatidiform mole or multiple pregnancy when the hCG titre is very much raised
   - Hyperoestrinism.
   - Progesterone excess leading to relaxation of the cardiac sphincter and simultaneous retention of gastric fluids due to impaired gastric motility.
   - Adrenocortical insufficiency.
2. **Psychogenic:** It probably aggravates the nausea once it begins. But neurogenic element sometimes plays a role, as evidenced by its subsidence after shifting the patient from the home surroundings.
3. **Dietetic deficiency:** Probably due to low carbohydrate reserve, as it happens after a night without food. Deficiency of vitamin B_6, vitamin B_1 and proteins may be the effects rather than the cause.
4. **Allergic:** May be related to some products secreted from the ovum.
5. **Immunological basis:** Vomiting, is probably aggravated by the neurogenic element. Unless it is not quickly rectified, features of dehydration and carbohydrate starvation supervene and a vicious cycle of vomiting appears—vomiting →carbohydrate starvation → ketoacidosis → vomiting.

Symptoms

1. Increased vomiting, retching and nausea persist in between vomiting. The vomitus may be coffee ground or even contain blood.

2. Decreased urine out put.
3. Constipation, at times, diarrhoea.
4. Epigastric pain.
5. Fatigue
6. Symptoms of complications
   • Wernicke's encephalopathy—mental apathy, restlessness, sleeplessness, convulsion or even coma.
   • Korsakoff's psychosis—mental confusion with loss of memory of recent events
   • Features of peripheral neuritis
   • Eye complications—diplopia, dimness of vision or even blindness.

Signs
1. Progressive emaciation with loss of weight
2. Anxious look
3. *Eyes:* Sunken, apathetic and becoming dull
4. Skin is lusterless and inelastic
5. *Tongue:* Dry, becoming brown, thickly coated or red and raw
6. *Teeth:* Covered with sordes
7. *Breath:* Acetone smell
8. Pulse rapid 100–120 or more per minute
9. *Blood pressure:* may be low, 100–110 mm of Hg systolic or less
10. *Temperature:* may be raised to 100°F or more
11. *Jaundice:* A late feature
12. Evidence of neurological manifestations—squint, nystagmus and palsies
13. Vaginal examination to confirm the diagnosis of pregnancy.

Investigations
• *Urinalysis*
  – Quantity—small
  – Dark colour
  – High specific gravity with acid reaction
  – Presence of acetone, occasional presence of protein and rarely bile pigments.
  – Diminished or even absence of chloride.
• *Biochemical and circulatory changes:* Routine and periodic estimation of the serum electrolytes (sodium, potassium and chloride) is helpful in the management of the case.

• Ophthalmoscopic examination is required if the patient is seriously ill. Retinal haemorrhage and detachment of the retina are the most unfavorable signs.
• ECG when there is abnormal serum potassium level.

Diagnosis
The pregnancy is to be confirmed first. Thereafter, all the associated causes of vomiting enumerated before are to be excluded by careful examination before pinpointing the diagnosis of hyperemesis gravidarum. In acute onset of vomiting, extra gestational causes are to be thought of more.

Complications
The majority of the clinical manifestations are due to the effects of dehydration and starvation with resulting ketoacidosis. The following complications may occur which are fortunately rare now-a-days.
1. Neurologic complications
   • Wernicke's encephalopathy
   • Peripheral neuritis
   • Korsakoff's psychosis
2. Stress ulcer in stomach
3. Jaundice

Prevention
The only prevention is to impart effective management to correct simple vomiting of pregnancy.

Management
The principles in the management are:
• To remove the neurogenic elements.
• To correct the fluids, electrolytes and other metabolic disturbances promptly and effectively.
• To prevent or to detect at the earliest, the ominous complications that may arise.

Hospitalisation
Whenever a patient is stamped as a case of hyperemesis gravidarum, it is desirable to

hospitalise the patient even in the early stage. Surprisingly, with the same diet and drugs used at home, the patient improves rapidly. The relatives may be too sympathetic or too indifferent. She should be cared by competent and tactful nurses. Visitors including the husband should be barred.

Fluids

Oral feeding is withheld for at least 24 hours after the cessation of vomiting. During this period fluid is given preferably through intravenous drip method.

Drugs

- **Adequate sedation** is obtained with the help of promazine or diazepam twice or thrice daily intramuscularly.
- **Antihistaminic and anti-emetic drugs such as** promethazine (phenergan) or prochlorperazine or trifluoperazine may be administered twice or thrice daily intramuscularly.
- **Vitamins** are administered to prevent neuropathy and to accelerate carbohydrate metabolism. Daily intramuscular injection of vitamin B_1 100 mg, vitamin B_6 (pyridoxine hydrochloride) 100 mg, vitamin C (ascorbic acid) 100 mg and vitamin B complex are given.
- **Hydrocortisone** 100 mg is given in the drip in case of severe hypotension.

Nursing care

Sympathetic but—firm handling of the patient is essential. Care of the teeth, gums and oral hygiene is to be taken.

To maintain a hyperemesis chart

A chart is to be maintained noting the progressive record of the vital features. *It includes*

1. Fluid intake and output (vomitus and urine) in 24 hours.
2. Character of the vomitus

3. Pulse, respiration; temperature and blood pressure at least twice daily or more frequently.
4. Urine examination at least twice daily for
   - Specific gravity
   - Acetone
   - Chloride and
   - Once daily for protein and bile
5. Blood biochemistry—on admission and as frequently as required if the facilities are available.
6. Weight of the patient on admission and again when out of bed.
7. ECG, to ascertain blood potassium status

Diet

The foods are given orally and if the patient can retain them. At first, dry carbohydrate foods like biscuits, bread and toast are given. The diet should be normalised quickly, as the stomach is more likely to retain solids than liquids. The meals are served at frequent intervals. Gradually full diet is restored.

Termination of pregnancy

The following are the indications for therapeutic termination.

1. A steady deterioration, in spite of therapy.
2. A rising pulse rate of 100/minute or over.
3. Temperature consistently above 38°C (100.4°F).
4. Gradually increasing oliguria and proteinuria.
5. Appearance of jaundice
6. Appearance of neurological complications. *The last two complications should not be allowed to occur when a patient is under observation.*

Method of termination

Below 12 weeks: Suction evacuation under paracervical block or slow dilatation of the cervix by laminaria tent followed by rapid dilatation of the cervix and evacuation.

Above 12 weeks: Abdominal hysterotomy preferably under local anaesthesia.

RH INCOMPATABILITY

Rh factor: It is an unknown antigen in the human red cells.Individuals having the antigen are called Rh positive and in whom not present Rh negative

Alternative Names

Rh induced hemolytic disease of the newborn

Definition of Rh incompatibility: Rh incompatibility is a condition that develops when a pregnant woman has Rh negative blood and the baby in her womb has Rh positive blood.

Causes: Factors that influence an Rh negative pregnant female's chances of developing Rh incompatibility include the following:

- Ectopic pregnancy
- Placenta previa
- Placental abruption
- Abdominal/pelvic trauma
- In uterofetal death
- Any invasive obstetric procedure (e.g. amniocentesis)
- Lack of prenatal care
- Spontaneous abortion

There are four blood types (A, B, AB, and O). Each of the four blood types is additionally classified according to the presence of another protein on the surface of red blood cells that indicates your Rh factor. If you carry this protein, you are Rh positive. If you do not carry the protein, you are Rh negative.

Most people, about 85%, are Rh positive. But if a woman who is Rh negative and a man who is Rh positive conceive a baby, there is the potential for incompatibility. The baby growing inside the Rh negative mother may have Rh positive blood, inherited from the father. Statistically, at least 50% of the children born to an Rh negative mother and an Rh positive father will be Rh positive.

MANIFESTATIONS OF THE HAEMOLYTIC DISEASE

Clinical manifestations of the haemolytic disease of the fetus and neonate are:

Hydrops fetalis

- Icterus gravis neonatorum
- Congenital anaemia of the newborn
- Hydrops fetalis

Excessive destruction of the fetal red cells leads to severe anaemia, tissue anoxaemia and metabolic acidosis.

Hyperplasia of the placental tissue occurs in an effort to increase the transfer of oxygen but the available fetal red cells (oxygen carrying cells) are progressively diminished due to haemolysis

As a result of fetal anoxaemia, there is damage to the liver leading to hypoproteinaemia which is responsible for generalised oedema (hydrops fetalis), ascites and hydrothorax.

Fetal death occurs sooner or later due to cardiac failure. The baby is either stillborn or macerated and even if born alive, dies soon after

ICTERUS GRAVIS NEONATORUM

The baby is born alive without evidences of jaundice but soon develops it within 24 hours of birth.

While the fetus is inutero, there is destruction of fetal red cells with liberation of unconjugated bilirubin which is mostly excreted through the placenta into the maternal system.

As the umbilical cord is clamped, with continuing haemolysis, the bilirubin concentration is increased. Sooner or later the baby becomes jaundiced.

If the bilirubin rises to the critical level of 20 mg per 100 ml (340 micromol/L—normal 30 micromol/L), the bilirubin crosses the blood-

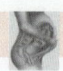

brain barrier to damage the basal nuclei of the brain permanently producing the clinical manifestation of kernicterus.

CONGENITAL ANAEMIA OF THE NEWBORN

The destruction of the red cells continues up to 6 weeks after which the antibodies are not available for haemolysis. The liver and spleen are enlarged.

Causes: Rh incompatibility occurs when a woman is Rh negative, but her fetus has inherited Rh positive blood from the father. It rarely occurs in a woman's first pregnancy. She only becomes sensitized to the fetus's Rh positive blood once she comes in contact with it. This is usually not until very late in pregnancy or during childbirth when fetal red blood cells can cross into the mother's blood system through the placenta or its attachment site to the uterus.

This can also occur during a miscarriage, induced abortion, or ectopic pregnancy. In rare cases, it can happen during an amniocentesis or other invasive testing procedures related to pregnancy.

A woman can also become sensitized to Rh positive blood if she receives an incompatible blood transfusion. In most cases of Rh incompatibility, there are not disease manifestations. If maternal antibodies develop against Rh positive proteins, then these antibodies could affect a current or future fetus during pregnancy. This is called Rh isoimmunization.

Risk factors include

- Pregnant woman with Rh negative blood who had a prior pregnancy with a fetus that was Rh positive
- Pregnant woman who had a prior blood transfusion or amniocentesis
- Pregnant woman with Rh negative blood who did not receive Rh immunization prophylaxis during a prior pregnancy with an Rh positive fetus

Symptoms of the fetus or newborn baby include

Anemia

Swelling of the body (also called hydrops fetalis), which may be associated with:

- Heart failure
- Respiratory problems
- Kernicterus (a neurological syndrome), which can occurs in stages:

Early

- High bilirubin level (greater than 18 mg/cc)
- Extreme jaundice
- Absent startle reflex
- Poor suck
- Lethargy

Intermediate

- High-pitched cry
- Arched back with neck hyperextended backwards (opisthotonos)
- Bulging fontanel (soft spot)
- Seizures

Late

- High-pitched hearing loss
- Intellectual disability
- Muscle rigidity
- Speech difficulties
- Seizures
- Movement disorder

Diagnosis

Blood test for Rh factor: If the blood test indicates that mother has developed Rh antibodies, assess the level of antibodies if the levels are high, an amniocentesis would be recommended to determine the degree of impact on the fetus.

Treatment

Since Rh incompatibility is almost completely preventable with the use of prophylactic

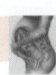

immunization (immune globulin injection of RhoGAM), prevention remains the best treatment.

Immune Globulin Injection

Give an injection of Rho immune globulin at week 28 of the pregnancy. This desensitizes mothers blood to Rh positive blood.

Injection of immune globulin within 72 hours after delivery (or miscarriage, induced abortion, or ectopic pregnancy). The injection further desensitizes your blood for future pregnancies.

Treatment to newborn

Treatment of a pregnancy or newborn depends on the severity of the condition.

Mild

- Aggressive hydration
- Phototherapy using bilirubin lights

Hydrops fetalis

- Amniocentesis to determine severity
- Intrauterine fetal transfusion
- Early induction of labour

A direct transfusion of packed red blood cells (compatible with the infant's blood) and also exchange transfusion of the newborn. This is done to rid the infant's blood of the maternal antibodies that are destroying the red blood cells.

Control of congestive failure and fluid retention

Kernicterus

- Exchange transfusion (may require multiple exchanges)
  - Phototherapy
  - Outcome
  - Full recovery is expected for mild Rh incompatibility.

Both hydrops fetalis and kernicterus represent extreme conditions caused by the break-

down of red blood cells, called hemolysis. Both have guarded outcomes; hydrops fetalis has a high-risk of mortality. Long-term problems can result from severe cases, including:

Cognitive delays

- Movement disorders
- Hearing loss
- Seizures

Possible complications include

- Brain damage due to high levels of bilirubin (kernicterus)
- Fluid buildup and swelling in the baby (hydrops fetalis)
- Problems with mental function, movement, hearing, speech, and seizures.

Prevention

Rh incompatibility is almost completely preventable. Rh negative mothers should be followed closely by their obstetricians during pregnancy.

Special immune globulins, called RhoGAM, are now used to prevent Rh incompatibility in mothers who are Rh negative. If the father of the infant is Rh positive or if his blood type cannot be confirmed, the mother is given an injection of RhoGAM during the second trimester.

If the baby is Rh negative, the mother will get a second injection within a few days after delivery.

These injections prevent the development of antibodies against Rh positive blood. However, women with Rh negative blood type must receive injections:

- During every pregnancy
- If they have a miscarriage or abortion
- After prenatal tests such as amniocentesis and chorionic villus biopsy
- After injury to the abdomen during pregnancy

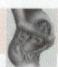
TO PREVENT OR MINIMISE FETOMATERNAL BLEED

- **Precautions during caesarean section (i):** To prevent blood spilling into the peritoneal cavity, (ii) manual removal of placenta should not be done as a routine.
- Prophylactic ergometrine with the delivery of the anterior shoulder should preferably be withheld, as it may facilitate more feto-placental bleed.
- Amniocentesis should be done after sonographic localisation of the placenta to prevent its injury.
- Forcible attempt to perform external version under anaesthesia should be avoided.
- Manual removal of placenta should be done gently.
- To refrain from abdominal palpation as far as possible in abruptio placentae

INFECTIONS IN PREGNANCY

Prenatal infections account for 2–3% of birth defects. These arise from spectrum of organisms taking varying modes of transmission. The composite term **TORCH** infections is used to describe these infections:

T-Toxoplasmosis
O-Others like syphilis
R-Rubella
C-Cytomegalovirus
H-Herpes simplex virus

TOXOPLASMOSIS

Toxoplasmosis is caused by *Toxoplasma gondii* (*T. gondii*) a protozoan parasite found in uncooked meat and cat and dog faeces. It derives its name from a North African rodent the gondii, from which it was first isolated in 1908. First case of a congenitally infected human baby was reported in 1923. Until 1969, life cycle of parasite was fully elucidated with the discovery of its definitive host, cats and other felines.

The major forms of the parasite are

- Oocysts (containing sporozoites), which are shed in the feces.
- Tachyzoites, rapidly multiplying organisms found in the tissues.
- Bradyzoites, slowly multiplying organisms found in the tissues.
- Tissue cysts: Walled structures, often found in the muscles and central nervous system (CNS), containing dormant *T. gondii* bradyzoites.

PARASITOLOGIC CONSIDERATIONS

T. gondii has two of hosts

- A definitive host—like cats and other felines
- An intermediate host—man and other .

It multiplies by sexual reproduction in the definitive hosts, and by asexual multiplication in definitive as well as intermediate hosts.

INCIDENCE DURING PREGNANCY

- Develop infection at least 6–9 months before pregnancy.
- within 2–3 months before conception—1% or below risk of transmission but a high-risk of miscarriage
- The first trimester—15% chance but severity of disease in neonate is more
- Second trimester—25% risk
- Third trimester—65% chance but severity of disease in neonate is less usually asymptomatic

RISK FACTORS

Eating uncooked or undercooked meats, having pets at home, poor hand hygiene, contact with infected material and soil, frequent consumption of raw vegetables.

Clinical signs

In immune competent non-pregnant individuals:

- Usually asymptomatic.
- App 10–20% develops lymphadenitis or a mild, flulike syndrome characterized by fever, malaise, myalgia, headache, sore throat, lymphadenopathy and rash. In some cases, may mimic infectious mononucleosis
- Symptoms usually resolve without treatment within weeks to months, although some cases may take up to a year.
- Severe symptoms, including myositis, myocarditis, pneumonitis and neurologic signs including facial paralysis, severe reflex alterations, hemiplegia and coma, are possible but rare.
- Ocular toxoplasmosis with uveitis, often unilateral, can be seen in adolescents and young adults; this syndrome is often the result of an asymptomatic congenital infection or the delayed result of a postnatal infection.

Congenital toxoplasmosis

- Up to 90 percent of infected babies appear normal at birth, 80 to 90 percent will develop sight-threatening eye infections months to years after birth. About 10 percent will develop hearing loss and/or learning disabilities, 60% of infected may suffer from long-term sequella. Mild cases with only slightly diminished vision. Ocular disease is usually bilateral. The most common symptom is chorioretinitis but strabismus, nystagmus and microphthalmia may also be seen. Infants infected late in gestation may have a fever, rash, hepatomegaly, splenomegaly, pneumonia or a generalized infection.

Transmission of the infection

- Occur as a result of ingestion of ocysts excreted in the faeces of cats or by ingestion of undercooked meat harboring tissue cysts.

- Approximately 5–35% of pork, 9–60% of lamb and 0–9% of beef contain *T. gondii*.
- Transplacental transmission to fetus from a mother infected during pregnancy is also a common occurrence.
- In days of modern medicine, the odes of transmission have attained a new perspective, like blood transfusion, leucocytes transfusion and organ transplantation.

TRANSMISSION CYCLE

Incubation period

- 10 to 23 days after ingesting contaminated meat,
- 5 to 20 days after exposure to infected cats.

DIAGNOSIS AND TREATMENT

It may be possible to identify all cases of congenital toxoplasmosis. Antenatally a combination of *T. gondii* polymerase reaction (PCR) and mouse inoculation of amniotic fluid most accurately predicts the infection, with sensitivity of 91%. Afterbirth, specific *T. gondii* IgA antibodies are more frequently detected than IgM.

Spiramycin is drug of choice can be given before 26 weeks which has no teratogenic effects. If fetus is infected there can be replaced by or addition of Sulfadiazine + Pyrimethamine. Clindamycin or Dapson : If patient has sulfa drug allergy.

Prevention

Providing information about toxoplasmosis is the most effective preventive strategy as health education can reduce the incidence of primary infection during pregnancy. Appropriate information includes advising women about proper hand washing, cleanliness, proper cooking the meats and avoiding the contact with cat and dog feaces.

Another preventive strategy is frequent serological screening during pregnancy. This assumes that treatment during pregnancy can

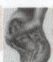

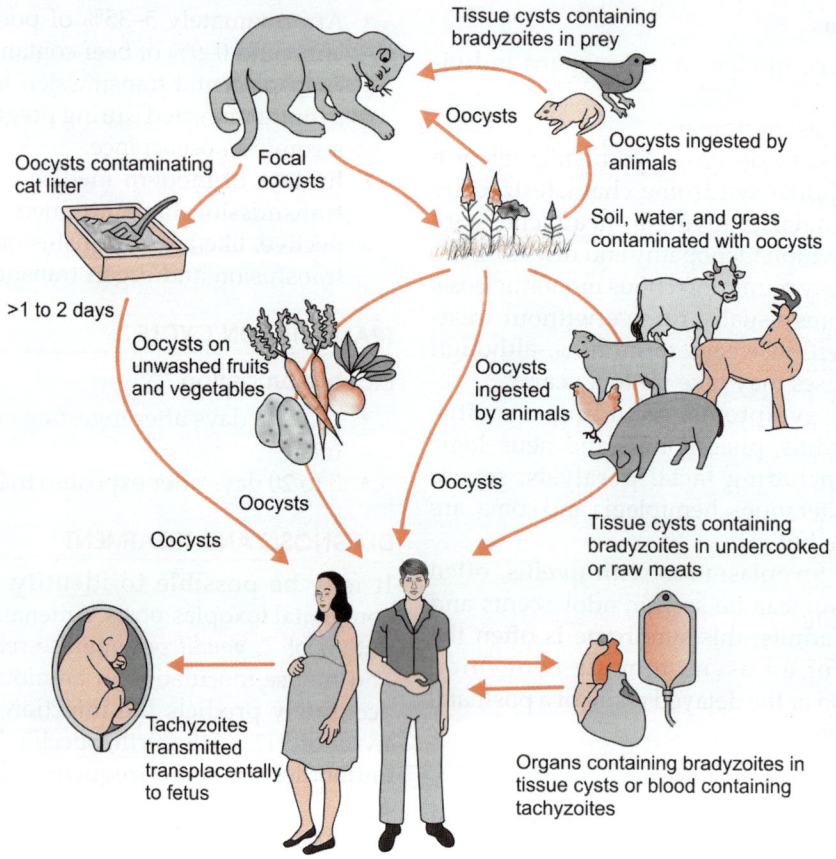

Tissue cysts containing bradyzoites in prey

Oocysts

Oocysts ingested by animals

Oocysts contaminating cat litter

Focal oocysts

Soil, water, and grass contaminated with oocysts

>1 to 2 days

Oocysts on unwashed fruits and vegetables

Oocysts ingested by animals

Oocysts

Oocysts

Oocysts

Tissue cysts containing bradyzoites in undercooked or raw meats

Tachyzoites transmitted transplacentally to fetus

Organs containing bradyzoites in tissue cysts or blood containing tachyzoites

Fig. 9.5: Transmission cycle

reduce the fetomaternal rate and result in improved infant outcome.

RUBELLA

Rubella or German measles (RNA virus) is transmitted by respiratory droplet exposure. Fetal transmission is by transplacental route throughout pregnancy. The risk of major anomalies when this infection occurs in first, second and third month is approximately 50%, 25% and 10% respectively. The virus predominantly affects the fetus and is extremely teratogenic if contracted in the first trimester. There is increased chance of abortion, stillbirth and congenitally malformed baby. Infants born with congenital rubella shed the virus for many months and are a source of infection to others.

INCIDENCE AND EFFECTS DURING PREGNANCY

Since 1988, in most industrialized countries the MMR vaccine has reduced the rubella incidence to a low endemic level. If primary rubella infection occurs during the first 12 weeks of pregnancy, maternal-fetal transmission rates are as high as 85%. First trimester infection can result in spontaneous abortion, and in surviving babies it can result in cataracts, sensorineural deafness, congenital heart diseases, microcephaly, thrombocytopenia and developmental delay.

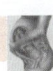

DIAGNOSIS AND TREATMENT

- A maternal history of a rash or contact with rubella.
- Serological screening of women for rubella-specific IgG and IgM antibodies.
- Cordocentesis to establish the presence of rubella IgM antibody in umbilical cord blood.
- The detection of viral RNA in chorionic villi, amniotic fluid or fetal blood.
- Ultrasonic examination of the neonate
- Specific antibody detection in the cord blood at birth.
- Isolation of the rubella virus from the throat, urine and CSF of the neonate
- Ongoing physical examination during early childhood.

Most women with first trimester infection require termination of pregnancy. Following the birth, management is mainly symptomatic and appropriate referrals to ensure best outcomes for the baby. Infants with congenital rubella syndrome (CRS) are highly infectious and should be isolated from other infants. Babies should always be followed up for several years, as some problems may not become apparent until they are old.

Prevention

Vaccination of the mother is advised before and after, but not during pregnancy. Susceptible individuals who works with pregnant women are also are offered rubella vaccine. Midwives need to emphasize the importance of avoiding contact with rubella infection, as re-infection during pregnancy has been reported despite previous vaccination.

CYTOMEGALOVIRUS (CMV) INFECTION

CMV is a DNA virus of the herpes family. It is so named because it has the effect of enlarging the cells that it infects. Transmission may be sexual, respiratory droplet or transplacental. Virus is also excreted in urine, cervix and breast milk. Fetus is affected by transplacental route in about 30–40% cases. Primary infection may cause generally mild mononucleosis-type symptoms such as malaise, myalgia and fever in immunocompetant adults whereas it is pathologic among immunosuppressed individuals, recipients of organ transplants, premature infants and patients with AIDS.

PREGNANCY AND CMV INFECTION

The incidence of vertical transmission with recurrent infections may vary between 0.5%–3% several studies suggests that primary infection occurs in all trimesters with about 37% of babies being born with congenital infection.

FETAL AND NEONATAL INFECTIONS

CMV is the most common intra uterine infection affecting from 0.45%–2.3% of all live births. Unlike rubella, which has the teratogenic effect, CMV allows fetal organs to develop normally but causes diseases by the secondary destruction of the cells. Up to 18% of infants born to mothers with primary infection may be symptomatic at birth. The prognosis is thus poor. More than 90% of all symptomatic patients develop sensorineural hearing loss, mental retardation, chorioretinitis and other more subtle complications in later years. Perinatal infections result from exposure to CMV in the maternal genital tract at delivery or to breast milk.

DIAGNOSIS AND TREATMENT

CMV infection can be diagnosed by direct methods of viral cultures (urine, saliva, breast milk, cervical secretions, and biopsy and autopsy samples) PCR and antigen detection. The best way to distinguish between congenital from perinatal infection is by isolating the virus during the first 2 weeks of life from urine or saliva. Primary infection is confirmed by simultaneous detection of the IgG and IgM

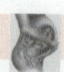
antibodies. IgG persists for life and rising titers may follow primary or recurrent infections. IgM antibodies can be demonstrated during the acute phase of infection. Other methods include radio immune assay, enzymes immune essay and IgM capture radioimmunoassay.

Ganciclovir and foscarnet is used in treatment of life threatening CMV infections in immunocompromised patients. Other measures such as the use of CMV—free blood and blood products, organs from donors free of CMV infections are the other important CMV preventive measure.

HERPES SIMPLEX VIRUS INFECTION

HSV is a genital tract infection which is inherited due to HSV-2. Infection may be primary non primary or recurrent. It is transmitted by sexual contact. Primary infection may occur during pregnancy or reactivation or recurrent infection occurs resulting in virus shedding with or without symptomatic lesions.

EFFECT ON PREGNANCY

Increased risk of abortion is inconclusive. If the primary infection is acquired in the last trimester there is chance of premature labour or IUGR. Transplacental infection is not usual. The fetus becomes affected by virus shed from the cervix or lower genital tract during vaginal delivery. The baby may be affected in utero from the contaminated liquor following rupture of membrane. Risk of fetal infection is high in primary genital HSV at term due to high virus shedding compared to a recurrent infection.

Treatment

Caesarean delivery is indicated in an active primary genital HSV infection. Acyclovir 200 mg five times daily for five days is the drug of choice when virus culture is positive.

Neonatal infection may be fatal, disseminated or localized or it may be asymptomatic. Diagnosis is made by detection of viral DNA by PCR. Neonatal infection is high following primary infection. It is manifested as chorioretinitis, microcephaly, mental retardation, seizures and death.

Prophylactic acyclovir 400 mg twice daily is recommended for women with recurrent infection. Breastfeeding is allowed provided mother avoids any contact between her lesions, her hands and the baby.

SYPHILIS

Syphilis is a sexually transmitted disease caused by Treponema pallidum. Incidence is rising due to upsurge of HIV infection and the IV drug use. Overall frequency of vertical transmission is high in primary (50%) and secondary (50%) syphilis. In tertiary syphilis it is about 10%. The symptoms may be suppressed in pregnancy.

Classification

(a) Acquired syphilis

- *Early Infectious:*
  - Primary—9–90 days after the exposure
  - Secondary—6 weeks—6 months (4–8 weeks after the primary lesion)
  - Latent—2 years after the exposure.
- *Late non-infectious*
  - Latent(late)-**e"** 2 years after the exposure without any signs and symptoms
  - Neurosyphilis, cardiovascular syphilis—3–20 years after the exposure.

(b) Congenital syphilis

Approximately two-thirds of live-born infected infants do not have any signs and symptoms at birth but they present over the following weeks or months or years. Lesions develop only after the 4th when immunological competence becomes established.

Clinical features

The primary lesion or chancre develops in 10–90 day after the infection. The typical primary lesion is circular and indurated, with

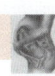

an eroded base, and there is marked edema of the surrounding tissues. It may develop on the labia majora or minora, at the fourchette, near the external urinary meatus, on the clitoris or on the cervix. An anal chancre may rarely occur following anal coitus. Superficial painless inguinal lymphadenopathy with discrete and rubbery glands develops in patients with chancres in all locations except cervix, followed by generalized lymphadenopathy in 3–6 weeks. The chancre persists for 1–5 weeks and then heals spontaneously. Serological tests for syphilis become reactive only 1–4 weeks after the chancre develops. In secondary syphilis, generalized bilateral symmetrical extra genital skin eruptions are seen; fever, papular lesions covered with scales or sodden white areas appear on the vulva. In the perianal region hypertrophic flat topped condylomas may be seen later and these may spread to the vulva and the thighs. These lesions may fuse to form large plaques and are very infectious. This stage lasts for 2–10 weeks. In late syphilis, gammatous lesions of the skin or mucus membrane may occur but are rarely seen on the genitalia.

EFFECTS ON PREGNANCY

Mother

Syphilis accelerates the course of HIV infection in pregnant.

Baby

The infection does not occur before the 4th month of pregnancy because treponemes from the maternal circulation are unable to pass through the Langhans cell layer (cytotrophoblast in the villi) of the early placenta. Once this layer begins to atrophy during the 4th month of pregnancy the fetus is exposed to the 1st risk of infection.

Diagnosis: mother

- Obstetric history in multigravidae: with serial pregnancies, there has been gradually improved obstetric performance.

- Clinical findings of various stages of syphilis usually suppressed during pregnancy.
- Investigations: serological test: this should be done as a routine in the 1st antenatal visit. VDRL (positive within 4 weeks of infection) is commonly done.

Clinical features of congenital syphilis

- Early: maculopapular rash, rhinitis, hepato-spleenomegaly, lymphadenopathy, chorio-retinopathy and pneumonia.
- Late: Hutchinson teeth. Deafness, saddle nose, hydrocephalus, mental retardation, intestinal keratitis and optic nerve atrophy.

If the baby is stillborn, spirochaetes may be detected from the fetal liver or spleen or from the intimal scraping of umbilical vein.

TREATMENT

Mother

Treatment may be started as soon as the diagnosis is made. For primary or secondary syphilis (<1 year)—benzathine penicillin intramuscularly single dose. If the patient is allergic to penicillin, oral erythromycin 2 gm daily for 15 days is given. If the treatment is given in early pregnancy it should be repeated in late pregnancy. Irrespective of the serological report, treatment should be repeated in subsequent pregnancies.

Baby

- Infected baby with positive serology reaction requires
  - Isolation from the mother
  - IM aqueous procaine penicillin
- Positive serological reaction without clinical evidences of the disease. The baby is treated with a single IM dose of penicillin.
- An apparently healthy child of a known syphilis mother: serological reaction should tested weekly for the first month and then monthly for 6 months.

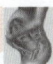

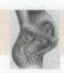

HUMAN IMMUNODEFICIENCY VIRUS (HIV) INFECTION AND ACQUIRED IMMUNO-DEFICIENCY SYNDROME (AIDS)

Acquired immunodeficiency syndrome (AIDS)

Aids is caused by a retrovirus known as human immunodeficiency virus (HIV).

Transmission of HIV infection is predominantly through three modes: (1) Person, (2) Parenteral exposure to infected blood or tissue, and (3) Perinatal exposure of an infected mother. The virus must enter the recipient's blood-stream to produce infection.

HIV infection is major challenge for the obstetric team and for midwifery care. There is a need to reduce the risk of vertical transmission to the fetus and to maintain optimal health of the mother. HIV causes an incurable infection that leads ultimately to terminal disease called AIDS. Worldwide 25–30% of infected patients are women and 90% of them are 20 to 49 years of age.

Human Immunodeficiency Virus (HIV) causes an incurable infection that leads ultimately to a terminal disease called *Acquired Immunodeficiency Syndrome* (AIDS). World wide 25–30% of infected patients are women and 90% of them are 20–49 years of age.

Incidence

Incidence is increasing both in developed and developing countries. It is now a global problem. The prevalence even in low-risk population in America is close to 1 in 100. *In most Asian countries the infection rate is less than 0.5%.*

The virus

HIV viruses (HIV 1 and HIV 2) are **RNA ritroviruses having the enzyme reverse transcriptase, which permits genomic RNA to be transcribed into double stranded DNA.**

The main modes of transmission of HIV are:

1. Sexual contact (homosexual or heterosexual)
2. Transplacental
3. Exposure to infected blood or tissue fluids
4. Through breast milk

Course of disease

Clinicians now recognize four relatively distinct stages of HIV infection (Barrick, 1991):

1. An early, or acute, stage, which produces high level viral replication and may include flu-like symptoms lasting a few weeks.
2. A middle, or asymptomatic, period of minor or no clinical problems, characterized by continuous, low level viral replication and T4 cell loss, lasting for years.
3. A transitional, intermediate—length period of symptomatic disease (previously referred to as AIDS—related complex, or ARC)
4. A late, or crisis period of symptomatic disease lasting months or years.

During stages 1 and 2, the infected person is termed HIV—positive; during stages 3 and 4, the immune system no longer offers adequate protection, and opportunistic diseases occur. The person is then said to have AIDS.

Perinatal transmission of HIV

Vertical transmission to the neonates is about 14–25%. Transplacental transmission may occur even in early (8–14 weeks) pregnancy, though *majority (40–80%) occur during the labour.*

Effects

Pregnancy got no effect on the disease progression in HIV positive women. Increased incidence of abortion, prematurity, IUGR and perinatal mortality in HIV seropositive mothers still remains inconclusive. Maternal mortality and morbidity are not increased by pregnancy.

Clinical presentation

Initial presentation of an infected patient may be fever, malaise, headache, sore throat, lymphadenopathy and maculopapular rash.

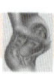

Primary illness may be followed by an asymptomatic period. Progression of the disease may lead to multiple opportunistic infections with candida, tuberculosis, pneumocystis and others. Patient may present with neoplasms such as cervical carcinoma, lymphomas (Hodgkin's and non-Hodgkin's) and Kaposi's sarcoma. *The median time from infection to AIDS is about 10 years.*

Diagnosis

The enzyme immunoassay (EIA) is used as a screening test for HIV antibodies.

MANAGEMENT

Prenatal care

1. *Voluntary serologic testing* for HIV infection to all pregnant women in the parental clinic should be offered
2. *In seropositive cases* the following additional tests should be done.
   - Test for other STDs—such as hepatitis B virus, gonorrhoea, syphilis, chlamydia and herpes.
   - Serologic testing for cytomegalovirus and toxoplasmosis.
   - Tuberculosis
   - Husband should be offered serologic testing for HIV.
3. *Counselling* about the risk of HIV transmission to the fetus and neonates should be made and termination offered. Women with AIDS are discouraged to become pregnant.
4. The patient should have T lymphocyte count in each trimester. If the count falls to less than 200 cells/mm^3 the patient should receive prophylaxis against *Pneumocystis carinii* and other opportunistic infections.
5. *Anti retroviral therapy* to HIV 1 positive women is highly effective in reducing the viral (HIV RNA) load. *Triple chemotherapy is preferred as a first line defence and to be started any time between 14 and 34 weeks and then continued throughout pregnancy, labour* and **postpartum period.**

Anti-HIV 1 drugs are grouped into

a. **Neucleoside analogs** (Zidovudine, Zalcitabine, Lamivudine, Stavudine).
b. **Protease inhibitors** (Indinavir, Saquinavir, Ritonavir)
c. Non-nucleoside analogs (Nevirapine, Delavirdine)

Treatment regimens change frequently. However recommended regimens (CDC-1998) are: Two from Group A plus one from either Group B or Group C. Zidovudine 100 mg given five times daily p.o. can reduce perinatal transmission from 25 to 7%.

Intrapartum care

- Zidovudine is given IV infusion starting at the onset of labour (vaginal delivery) or 4 hours before caesarean section. Loading dose 2 mg/kg/hr, maintenance dose 1 mg/kg/hr *until cord clamping is given.*
- Elective caesarean delivery reduces the risk of vertical transmission by about 50%. The combination of anteretroviral therapy reduces the risk to only 2%. Cord should be clamped as early as possible. Baby should be bathed immediately.
- High viral load, lower CD4 count, rupture of membranes > 4 hrs and breastfeeding double the risk of MTCT. A maternal sample for plasma viral load should be taken at delivery.
- To avoid procedures that might result in break in the skin or mucous membrane of the infants. Amniotomy, attachment of scalp electrode and determination of scalp blood pH should best be avoided.
- Long term safety of anti-retroviral drugs is unknown. Neuropathy, myopathy, lactic acidosis, pancreatitis, hepatitis and mitochondrial toxicity have been observed.

 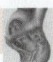

Universal precautions

Universal precautions to reduce the risk of STDs' including risk of HIV infection.

Body fluids of high-risk (all universal precautions apply):

Blood, semen, vaginal secretions, amniotic fluid, tears, saliva, cerebrospinal fluid.

Breast milk is source of perinatal transmission; health care worker may wish to ware gloves if exposed. Body fluids of low risk (all universal precautions may not apply):

Feces nasal secretions, sweat, urine and vomitus precautions.

1. Use appropriate barrier precautions to prevent skin and mucous membrane contact with bodily fluids.
2. When caring for all patients, gloves should be worn for:
   Contact with blood (venipuncture; finger stick; changing perineal pads, chux, or linen).
   Contact with bodily fluids (changing any saturated pad, chux, or linen; saturation after rupture of membranes).
   Contact with mucous membranes (vaginal, etc.).
   Contact with nonintact skin. Handling things soiled, with blood or bodily fluids (soiled pads, chux, bedding or clothing).
3. Gloves should be changed after contact with patients and between patient contacts.
4. Medical gloves (vinyl or latex sterile or non sterile) should not be washed and reused.
5. Masks protective eyewear, or face protections should be worn during procedures that causes splashes of blood or bodily fluids on mucous membranes of eyes, nose, or mouth, e.g.:
   - Vaginal or cesarean birth
   - Cutting or umbilical cord
   - Rupture of membranes underpressure
6. Fluid-resistant gowns and aprons should be worn during procedures likely to cause splashes of bodily fluids:
   - Vaginal or caesarean birth
   - Artificial rupture of membranes
7. Gowns and gloves should be worn by health acre workers handling placenta or infant until blood and amniotic fluid have been removed from infant's skin; gloves should be worn for care of umbilical cord after delivery.
8. Removal of infant nasopharyngeal secretion at birth should not be done by mouth but by mechanical suction. Resuscitation should be done by ventilation equipment.
9. Gloves torn or punctured by needle stick or other injury should be removed and replaced promptly.
10. Precautions should be taken to prevent injury from needles and surgical instruments.
    - Needles should not be recapped, bent or removed from disposal syringes by hands.
    - After use, needles and other sharp items should be placed in puncture—resistant containers for disposal
    - Surgical instruments should be carefully cleaned to avoid injury
11. Health care workers who have frequent exposure to breast milk may wear gloves.

Postpartum care

- *Breast feeding*—where alternative forms of infant nutrition are not safe, the minor risk associated with breast feeding may be accepted. Mother is counselled as regard the risks and benefits. She is helped to make an informed choice.
- *Zidovudine syrup*—2 mg/kg, is given to the neonate 4 times daily for first 6 weeks of life.

Contraception

Barrier methods of contraception (condom or female condom) is effective in preventing transmission of the virus. *Thus, the disease*

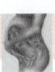

could be prevented predominantly by health edu-cation and by practice of safer sex.

Counselling

Pre-pregnancy and early pregnancy counselling for HIV infected patient is essential. The counsellor must provide up-to-date knowledge which enables the patient to make an informed choice.

NURSING MANAGEMENT

While taking the care of HIV/AIDS clients the nurse has to follow some standards of care guidelines, i.e.

- Utilize universal precautions
- Protect confidentiality
- Educate the patient about methods for the prevention of HIV transmission
- Perform a psychosocial assessment
- Develop adherence strategies for patients taking antiviral therapy.
- Provide education and interventions for HIV symptom management.

PARASITIC AND PROTOZOAL INFESTATIONS IN PREGNANCY

Malaria

Malaria is predominantly a tropical disease. In India and other south east Asian countries there is incidence of malaria. The diagnosis is confirmed by the detection of malaria parasites in peripheral thick blood smear.

The fetal effects are due to *high fever* or due to **placental parasitization.** The intervillous spaces become blocked with macrophages and parasites and there is diminished placental blood flow. This is mostly seen with *P. falciparum infection and in the second half of pregnancy. Congenital malaria is rare (< 5%) unless the placenta is damaged.*

Effects of pregnancy on malaria

- Risk and severity of infection are high due to immunocompromised state.
- Complications are high.

Management

Prevention from mosquito bites using mosquito nets and repellents. Prophylaxis with chloroquine (300 mg base) orally once a week when a pregnant woman is travelling to endemic areas.

Treatment

Risks of malaria is life threatening in pregnancy. So benefits of treatment outweigh the potential risk of antimalarial drugs. Chloroquine for radical cure, primaquin should be postponed until pregnancy is over. Parasites resistant to chloroquine should be given quinine (10 mg salt/kg p.o. every 8 hours for 7 days) under supervision. Patients with severe anaemia may need blood transfusion. The antimalarial drugs when given in therapeutic doses, have got no effect on uterine contraction unless the uterus is irritable. Folic acid 10 mg should be given daily to prevent megaloblastic anaemia.

ASSESSMENT AND SCREENING OF HIGH-RISK PREGNANCY

RISK APPROACH OF OBSTETRIC NURSING CARE

Pregnancy should be considered a unique physiologically normal episode in a woman's life. However, pre-existing disease or unexpected illness of the mother or fetus can complicate the pregnancy.

Risk is a reflection of the incidence of an adverse health outcome arising in a defined population during a given period.

Definition

A high-risk pregnancy is one in which some condition puts the mother, the developing fetus, or both at higher-than-normal risk for complications during or after the pregnancy and birth.

Or

A high-risk pregnancy is one in which some conditions put the mother, the developing fetus

or both at higher than normal risk for complications during or after the pregnancy and birth.
Or

According to D. El. Mowafi, high-risk pregnancy is the one in which the mother, the fetus and or the newborn are at risk of morbidity or mortality during pregnancy labour and or postpartum.

Risk approaches

A pregnancy can be considered a high-risk pregnancy for a variety of reasons. Some of the factors are:

1. Maternal factors include

- **Prenatal factors**
  - History of any of the following conditions
  - Complications during previous pregnancies (including stillbirth, fetal loss, preterm labour and/or delivery, small-for-gestational age baby, large baby, pre-eclampsia or eclampsia)
  - Grandmulti
  - Bleeding during the third trimester;
  - Abnormalities of the reproductive tract
  - Medical disorders complicating pregnancy
  - Rh incompatability
  - Infections of the genital tract
  - Any abdominal surgery
  - Post-term pregnancy
  - Chronic illness
  - Lack of antenatal care
  - Conception within two months of previous pregnancy
  - Hereditary abnormality such as downs syndrome
  - Prolonged infertility
- **Diagnosis of any of the following factors**
  - Age (younger than age 15, older than age 35)
  - Weight (pre-pregnancy weight under 100 lb or obesity)

  - Height (under five feet)
  - Obstetric complications such as pre-eclampsia, eclampsia, multiple pregnancy
  - Abnormal presentation
  - IUGR
- **During labour and neonatal factors**
  The period after delivery especially the first hour may be critical for the infant who must quickly and effectively adapt to extra-uterine life. The following associations identified before and immediately after-birth place the infant at risk for complications and demand special observation
  1. Maternal
     - Prolonged rupture of membranes
     - Abnormal presentation and delivery
     - Prolonged or precipitate labour
     - Prolapsed cord
  2. Birth asphyxia
  3. Preterm birth
  4. Postterm birth
  5. Small for date infants
  6. Large for date infants
  7. Any respiratory distress of the newborn
  8. Obvious congenital anomalies
  9. Convulsions
  10. Distension and vomiting in newborn
- **Postpartum factors**
  - Low birth weight
  - Hypoglycemia
  - Anemia
  - Major congenital anomalies
  - Convulsions
  - Fetal infection
  - Jaundice during the first 24 hours or bilirubin levels above 15 mg/100 ml
  - Respiratory distress syndrome
  - Persistent cyanosis
  - Haemorrhage
- **Risks for mother and neonate**
  - Placenta previa
  - Premature rupture of membrane

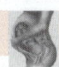

– Preterm labour
– Infection
– Epilepsy
– IUGR
– Obstructed labour
– CPD
– Haemorrhage
– Eclampsia
– Shock
– Death

Management

- **Prenatal**
  – Good antenatal care and screening for high-risk cases
  – Education of the mother regarding understanding of the risk and taking appropriate measures
) Immunization
) Moniter maternal weight gain—over weight or underweight
) Iron and folic acid supplements
) Fetal monitoring
) Antenatal exercises
) Choice of birth setting
) Preparation towards new parental roles
) Counselling
- **Intranatal**
  – Institutionalized birth
  – Well trained personnels should be available at all times to meet any emergency.
  – Monitoring of the mother and fetus throughout the labour process.
  – good referral system should be available as needed
  – liberal episiotomy under local anesthesia should be given to the mother
  – interventions as per the condition of the mother
  – breathing exercises should be taught to the mother to help her cope with the labour pains.

– apgar score should be checked immediately after the birth of the baby
- **Postnatal**
  – Initiate breastfeeding within half an hour of birth if mothers condition is stable
  – Moniter the condition of the mother and baby
  – Watch for maternal PPH
  – contraception should be adviced to the mother.
  – Immunization of the baby should be done according to the national immunization schedule.

2. Maternal weight and weight gain

- Although routine weighing of pregnant women has become an important feature of prenatal care, surprising little is known about the effectiveness of weighing as a screening procedure for predicting fetal demise or about the clinical and practical implications of abnormal weight changes in pregnancy
- Some mothers are overweight or underweight
- Body mass index is also known as quetelets Index (weight in kg/height (m)^2.

Risk

Nutritional deprivation has a negative effect on birth weight.

MANAGEMENT

Pre pregnancy

Women who had anorexia or bulimia and wish to become pregnant are advised to wait until the eating disorder is well treated.

Prenatal

- Woman who have anorexia or bulimia and wish to become pregnancy should seek medical fitness before deciding to become pregnant.

- Careful dating of gestation
- Adequate weight gain should be ensured

Labour and delivery

- If fetal growth restriction is suspected, the patient should be admitted to a specialist unit
- Continuous fetal heart sound monitoring
- Emergency resuscitation equipments should be kept ready
- **Over weight women**
- *Risk*

  Hypertensive disorders during pregnancy are more common in women with excessive weight

Management

- Maternal height and weight should be well recorded
- Monitor BP regularly
- Ultrasonic examination to know fetal condition

3. Social factors

- Low socioeconomic status
  - Risks
  - Teenage pregnancy: The number of teenage pregnancies are increasing. The teenage mother married or unmarried suffers from lack of emotional, intellectual and physical maturity. The pregnant teenager has more problems then the average married women
  - Perinatal mortality
  - Preterm birth
  - Low birth weight

Management

- *Prenatal*
  - Widespread antenatal health education
  - Anti smoking measures
  - Competent care at low cost at the grass root level
  - Registration of pregnancy at the anganwadi
  - Minimum 3 antenatal check-ups

- **Labour**
  - Depends on the condition of the mother
  - No modification from normal labour if risk factors are absent
- **Postnatal**
  - Encourage breastfeeding
  - Contraception methods

4. Paternal factors

- Cigarette smoker or a diabetes patient
  - Risk
  - The incidences of congenital anomalies is slightly elevated when the father is a smoker
  - Certain inheritable disorders such as Rh-D isoimmunization are traceable to the father.

Management

- Avoid smoking when a pregnant lady is around
- Counseling of the couple regarding smoking and its ill effects on health, pregnancy and the fetus.

5. Fetal factors include

- Exposure to infection
- Exposure to damaging medications (especially phenytoin, folic acid antagonists, lithium, streptomycin, tetracycline, thalidomide, and warfarin)
- Exposure to addictive substances (cigarette smoking, alcohol intake, and illicit or abused drugs)
- A pregnancy is also considered high-risk when prenatal tests indicate that the baby has a serious health problem (for example, a heart defect).

Risk

- Viral hepatitis
- Mumps
- Varicella
- Syphilis
- TORCH

- Infections caused by coxsackie virus
- Asphyxia
- Congenital anomaly
- Mental retardation

Management
- The mother will need special tests
- Avoid over the counter medication
- Carry the baby safely through to delivery
- Certain maternal or fetal problems may prompt a physician to deliver a baby early
- Choose a surgical delivery (cesarean section) rather than a vaginal delivery depending on the condition.

6. Genetic factors
- Previous child affected with a single gene disorder
- Family history of single gene disorder
- Parent with chromosomal anomaly
- Structural abnormalities found on ultrasound examination.

7. Environmental factors
- *Chemicals:* Exposure to polychlorinated biphenyls (PCBs), dioxins and pesticides including fungicides, herbicides, insecticides and rodenticides. Exposure to pesticides may lead to birth defects
- *Prescribed drugs:* The safety of half the medications for the mother and the fetus remain unknown
- Most pregnant mothers are exposed to medications such as vitamins, laxatives, antibiotics before pregnancy is recognized
- Sometimes medications are necessary to manage life threatening diseases
- **Medications known or suspected to be human teratogens:** retinoids (vit A), hormones (androgens), anticoagulants (warfarin), antineoplastics (methotrexate), anticonvulsants (phenytoin), trimethadione and paramethadione (fluconazole) other drugs like lithium and danazol

- **Drug abuse, cigarette smoking and alcohol:** Maternal smoking increases all placental complications which include placental abruption, placental insufficiency, placenta previa and low birth weight. Excessive consumption of alcohol is detrimental. The main features include:
  - CNS disturbances
  - Abnormal facial characteristics especially low set ears, an elongated mid face and a small head and a short up turned nose.
  - Malformation of major organs especially the heart and skeletal deformities.

Drug abuse, e.g. heroin. Their use decreases the ability of the mother to care for the baby. Opiates are not teratogenic but their use is associated with intrauterine growth retardation.

- Vaccines such as live attenuated measles, mumps, rubella should be avoided during pregnancy.
- Ionizing radiation have 2 effects:
  - Deterministic effect pertains to decrease in or loss of organ function as a result of cell damage or cell killing.
  - Stochastic effect are those that result from radiation changes in the cell that retain their ability to divide.
- Diagnostic factors like magnetic reso-nance imaging, ultrasound and video display terminals.

The use of contrast may produce side effects, claustrophobia and temporary hearing loss as a result of acoustic noise generated by an MRI.

No association between ultrasound and video display terminal exposure in pregnancy and adverse effects on the fetus.

Risk
- **Loss of organ function as a result of cell damage leading to**
  - Fetal malformation
  - Mental retardation
  - Death

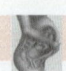

Management

- Every woman of child bearing age who is undergoing X-ray should be asked whether she might be pregnant or missed a period
- Use alternative diagnostic measures
- Reduction of radiation dose by lead shielding the abdomen
- Avoid unnecessary exposure to radiations
- Termination of pregnancy should be considered if the radiation dose would lead to severe deterministic effects
- Avoid using contrast medias during MRI if the woman is pregnant
- MRI is not recommended during the first trimester
- USG is the modality of choice to evaluate obstetric patients
- USG should be carried out with care in the first trimester with careful control of output level and exposure times as with increased mineralization of the fetal bones as the fetus develops, the possibility fetal bone heating increases
- Use USG cautiously in febrile patients

8. Nutritional factors

- *Caffeine:* Its effect on pregnancy is controversial. Risks associated with maternal caffeine consumption during pregnancy and perinatal outcomes have proved difficult to estimate
- *Folate:* Deficiency during pregnancy may lead to neural tube defects
- *Vitamin A:* High doses during pregnancy may cause heart defect
- *Vitamin B_6:* it is involved in many enzymatic activity
- *Vitamin B_{12}:* Deficiency results in macrocytic anaemia and neurologic abnormalities
- *Vitamin C:* Required for collagen synthesis and a deficiency of this results in bruising and early bleeding

- *Vitamin D:* No evidence that vitamin D deficiency causes any adverse pregnancy outcomes
- *Vitamin E:* It is assumed and not proved that vitamin E requirement increases during pregnancy
- *Vitamin K:* Newborn infants are at risk for deficiency due to poor placental transfer, lack of intestinal bacteria and low content in breast milk
- *Iodine and zinc:* Deficiencies are implicated in low birth weight, perinatal mortality, mental retardation, childhood speech and hearing disorders and birth defects
- *Iron:* deficiency causes anaemia and increases risk for labour complications.

9. Occupational factors

Womens occupations are usually multidimensional.

- Household work
  - Exposure to toxic chemicals like cleaning fluids, bleach, detergents, insecticides and pesticides
- Poor working environment
  - Problems of isolation, stress, tiredness and depression
  - Physical harassment
- Poverty and employment
  - Work in sex industry
  - Increased risk of sexually transmitted diseases

10. Medical factors

- Bleeding and pain in early pregnancy
- Spontaneous abortion or miscarriage
- Ectopic pregnancy
- Gestational trophoblastic disease
- Rhesus prophylaxis

11. Miscellaneous factors

- Physical activity
- Air travel during pregnancy
- Accident during pregnancy

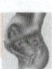

Diagnosis

General physical examination

Height: Below 150 cm particularly below 145 cm in India

- Overweight or underweight
- High blood pressure
- Anemia
- Cardiac or pulmonary disease
- Orthopedic problems

Pelvic examination

Uterine size: Disproportionately smaller or bigger

- Genital prolapse
- Lacerations or dilatation of the cervix
- Associated tumors
- Pelvic inadequacy

Identification of high-risk factors

The following laboratory screening studies should be obtained as early as possible in pregnancy

1. Haemocrit and haemoglobin
2. WBC
3. Differential blood count
4. Urinalysis
5. Urine culture
6. Serology tests for pregnancy
7. Rubella antibody titer
8. Toxoplasmosis antibody titer
9. Blood grouping and Rh determination
10. Screening test for isoimmunization antibodies.

Pregnant patients 35 years of age or older have an increased incidence of bearing children with down syndrome. For this reason an amniocentesis should be performed at the 14th to 16th week of pregnancy to identify or exclude this genetic problem by tissue culture of fetal cells and chromosomal analysis. If down syndrome is diagnosed the couple should be given the option of therapeutic abortion

Periodic screening

The following timing may be employed:

- Initial pregnancy screening examination
- Antenatal screening at the time of office or clinic visits
- Intranatal screening when the patient is admitted to the hospital
- delivery evaluation both maternal and fetal
- postnatal appraisal both maternal and fetal

The patients at risk are then identified by an established criteria at each checkpoint. The criteria for diagnosis of high-risk pregnancy are as follows:

A. Biologic and maternal factors

1. High-risk
   a. Maternal age of 15 years or younger
   b. Maternal age of 35 years or older
   c. Massive obesity
2. Moderate risk
   a. Maternal age of 15–19 yrs
   b. Maternal age of 30–34 yrs
   c. Nonwhite
   d. Single
   e. Obesity
   f. Malnutrition
   g. Short stature (60 inches or less)

B. Obstetric history

1. High-risk
   a. Previously diagnosed genital anomalies
   b. Two or more previous abortions
   c. Previous stillbirth or neonatal loss
   d. Two previous premature labours or low birth weight infants
   e. Two excessively large previous births
   f. Maternal mallignancy
   g. Uterine leiomyomata
   h. Ovarian mass
   i. Parity of 8 or more
   j. History of eclampsia, etc.
   k. Previous birth damaged infant
   l. Previous MTP

2. Moderate risk
   a. Previous premature labour
   b. One excessively large infant
   c. Previous operative delivery
   d. Previous prolonged labour
   e. Previous emotional problems associated with pregnancy and delivery
   f. Previous uterine or cervical operations
   g. Primigravidae
   h. Parity of 5 to 8
   i. Involuntary sterility
   j. Prior ABO incompatibility
   k. Prior fetal malpresentation
   l. History of endometriosis
   m. Pregnancy within 3 months of previous delivery

C. Medical and surgical history

1. High-risk
   a. Moderate to severe chronic hypertension
   b. Moderate to severe renal disease
   c. Severe heart disease
   d. Diabetes
   e. Previous endocrine disorders
   f. Abnormal cervical cytology
   g. Sickle cell disease
   h. Drug addiction
   i. History of tuberculosis
   j. Pulmonary disease
   k. Malignancy
   l. GI or liver disease

2. Moderate risk
   a. Mild chronic hypertension
   b. Mild renal disease
   c. Mild heart disease
   d. History of mild hypertensive states during pregnancy
   e. History of pyelitis
   f. Diabetes
   g. Thyroid disease
   h. Positive serology
   i. Excessive use of drugs

Screening of high risk cases

The cases are assessed in first trimester of pregnancy. The WHO recommends referral system for high risk cases to prevent maternal mortality

INITIAL SCREENING

Maternal age: Pregnancy below the age 20 and above 35 caries high-risk.

Reproductive history

The high risk checklist includes the following:
- Age less than 17 and more than 35 yrs
- Height less then 145 cm
- Weight less then 40 kg or more then 70 kg
- History of APH or PPH in previous pregnancy
- History of twin delivery
- History of repeated abortions, stillbirths or early neonatal deaths
- Previous delivery of small or large babies
- History of preterm delivery
- History of medical diseases as heart diseases, diabetes, hypertension, renal disease, tuberculosis
- Pre-eclampsia, eclampsia in previous pregnanacy
- Abnormal presentation
- Overdistension of abdomen due to twins or hydramnios
- APH in present pregnancy

Labour complications

- Patient having no antenatal care
- Anaemia, pre-eclampsia, eclampsia
- Premature prolonged rupture of membranes
- Meconium stained liquor
- Abnormal presentation and position
- Disproportion, floating head in labour
- Multiple pregnancy
- Abnormal fetal heart rate
- Rupture of uterus

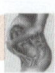

- Patients having induction or acceleration of labour
- Difficult forceps or breech delivery
- Need to deliver under general anaesthesia

Postpartum complications
- Retained placenta
- Sepsis
- Shock
- Uterine inversion
- Cervical and vaginal tears

Neonatal complications
- Apgar score below 7
- Birth weight less than 2.5 kg or more than 4 kg
- Major congenital anomalies
- Anaemia
- Fetal infection
- Jaundice
- Hypoglycaemia
- Persistent cyanosis
- Convulsions
- Haemorrhagic disease
- Respiratory distress syndrome

Management
1. *Pre pregnancy management*
   Provide education, screening and counseling for communities at specific risk
2. *Prenatal risk management*
   A woman with a high-risk pregnancy will need closer monitoring than the average pregnant woman. Such monitoring may include:
   - A carefully detailed history
   - More frequent visits with the primary caregiver
   - Antenatal care
   - Blood and urine analysis
   - Serial ultrasound examination
   - Fetal monitoring or assessment
   - **Once the diagnosis of a high-risk pregnancy is made** the following considerations are most important

   - The obstetrician must anticipate the worst possible eventuality and prepare for this in the hope that this turn of events may not ensure
   - All aspects of the case must be appraised with realization that the studies must be appropriate in the overall management.
   - No single test report must justify sudden conclusive action
3. *Labour risk management*
   - transfer of patient to a maternity centre should be arranged if a maternal fetal intensive care unit is not available in the physicians local community
   - intranatal monitoring
   - supportive companion during labour and delivery
   - elective LSCS in case of a high-risk case is evident
   - some cases labour is induced after 37–38 completed weeks of gestation
4. *Postnatal risk management*
   - Continuous monitoring of mother and baby
   - Babies who are high-risk are shifted to NICU for observation
   - Encourage breastfeeding
   - Offer contraceptive advice taking account of individual sociocultural norms and values

Prognosis
The prognosis depends in large part on the specific medical condition. Some medical conditions make it difficult to get pregnant and lead to a higher risk of problems in the baby.

Prevention of high-risk cases
- Strengthen midwifery skills, community participation and referral system
- Proper training of resident, nursing personnel and community health workers

- Arranging periodic seminars, refresher courses with participation of workers involved in care of these cases
- Concentration of these cases in specialized centres for management
- Community participation, proper utilization of health care manpower and financial resources where it is mostly needed
- Availability of prenatal laboratory for necessary investigations, availability of a good paediatric services
- Lastly improvement of the economic status, literacy and health awareness of the community.

Cases having a previous unsuccessful pregnancy should be seen and investigated before another conception occurs. Investigation like hysterogram, hysteroscopy, laproscopy or TVS should be performed to rule out mullerian abnormality. Complete investigations for hypertension, diabetes, kidney disease or thyroid disease should be undertaken and proper treatment instituted in the non pregnant state. Sexually transmitted disease should be treated before entering to another pregnancy. Cervical tear should also be repaired in the non pregnant state. Serology for toxoplasma IgG, IgM and antiphospholipid antibodies should be done and corrected appropriately when found positive.

Folic acid (4 mg/day) therapy should be started in the pre pregnant state and is continued throughout the pregnancy. Early in pregnancy after the initial clinical examination, routine and special laboratory investigations should be undertaken. Necessary advice should be given regarding diet activities rest and medicines. Minimum medicines should be taken during pregnancy particularly in the early months.

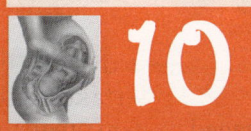

10

Malpositions and Malpresentations

OUTLINE

- Occipitoposterior position
- Breech presentation
- Face presentation
- Brow presentation
- Transverse lie
- Unstable lie
- Compound presentation
- Shoulder dystocia
- Cord prolapse

Malposition and malpresentations present the midwife with a challenge of recognition and diagnosis both in the antenatal period and labour.

OCCIPITOPOSTERIOR POSITION

In a vertex presentation where the occiput is placed posteriorly over the sacroiliac joint or directly over the sacrum, it is called an occipitoposterior position. When the occiput is placed over the right sacroiliac joint, the position is called right occipitoposterior (ROP) and when placed over the left sacroiliac joint, is called left occipitoposterior (LOP) and when it points towards the sacrum, is called direct occipitoposterior (Fig. 10.1).

Occipitoposterior is an abnormal position of the vertex rather than an abnormal presentation. In the majority of cases (90%), anterior rotation of the occiput occurs and follows the course like that of an occipitoanterior and moreover, in certain type of pelvis (anthropoid), it is a favourable position.

Incidence

At the onset of labour, the incidence is about 10% of all the vertex presentations. Right occipitoposterior is 5 times more common than the left occipitoposterior. Dextrorotation of the uterus and the presence of the sigmoid colon on the left, disfavour LOP position.

Cause

In the majority, the cause of the abnormal position is not clear. The following are the responsible factors:

- *Shape of the pelvic inlet:* In more than 50%, the occipitoposterior position is associated with either an anthropoid or android pelvis.

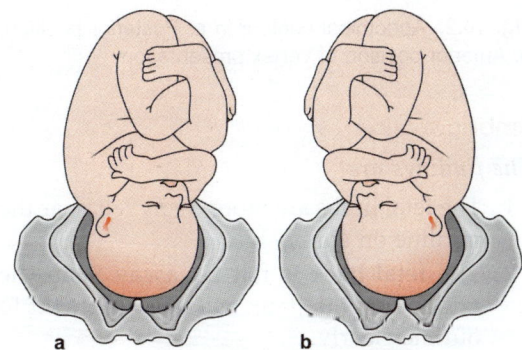

Fig. 10.1: a. Right occipitoposterior position, **b.** Left occipitoposterior position

- *Fetal factors:* Marked deflection of the fetal head, too often favours posterior position of the vertex. The causes of deflection are:
  - High pelvic inclination
  - Attachment of the placenta on the anterior wall of the uterus
  - *Primary brachycephaly:* This shortens the length of the lever from the frontal to atlantooccipital deflection and occipito-posterior position.
- *Uterine factor:* Abnormal uterine contraction which may be the cause or effect leads to persistent deflexion and occipito-posterior position.

DIAGNOSIS

ABDOMINAL EXAMINATION

Inspection

There is a saucer-shaped depression at or just below the umbilicus. This dip is created by the 'dip' between the head and the lower limbs of the fetus (Fig. 10.2).

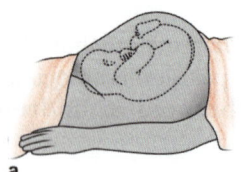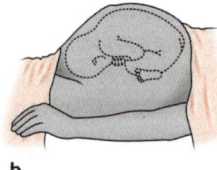

a   b

Fig. 10.2: Abdominal contour in **a.** Posterior position, **b.** Anterior position of vertex presentation

Umbilical grip

The findings are

1. The fetal limbs are more easily felt near the midline on either side.
2. The fetal back is felt far away from the midline on the flank and often difficult to outline clearly.
3. The anterior shoulder lies far away from the midline.

Pelvic grips

The findings is

1. The head is not engaged.

Auscultation

The maximum intensity of the fetal heart sound is heard on the flank. The fetal back is not well flexed, the fetal chest is thrust forward, therefore the fetal heart can be heard in the midline.

VAGINAL EXAMINATION

The findings in early labour are

1. Elongated bag of membranes which is likely to rupture during examination.
2. The sagittal suture occupies any of the oblique diameters of the pelvis.
3. Posterior fontanelle is felt near the sacro-iliac joint.
4. The anterior fontanelle is felt more easily.

   In late labour, the diagnosis is often difficult because of caput formation which obliterates the sutures and fontanelles.

Mechanism of right occipitoposterior position (long rotation) (Figs 10.3 to 10.6)

- The lie is longitudinal.
- The attitude of the head is deflexed.
- The presentation is vertex.
- The position is right occipitoposterior.
- The denominator is the occiput.
- The presenting part is the middle or anterior area of the left parietal bone.
- The occipitofrontal diameter, 11.5 cm, lies in the right oblique diameter of the pelvic brim. The occiput points to the right sacro-iliac joint and the sinciput to the left iliopectineal eminence (Fig. 10.7).

Flexion

Descent takes place with increasing flexion. The occiput becomes the leading part.

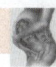

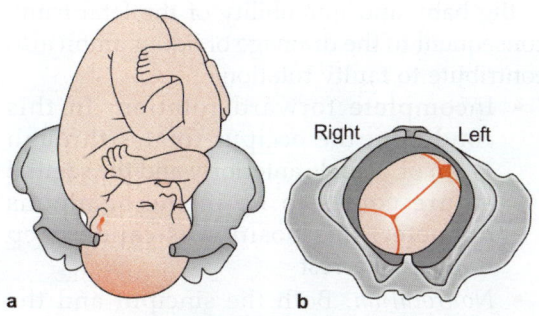

Fig. 10.3: Head descending with increased flexion. Sagittal suture in right oblique diameter of the pelvis

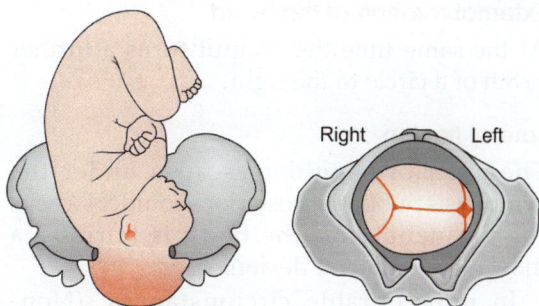

Fig. 10.4: Occiput and shoulders have rotated 1/8th of a circle forwards. Sagittal suture in transverse diameter of the pelvis

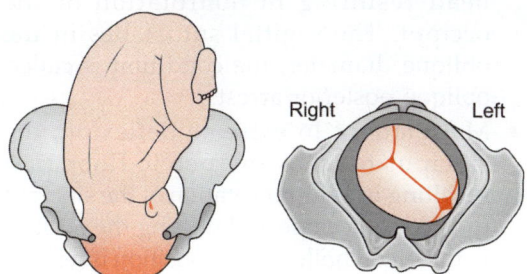

Fig. 10.5: Occiput and shoulders have rotated 2/8th of a circle forwards. Sagittal suture in the left oblique diameter of the pelvis. The position is right occipitoanterior

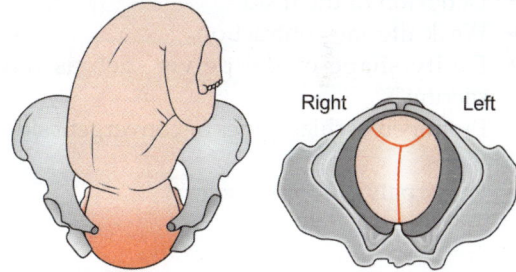

Fig. 10.6: Occiput has rotated 3/8th of a circle forwards. Note the twist in the neck. Sagittal suture in the anteroposterior diameter of the pelvis

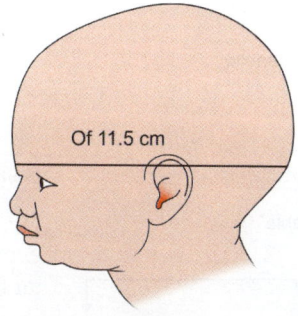

Fig. 10.7: Engaging diameter of a deflexed head, occipitofrontal (OF) 11.5 cm.

Internal rotation of the head

The occiput reaches the pelvic floor first and rotates forwards 3/8th of a circle along the right side of the pelvis to lie behind the symphysis pubis. The shoulders follow, turning 2/8th of a circle from the left to the right oblique diameter.

Crowning

The occiput escapes under the symphysis pubis and the head is crowned.

Extension

The sinciput, face and chin sweep the perineum and the head is born by a movement of extension.

Restitution takes place and the occiput turns 1/8th of a circle to the right and the head rights itself with the shoulders.

Internal rotation of the shoulders

The shoulders enter the pelvis in the right oblique diameter, the anterior shoulder reaches the pelvic floor first and rotates forwards 1/8th of a circle to lie behind the symphysis pubis.

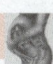

External rotation of the head

At the same time the occiput turns a further 1/8th of a circle to the right.

Lateral flexion

The anterior shoulder escapes under the symphysis pubis, the posterior shoulder sweeps the perineum and the body is born by a movement of lateral flexion.

In unfavourable circumstances: (Non-rotation or malrotation)—10%

In certain circumstances, the occiput fails to rotate as described previously (Fig. 10.8). The causes are:

- Deflexion of the head
- Weak uterine contraction
- Faulty shape of the pelvis such as flat sacrum
- Prominent ischial spines or convergent side walls
- Weak pelvic floor muscles

Big baby and immobility of the fetal trunk consequent to the drainage of liquor amnii also contribute to faulty rotation.

- Incomplete forward rotation: In this condition, the occiput rotates through 1/8th of a circle anteriorly and the sagittal suture comes to lie in the bispinous diameter, this position is called deep transverse arrest.
- *Nonrotation:* Both the sinciput and the occiput touch the pelvic floor simultaneously due to moderate deflexion of the head resulting in nonrotation of the occiput. The sagittal suture lies in the oblique diameter, the condition is called oblique posterior arrest.
- Malrotation: In extreme deflexion, the sinciput touches the pelvic floor first resulting in anterior rotation of the sinciput to 1/8th of a circle and putting the occiput to the sacral hollow. This position is termed

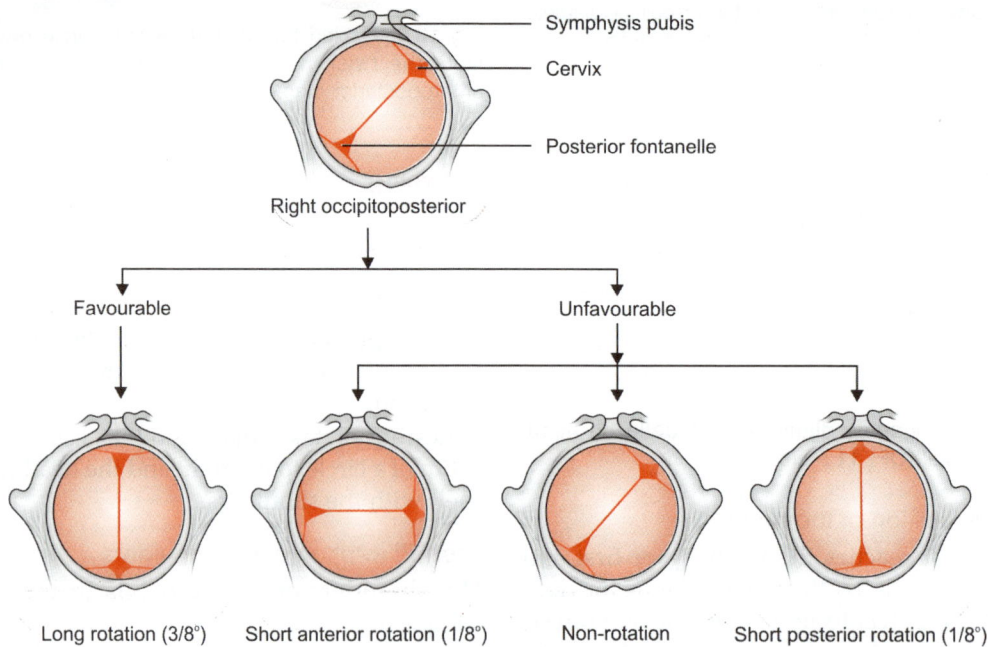

Fig. 10.8: Diagrammatic representation showing favourable and unfavourable rotation of occipitoposterior position

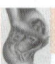

as occipitosacral position. This is, in the true sense, "Persistent occipitoposterior (POP) position" of the vertex. In favourable circumstances, i.e. with an average size baby, good uterine contractions and an adequate pelvis such as an anthropoid or spacious gynaecoid—spontaneous delivery may occur as "face to pubis". In unfavourable circumstances, when arrest occurs, it is called occipitosacral arrest (Fig. 10.9).

Mechanism of face to pubis delivery
(Fig. 10.10)

- Further descent occurs until the root of the nose, hinges under the symphysis pubis.
- Flexion occurs, releasing successively the brow, vertex and occiput out of the stretched perineum and then the face is born by extension.
- Restitution: The head moves 1/8th of a circle in the opposite direction of internal

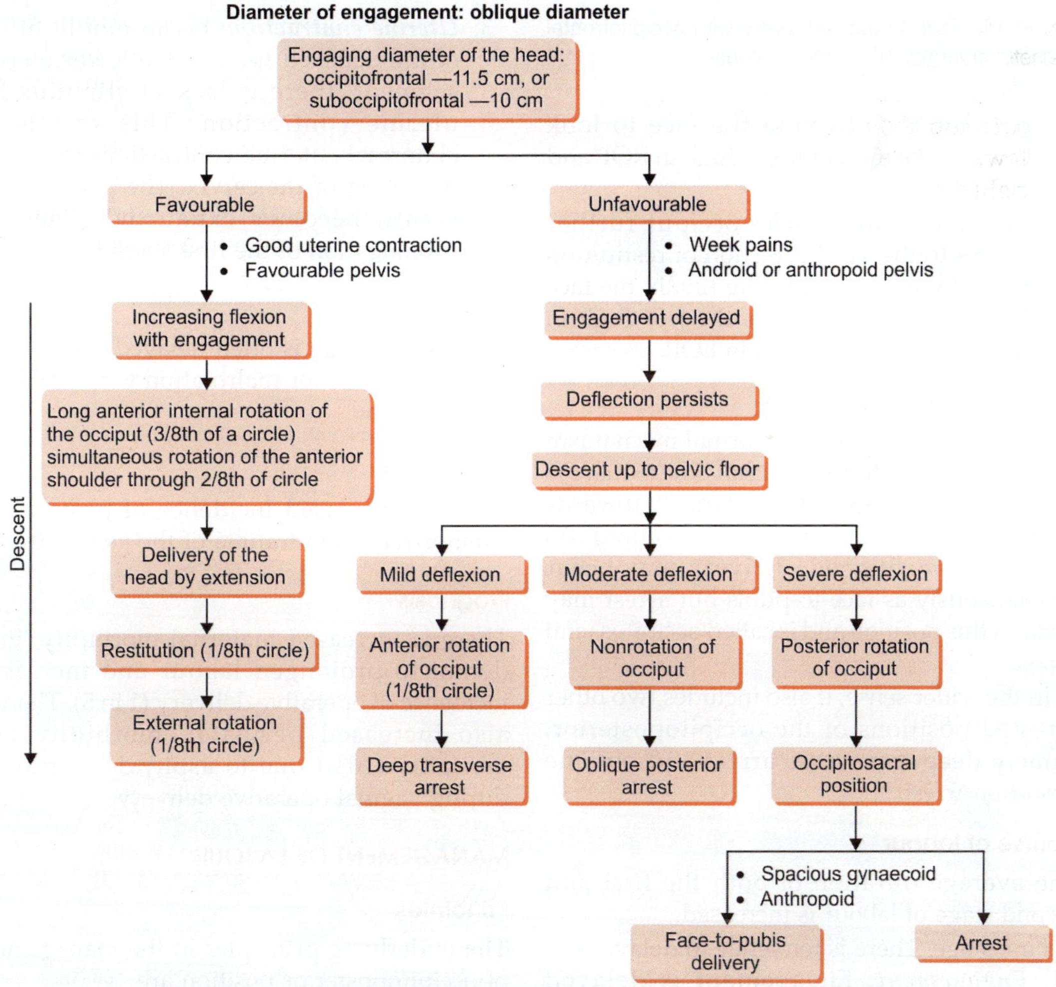

Diameter of engagement: oblique diameter

Engaging diameter of the head:
occipitofrontal —11.5 cm, or
suboccipitofrontal —10 cm

Favourable
- Good uterine contraction
- Favourable pelvis

Increasing flexion with engagement

Long anterior internal rotation of the occiput (3/8th of a circle) simultaneous rotation of the anterior shoulder through 2/8th of circle

Delivery of the head by extension

Restitution (1/8th circle)

External rotation (1/8th circle)

Descent

Unfavourable
- Week pains
- Android or anthropoid pelvis

Engagement delayed

Deflection persists

Descent up to pelvic floor

Mild deflexion | Moderate deflexion | Severe deflexion

Anterior rotation of occiput (1/8th circle) | Nonrotation of occiput | Posterior rotation of occiput

Deep transverse arrest | Oblique posterior arrest | Occipitosacral position

- Spacious gynaecoid
- Anthropoid

Face-to-pubis delivery | Arrest

Fig. 10.9: Scheme of mechanism of labour in occipitoposterior position

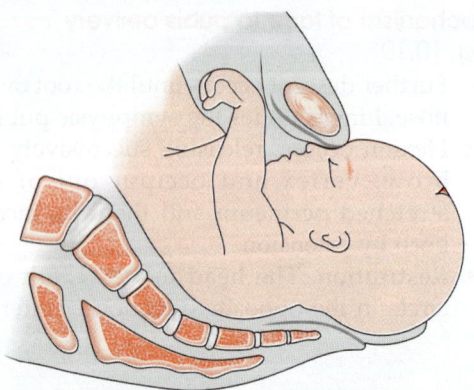

Fig. 10.10: Face to pubis delivery with occipitofrontal diameter emerges out of the introitus

rotation thus turning the face to look towards the mother's left thigh in ROP and right thigh in LOP.

- External rotation: The occiput further rotates to the same direction of restitution to 1/8th of a circle placing finally the face looking directly towards the left thigh in ROP and the right thigh in LOP.

Persistent occipitoposterior

In the true sense, it is an abnormal mechanism of the occipitoposterior position where there is malrotation of the occiput posteriorly towards the sacral hollow (occipitosacral position). As previously mentioned, delivery may occur spontaneously as face-to-pubis but arrest may occur in this position and is called occipitosacral arrest.

In the wider sense, it also includes two other arrested positions of the occipitoposterior, namely deep transverse arrest and oblique posterior arrest.

Course of labour

The average duration of both the first and second stage of labour is increased.

First stage: There is tendency to delay.

1. *Engagement:* Engagement is delayed due to:

- Persistence of deflexion of the head thereby increasing the diameter of engagement [occipitofrontal—11.5 cm (4½")].
- The driving force transmitted through the fetal axis is not in alignment with the axis of the inlet.

2. *Membrane status:* Deflexed head becomes ovoid and this cannot fit well the spherical lower segment →loss of ball valve action during uterine contraction →early rupture of the membranes and drainage of liquor.

3. *Uterine contraction:* Because of ill fitting of the deflexed head to the lower uterine segment, there is lack of stimulus for uterine contraction. This results in abnormal uterine contraction with slow dilatation of the cervix. The patient, as a result, becomes exhausted. There is prolongation of the first stage.

Second stage

The second stage is often delayed due to long internal rotation or malrotation with, at times, arrest of head.

Third stage

There is increased incidence of postpartum haemorrhage and trauma of the genital tract.

Prognosis

There is increased maternal morbidity, incidental to prolonged labour and increased incidence of operative delivery (1 in 5). There is also increased perinatal, morbidity and mortality (10%) due to asphyxia or trauma during vaginal operative delivery.

MANAGEMENT OF LABOUR

Principles

The underlying principles in the management of occipitoposterior position are:

1. Early diagnosis

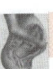

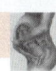

2. Strict vigilance with watchful expectancy hoping for descent and anterior rotation of the occiput
3. Judicious and timely interference.

Diagnosis and evaluation: Fetal back on the flank with the FHS not being easily located, early rupture of the membranes should arouse suspicion. Internal examination is confirmatory.

Pelvic adequacy is assessed clinically. Inclination of the pelvis, configuration of the inlet, sacrum, ischial spines and the side walls are to be noted.

Early caesarean section: Pelvic inadequacy or its unfavourable configuration, along with obstetric complications such as pre-eclampsia, post-caesarean pregnancy, big baby usually need caesarean section.

First stage

In otherwise uncomplicated cases, the labour is allowed to proceed in a manner similar to normal labour.

The following are the special instructions

- Anticipating prolonged labour, intravenous infusion line is sited and Ringer's solution drip is started.
- Progress of labour is judged by:
  - Progressive descent of the head
  - Rotation of the back and the anterior shoulder towards the midline
  - Increasing flexion of the head
  - Position of the sagittal suture on vaginal examination
  - Cervical dilatation
- Weak pain, persistence of deflexion and non-rotation of the occiput. In such a situation, oxytocin infusion is started for augmentation of labour.
- Indication of caesarean section
  - Arrest of labour (failure of rotation)
  - Incoordinate uterine action
  - Fetal distress

Second stage

In majority anterior rotation of the occiput is completed and the delivery is either spontaneous or can be accomplished by low forceps or ventouse.

In minority (unrotated and malrotated)

Provided the fetal and maternal conditions permit, one should take a watchful expectancy for the anterior rotation of the occiput and descent of the head. In occipitosacral position, spontaneous delivery as face-to-pubis may occur. Owing to the larger presenting diameters, perineal trauma is common and the midwife should watch for signs of rupture in the centre of the perineum ('button hole' tear).

In such cases, proper conduct of delivery and liberal episiotomy should be done to prevent complete perineal tear.

Third stage (Fig. 10.11)

Because of prolongation of labour, tendency of postpartum haemorrhage can be prevented by prophylactic intravenous ergometrine 0.25 mg with the delivery of anterior shoulder. Following vaginal operative delivery meticulous inspection of the cervix and lower genital tract should be made to detect any injury.

COMPLICATIONS ASSOCIATED WITH OCCIPITOPOSTERIOR POSITIONS

Apart from prolonged labour risks to mother and fetus and the increased likelihood of instrument delivery, the following complications may occur:

Obstructed labour

This may occur when the head is deflexed or partially extended and becomes impacted in the pelvis.

Maternal trauma

Forceps delivery may result in perineal bruising and trauma. Delivery of a fetus in the persistent

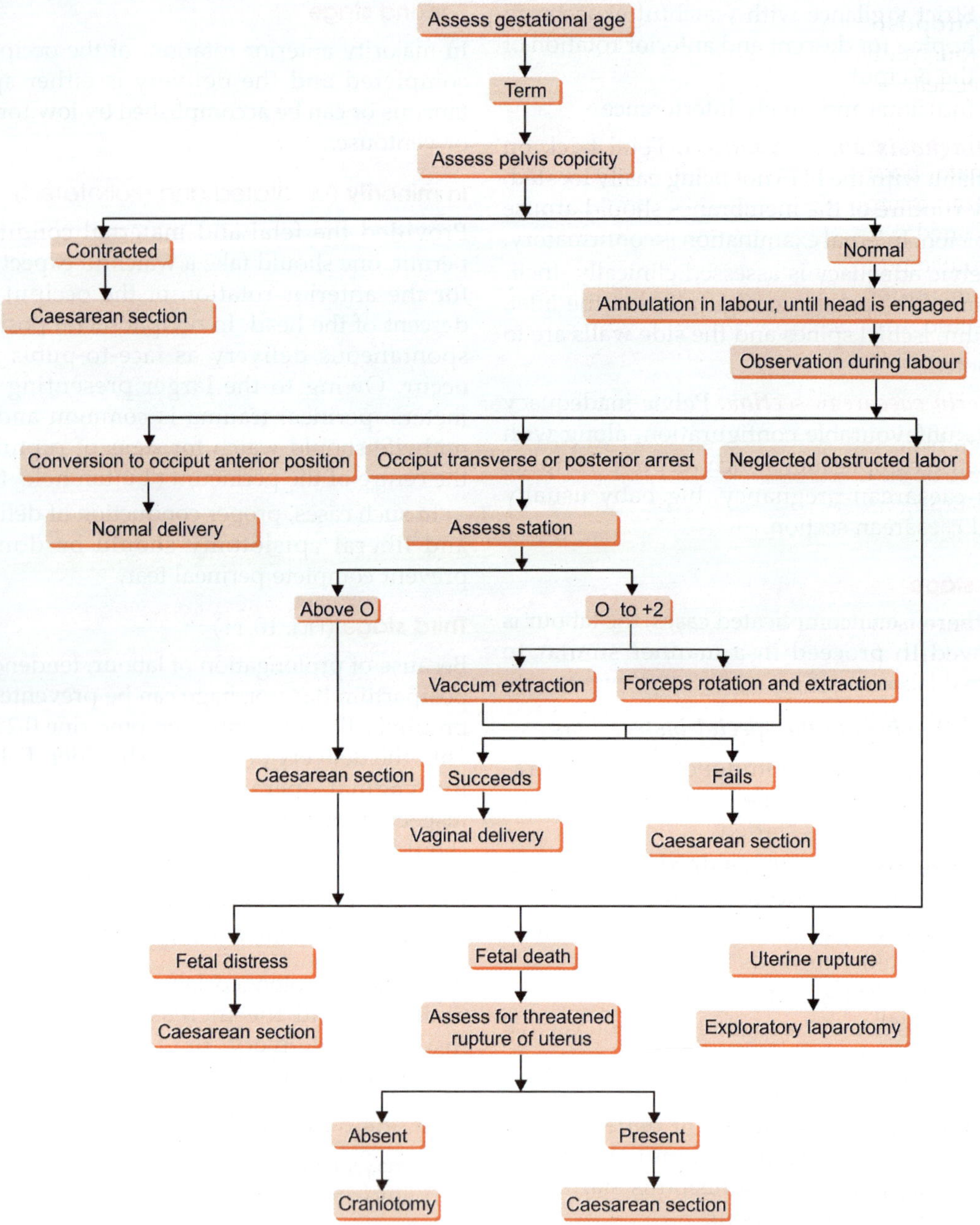

Assess gestational age

↓

Term

↓

Assess pelvis copicity

↓

Contracted — Normal

Contracted → Caesarean section

Normal → Ambulation in labour, until head is engaged

↓

Observation during labour

↓

Conversion to occiput anterior position — Occiput transverse or posterior arrest — Neglected obstructed labor

Conversion to occiput anterior position → Normal delivery

Occiput transverse or posterior arrest → Assess station

↓

Above O — O to +2

Above O → Caesarean section

O to +2 → Vaccum extraction / Forceps rotation and extraction

Vaccum extraction / Forceps rotation and extraction → Succeeds / Fails

Succeeds → Vaginal delivery

Fails → Caesarean section

Fetal distress — Fetal death — Uterine rupture

Fetal distress → Caesarean section

Fetal death → Assess for threatened rupture of uterus

Uterine rupture → Exploratory laparotomy

Assess for threatened rupture of uterus → Absent / Present

Absent → Craniotomy

Present → Caesarean section

Fig. 10.11: Scheme of management of occipitoposterior position

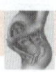

occipitoposterior position, particularly if previously undiagnosed, may cause a third-degree tear.

Neonatal trauma

Neonatal trauma occurring following delivery from an occipitoposterior position has been associated with forceps or ventouse delivery. The outcome for a neonate delivered from an occipito posterior position is comparable to that expected for an infant delivered from an occipitoposterior position.

Cord prolapse

A high head predisposes to early spontaneous rupture of the membranes which, together with an ill-fitting presenting part, may result in cord prolapse.

Cerebral haemorrhage

The unfavourable upward moulding of the fetal skull, found in an occipitoposterior position, can cause intracranial haemorrhage, due to the falx cerebella being pulled away from the tentorium cerebri. The larger presenting diameters also predispose to a greater degree of compression. Cerebral haemorrhage may also result from chronic hypoxia which may accompany prolonged labour.

BREECH PRESENTATION

In breech presentation, the lie is longitudinal and the podalic pole presents at the pelvic brim. The presenting diameter is the bitrochanteric (10 cm) and the denominator is sacrum. It is the commonest malpresentation.

Incidence

The incidence is about 1 in 5 at 28th week and drops to 5% at 34th week and 3% at term.

VARIETIES

There are two varieties of breech presentation (Fig. 10.12):

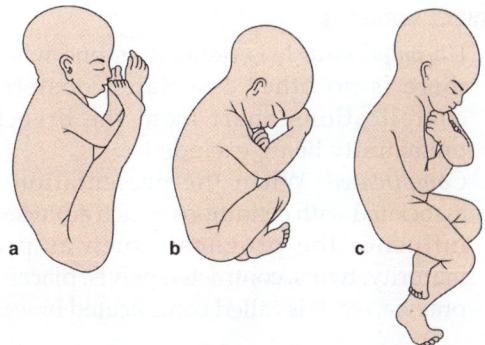

Fig. 10.12: Varieties of breech presentation. **a.** Breech with extended legs (frank breech), **b.** Flexed breech (complete breech), **c.** Footling presentation

- Complete
- Incomplete

Complete (flexed breech)

The normal attitude of full flexion is maintained. The thighs are flexed at the hips and legs at the knees. The presenting part consists of two buttocks, external genitalia and two feet. It is commonly present in multiparae.

Incomplete

This is due to varying degrees of extension of thighs or legs at the podalic pole. Three varieties are possible:

- *Breech with extended legs (frank breech):* In this condition, the thighs are flexed on the trunk and the legs are extended at the knee joints. The presenting part consists of the two buttocks and external genitalia only. *It is commonly present in primigravidae,* about 70%. The increased prevalence in primigravidae is due to a tight abdominal wall, good uterine tone and early engagement of breech.
- *Footling presentation:* Both the thighs and the legs are partially extended bringing the legs to present at the brim.
- *Knee presentation:* Thighs are extended but the knees are flexed, bringing the knees down to present at the brim.

 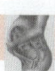

Clinical varieties

1. *Uncomplicated:* It is defined as one where there is no other associated obstetric complications apart from the breech, prematurity being excluded.
2. *Complicated:* When the presentation is associated with conditions which adversely influence the prognosis such as prematurity, twins, contracted pelvis, placenta praevia, etc. It is called complicated breech.

Etiology

The following are the known factors responsible for breech presentation. In a significant number of cases, the cause remains obscure.

- *Prematurity:* It is the commonest cause of breech presentation.
- *Factors preventing spontaneous version*
  - Breech with extended legs
  - Twins
  - Oligohydramnios
  - Congenital malformation of the uterus such as septate or bicornuate uterus
  - Short cord
  - Intrauterine death of fetus
- *Favourable adaptation*
  - Hydrocephalus
  - Placenta praevia
  - Contracted pelvis
- *Undue mobility of the fetus*
  - Hydramnios
  - Multiparae with lax abdominal wall.
- *Fetal abnormality:* Trisomies 13, 18, 21.

Recurrent or habitual breech

On occasion, the breech presentation recurs in successive pregnancies. The probable causes are congenital malformation of the uterus, septate or bicornuate and repeated cornuated attachment of the placenta.

Diagnosis

- Clinical
- Sonography
- Radiology

Clinical

The diagnostic features of a complete breech and a frank breech are given in a tabulated form (Table 10.1).

Ultrasonography is most informative

1. It confirms the clinical diagnosis, especially in primigravidae with engaged frank breech or with tense abdominal wall and irritable uterus.
2. It can detect fetal congenital abnormality and also congenital anomalies of the uterus.
3. It measures biparietal diameter, gestational age and approximate weight of the fetus.
4. It also localizes the placenta.
5. Assessment of liquor volume.
6. Attitude of the head flexion or hyperextension.

Radiology: a straight X-ray is rarely done

1. To confirm the clinical diagnosis
2. To exclude bony congenital malformation (hydrocephalus).
3. To note the size of the baby
4. To note the position of the limbs and the head.

Positions

The sacrum is the denominator of breech and there are four positions.

The positions are

1. Ist position—left sacroanterior (LSA) being the commonest
2. 2nd position—right sacroanterior (RSA)
3. 3rd position—right sacroposterior (RSP)
4. 4th position—left sacroposterior (LSP).

MECHANISM OF LEFT SACROANTERIOR POSITION

- The lie is longitudinal
- The attitude is one of complete flexion
- The presentation is breech

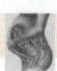

Table 10.1: Diagnostic features of a complete breech and a frank breech

	Complete breech	Frank breech
Per abdomen Fundal grip	• Head—suggested by hard and globular mass	• Head—Irregular small parts of the feet may be felt by the side of the head
	• Head is ballottable	• Head is non-ballottable due to splitting action of the legs on the trunk
Lateral grip	• Fetal back is to one side and the irregular limbs to the other	• Irregular parts are less felt on the side
Pelvic grip	• Breech—suggested by soft, broad and irregular mass	• Small, hard and a conical mass is felt
	• Breech is usually not engaged during pregnancy	• The breech is usually engaged
FHS Per vaginum	• Usually located at a higher level round about the umbilicus	• Located at a lower level in the midline due to early engagement of the breech
During pregnancy	• Soft and irregular parts are felt through the fornix	• Hard feel of the sacrum is felt, often mistaken for the head
During labour	• Palpation of ischial tuberosities, anal opening, sacrum and the feet by the sides of the buttocks. The foot felt is identified by the prominence of the heel and lesser mobility of the great toe	• Palpation of ischial tuberculosities, anal opening and sacrum only

- The position is left sacroanterior
- The denominator is the sacrum
- The presenting part is the anterior (left) buttock
- The bitrochanteric diameter, 10 cm, enters the pelvis in the left oblique diameter of the brim.
- The sacrum points to the left iliopectineal eminence.

Compaction

Descent takes place with increasing compaction, owing to increased flexion of the limbs.

- *Internal rotation of the buttocks:* The anterior buttock reaches the pelvic floor first and rotates forwards 1/8th of a circle along the right side of the pelvis to lie behind the symphysis pubis. The bitrochanteric diameter is now in the antero-posterior diameter of the outlet.

- *Lateral flexion of the body:* The anterior buttock escapes under the symphysis pubis, the posterior buttock sweeps the perineum and the buttocks are born by a movement of lateral flexion.

- *Restitution of the buttocks:* The anterior buttock turns slightly to the mother's right side.

- *Internal rotation of the shoulders:* The bisacromial diameter (12 cm) engages in the same oblique diameter as the buttocks, the left oblique. The anterior shoulder rotates forwards 1/8th of a circle along the right side of the pelvis and escapes under the symphysis pubis, the posterior shoulder sweeps the perineum and the shoulders are born.

- *Internal rotation of the head:* Descent with increasing flexion occurs the head enters

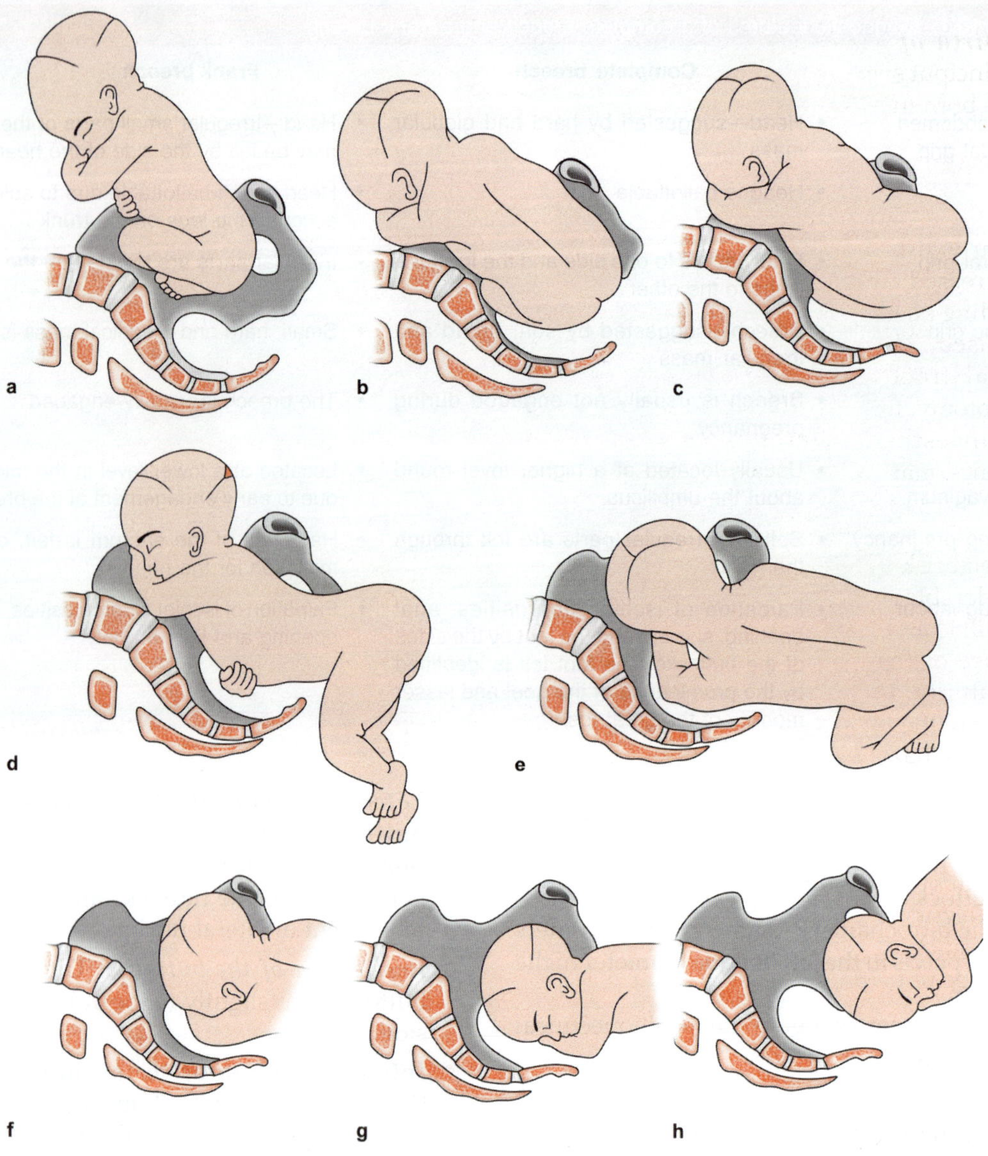

a

b

c

d

e

f

g

h

Fig. 10.13: Mechanism of labour in breech (RSA)

the pelvis with the sagittal suture in the transverse diameter of the brim. The engaging diameter of the head is sub-occipitofrontal (10 cm). The occiput rotates forwards 1/8th or 2/8th of a circle placing the occiput behind the symphysis pubis along the left side and further descent occurs until the subocciput hinges under the symphysis pubis.

- **External rotation of the body:** At the same time the body turns so that the back is uppermost.

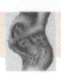

- *Birth of the head:* The chin, face and sinciput sweep the perineum and the head is born in a flexed attitude.

PROGNOSIS

Maternal

Labour is usually not prolonged. But because of increased frequency of operative delivery including caesarean section, the morbidity is increased. The risks include trauma to the genital tract, operative vaginal delivery (episiotomy, forceps), caesarean section, sepsis and anaesthetic complications. As a consequence, maternal morbidity is slightly raised.

Fetal

The fetal risk in terms of perinatal mortality is considerable in vaginal breech delivery. It is difficult to assess the magnitude of the real risk, because of the complicating factors such as prematurity, birth trauma, congenital malformation of the fetus that contribute significantly to the fetal hazards. The overall perinatal mortality in breech still remains 9–25% compared with 1–2% for nonbreech deliveries. The factors which significantly influence the fetal risks are:

1. Skill of the obstetrician
2. Weight of the baby
3. Position of the legs
4. Type of pelvis

The fetal dangers

The fetal dangers in breech delivery are as follows:

1. *Intracranial haemorrhage:* Compression followed by decompression during delivery of the unmoulded after coming head results in tear of the tentorium cerebelli and haemorrhage in the subarachnoid space. The risk is more with preterm babies.

2. *Asphyxia: It is due to*
   - Cord compression soon after the buttocks are delivered and also when the head enters into the pelvis.

- Retraction of the placental site
- Premature attempt at respiration while the head is still inside
- Delayed delivery of the head
- Cord prolapse

3. *Injuries:* The following injuries are inflicted during manipulative deliveries:
   - *Haematoma:* Over the sternomastoid or over the thighs.
   - *Fractures:* The common sites are femur, humerus, clavicle, odontoid process. There may be dislocation of the hip joint, mandible or 5th and 6th cervical vertebrae.
   - Visceral injuries include rupture of the liver, kidneys, suprarenal glands, lungs and haemorrhage in the testicles.
   - *Nerve:* Spinal cord injury, stretching of the brachial plexus to cause either Erb's or Klumpke's palsy.

Some of the injuries may prove fatal and contribute to perinatal mortality. Long-term (neurological) morbidity of the surviving infants should not be under estimated.

Prevention of the fetal hazards

- The incidence of breech can be minimized by external cephalic version where possible.
- If the version fails or is contraindicated, delivery is done by elective caesarean section.
- Vaginal breech delivery should be conducted by a skilled obstetrician along with an organized team consisting of a skilled anaesthesist and an assistant.
- Vaginal manipulative delivery should be done by a skilled person with utmost gentleness, especially during delivery of the head.

ANTENATAL MANAGEMENT

Antenatal management in breech presentation consists of:

- Identification of the complicating factors related to breech presentation.

- External cephalic version, if not contra-indicated.
- Formulation of the line of management, if the version fails or is contraindicated.

Identification of complicating factor

It can be detected by clinical examination, supplemented by sonography. Sonography is particularly useful to detect congenital malformations of the fetus, the precise location of the placental site and congenital anomalies of the uterus.

External cephalic version (ECV)

There are protagonists and antagonists to external version. As such, in an institution or to an individual where the perinatal mortality in vaginal breech delivery is appreciably high, there is enough justification for its use. The success rate of version is about 60%. Successful version reduces the risk of caesarean section significantly. Prior sonography should be a routine. Cardiotocography (CTG) should ideally be done before and after the procedure.

Time of version

ECV has been considered at 35–37 weeks but can be attempted at any time thereafter up to early labour. While version in the early weeks is easy but chance of reversion is more. Late version may be difficult because of increasing size of the fetus and diminishing volume of liquor amnii.

Benefits of ECV are

1. Reduction in the incidence of breech presentation at term.
2. Reduction in the incidence of breech delivery (vaginal or caesarean) and the associated complications.
3. Reduction in the incidence of caesarean delivery by 5%.

Successful version is likely in cases of

1. Complete breech
2. Non-engaged breech

3. Sacroanterior position (fetal back anteriorly)
4. Adequate liquor
5. Non-obese patient

Causes of failure of version

1. Breech with extended legs difficult to disimpact because of early engagement and difficult to flex the trunk because of splinting action of the limbs.
2. Scanty liquor or big size baby.
3. Mechanical obesity, increased tone of the abdominal muscles and irritable uterus.
4. Short cord—either relative (common) or absolute.
5. Uterine malformations—septate or bicornuate.

Dangers of version

The dangers of version are
1. Premature onset of labour.
2. Premature rupture of the membranes.
3. Placental separation and bleeding.
4. Entanglement of the cord round the fetal part or formation or a true knot leading to impairment of fetal circulation and fetal death.
5. Increased chance of fetomaternal bleed.
6. Amniotic fluid embolism.

Immunoprophylaxis with anti-D gamma globulin is to be administered in nonimmunized Rh negative mother.

Management, if version fails or is contraindicated

The pregnancy is to be continued with usual check up and unexpectedly, one may find that spontaneous version has occurred. But if the breech persists, the assessment of the case is to be done with respect to:

1. Age of the mother especially in primigravidae
2. Associated complicating factors
3. Size of the baby and
4. Pelvic capacity

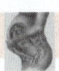

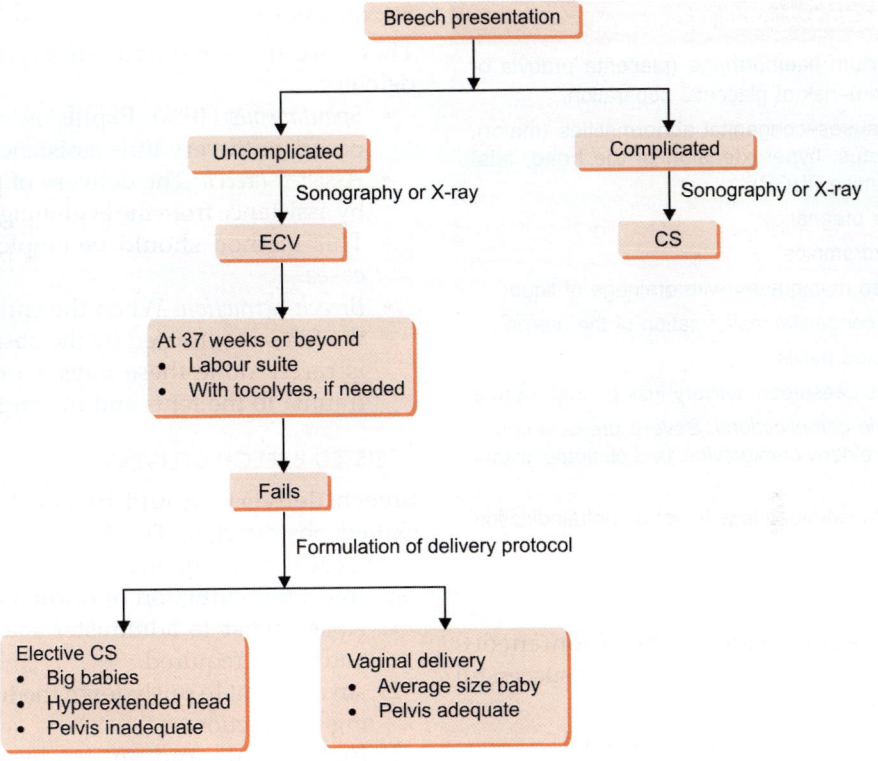

Fig. 10.14: Scheme of management of breech presentation

Clinical assessment of the pelvis should be done in all primigravidae and in selected multigravidae with previous history suggestive of pelvic inadequacy. Ultrasonographic examination is done and delivery can be planned:

- To perform an elective caesarean section.
- To allow spontaneous labour to start and vaginal breech delivery to occur.

Elective caesarean section

The indications of CS in breech are:
- Big baby (estimated fetal weight > 3.5 kg)
- Hyperextension of the head
- Footling presentation (risk of cord prolapse)
- Suspected pelvic contraction.

Any associated complication (obstetric or medical) is often considered for CS in breech.

The overall incidence of caesarean section in breech ranges from 15–50%, out of which about 80% is elective. Delivery of preterm breech (weight < 1500 gm) by caesarean section is commonly done but it should be reserved in selected centres, equipped with intensive neonatal care unit.

Vaginal breech delivery is considered in cases with adequate pelvis, average fetal weight (between 1.5 and 3.5 kg), flexed head and without any other complications. Frank breech is preferred.

MANAGEMENT OF VAGINAL BREECH DELIVERY

First stage

The management protocol is similar to that mentioned in normal labour. The following are

- Antepartum haemorrhage (placenta praevia or abruption)–risk of placental separation.
- Fetal causes–congenital abnormalities (major), dead fetus, hyperextension of the head, fetal compromise (IUGR).
- Multiple pregnancy
- Oligohydramnios
- Ruptured membranes–with drainage of liquor
- Known congenital malformation of the uterus
- Contracted pelvis
- Previous caesarean delivery–risk of scar rupture
- *Obstetric complications:* Severe pre-eclampsia, obesity, elderly primigravida, bad obstetric history (BOH).

Breech with extended legs is not a contraindication for version.

the important considerations. Spontaneous onset labour increases the chance of successful vaginal delivery.

- Vaginal examination is indicated
  - At the onset of labour for pelvic assessment,
  - Soon after rupture of the membranes to exclude cord prolapse.
- An intravenous line is sited with Ringer's solution, oral intake is avoided, blood is sent for group and cross matching.
- Adequate analgesia is given, epidural is preferred.
- Fetal status and progress of labour are monitored.
- Oxytocin infusion may be used for augmentation of labour.

Indications of caesarean section (CS)

- Cases seen for the first time in labour with presence of complications.
- Arrest in the progress of labour
- Non-reassuring FHR pattern (fetal distress)
- Cord presentation or prolapse

Second stage

There are three methods of vaginal breech delivery:

- *Spontaneous (10%):* Expulsion of the fetus occurs with very little assistance.
- *Assisted-breech:* The delivery of the fetus is by assistance from the beginning to the end. This method should be employed in all cases.
- *Breech extraction:* When the entire body of the fetus is extracted by the obstetrician. It is rarely done these days as it produces trauma to the fetus and the mother.

ASSISTED BREECH DELIVERY

Breech delivery should be conducted by a skilled obstetrician. The following are to be kept ready beforehand, in addition to those required for conduction of normal labour:

1. Anaesthetist–to administer anaesthesia as and when required.
2. An assistant to push down the fundus during contraction.
3. Instruments and suture materials for episiotomy.
4. A pair of obstetric forceps for the after-coming head, if required.
5. Appliances for revival of the baby, if asphyxiated.

Principles in conduction

1. Never to rush
2. Never pull from below, but push from above
3. Always keep the fetus with the back anteriorly.

Steps

1. The patient is brought to the table when the anterior buttock and fetal anus are visible. She is placed in lithotomy position when the posterior buttock distends the perineum.
2. Antiseptic cleaning is done, bladder is emptied with an 'in and out' catheter.

3. Episiotomy: It should be done in all cases of primigravidae and selected multiparae. Its advantages are:
   - To straighten the birth canal which specially facilitates the delivery of breech with extended legs where lateral flexion is inadequate.
   - To facilitate intravaginal manipulation and for forceps delivery.
   - To minimize compression of the after coming head. The best time for episiotomy is when the perineum is distended and thinned by the breech as it is 'climbing' the perineum.

4. The patient is encouraged to bear down as the expulsive forces from above ensure flexion of the fetal head and safe descent. The 'no touch of the fetus' policy is adopted until the buttocks are delivered along with the legs in flexed breech and the trunk slips upto the umbilicus.

5. Soon after the trunk upto the umbilicus is born the baby is wrapped with a sterile towel to prevent slipping when held by the hands and to facilitate manipulation, if required.

6. *Delivery of the arms:* The assistant is to place a hand over the fundus and keep a steady pressure during uterine contractions to prevent extension of the arms. Soon, the anterior scapula is visible. The position of the arm should be noted. The arms are delivered one after the other only when one axilla is visible, by simply hooking down each elbow with a finger. It is immaterial as to which arm is to be delivered first. The baby should be held by the feet over the sterile towel while the arms are delivered (Fig. 10.15).

7. *Delivery of the aftercoming head:* This is the most crucial stage of the delivery. The time between the delivery of umbilicus and delivery of mouth should preferably be 5 to 10 minutes. There are various methods

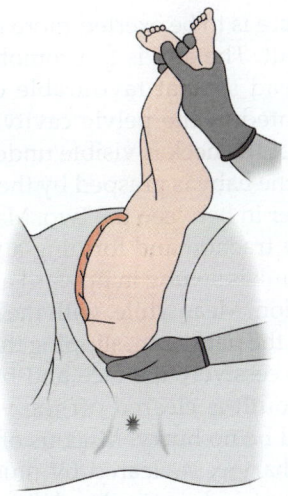

Fig. 10.15: Delivery of the posterior arm

of delivery for the aftercoming head. The following are the common methods employed:

- *Burns-Marshall method (Fig. 10.16):* The baby is allowed to hang by its own weight. The assistant is asked to give suprapubic pressure with the flat of hand in a downward and backward direction, the

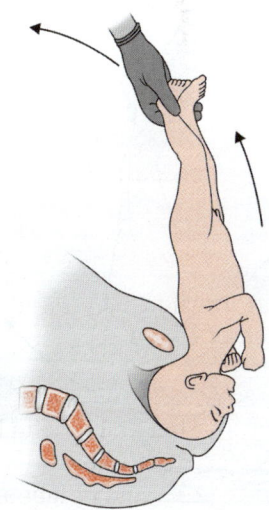

Fig. 10.16: Burns-Marshall method

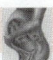

pressure is to be exerted more towards the sinciput. The aim is to promote flexion of the head so that favourable diameter is presented to the pelvic cavity. When the nape of the neck is visible under the pubic arch, the baby is grasped by the ankle with a finger in between the two. Maintaining a steady traction and forming a wide circle, the trunk is swung in upward and forward direction. Meanwhile, with the left hand to guard the perineum, slipping the perineum off successively the face and brow. When the mouth is cleared off the vulva, there should be no hurry. Mucous of the mouth and pharynx is cleared by mucus sucker. The trunk is depressed to deliver rest of the head.

- Forceps delivery can be used as a routine (Fig. 10.17).
- *Malar flexion and shoulder traction (modified Mauriceau-Smellie-Veit technique):* The technique is named after the three great obstetricians who described the use of the grip independently. The baby is placed on the supinated left forearm (preferred) with the limbs hanging on

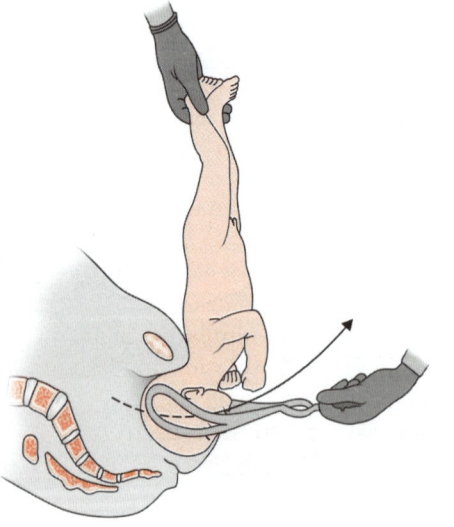

Fig. 10.17: Delivery of the aftercoming head by forceps

either sides. The middle and the index fingers of the left hand are placed over the malar bones on either sides (modification of the original method, where the index finger was introduced inside the mouth). This maintains flexion of the head. The ring and little fingers of the pronated right arm are placed on the child's right shoulder, the index finger is placed on the left shoulder and the middle finger is placed on the suboccipital region. Traction is now given in downward and backward direction till the nape of the neck is visible under the pubic arch. The assistant gives suprapubic pressure during the period to maintain flexion. Thereafter, the fetus is carried in upward and forward direction towards the mother's abdomen releasing the face, brow and lastly, the trunk is depressed to release the occiput and vertex (Fig. 10.18).

Third stage

The third stage is usually uneventful. The placenta is usually expelled out soon after delivery of the head. The prophylactic ergometrine is to be given, it should be administered intravenously with the crowning of the head.

MANAGEMENT OF COMPLICATED BREECH DELIVERY

When a woman presents in advanced labour it may be difficult to decide what would be ideal mode of delivery. However, if breech is not visible at the perineum it may be possible to deliver the baby by C.S. unless the attending staff has the necessary expertise for vaginal breech delivery.

Frank breech extraction (Pinard's maneuver)

It is done by intrauterine manipulation (for breech decomposition) to convert a frank breech to a footling breech. This is possible when the membranes have ruptured recently. In Pinard's maneuver the middle and the index fingers are

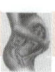

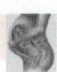

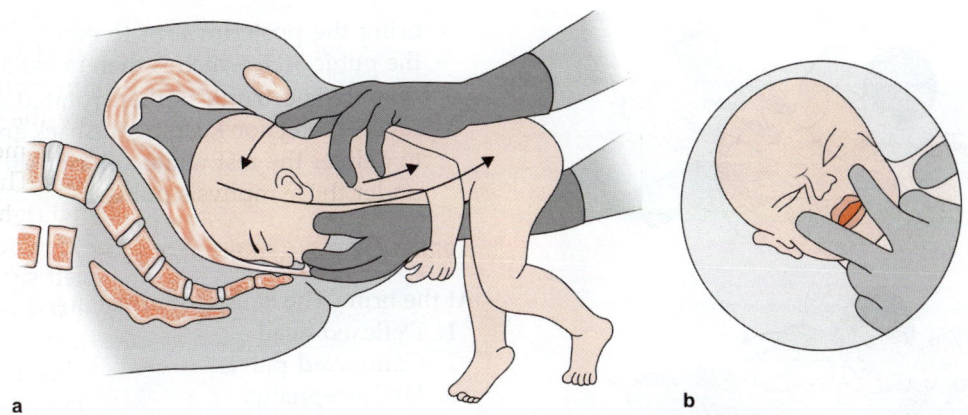

Fig. 10.18: Delivery of the aftercoming head by malar flexion and shoulder traction. **a.** Original Mauriceau-Smellie-Veit, **b.** Modification (preferred)

carried up to the popliteal fossa. It is then pressed and abducted so that the fetal leg is flexed. The fetal foot is then grasped at the ankle and breech extraction is accomplished (Fig. 10.19).

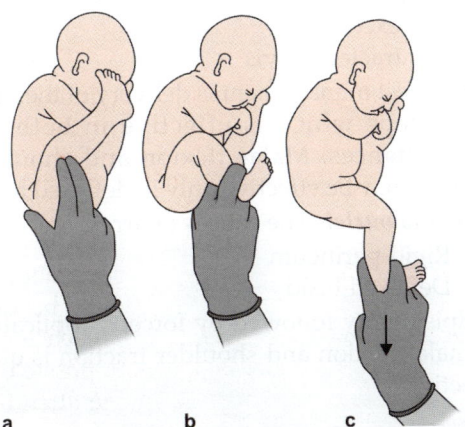

Fig. 10.19: Pinard's manoeuvre. **a.** Flexion and abduction of popliteal fossa, **b.** To catch hold the ankle, **c.** To pull down by movement of abduction

Extended arms

One or both arms may be fully stretched along the side of the head or lie behind the neck (nuchal displacement). The cause is usually the faulty technique in delivery, using unnecessary traction, forgetting the principle of 'never pull but push from above'. Arrest occur with the delivery of the trunk upto the costal margins. The diagnosis is made by noting the winging of the scapula and absence of the flexed limbs in front of the chest.

Management

The management calls for the urgent delivery of the arms, first the posterior and then the anterior one. The delivery of the arm may be accomplished by adopting the following method:

Lovset's manoeuvre (Fig. 10.20)

It is widely practised in preference to the classical method of bringing down an arm. The following are the advantages:

1. Wider applicability: It can be applied even when the classical method becomes difficult.
2. Intrauterine manipulation is nil.
3. A single manipulation is effective to all types of displacement of the arms.
4. General anaesthesia is usually not needed.

Principles

Because of the curved birth canal, when the anterior shoulder remains above the symphysis

 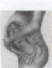

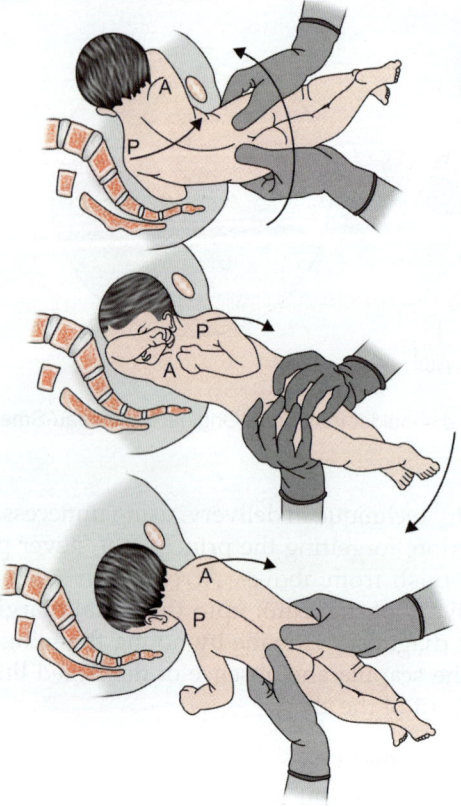

Fig. 10.20: Lovset's manoeuvre

pubis, the posterior shoulder will be below the sacral promontory. If the fetal trunk is rotated keeping the back anterior and maintaining a downward traction, the posterior shoulder will appear below the symphysis pubis.

Procedure: The baby (wrapped in a warm dry towel) is grasped, using both hands by femoro-pelvic grip keeping the thumbs parallel to the vertebral column. The manoeuvre should start only when the inferior angle of the anterior scapula is visible underneath the pubic arch.

- *Step 1:* The baby is lifted slightly to cause lateral flexion. The trunk is rotated through 180° keeping the back anterior and maintaining a downward traction. This will

bring the posterior arm to emerge under the pubic arch which is then hooked out.
- *Step 2:* The trunk is then rotated in the reverse direction keeping the back anterior to deliver the rest while anterior shoulder under the symphysis pubis.

ARREST OF THE AFTERCOMING HEAD

At the brim: The causes of arrest are:
1. Deflexed head
2. Contracted pelvis
3. Hydrocephalus

Management

If the arrest is due to a deflexed head, the delivery is to be completed by malar flexion and shoulder traction along with suprapubic pressure by the assistant. The head is to be negotiated through the brim in the transverse diameter and rotated in the cavity.

In the cavity: The causes of arrest of the head in the cavity are:
1. Deflexed head
2. Contracted pelvis

The best management is delivery of the head by forceps which is effective in both the circumstances. Malar flexion and shoulder traction may be effective only in deflexed head.

At the outlet: The causes of arrest are:
1. Rigid perineum
2. Deflexed head

Episiotomy followed by forceps application or malar flexion and shoulder traction is quite effective.

FACE PRESENTATION

Face is a rare variety of cephalic presentation where the presenting part is the face. The attitude of the fetus shows complete flexion of the limbs with extension of the spine. There is complete extension of the head so that the occiput is in contact with its spine or back. The denominator is mentum (Fig. 10.21).

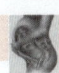

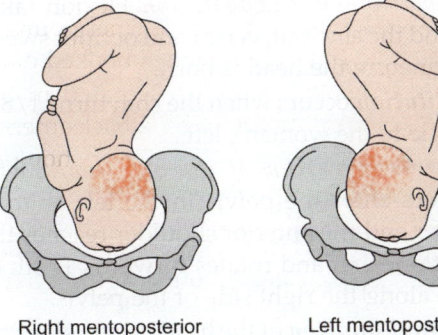

Right mentoposterior	Left mentoposterior

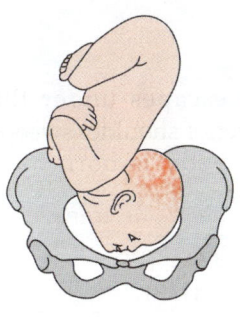 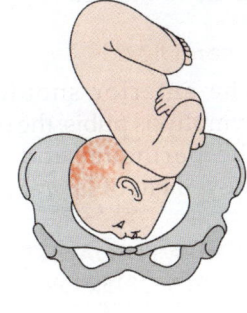

Right mentolateral	Left mentolateral

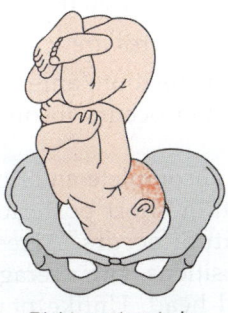 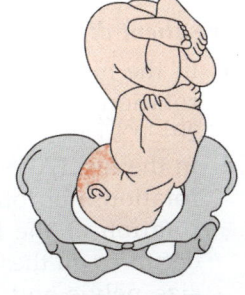

Right mentoanterior	Left mentoanterior

Fig. 10.21: Six positions of face presentation

The commonest position is left mento-anterior (LMA): As the ROP position is 5 times more common than LOP and as the conversion of face occurs from deflexed OP, LMA is the commonest. Overall anterior positions are more frequent than the posterior one.

Incidence

Its frequency is about 1 in 500 births. Face presentation present during pregnancy (primary face presentation) is rare while that developing after the onset of labour (secondary face presentation) is common. It occurs more frequently in multiparae (70%).

Etiology

The cause of extreme extension of the head is not clear in all the cases. The following are the factors which are often associated:

Maternal

1. Multiparity with pendulous abdomen.
2. Lateral obliquity of the uterus, especially if it is directed to the side towards which the occiput lies.
3. Contracted pelvis is associated in about 40% cases. Flat pelvis favours face presentation.

Fetal

1. Congenital malformations (15%)
   a. The commonest one is anencephaly. The almost nonexistent neck with absence of the cranium makes it easy to feel the facial structure even with semiextended head.
   b. Congenital goitre, prevalent in endemic areas
   c. Congenital bronchocele
2. Twist of the cord several turns round the neck
3. Increased tone of the extensor group of neck muscles

MECHANISM OF A LEFT MENTOANTERIOR POSITION

- The engaging diameter of the head is submentobregmatic 9.5 cm.
- The lie is longitudinal
- The attitude is one of extension of head and back.

- The presentation is face.
- The position is left mentoanterior.
- The denominator is the mentum.
- The presenting part is the left malar bone.

Extension: Descent takes place with increasing extension. The mentum becomes the leading part.

Internal rotation of the head: Occurs when the chin reaches the pelvic floor and rotates forwards 1/8th of a circle. The chin escapes under the symphysis pubis (Fig. 10.22).

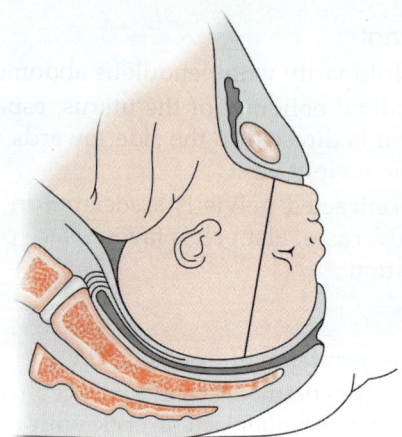

a

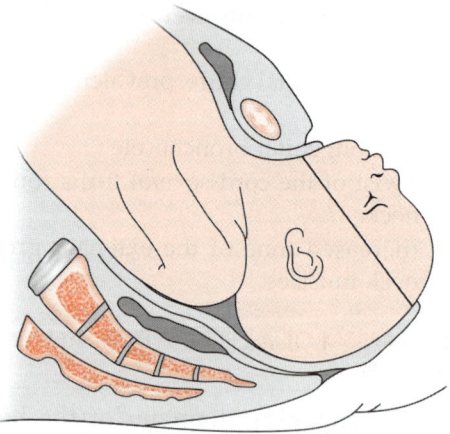

b

Fig. 10.22: Birth of head in mentoanterior position. **a.** The chin escapes under symphysis pubis. Submento-bregmatic at outlet, **b.** The head is born by movement of flexion

Delivery of the head by flexion: Flexion takes place and the sinciput, vertex and occiput sweep the perineum; the head is born.

Restitution occurs when the chin turns 1/8th of a circle to the woman's left.

Internal rotation of the shoulders: The shoulders enter the pelvis in the left oblique diameter and the anterior shoulder reaches the pelvic floor first and rotates forwards 1/8th of a circle along the right side of the pelvis.

External rotation of the head occurs simultaneously. The chin moves a further 1/8th of a circle to the left.

Lateral flexion

The anterior shoulder escapes under the symphysis pubis, the posterior shoulder sweeps the perineum and the body is born by a movement of lateral flexion.

RIGHT MENTOANTERIOR (RMA), LEFT MENTOPOSTERIOR (RMP OR LMP)

The cardinal movements in the mechanism of mentoposterior positions are like those of occipitoposterior position.

The salient differentiating features are

1. In the mentoposterior position/anterior rotation of the mentum occurs in only 20–30% cases.
2. In the rest (70–80%), incomplete anterior rotation, nonrotation or short posterior rotation of the mentum occurs. Arrest occurs in all these positions with average size pelvis and fetal head. Unlike persistent occipitoposterior, where occasional face to pubis delivery occurs, there is no possibility of spontaneous delivery in persistent mentoposterior.

Diagnosis

Antenatal diagnosis is rarely made. Diagnosis is made only during labour but in about half, the detection is made at the time of delivery.

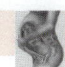

ABDOMINAL FINDINGS

Inspection

Because of 'S' shaped spine, there is no visible bulging of the flanks.

Palpation

The diagnostic features in mentoanterior and mentoposterior are tabulated below in Table 10.2.

VAGINAL EXAMINATION

The diagnostic features are palpating the mouth with hard alveolar margins, nose, malar. In early labour, because of high head and sausageshaped bag of membranes, the parts are not clearly defined. The distinguishing features are:

1. The mouth and the malar eminences are not in a line; but in breech, the anus and the ischial tuberosities are in one line.
2. Sucking effect of mouth
3. Hard alveolar margins
4. Absence of meconium staining on the examination fingers. The examination should be conducted gently, as there is chance of injury to the eyes. Assessment of the pelvis should be done as a routine.

Sonography/Radiography

This should be done to confirm the diagnosis, to exclude bony congenital malformation of the fetus and to note the size of the baby.

Clinical course

In spite of the fact that the engaging diameter of the head in flexed vertex and the extended face presentation is the same, 9.5 cm (3 ¾"), the clinical course of the latter is adversely affected because of the following:

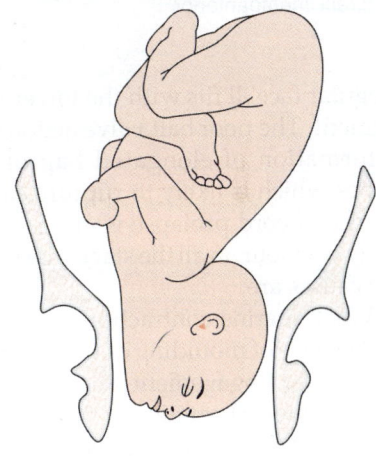

Fig. 10.23: Chief features to be recognised on abdominal examination in face presentation

Table 10.2: Diagnostic features of mentoanterior and mentoposterior		
	Mentoanterior	**Mentoposterior**
Lateral grip	1. Fetal limbs are felt anteriorly 2. Back is on the flank and is difficult to palpate. 3. The chest is thrown anteriorly against the uterine wall and is often mistaken for back.	Back is felt to the front and better palpated only towards the podalic ple because of extension of spine.
Pelvic grip	1. Head seems big and is not engaged. 2. Cephalic prominence is to the side towards which back lies. 3. Groove between the head and back is not so prominent.	1. Same 2. Same 3. The groove is prominent
Auscultation	FHS is distinctly audible anteriorly through the chest wall of the fetus towards the side of limbs.	FHS is not so distinct and is audible on the flank towards the side of limbs

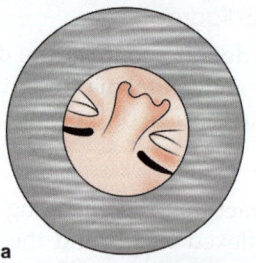 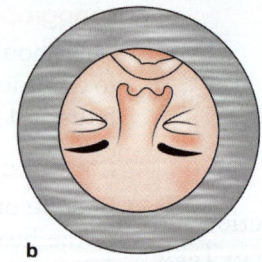 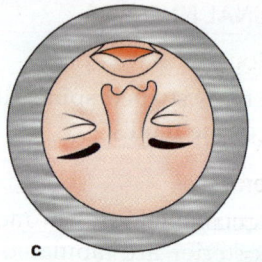

a   b   c

Fig. 10.24: Vaginal touch pictures of left mentoanterior position. **a.** The mentum is felt to left and anteriorly. Orbital ridges in left oblique diameter of the pelvis, **b.** Following increased extension of the head, the mouth can be felt. **c.** The face has rotated 1/8th of a circle forwards. Orbital ridges in transverse diameter of the pelvis. Position direct mentoanterior

1. Irregular face ill fits with the lower uterine segment. The poor ball valve action results in formation of elongated bag of membranes which is likely to rupture early.
2. Chance of cord prolapse is more.
3. Delay of labour, in all the stages, is common. The causes are:
   - Weak uterine contractions
   - Absence of moulding of the facial bones
   - Delayed engagement
   - Late internal rotation
4. Chance of perineal damage is more because a wide biparietal diameter—9.5 cm (3 ¾") stretches the perineum and submento-vertical diameter 11.5 cm (4 ½") emerges out of the introitus (Fig. 10.25).

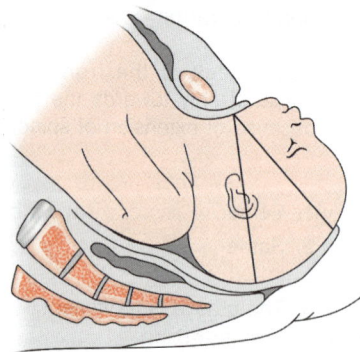

Fig. 10.25: Submentovertical diameter (11.5 cm or 4½") emerges out of the introitus

5. Postpartum haemorrhage is more likely due to atonic uterus and trauma following operative delivery.

PROGNOSIS

Maternal

In mentoanterior, the maternal risk is not much increased. However, there is increased morbidity due to operative delivery and vaginal manipulation. In neglected cases, the risks of impacted mentoposterior leading to obstructed labour and rupture uterus are not uncommon.

Fetal

Fetal prognosis is, however, adversely affected due to:

1. Cord prolapse
2. Increased operative delivery
3. Cerebral congestion due to poor venous return from the head and neck.
4. Neonatal infection due to bacterial contamination within the vagina.

Caput and moulding

Due to poor venous return from the head and neck, marked caput forms distorting the entire face. The lips and the eyelids are markedly swollen with considerable appearance of bruising.

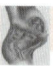

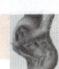

Management

Overall assessment of the case is to be done to note:

1. Pelvic adequacy
2. Size of the baby
3. Associated complicating factors, if any, like elderly primigravidae, severe pre-eclampsia, post caesarean pregnancy and post-maturity
4. Congenital fetal malformation
5. Position of the mentum.

Indications of elective or early caesarean section

1. Contracted pelvis
2. Big baby
3. Associated complicating factors

MANAGEMENT OF LABOUR

Mentoanterior

First stage

In uncomplicated cases/a wait and watch policy is adopted. Labour is conducted in the usual procedure and the special instructions, as laid down in occipitoposterior positions, are to be followed.

Second stage

One should wait for spontaneous delivery to occur. When the face appears at the vulva, extension must be maintained by holding the back, the sinciput and permitting the mentum to escape under the symphysis pubis before the occiput is allowed to sweep the perineum. In this way the submentovertical diameter (11.5 cm) distends the vaginal orifice instead of the mentovertical diameter (13.5 cm). Because the perineum is also distended by the biparietal diameter 9.5 cm, it should be protected with liberal mediolateral episiotomy. In case of delay, forceps delivery is done.

Mentoposterior

First stage

In uncomplicated cases, vaginal delivery is allowed with strict vigilance hoping for spontaneous anterior rotation of the chin.

Second stage

1. If anterior rotation of the chin occurs, spontaneous or forceps delivery with episiotomy is all that is needed.
2. *In incomplete or malrotation:* Early decision for the method of delivery is to be taken soon after full dilatation of the cervix. The following methods may be employed to expedite the delivery:
   - Caesarean section is the preferred method and is commonly done these days.
   - Manual rotation of the chin anteriorly followed by immediate forceps extraction is rarely done these days. The principles and the methods are similar to those employed in unrotated occipitoposterior position.

BROW PRESENTATION

Brow is the rarest variety of cephalic presentation where the presenting part is the brow and the attitude of the head is short of that degree of extension necessary to produce face presentation, i.e. the head lies in between full flexion and full extension. The presenting diameter is the mentovertical 13.5 cm which exceeds all diameters in an average size pelvis (Fig. 10.26).

Incidence

The incidence of brow is very rare, about 1 in 1000 births.

Causes

The causes of persistent brow are more or less the same as those of face presentation. The position is commonly unstable and converts to either vertex or face presentation.

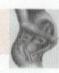

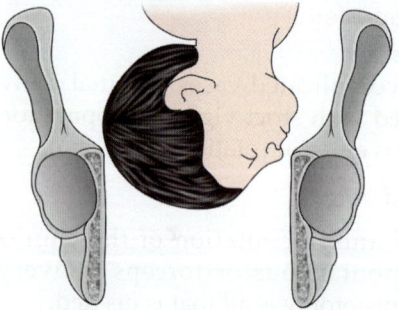

Fig. 10.26: Brow presentation

Diagnosis

Antenatal diagnosis is rarely made. The findings are more or less like those of face presentation. The cephalic prominence and the groove between it and the back are less prominent. The head feels very big and is nonengaged.

Vaginal examination

The position is to be confirmed on vaginal examination by palpating supra orbital ridges and anterior fontanelle. In late labour, the landmarks may be obscured by caput formation.

Sonography/Radiography

It is confirmatory and also helps in excluding bony congenital malformation of the fetus.

MECHANISM OF LABOUR

Diameter of engagement is through the oblique diameter with the brow anterior or posterior. As the engaging diameter of the head is mentovertical (13.5 cm) there is no mechanism of labour in an average size baby with normal pelvis. However, if the baby is small and the pelvis is roomy with good uterine contractions, delivery can occur in mentoanterior brow position. The brow descends until it touches the pelvic floor. Internal rotation and descent occur till the root of the nose hinges under the symphysis pubis. The brow and the vertex are delivered by flexion followed by extension to deliver the face. The mechanism is more or less the same as face-to-pubis delivery. Usual

restitution and external rotation occur. There is no mechanism in posterior brow position (Fig. 10.27).

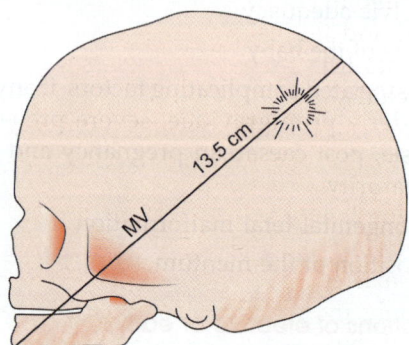

Fig. 10.27: Brow presentation. The mentovertical (MV) diameter, 13.5 cm, lies at the pelvic brim

Course and prognosis

In case of persistent brow presentation there is a chance of obstructed labour. It is an important cause of rupture of uterus in multiparae. On occasion (10%), there may be spontaneous conversion of brow into face or vertex presentation.

MANAGEMENT

During pregnancy

If the presentation is diagnosed during pregnancy and there is no other contraindications for vaginal delivery, nothing is to be done. Contracted pelvis and congenital malformation of the fetus are to be excluded. Spontaneous correction into face is likely to occur.

Elective caesarean section: Cases with persistent brow presentation are delivered by elective caesarean section.

During labour

1. In uncomplicated cases, if spontaneous correction to either vertex or face, fails to occur early in labour, caesarean section is the best method of treatment.

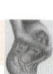

2. Manual correction to face with full dilatation of cervix is seldom practised now-a-days.
3. Craniotomy: If the labour becomes obstructed and the baby is dead, craniotomy is done. Rupture of the uterus should be excluded.

TRANSVERSE LIE

When the long axis of the fetus lies perpendicularly to the maternal spine or centralized uterine axis, it is called transverse lie. But more commonly, the fetal axis is placed oblique to the maternal spine and is then called oblique lie. In either of the conditions, the shoulder usually presents over the cervical opening during labour and as such both are collectively called shoulder presentations.

Position

The position is determined by the direction of the back, which is denominator. The position may be:
1. Dorsoanterior, which is the commonest (60%).
2. Dorsoposterior
3. Dorsosuperior
4. Dorsoinferior
   The last two are rare (Fig. 10.28).

Incidence

The incidence is about 1 in 200 births. It is common in premature and macerated fetuses, 5 times more common in multiparae than primigravidae. Transverse lie in twin pregnancy is found in 40% of cases.

Etiology

The causes are
1. Multiparity—lax and pendulous abdomen, imperfect uterine tone and extreme uterine obliquity are the responsible factors.
2. Prematurity

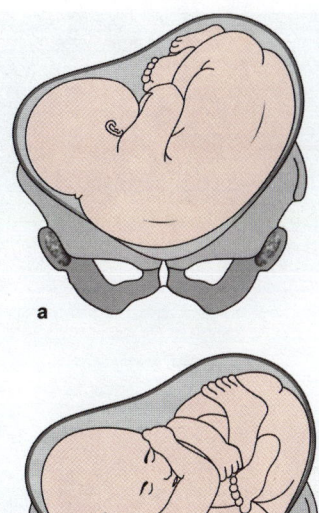

Fig. 10.28: Positions of transverse lie. **a.** Dorsoanterior, **b.** Dorsoposterior

3. Twins—it is more common for the second baby than the first one to be in transverse position.
4. Hydramnios
5. Contracted pelvis
6. Placenta praevia
7. Pelvic tumours
8. Congenital malformation of the uterus—arcuate or subseptate
9. Intrauterine death

DIAGNOSIS

Abdominal examination

Inspection

The uterus looks broader and often asymmetrical, not maintaining the pyriform shape.

Palpation

- The fundal height is less than the period of amenorrhoea.

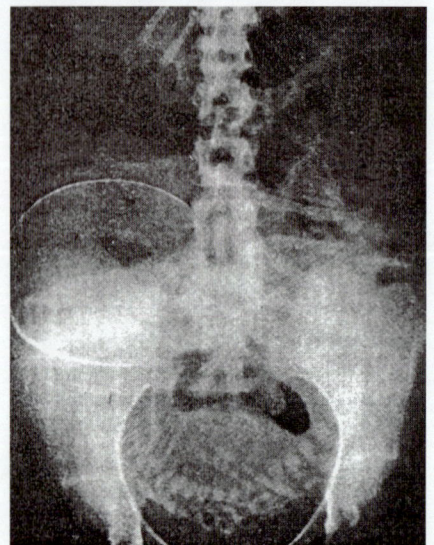

Fig. 10.29: Straight X-ray abdomen showing single fetus with transverse lie

- *Fundal grip:* Fetal pole (breech or head) is not palpable.
- Lateral grip
  a. Soft, broad and irregular breech is felt to one side of the midline and smooth, hard and globular head is felt on the other side. The head is usually placed at a lower level on one iliac fossa.
  b. The back is felt anteriorly across the long axis in dorsoanterior or the irregular small parts are felt anteriorly in dorsoposterior.
- *Pelvic grip:* The lower pole of the uterus is found empty. This, however, is evident only during pregnancy but during labour, it may be occupied by the shoulder.

Auscultation

FHS is heard easily much below the umbilicus in dorsoanterior position. FHS is, however, located at a higher level and often indistinct in dorsoposterior position.

Ultrasonography or radiography confirms the diagnosis.

Vaginal examination

During pregnancy, the presenting part is so high that it cannot be identified properly but one can feel some soft parts.

During labour, elongated bag of the membranes can be felt if it does not rupture prematurely. The shoulder is identified by palpating the following parts: acromion process, the scapula, the clavicle and axilla. The characteristic landmarks are the feeling of the ribs and intercostal spaces. On occasion, the arm is found prolapsed. It should be remembered that the findings of a prolapsed arm is confined not only to transverse lie but it may also be associated with compound presentation.

Determination of position

The thumb of the prolapsed hand, when supinated, points toward the head, the palm corresponds to the ventral aspect. The angle of the scapula, if felt, indicates the position of the back. The side to which the prolapsed arm belongs, can be determined by shaking hands with the fetus. If the right hand is required for this, the prolapsed arm belongs to right side and vice versa.

CLINICAL COURSE OF LABOUR

There is no mechanism of labour in transverse lie and an average size baby fails to pass through an average size pelvis. If the lie remains

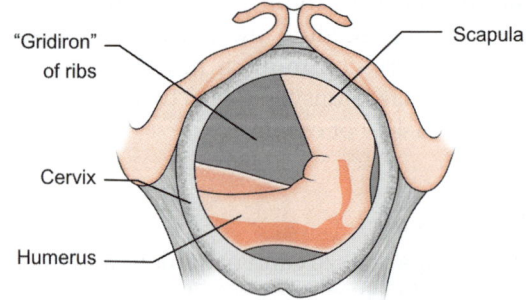

Fig. 10.30: Vaginal touch picture showing identified landmarks in shoulder presentation

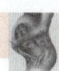

uncorrected and the labour is left uncared for, the following sequence of events may occur:

UNFAVOURABLE EVENTS (MOST COMMON)

There may be premature rupture of the membranes with escape of good amount of liquor because of absence of ball valve action of the presenting part. The hand of the corresponding shoulder may be prolapsed with or without a loop of cord. The cord may be prolapsed in isolation. There is increased chance of ascending infection from the lower genital tract. With increasing uterine contractions, the shoulder becomes wedged and impacted into the pelvis and the prolapsed arm becomes swollen and cyanosed. Gradually, features of obstructed labour supervene.

There is formation of a pathological retraction ring (Fig. 10.31).

The mother gets exhausted and features of dehydration and ketoacidosis develop; evidences of sepsis usually become apparent. In primigravidae, in response to obstruction, the uterus becomes inert and features of exhaustion and sepsis are only evident. But in multiparae,

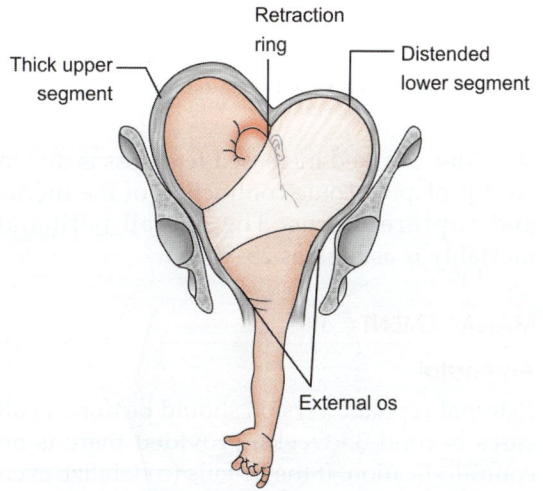

Fig. 10.31: Pathologic anatomy of the uterus in neglected shoulder presentation

the uterus reacts vigorously in response to obstruction and ultimately, the lower segment gives way as a result of marked thinning of its wall.

Neglected shoulder

By neglected shoulder is meant the series of complications that may arise out of shoulder presentation when the labour is left uncared. Such complications are impacted shoulder → obstructed labour → rupture uterus with clinical evidences of dehydration, ketoacidosis, shock and sepsis. These put the mother and the fetus at risk.

FAVOURABLE EVENTS (VERY RARE)

The following are the favourable events that may occur:
1. Spontaneous rectification or version
2. Spontaneous evolution
3. Spontaneous expulsion (conduplicate corpore). These events are very rare and occur only when the baby is premature or macerated.

Spontaneous rectification or version: It usually occurs in early labour with good amount of liquor and the baby is small and movable. Contracting uterus forces the head or the breech lying in the iliac fossa to lie in alignment to the brim. Thus, the lie may be changed from oblique to longitudinal with vertex presentation, when it is called rectification or with breech presentation when it is called version.

Spontaneous evolution: The arm is usually prolapsed, the head lies on one iliac fossa, the trunk and breech are forced into the cavity, the neck is markedly elongated. Breech and the trunk are expelled first followed by delivery of the head. This requires very strong uterine contractions.

Spontaneous expulsion: It is extremely rare and occurs only in premature and macerated fetus. Fetus is expelled doubled up, with chest

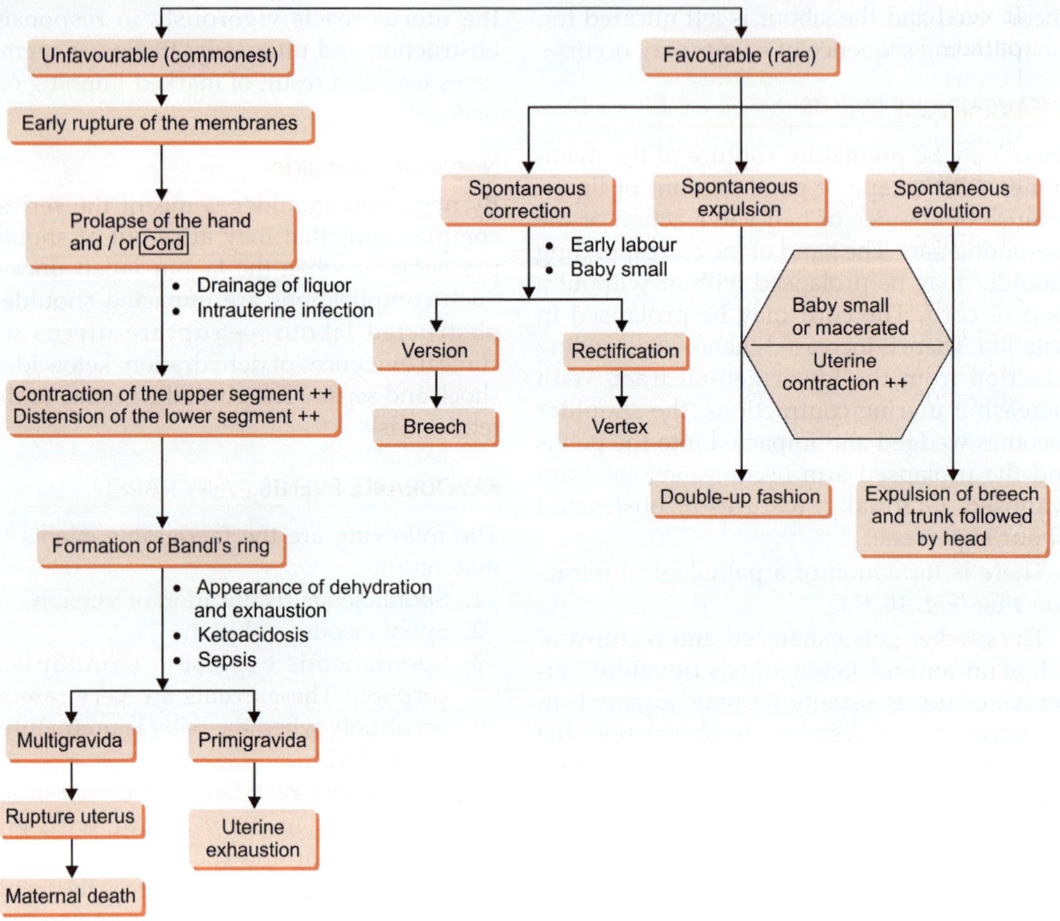

Fig. 10.32: Scheme of clinical course of labour in transverse lie left uncared for

and abdomen apposed. The head and the feet are delivered last.

Prognosis

In a well supervised pregnancy and labour, the maternal and the fetal outlook is not much unfavourable with the extended use of caesarean section. But in uncared pregnancy and labour, the outlook of the mother and the fetus is very much unpredictable. The maternal risk is increased due to dehydration, ketoacidosis, septicaemia, rupture uterus, haemorrhage, shock and peritonitis—sequences of neglected

shoulder. Marked increased fetal loss is due to cord prolapse. Tonic contraction of the uterus and rupture uterus. The overall perinatal mortality is as high as 25–50%.

MANAGEMENT

Antenatal

External cephalic version should be done in all cases beyond 35 weeks, provided there is no contraindication. If the lie fails to stabilize even at 36th week, the case is to be managed as outlined in unstable lie.

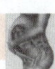

- If version fails or is contraindicated the patient is to be admitted at 37th week, because risk of early rupture of the membranes and cord prolapse is very much there. Elective caesarean section is the preferred method of delivery.
- Vaginal delivery may be allowed in a dead or congenitally malformed (small size) fetus. The labour may be allowed to continue under supervision till full dilatation of the cervix, when the baby can be delivered by internal version or destructive operation.

PATIENT SEEN IN LABOUR

The principles in management are as follows:

Early labour

- *External cephalic version:* Provided there is good amount of liquor amnii and there is no contraindication.
- *Caesarean section:* It is the preferred method of delivery, if version fails or is contraindicated.

Late labour

- *Baby alive:* There is hardly any scope of external version in late labour because of invariable rupture of the membranes and drainage of liquor. If the baby is mature and the fetal condition is good, it is preferable to do caesarean section in all cases.

  Internal version: In a singleton fetus, the risk of internal version is high. Not only it might inflict injury to the uterus (rupture uterus) but the fetal mortality is also increased to the extent of about 50%.
- *Baby dead:* Caesarean section even in such cases, is much safer in the hands of those who are not conversant with destructive operations. Following destructive operation, the uterine cavity is to be explored to exclude rupture of the uterus. Internal version should not be done.

This is a condition where the presentation of the fetus is constantly changed even beyond 36th week of pregnancy when it should have been stabilized.

Causes

The causes are those which prevent the presenting part to remain fixed in the lower pole of the uterus. Such conditions are:

1. Grand multipara with lack of uterine tone and pendulous abdomen—commonest cause.
2. Hydramnios
3. Contracted pelvis
4. Placenta praevia
5. Pelvic tumour

MANAGEMENT

Antenatal

At each antenatal visit, the presentation and the lie are to be checked. If there is no contraindication, external version is to be done to correct the malpresentation.

Hospitalization

The patient is to be admitted at 37th week. Premature or early rupture of the membranes with cord prolapse is the real danger with the lie remaining oblique. After admission, the investigation is directed to exclude placenta praevia, contracted pelvis or congenital malformation of the fetus with the help of sonography for localization of the placenta.

FORMULATION OF THE LINE OF TREATMENT

- Elective caesarean section is done in majority of the cases especially in the presence of complicating factors like pre-eclampsia, placenta praevia, contracted pelvis, etc.
- Stabilizing induction of labour.

 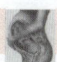

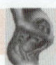

Procedure

Presentation is to be checked and external cephalic version is done, if necessary. Oxytocin drip is then started until effective uterine contraction occurs. After about 1 hour, internal examination is done to exclude cord presentation and then low rupture of the membranes is done. The possibility of change of lie is far and remote and the labour is expected to continue normally with usual management.

COMPOUND PRESENTATION (SYN: COMPLEX PRESENTATION)

When a cephalic presentation is complicated by the presence of a hand or a foot or both alongside the head or presence of one or both hands by the side of the breech, it is called compound presentation. The commonest one being the head with hand. The incidence is about 1 in 600.

Etiology

Conditions preventing engagement of the head can result in slipping of either upper or lower limbs by the side of the head. Prematurity (commonest), contracted pelvis, pelvic tumours, multiple pregnancy, macerated fetus, high head with premature or early rupture of the mem-

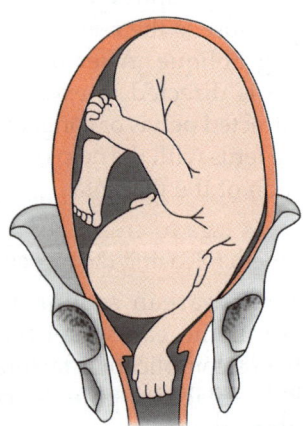

Fig. 10.33: Compound presentation: head with hand

branes and hydramnios are the known etiological factors.

Diagnosis

The diagnosis is not difficult when the cervical os is sufficiently dilated to feel the limb by the side of the presenting part, especially after rupture of the membranes. Cord prolapse is to be excluded because of its frequent association 10–15%.

Management

Factors to be considered are:
1. Stage of labour
2. Maturity of the fetus
3. Singleton or twins
4. Pelvic adequacy
5. Associated cord prolapse

Indication of caesarean section

Mature singleton fetus associated with contracted pelvis or cord prolapse with the fetus alive should be safely delivered by caesarean section.

Expectant treatment

In otherwise uncomplicated cases, an attitude of wait and watch policy is preferable. Elevation of the prolapsed limb with descent of the presenting part usually takes place spontaneously.

SHOULDER DYSTOCIA

The term shoulder dystocia is the failure of the shoulders to transverse the pelvis spontaneously after delivery of the head.

The anterior shoulder becomes trapped behind or on the symphysis pubis, whilst the posterior shoulder may be in the hollow of the sacrum or high above the sacral promontory (Fig. 10.34). This is, therefore, a bony dystocia and traction at this point will further impact the anterior shoulder, impeding attempts at delivery.

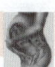

Incidence

Shoulder dystocia is not a common emergency, the incidence is reported as varying between 0.37% and 1.1%.

Risk factors

Antenatally, these risk factors include post-term pregnancy, high parity, maternal age over 35 and maternal obesity (weight over 90 kg at delivery).

Fetal macrosomia (birth weight over 4000 g) has been associated with an increased risk of shoulder dystocia.

Maternal diabetes and gestational diabetes have been identified as important risk factors. In diabetic women a previous delivery complicated by shoulder dystocia increases the risk of recurrence to 9.8%; this compares with a risk of recurrence of 0.58% in the general population.

In labour, risk factors that have been consistently linked with shoulder dystocia include oxytocin augmentation, prolonged labour, prolonged second stage of labour and operative deliveries.

Warning signs and diagnosis

The delivery may have been uncomplicated initially but the head may have advanced slowly and the chin may have had difficulty in sweeping over the perineum. Once the head is

delivered it may look as if it is trying to return into the vagina, which is caused by reverse traction. Shoulder dystocia is diagnosed when maneouvres normally used by the midwife, fail to accomplish delivery.

MANAGEMENT

Upon diagnosing shoulder dystocia the midwife must summon help immediately. An obstetrician, an anaesthetist and a person proficient in neonatal resuscitation should be called.

Noninvasive procedures

Change in maternal position: Any change in the maternal position may be useful to help release the fetal shoulders. However, certain manoeuvres have proved useful and are described below:

The McRoberts manoeuvre: This manoeuvre involves helping the woman to lie flat and to bring her knees up to her chest as far as possible (Fig. 10.35).

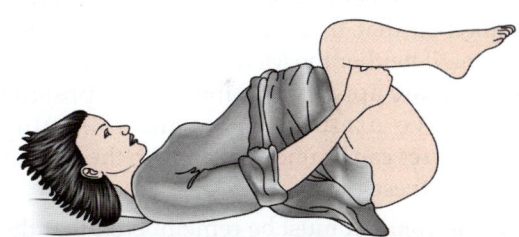

Fig. 10.35: The McRoberts manoeuvre position

This manoeuvre will rotate the angle of the symphysis pubis superiorly and use the weight of the mother's legs to create gentle pressure on her abdomen, releasing the impaction of the anterior shoulder.

Suprapubic pressure: Pressure should be exerted on the side of the fetal back and towards the fetal chest. This manoeuvre may help to adduct the shoulders and push the anterior shoulder away from the symphysis pubis (Fig. 10.36).

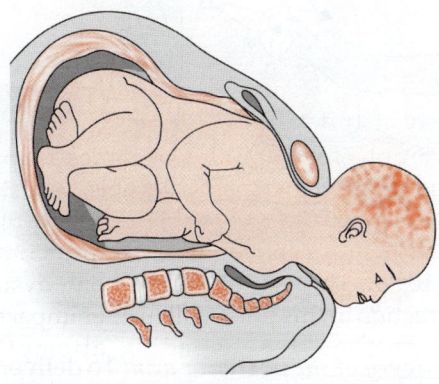

Fig. 10.34: Shoulder dystocia

 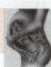

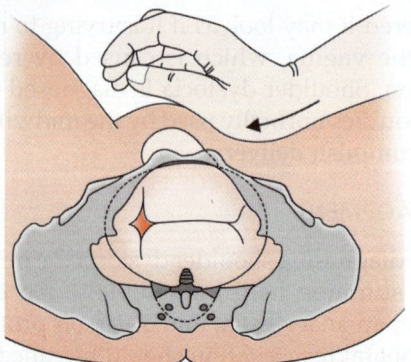

Fig. 10.36: Correct application of suprapubic pressure for shoulder dystocia

MANIPULATIVE PROCEDURES

Where non-invasive procedures have not been successful, direct manipulation of the fetus must now be attempted.

Positioning of the mother: The McRoberts position as detailed above can be used, or the mother could be placed in the lithotomy position with her buttocks well over the end of the bed so that there is no restriction on the sacrum. If neither the McRoberts nor lithotomy positions are appropriate, the all-four position may prove useful. Any of the following manoeuvres can be undertaken with the mother in one of these positions.

Episiotomy: It must be remembered that the problem facing the midwife is an obstruction at the pelvic inlet and is a bony dystocia, not an obstruction caused by soft tissue. Although episiotomy will not help to release the shoulders per se, the midwife should nevertheless perform one to gain access to the fetus without reaching the perineum and vaginal walls.

Rubin's manoeuvre: This manoeuvre requires the midwife to identify the posterior shoulder on vaginal examination, then to push the posterior shoulder in the direction of the fetal chest, thus rotating the anterior shoulder away from the symphysis pubis. By adducting the

shoulders, this manoeuvre reduces the 12 cm bisacromial diameter (Fig. 10.37).

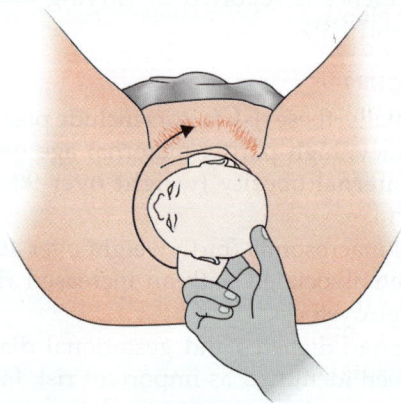

Fig. 10.37: The Rubin manoeuvre

Wood's manoeuvre: Wood's manoeuvre requires the midwife to insert her hand into the vagina and identify the fetal chest. Then, by exerting pressure on to the posterior shoulder, rotation is achieved. Although this manoeuvre does abduct the shoulders, it will rotate the shoulders into a more favourable diameter and enable the midwife to complete the delivery (Fig. 10.38).

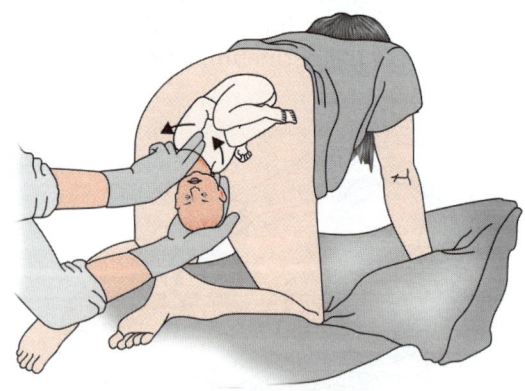

Fig. 10.38: The Wood's manoeuvre

Delivery of the posterior arm: To deliver the posterior arm the midwife has to insert her

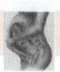

hand into the vagina making use of the space created by the hollow of the sacrum. Then two fingers splint the humerus of the posterior arm, flex the elbow, and sweep the forearm over the chest to deliver the hand. If the rest of the delivery is not then accomplished, the second arm can be delivered following rotation of the shoulder using either Wood's or Rubin's manoeuvre or by reversing the Lovset's manoeuvre (Figs 10.39a to d).

Zavanelli manoeuvre: If the manoeuvres described above have been unsuccessful, the obstetrician may consider the Zavanelli manoeuvre (Sandberg 1985) as a last hope for delivery of a live infant.

The Zavanelli manoeuvre requires the reversal of the mechanisms of delivery so far and reinsertion of the fetal head into the vagina. Delivery is then completed by caesarean section.

Method: The head is returned to its pre-restitution position. Pressure is then exerted on to the occiput and the head is returned to the vagina (Figs 10.40a and b). Prompt delivery by caesarean section is then required.

Symphysiotomy: Symphysiotomy is the surgical separation of the symphysis pubis and is used to enlarge the pelvis for delivery. It is usually performed in cases of cephalopelvic disproportion and is used more routinely in Third World countries.

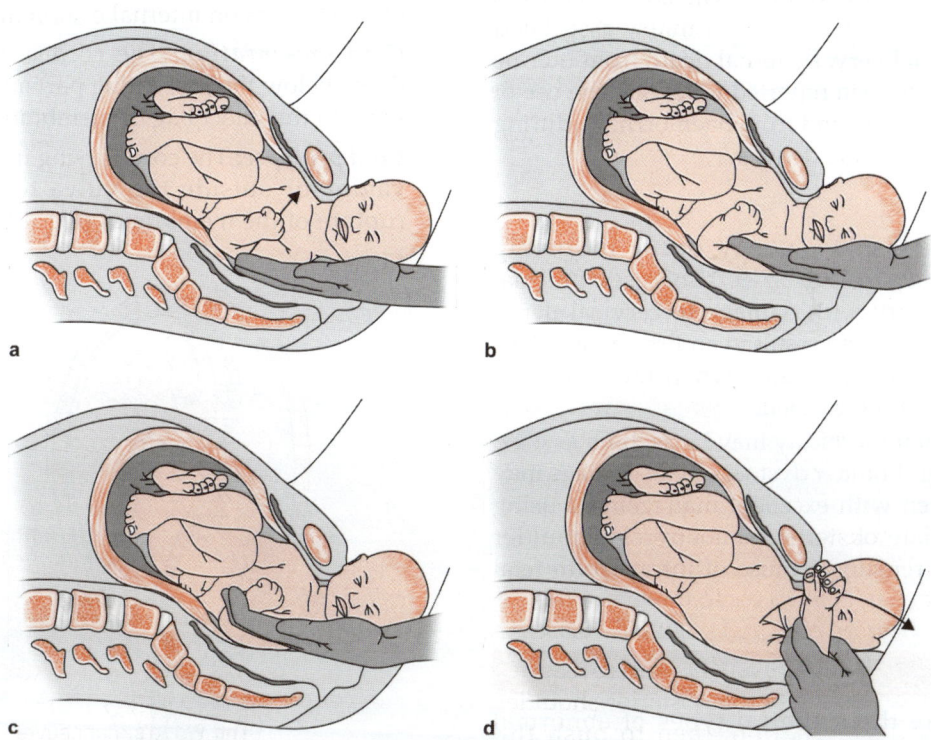

Fig. 10.39: Delivery of the posterior arm. **a.** Location of the posterior arm, **b.** Directing the arm into the hollow of the sacrum, **c.** Grasping and splinting the wrist and forearm, **d.** Sweeping the arm over the cheats and delivering the hand

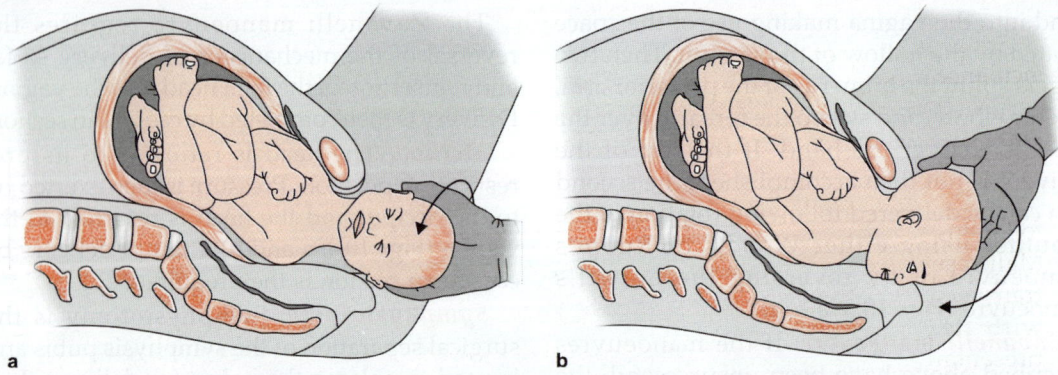

Fig. 10.40: The Zavanelli manoeuvre. **a.** Head being returned to direct anteroposterior (pre-restitution) position, **b.** Head being returned to vagina

OUTCOMES FOLLOWING SHOULDER DYSTOCIA

Approximately two-thirds will have a blood loss of more than 1000 ml from injury associated with the delivery. Maternal death from uterine rupture has been reported following the use of fundal pressure and from haemorrhage during and following the delivery.

Fetal

Neonatal asphyxia may occur following shoulder dystocia in 5.7–9.7% of cases. Brachial plexus injury with damage to cervical nerve roots 5 and 6 may result in an Erb's palsy. This is commonly associated when the head and neck have been twisted.

Neonatal morbidity may be as high as 4.2% following shoulder dystocia. Fetal damage may occur even with excellent management using appropriate obstetric manoeuvres. Shoulder dystocia remains a cause of intrapartum fetal death.

CORD PROLAPSE

There are three clinical types of abnormal descent of the umbilical cord by the side of the presenting part. All these are placed under the heading cord prolapse.

- *Occult prolapse:* The cord is placed by the side of the presenting part and is not felt by the fingers on internal examination.
- *Cord presentation:* The cord is slipped down below the presenting part and is felt lying in the intact bag of membranes.
- *Cord prolapse:* The cord is lying inside the vagina or outside the vulva following rupture of the membranes (Fig. 10.41).

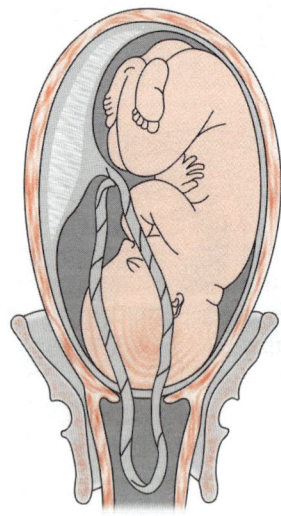

Fig. 10.41: Cord prolapse with ruptured membranes

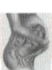

Incidence

The incidence of cord prolapse is about 1 in 300 deliveries. It is mostly confined to parous women.

Etiology

The following are the associated factors:

1. Malpresentations: the commonest being transverse (1 in 5) and breech, especially with flexed legs (1 in 20) or footling presentation
2. Contracted pelvis
3. Prematurity
4. Twins
5. Hydramnios
6. Placental factor: Minor degree of placenta praevia with marginal insertion of the cord or long cord
7. Iatrogenic: Low rupture of the membranes, manual rotation of the head and version.

Diagnosis

Occult prolapse: It is difficult to diagnose. The possibility should be suspected if there is persistence of variable deceleration of fetal heart rate pattern. Cord presentation. The diagnosis is made by feeling the pulsation of the cord through the intact membranes. Cord prolapse. The cord is palpated directly by the fingers and its pulsation can be felt if the fetus is alive.

PROGNOSIS

Fetal

The fetus is at risk of anoxia from the moment cord is prolapsed. The hazards to the fetus are more in vertex presentation, especially when the cord is prolapsed through the anterior segment of the pelvis or when the cervix is partially dilated. The overall perinatal mortality is about 50%.

Maternal

The maternal risks are incidental due to emergency operative delivery, especially through the vaginal route. Operative delivery involves the risk of anaesthesia, blood loss and infection.

Management

Cord presentation: The aim is to preserve the membranes and to expedite the delivery.

- Once the diagnosis is made, no attempt should be made to replace the cord, as it is not only ineffective but also the membranes inevitably rupture leading to prolapse of the cord.
- If immediate vaginal delivery is not possible or contraindicated, caesarean section is the best method of delivery. During the time of preparing the patient for operative delivery, she is kept in exaggerated Sim's position to minimize cord compression.
- A rare occasion is a multipara with longitudinal lie having good uterine contractions with the cervix three-fourths (7–8 cm) dilated, without any evidence of fetal distress. Watchful expectancy can be adopted till full dilatation of the cervix, when the delivery can be completed by forceps or breech extraction.

Management protocol is to be guided by

1. Baby living or dead
2. Maturity of the baby
3. Degree of dilatation of the cervix

Baby living

Immediate safe vaginal delivery is not possible or is contraindicated.

- *First aid management:* The aim is to minimize pressure on the cord till such time when the patient is prepared for assisted delivery or is transferred to an equipped hospital. If an oxytocin infusion is on, this should be stopped. At this time intravenous fluid and O_2 by face mask is given.
  - Bladder filling has been done to raise the presenting part off the compressed

cord till such time that patient is delivered (either by C.S. or vaginally). Bladder is filled with 400–750 ml of normal saline with a Foley's catheter, the balloon is inflated and the catheter is clamped. Bladder is emptied before caesarean delivery.

– To lift the presenting part off the cord, by the gloved fingers introduced into the vagina. The fingers should be placed inside the vagina till definitive treatment is instituted.

– Postural treatment—exaggerated and elevated Sim's position a with pillow or wedge under the hip or high Trendelenburg or knee-chest position has been traditionally mentioned but may be tiring to the patient.

– To replace the cord into the vagina to minimize vasospasm due to irritation.
• Definitive treatment
– *Caesarean section:* It is the best treatment when the baby is sufficiently mature enough to survive.

Immediate safe vaginal delivery is possible

• If the head is engaged, delivery is to be completed by forceps.
• If breech, the delivery is to be completed by breech extraction and in transverse lie, it should be completed by internal version followed by breech extraction.

Baby dead

Labour is allowed to proceed awaiting spontaneous delivery.

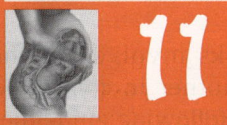

11

Abnormal Labour

OUTLINE

- Preterm labour
- Premature rupture of the membrane
- Obstructed labour
- Induction of labour
- Prolonged labour
- Abnormal uterine action
- Amniotic fluid embolism
- Blood coagulation disorders
- Fetal distress
- Obstetric shock
- Contracted pelvis
- Rupture of uterus
- Cervical dystocia
- DIC

PRETERM LABOUR
(SYN : PREMATURE LABOUR)

Definition

Preterm labour is defined as one where the labour starts before the 37th completed week (<259 days), counting from the first day of the last menstrual period.

Incidence

The prevalence widely varies and ranges between 5 and 10%.

Etiology

In more than 50%, the cause of preterm onset of labour is not known. The following are however, related with increased incidence of preterm labour.

High-risk factors

a. *History:* There is an increased incidence of preterm labour in cases such as:
   1. Previous history of induced or spontaneous abortion or preterm delivery
   2. Asymptomatic bacteriuria or recurrent urinary tract infection
   3. Smoking habits
   4. Low socioeconomic and nutritional status.

b. *Complications in present pregnancy:* Preterm labour may be due to a direct consequence of maternal/fetal/placental complicating factors or may be induced.

   1. **Maternal**
      - Pregnancy complications—such as pre-eclampsia, antepartum haemorrhage, premature rupture of the membranes, polyhydramnios.
      - **Uterine anomalies** such as, cervical incompetence, malformation of uterus
      - **Medical and surgical illness**—acute fever, acute pyelonephritis, diarrhoea, acute appendicitis, toxoplasmosis and abdominal operation. Chronic diseases such as hypertension, nephritis, diabetes, severe anaemia.
      - **Genital tract infection**—bacterial vaginosis, beta-haemolytic streptococcus, bacteroides, chlamydia, mycoplasma.

2. **Fetal:** Multiple pregnancy, congenital malformations, intrauterine death.
3. **Placental:** Infarction, thrombosis, placenta praevia or abruption.
c. *Iatrogenic:* Elective induction with wrong estimation of gestational period.
d. *Idiopathic (majority):* Premature effacement of the cervix with hyperirritable uterus and early engagement of the head are often associated. In the absence of any complicating factors, it is presumed that there is premature activation of the same systems involved in initiating labour at term.

Diagnosis

1. Regular uterine contractions with or without pain (at least one in every 10 minute).
2. Dilatation (> 2 cm) and effacement (80%) of the cervix.
3. Pelvic pressure, backache or vaginal discharge. It is better to overdiagnose preterm labour than to ignore the possibility of its presence.

MANAGEMENT

The objectives of management

1. To minimize the risk of perinatal mortality and morbidity
2. To preserve maternal health.

The management includes

1. To prevent preterm onset of labour, if possible
2. To arrest preterm labour, if not contraindicated
3. Appropriate management of labour
4. Effective neonatal care

PREVENTION

In about 50%, the cause remains unknown. Among the remaining complicated groups, decision has to be taken whether to allow the pregnancy to continue or not. The risk of delivery of a low birth weight baby has to be weighed against the risks involved to the unborn and/or to the mother in continued pregnancy. However, the following guidelines are adopted.

- Identification of risk factors is to be ascertained from the history and the defects are to be rectified as far as possible by:
  - Adequate rest
  - Nutritional supplement
  - Avoidance of smoking
  - Encirclage operation, if required
- Premature effacement of the cervix with irritable uterus and early engagement of the head should be viewed with concern. The patients are to be put to bed rest and tocolytic agents may be administered.
- Be sure about the gestational age before induction.
- Selective continuation of complicated pregnancy such as twins, polyhydramnios, placenta praevia, pre-eclampsia etc. with rest and appropriate therapy. These patients should be admitted in the hospital for close supervision.

Investigations

1. Full blood count
2. Urine for routine analysis, culture and sensitivity
3. Endocervical swab for any causative organism
4. Ultrasonography for fetal well being, cervical length and placental localization
5. Serum electrolytes and glucose levels when tocolytic agents are to be used.

TO ARREST PRETERM LABOUR

The following regime may be instituted in an attempt to arrest premature labour.

- *Absolute rest in bed is imposed:* The patient is to lie preferably in left lateral position
- *Adequate sedation:* is ensured with tablet diazepam 5 mg or phenobarbitone 30–60 mg—twice or thrice daily.

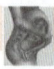

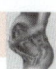

- *Adequate hydration* is maintained. Pro-phylactic antibiotic is not routinely given. It is recommended when infection is evident or culture report suggests.
- *Tocolytic agents:* Various drugs are used like MgSO$_4$, Ritrodine, Duadilan and Terbutaline. These drugs inhibit uterine contractions. The tocolytic agents can be used as short-term (1–3 days) or long-term therapy.

Short-term therapy: The objectives are:

1. To delay delivery for at least 24 hours for glucocorticoid therapy to the mother to enhance fetal lung maturation, if premature labour starts before 34th week.
2. In utero transfer of the patient to a unit more able to manage a preterm neonate.

Contraindications

1. *Maternal:* Diabetes, thyrotoxicosis, severe hypertension, cardiac disease, haemor-rhage in pregnancy, e.g. placenta praevia or abruption.
2. *Fetal:* Fetal distress, fetal death, congenital malformation, pregnancy beyond 34 weeks.
3. *Others:* Rupture of membranes, chorio-amnionitis, cervical dilatation more than 4 cm.

Long-term use: It is not so effective. *It is said to be successful* if the pregnancy can be continued for atleast one week following established onset of labour prior to 34th week.

Glucocorticoid therapy: Maternal adminis-tration of glucocorticoids is advocated where the pregnancy is less than 34 weeks. This helps in fetal lung maturation so that the incidence of respiratory distress syndrome can be mini-mized. This is beneficial only when the delivery is delayed beyond 24 hours but less than 7 days. Either betamethasone (Betnesol) 12 mg IM every 12 hrs for two doses or dexamethasone (Decadron) 8 mg IM every 12 hrs. for 3 doses is given. If the delivery is delayed for more than 7 days after the first injection, treatment must be repeated.

Contraindications of its use

1. Premature rupture of the membranes specially with evidence of infection
2. Severe pre-eclampsia
3. Estimated delivery time is outside the "24 hours–7 days" interval.

MANAGEMENT OF PRETERM LABOUR

The principles in management of preterm labour are:

1. To prevent asphyxia which makes the baby more susceptible to RDS.
2. To prevent birth trauma.

First stage

- *The patient is put to bed* to prevent early rupture of the membranes.
- *To ensure adequate fetal oxygenation* by giving oxygen to the mother by mask.
- *Strong sedative or acceleration of labour* should be avoided. Epidural analgesia is of choice.
- *Labour should be watched* by intensive clinical monitoring in the absence of continuous electronic monitoring.
- **In case of delay or anticipating a tedious traumatic vaginal delivery,** it is better to deliver by caesarean section.

Second stage

- The birth should be gentle and slow to avoid rapid compression and decom-pression of the head.
- Liberal episiotomy should be done under local anaesthesia with 1% lignocaine—specially in primigravidae to minimize head compression.
- Tendency to delay is curtailed by low forceps. As such, routine forceps is not indicated.
- The cord is to be clamped immediately at birth to prevent hypervolaemia and hyper-bilirubinaemia to develop.

- Remain on bed rest except to use the bathroom
- Drink eight to ten glasses of fluid daily (keep a pitcher by your bed so you do not have to get up to get some
- Be certain to take your prescribed tocolytic medication on time to maintain a constant blood level. Set an alarm clock as necessary, especially at night
- Monitor fetal heart rate and uterine contractions daily
- Keep mentally active by reading to prevent boredom
- Avoid activities that could stimulate labour such as nipple stimulation
- Consult your primary care provider as to whether sexual relations should be restricted
- Immediately report signs of ruptured membranes (sudden gush of vaginal fluid) or vaginal bleeding
- Report signs of urinary tract or vaginal infection (burning on and frequency of urination, vaginal itching or pain)
- Report symptoms of pulmonary congestion (cough and difficulty breathing unless upright) which can be effects of tocolytic drugs
- Keep appointments for prenatal care

If uterine contractions recur
- Empty your bladder to relieve pressure on the uterus
- Lie down on your left or right side to encourage blood return to the uterus
- Attach the fetal and uterine contraction monitor
- Drink two to three glasses of fluid to increase hydration

- To place the baby in the intensive neonatal care unit under the care of a neonatologist.

Place of caesarean section: Preterm fetuses before 34 weeks presented by breech are generally delivered by caesarean section. Lower segment vertical or 'J' shaped incision may have to be made to minimize trauma during delivery. This is due to poor formation of lower uterine segment.

PRETERM RUPTURE OF THE MEMBRANES (PROM)

Definition

Spontaneous rupture of the membranes any time beyond 28th week of pregnancy but before the onset of labour is called prelabour rupture of the membranes (PROM). When rupture of membranes occur beyond 37th week but before the onset of labour it is called **term PROM.**

Incidence

PROM occurs in approximately 10% of all pregnancies.

Causes

In majority, the causes are not known. *The possible causes are:*
1. Increased friability of the membranes
2. Decreased tensile strength of the membranes
3. Polyhydramnios
4. Cervical incompetence
5. Multiple pregnancy
6. Infection—chorioamnionitis, urinary tract infection and lower genital tract infection.

Diagnosis

The only subjective symptom is escape of watery discharge per vaginum either in the form of a gush or slow leak.

Confirmation of diagnosis
1. Speculum examination is done taking aseptic precautions to inspect the liquor escaping out through the cervix.
2. To examine the collected fluid from the posterior fornix (vaginal pool) for
   - Detection of pH by litmus or Nitrazine paper. The pH becomes 6–6.2 (normal vaginal pH during pregnancy is 4.5– 5.5 whereas that of liquor amnii is 7–7.5).
   - To note the characteristic ferning pattern when a smeared slide is examined under microscope.

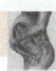

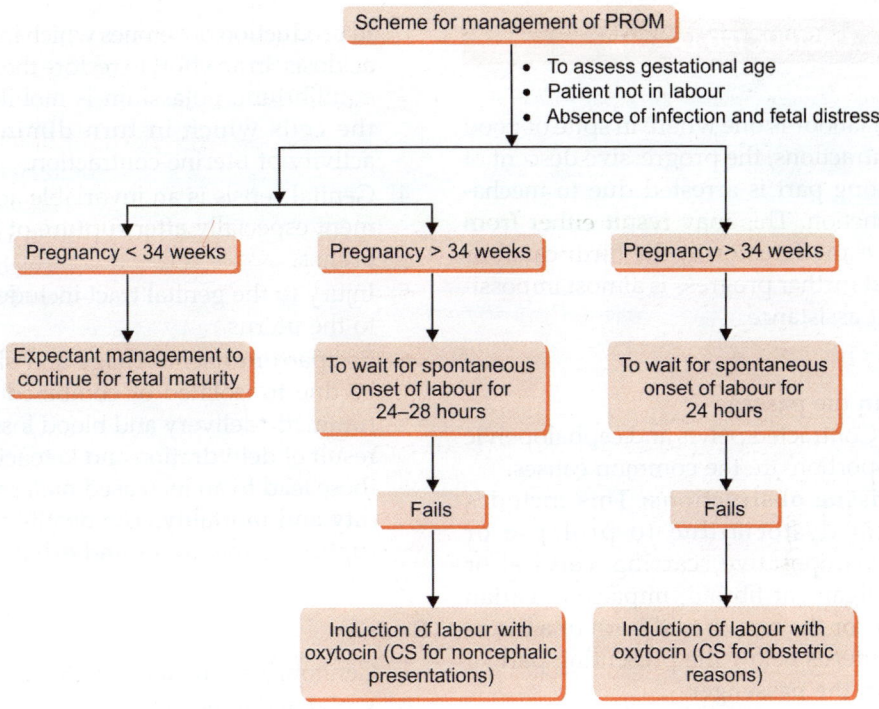

Fig. 11.1: Scheme of management of premature rupture of the membranes

- Ultrasonography is to be done not only to support the diagnosis but also to assess the fetal well-being.

Investigations

1. Full blood count
2. Urine for routine analysis and culture
3. High vaginal swab for culture
4. Ultrasonography for fetal biophysical profile.

MANAGEMENT

Preliminaries

1. Aseptic examination with a sterile speculum is done not only to confirm the diagnosis but also to note the state of the cervix and to detect any cord prolapse.
2. Vaginal digital examination is generally avoided.
3. Patient is put to bed rest and sterile vulval pad is applied to observe any further

leakage. Once the diagnosis is confirmed, management depends on:

- Gestational age of the fetus
- Whether the patient is in labour or not
- Any evidence of sepsis
- Prospect of fetal survival in that institution, if delivery occurs. Maternal pulse, temperature and fetal heart rate are monitored 4 hourly.

Use of antibiotics

Prophylactic antibiotics are given to minimise maternal and perinatal risks of infection. Oral ampicillin 500 mg is given for 3 days.

Corticosteriods to stimulate surfactant against RDS in preterm neonates are favoured. As such PROM alone accelerate fetal lung maturation. Moreover, use of corticosteroids enhances the risk of infection.

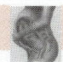

OBSTRUCTED LABOUR

Definition

Obstructed labour is one where in spite of good uterine contractions, the progressive descent of the presenting part is arrested due to mechanical obstruction. This may result either from the faults in the fetus or in the birth canal or both, so that further progress is almost impossible without assistance.

Causes

- **Fault in the passage**
- **Bony:** Contracted pelvis and cephalopelvic disproportion are the common causes.
- **Soft tissue obstructions:** This includes cervical dystocia due to prolapse or previous operative scarring, cervical or broad ligament fibroid, impacted ovarian tumour or the non-gravid horn of a bicornuate uterus below the presenting part.
- **Fault in the passenger**
- Transverse lie
- Brow presentation
- Congenital malformations of the foetus—hydrocephalus (commonest), foetal ascites, double monsters
- Big baby especially in high parity associated with deflexed head and occipitoposterior position
- Impacted mentoposterior
- Big breech with pendulous abdomen
- Compound presentation
- Locked twins.

Effects on mother

Immediate

1. Exhaustion is due to a constant agonising pain and anxiety.
2. Dehydration is due to increased muscular activity without adequate fluid intake.
3. Metabolic acidosis is due to accumulation of lactic acid produced by the contractile uterine and voluntary muscles—catabolism of fat in the absence of carbohydrate leads

to production of ketones which increase the acidosis. In an effort to restore the acid–base equilibrium, potassium is mobilised from the cells which in turn diminishes the activity of uterine contraction.

4. Genital sepsis is an invariable accompaniment especially after rupture of the membranes.
5. Injury to the genital tract includes rupture to the uterus.
6. Postpartum haemorrhage and shock may be due to isolated or combined effects of traumatic delivery and blood loss or as—a result of dehydration and ketoacidosis. All these lead to an increased maternal morbidity and mortality. The deaths are due to rupture of the uterus and exhaustion with sepsis.

Remote

1. Genitourinary fistula or rectovaginal fistula
2. Variable degree of vaginal atresia
3. Secondary amenorrhoea following removal of uterus or due to Sheehan's syndrome.

Effects on the fetus

1. Asphyxia results from tonic uterine contraction which interferes with the uteroplacental circulation or due to cord prolapse specially in shoulder presentation.
2. Acidosis is the result of maternal acidosis.
3. Intracranial haemorrhage is due to supermoulding of the head leading to tentorial tear or due to traumatic delivery
4. *Infection:* All these lead to increased perinatal loss; the causes are asphyxia, intracranial haemorrhage and neonatal infection.

Clinical features

1. Patient is in agony from continuous pain and discomfort and becomes restless.
2. Features of exhaustion and ketoacidosis are evident.

3. Abdominal palpation reveals
   - Upper segment is hard and tender. Lower segment is distended and tender.
   - The pathological retraction ring is placed obliquely between the umbilicus and symphysis pubis and rises upwards in course of time.
   - Taut tender round ligaments may be felt on either side. This is because; the uterine attachments of the round ligaments have been raised by the shortening of the upper segment and distension of the lower segment.
   - Fetal parts may not be well defined.
   - F.H.S. is usually absent
4. Internal examination reveals
   - Vagina is dry and hot and the discharge is offensive
   - Cervix fully dilated.
   - Membranes are absent
   - Cause of obstructed labour is revealed.

Prevention

- *Antenatal:* Intelligent anticipation of the case 'likely to develop obstructed labour and appropriate management in an equipped hospital are the positive measures to prevent the tragedy to occur.
- *Intranatal:* Continuous vigilance, use of partograph and timely intervention of a prolonged labour.

Actual treatment

The underlying principles are:
1. To relieve the obstruction at the earliest by a safe procedure
2. To combat dehydration and keto-acidosis
3. To control sepsis.

Preliminaries

1. The patient should be sedated by intramuscular pethidine 75–100 mg, if prompt delivery for fetal interest is not undertaken.
2. Dehydration and ketoacidosis are to be energetically corrected by rapid infusion of Ringer's solution; at least one litre is to be given in running drip.
3. Parenteral ampicillin 500 mg is administered and then repeated at 6 hourly interval.
4. Blood sample is sent for group and cross matching and a bottle blood should be at hand prior to operative interferences.
5. A vaginal swab is taken and sent for culture and sensitivity test

Obstetric management

Before proceeding for definitive operative treatment, rupture of the uterus must be excluded. There is no place of 'wait and watch' neither any scope of using oxytocin to stimulate uterine contraction.

Vaginal delivery

The baby is invariably dead in most of the neglected cases and destructive operation is the best choice to relieve the obstruction. If, however, the head is low down and vaginal delivery is not risky, forceps extraction may be done in a living baby. After completion of the delivery and expulsion of the placenta, exploration of the uterus and the lower genital tract should be done to exclude uterine rupture or tear.

Caesarean section

If the case is detected early with good fetal condition, caesarean section gives good results.

INDUCTION OF LABOUR

Definition

Induction of labour means deliberate termination of pregnancy beyond 28 weeks (period of viability) by any method which aims at initiation of labour and a vaginal delivery.

Indications

The indications are broadly grouped into
- Fetal
- Maternal
- Combined

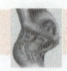

Fetal: Continuation of pregnancy may adversely affect the fetal prognosis.

- Postmaturity
- Previous history of unexplained intrauterine death. Timely intervention provides an opportunity to avert repetition of the disaster.
- Diabetes mellitus
- Chronic placental insufficiency leading to growth retardation of the fetus.
- Rh isoimmunisation
- Unstable lie after correcting into longitudinal lie

Maternal: Continuation of pregnancy may adversely affect the maternal outlook.

- Intrauterine death of the fetus
- Chronic polyhydramnios with maternal distress
- Congenital malformation of the fetus

Combined: Continuation of pregnancy adversely affects both the mother and the baby.

- Pre-eclampsia and eclampsia
- Minor degree of placenta praevia
- Abruptio placentae—early termination saves the mother from untoward complications like blood coagulation disorders and anuria. The baby can also be saved.
- Premature rupture of the membranes
- Chronic hypertension
- Chronic renal diseases

Elective induction

The term elective induction means deliberate termination of pregnancy 'at term' for the convenience of the patient (usually parous), obstetrician or hospital.

Common indications of induction in practice are

1. Postmaturity
2. Pre-eclampsia–eclampsia
3. Intrauterine fetal death
4. Antepartum haemorrhage
5. Premature rupture of the membranes

6. Chronic hydramnios
7. Congenital malformation of the fetus

Contraindications

The following are the contraindications of induction:

1. Contracted pelvis and cephalopelvic disproportion
2. Persistent mal presentation
3. Pregnancy with previous caesarean section.
4. Elderly primigravida specially associated with complicating factors (obstetric or medical).
5. Heart disease
6. High-risk pregnancy with compromised foetus.
7. Pelvic tumour

Dangers

- Maternal
- Fetal

Maternal

1. Psychologic upset, more so, when there is failure for which caesarean section is contemplated.
2. Tendency of prolonged labour due to abnormal uterine action.
3. Increased need of analgesia during labour
4. Increased operative interference
5. Increased morbidity.

Fetal

1. Iatrogenic prematurity
2. Hypoxia due to disordered uterine action, prolonged labour and operative interference.

PREINDUCTION SCORING

Amongst many a scoring system. Bishop's scoring still maintains popularity. The scoring system takes into consideration of the cervical factor arid station of the head. **The dilatation of the cervix is, however, the single factor of great importance.**

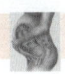

But it is to be borne in mind that, while the poor scoring is likely to be unfavourable for induction, the induction should not be deferred because of poor score (Table 11.1).

METHODS OF INDUCTION

- Medical
- Surgical
- Combined

MEDICAL INDUCTION

Indications

The following are the conditions where the medical induction is specially indicated.

- Exclusive
  - Intrauterine death
  - Premature rupture of the membranes
- In cases of failure of surgical induction as an alternative to caesarean section
- Along with surgical induction to shorten the induction—delivery interval (commonly done).

Drugs used

Oxytocin and prostaglandins

Oxytocin

Effectiveness

The drug is effective in most of the cases either with single or repeat infusions. However, oxytocin is less effective in cases of intrauterine death, elderly primigravidae or early gestational period with unfavourable cervix.

Advantages

The following are the advantages
1. Wider availability
2. Less systemic side-effects
3. Major catastrophe is a rarity

Prostaglandins

The topical application of prostaglandin E_2 intravaginally in a viscus base, is an effective, safe and highly acceptable method.

Effectiveness

The drug is equally effective as that of oxytocin. It is, however, more effective in cases of intrauterine death or early gestational period with unfavourable cervix where oxytocin is less effective.

Advantages

1. Effective method in intrauterine death or in cases with unfavourable cervix.
2. No antidiuretic effect

SURGICAL INDUCTION

The initiation at labour is attempted by surgical method and is almost exclusively done by rupture of the membranes.

Table 11.1: Bishop's pre-induction cervical scoring system (modified)

Parameters	Score			
	0	1	2	3
Cervix				
Dilatation	Closed	1–2	3–4	5+
Cervical length (cm)	3	2	1	0
Consistency	Firm	Medium	Soft	–
Position	Posterior	Midline	Anterior	–
Head: Station	–3	–2	–1, 0	+1, +2

Total score = 13   Favourable score = 6–13   Unfavourable score = 0–5

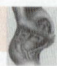

Contraindication

Intrauterine fetal death

Limitation

It cannot be employed in an unfavourable cervix (long, firm cervix with os closed). The cervix should be at least one finger dilated.

Effectiveness depends on

1. State of the cervix
2. Station of the presenting part.

Methods

- Artificial rupture of the membranes (ARM)
- Stripping the membranes
- Low rupture of the membranes (LRM)
- High rupture of the membranes (HRM)

Hazards of ARM

Once the procedure is adopted, there is no scope of retreating from the decision of termination. The cases are, therefore, to be judiciously selected with genuine indi-cations.

LOW RUPTURE OF THE MEMBRANE (LRM)

It is widely practised now-a-days with high degree of success. The membranes below the presenting part overlying the internal os are ruptured to drain some amount of amniotic fluid.

PROCEDURES

Preliminaries

The lower bowel is emptied, if necessary by enema. The patient is asked to empty her bladder.

Steps

- The patient is placed in lithotomy position.
- Full surgical asepsis is to be taken. Perineal and vaginal toileting with antiseptic solution and usual draping with sterile towels are to be done. The surgeon should wear sterile mask, gowns and gloves.

- Two fingers arc introduced into the vagina smeared with antiseptic ointment. The index finger is passed through the cervical canal beyond the internal os. The membranes are swept free from the lower segment as far as reached by the finger.
- With one or two fingers still in the cervical canal with the palmar surface upwards, a long Kocher's forceps with the blades closed, is introduced along the palmar aspect of the fingers upto the membranes.
- *The blades are opened to seize the membranes and are torn by twisting movements.* This is followed by visible escape of amniotic fluid.
- After the membranes rupture, the following are to be noted:
  a. Colour of the amniotic fluid
  b. Status of the cervix
  c. Station of the head
  d. Presence or absence of cord prolapse
  e. Quality of FHR.
- After being fully satisfied, a sterile vulval pad is placed and the patient is returned to her bed, Prophylactic antibiotic may be prescribed.

Hazards

1. Cord prolapse
2. Uncontrolled escape of amniotic fluid
3. Injury to the cervix or the presenting part
4. Rupture of vasa-praevia leading to fetal blood loss
5. Amnionitis

HIGH RUPTURE OF THE MEMBRANES (HRM)

It is a procedure where, the puncture of the hind waters above the presenting part, is made by a special instrument—Drew-Smythe catheter.

Indications

It is almost obsolete now-a-days. However, it was used in chronic hydramnios specially associated with congenital malformation of the

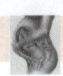

fetus or with floating head where regulated escape of liquor amnii facilitates settling down of the presenting part. Slow decompression also prevents premature placental separation.

Conditions to be fulfilled

1. Cervix should be at least 1 finger dilated
2. Vertex must be presenting
3. Forewaters must be present.

Contraindications

It is contraindicated in APH and severe pre-eclampsia or eclampsia.

Hazards

1. Injury to the placenta by the tip of the instrument
2. Accidental injury to the uterine wall
3. Injury to the fetal parts specially to the eye
4. Displacement of the presenting part
5. Intra-amniotic infection is possible

STRIPPING THE MEMBRANES

As an isolated procedure, stripping the membranes off from its attachment from the lower segment is an effective procedure for induction provided cervical score is favourable.

COMBINED METHOD

The combined medical and surgical methods are commonly used to increase the efficicacy of induction by reducing the induction-delivery interval. The oxytocin infusion is started either prior to or following rupture of the membranes depending mainly upon the state of the cervix and head brain relation. With the head non-engaged, it is preferable to induce with prostaglandin gel or to start oxytocin infusion followed by ARM.

The advantages of the combined methods are

1. More effective than any single procedure
2. Shortens the induction-delivery interval and thereby

a. Minimises the risk of infection
b. Lessens the period of observation.

PROLONGED LABOUR

Definition

The labour is said to be prolonged when the combined duration of the first and second stage is more than the arbitrary time limit of 18 hours. Labour is considered prolonged when the cervical dilatation rate is less than 1 cm/hr and descent of the presenting part is <1 cm/hr for a period of minimum 4 hours observation.

Causes of prolonged labour

Any one or combination of the factors in labour could be responsible

First stage: Failure to dilate the cervix is due to:

- *Fault in power:* Abnormal uterine contraction such as uterine inertia (common) or incoordinate uterine contraction.
- *Fault in the passage:* Contracted pelvis, cervical dystocia, pelvic tumour, or even full bladder.
- *Fault in the passenger:* Malposition and malpresentation. Congenital anomalies of the fetus (hydrocephalus).
- *Others:* Injudicious (early) administration

BOX 11.2: Nursing diagnoses during dysfunctional labour

- Anxiety related to slow progress of labour.
- Fatigue related to the length of labour.
- Individual coping, ineffective, related to inability to relax.
- Risk for fluid volume deficit, related to lack of fluid intake.
- Risk for infection, related to prolonged labour
- Sleep pattern disturbance related to maternal exhaustion and inability to relax.
- Knowledge deficit related to potential fetal distress and fetal sepsis.

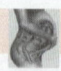

of sedatives and analgesics before the active labour begins.

Second stage: Sluggish or non-descent of the presenting part in the second stage is due to:

- *Fault in power*
  - Uterine inertia
  - Inability to bear down
  - Epidural analgesia
  - Constriction ring
- *Fault in the passage*
  - Cephalopelvic disproportion, android pelvis, contracted pelvis.
  - Undue resistance of the pelvic floor or perineum due to spasm or old scarring.
  - Soft tissue pelvic tumour
- *Fault in the passenger*
  - Malposition (occipitoposterior)
  - Malpresentation
  - Big baby
  - Congenital malformation of the baby

Diagnosis

During vaginal examination, if a finger is accommodated in between the cervix and the head during uterine contraction pelvic adequacy can be reasonably established. Intranatal imaging (radiography, CT or MRI) is of help in determining the fetal station and position as well as pelvic shape and size.

First stage

First stage of labour is considered prolonged when the duration is more than 12 hours. The rate of cervical dilatation is < 1 cm/hr in a primi and < 1.5 cm/hr in a multi. The rate of descent of the presenting part is slow < 1 cm/hr in a primi and < 2 m/hr in a multi. Cervical dilatation rate (cervicograph) is plotted in relation to alert line and action line. Labour considered abnormal when cervicograph crosses the alert line and falls on zone 2 and intervention required when it crosses the action line and falls on zone 3 (Fig. 11.2).

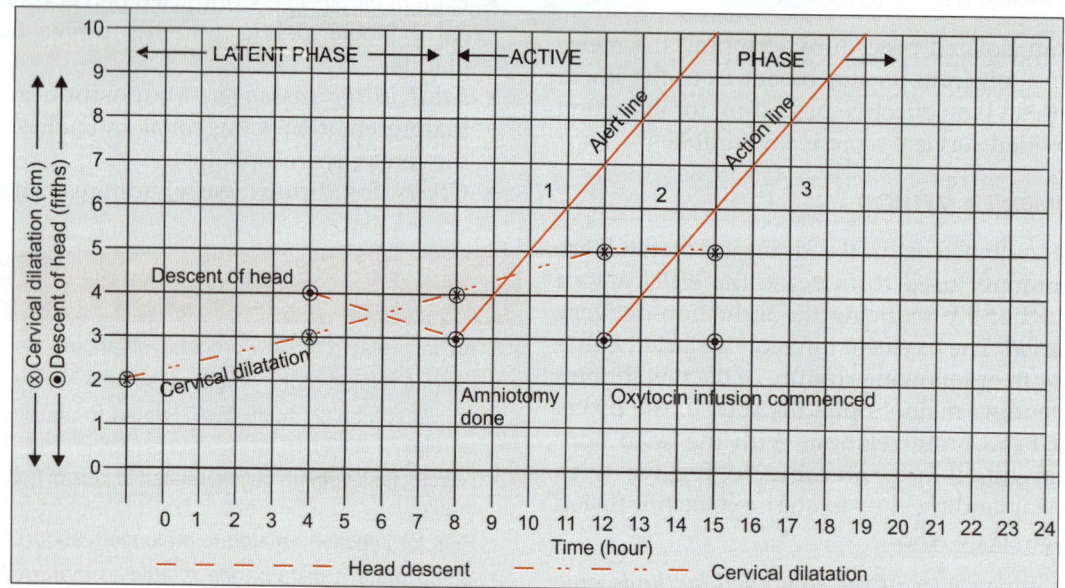

Fig. 11.2: Cervicograph showing slow cervical dilatation and descent of the presenting part. Oxytocin infusion was started following amniotomy. Partograph showed arrest in the progress in spite of adequate contractions. Labour was terminated by caesarean section

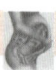

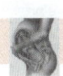

Secondary arrest is defined when the active phase of labour (cervical dilatation) commences normal but stops or slows significantly for 2 hours or more prior to full dilatation of the cervix. It is commonly due to malposition or CPD.

Second stage

The second stage is considered prolonged if it lasts for more than 2 hours in primi and 1 hour in multi. The diagnostic features are:
- Sluggish or non descent of the presenting part even after full dilatation of the cervix.
- Variable degrees of moulding and caput formation in cephalic presentation.
- Identification of the cause of prolongation.

Dangers

Fetal

The fetal risk is increased due to the combined effects of
1. Hypoxia due to diminished uteroplacental circulation.
2. Intrauterine infection
3. Intracranial stress of haemorrhage
4. Increased operative delivery

Maternal

There is increased incidence of
1. Distress
2. Postpartum haemorrhage
3. Trauma to the genital tract—concealed or revealed such as cervical tear, rupture uterus

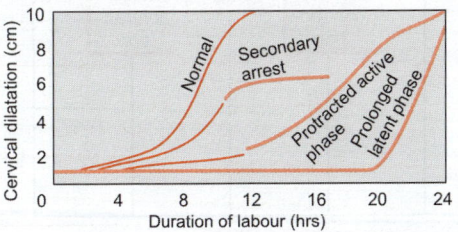

Fig. 11.3: Partograph analysis of labour to detect types of prolonged labour—protracted latent phase, protracted active phase and secondary arrest

4. Increased operative delivery
5. Puerperal sepsis
6. Subinvolution

Treatment
Prevention
- Antenatal or early intranatal detection of the factors likely to produce prolonged labour (big baby, malpresentation or position).
- Use of partograph helps in early detection.
- Selective and judicious augmentation of labour by low rupture of the membranes followed by oxytocin drip.
- Change of posture in labour other than supine to increase uterine contractions, avoidance of dehydration in labour and use of adequate analgesia for pain relief.

Actual treatment

Careful evaluation is to be done to find out:
- Cause of prolonged labour
- Effect on the mother
- Effect on the fetus

In a nulliparous patient inadequate uterine activity is the most common cause of primary dysfunctional labour. Whereas in a multiparous patient, cephalopelvic disproportion (due to malposition) is the most common cause.

Preliminaries: Correction of ketoacidosis should be made urgently by rapid intravenous infusion of Ringer's solution.

Definitive treatment: First stage delay—vaginal examination is done to verify the fetal presentation position and station. Clinical pelvimetry is done. If only uterine activity is suboptimal.
- Amniotomy and or oxytocin infusion is adequate.
- Effective pain relief is given by intramuscular pethidine or by regional (epidural) analgesic. For the management of secondary arrest specially in multipara one should be very careful to use oxytocin.

 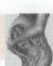

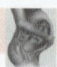

- Caesarean section is done when vaginal delivery is unsafe (malpresentation, malposition, big baby or COPD).

Second stage delay: Short period of expectant management is reasonable provided the FHR (electronic monitoring) is reassuring and vaginal delivery is imminent. Otherwise assisted delivery vaginal (forceps, ventouse) or abdominal (caesarean) should be done.

ABNORMAL UTERINE ACTION

Any deviation of the normal pattern of uterine contractions affecting the course of labour is designated as disordered or abnormal uterine action.

Types

The different varieties of abnormal uterine actions are described in Fig. 11.4.

Etiology

The following clinical conditions are often associated.

- Prevalent in the first birth specially with advancing age of the mother
- Prolonged pregnancy
- Over distension of the uterus due to twins and/or hydramnios
- Psychologic factor
- Contracted pelvis, malpresentation and deflexed head, full bladder are often associated too. All these lead to ill fitting of the presenting part into the lower uterine segment.
- Injudicious administration of sedatives, analgesics and oxytocics.
- Premature attempt at vaginal delivery or attempted instrumental vaginal delivery under light anaesthesia.

Uterine activity (contraction) is measured by noting basal tone, active (peak) pressure and frequency. Assessment is usually done by:

- Clinical palpation—inaccurate
- Tocodynamometer with external transducer
- Using intrauterine pressure catheter (accurate). Normal baseline tonus is between 5 and 20 mm of Hg and peak pressure is around 60 mm of Hg (8 KPa).

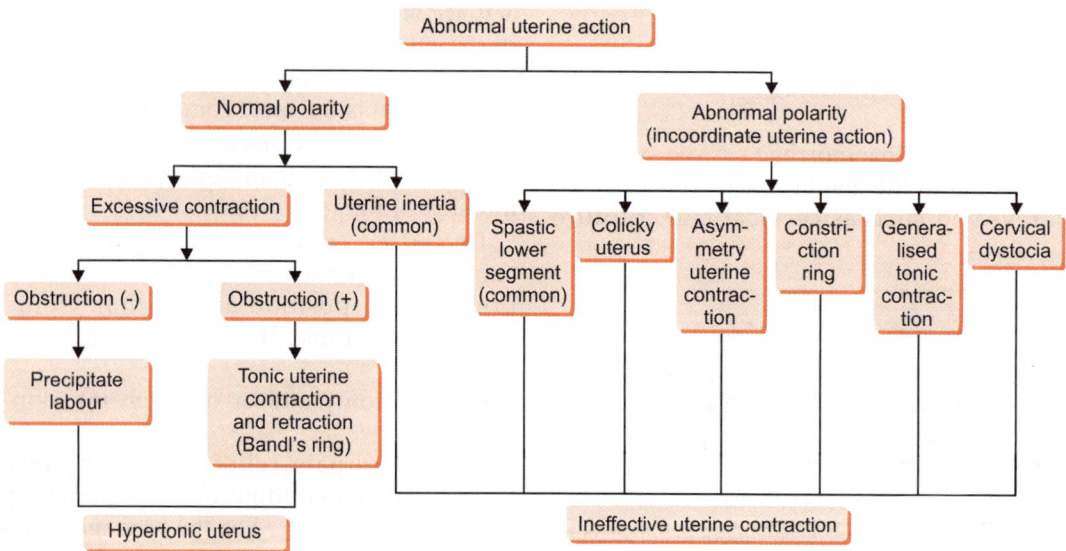

Fig. 11.4: Different varieties of abnormal uterine action

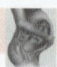

UTERINE INERTIA (HYPOTONIC ACTIVITY)

Uterine inertia is the hypotonic activity of the uterus where there is good relaxation between contractions, but are present for a prolonged interval.

Uterine contraction

The intensity is diminished, duration is shortened, good relaxation in between contractions and the intervals are increased. General pattern of uterine contraction of labour is maintained but intrauterine pressure during contraction hardly rises above 25 mm Hg.

Diagnosis

1. Patient feels less pain during uterine contraction
2. Hand placed over the uterus during contraction reveals less hardening of the uterus.
3. Uterine wall is easily indentable at the acme of a pain.
4. Uterus becomes relaxed after the contraction, fetal parts are well palpable and fetal heart rate remains good.
5. Internal examination reveals
   - Poor dilatation of the cervix
   - Associated presence of contracted pelvis, malposition, deflexed head or malpresentation may be evident.
   - Membranes usually remains intact.

EFFECTS ON THE MOTHER AND FETUS

Maternal exhaustion and or fetal distress are unusual and appear late.

Management

Case is reassessed to exclude cephalopelvic disproportion or malpresentation.

Indications of caesarean section

1. Presence of contracted pelvis
2. Malpresentation
3. Evidences of fetal or maternal distress

Contemplating vaginal delivery

General measures

- To keep up the morale of the patient
- Posture of the woman is changed. Supine position is avoided.
- To empty the bladder by catheterization if needed.
- To maintain hydration by infusion of Ringer's solution.
- Adequate pain relief by intramuscular pethidine 100 mg or combination of pethidine 75 mg and sparine 50 mg.

Active measures

Acceleration of uterine contraction can be brought about by low rupture of the membranes followed by oxytocin drip. The drip rate is gradually increased until effective contractions are set up.

INCOORDINATE UTERINE ACTION

The hypertonic state of the uterus arises from any of the conditions such as spastic lower uterine segment, colicky uterus, asymmetrical uterine contraction, constriction ring or generalized tonic contraction of the uterus and all these states are collectively called incoordinate uterine action. Increased frequency and or duration of uterine contractions cause rise in base line tone and thereby diminish circulation in the placental intervillous space. This results in fetal hypoxia in labour. Uterine hyperstimulation due to oxytocics (oxytocin, prostaglandins) are often associated with fetal tachycardia (fetal adrenergic activity) due to fetal stress.

CONSTRICTION RING

It is one form of incoordinate uterine action where there is localised spastic contraction of a ring of circular muscle fibres of the uterus. It is usually situated at the junction of the upper and lower segment around a constricted part of the fetus usually around the neck in cephalic presentation. It may appear in all the stages of labour.

Its occurrence is associated with

1. Injudicious administration of oxytocics
2. Premature rupture of the membranes and
3. Premature attempt at instrumental delivery specially under light anaesthesia.

Diagnosis

It is revealed during caesarean section in the first stage, during forceps application in the second stage and during manual removal in the third stage (hour-glass contraction).

Treatment

The outline of treatment protocol is based on the stage at which the diagnosis is made.

- *First stage:* The diagnosis is made during caesarean section after opening the uterine cavity. The ring may have to be cut vertically to deliver the baby.

- *Second stage:* Failure to deliver the head even after correct and judicious application of forceps raises the suspicion of constriction ring. The confirmation is done by palpating the ring after removing the forceps blades. Caesarean section should be performed even at this stage.

- *Third stage:* The diagnosis is made during attempted manual removal. Deepening the plane of anaesthesia is usually effective.

GENERAL TONIC CONTRACTION (SYN: UTERINE TETANY) (Fig. 11.5)

In this condition, pronounced retraction occurs involving whole of the uterus up to the level of internal os. Thus, there is no physiological differentiation of the active upper segment and the passive lower segment of the uterus. As there is no thinning of the lower segment, there is no chance of rupture of the uterus. The uterine contraction ceases and the whole uterus undergoes a sort of tonic muscular spasm holding the fetus inside (active retention of the fetus).

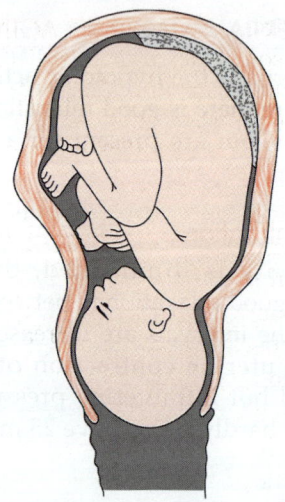

Fig. 11.5: Generalised tonic contraction of the uterus

Causes

1. Failure to overcome the obstruction by powerful contractions of the uterus.
2. Injudicious administration of oxytocics.

Clinical features

The patient is in prolonged labour having severe and continuous pain. Abdominal examination reveals the uterus to be somewhat smaller in size, tense and tender. Fetal parts are neither well defined, nor is the fetal heart sound audible. Vaginal examination reveals jammed head with big caput; dry and oedematous vagina.

Treatment

- Correction of dehydration and ketoacidosis by rapid infusion of Ringer's solution.
- Antibiotic to control infection
- Adequate pain relief

Caesarean delivery is done in majority of the cases specially when obstruction is suspected.

PRECIPITATE LABOUR

A labour is called precipitate when the combined duration of the first and second stage is less than two hours. It is common in multiparae. Rapid expulsion is due to the combined effect of hyper-

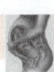

active uterine contractions associated with diminished soft tissue resistance. Labour is short as the rate of cervical dilatation is 5 cm/hour or more for the nulliparous women.

Maternal risk include

1. Extensive laceration of the cervix, vagina and perineum (to the extent of complete perineal tear).
2. PPH due to uterine hypotonia that develops subsequently
3. Inversion
4. Uterine rupture
5. Infection
6. Amniotic fluid embolism

The fetal risk include intracranial stress and haemorrhage because of rapid expulsion without time for moulding of the head. The baby may sustain serious injuries if delivery occurs in standing position, bending from the torn cord and direct hit on the skull are real hazards.

Treatment

The patient having history of precipitate labour should be hospitalized prior to labour. During labour, the uterine contraction may be suppressed by administering ether or magnesium sulphate during contractions. Delivery of the head should be controlled. Episiotomy should be done liberally. Elective induction of labour by low rupture of the membranes and careful conduction of controlled delivery may be advantageous. Oxytocin augmentation should be avoided.

TONIC UTERINE CONTRACTION AND RETRACTION

This type of uterine contraction is predominantly due to obstructed labour.

Pathologic anatomy of the uterus

There is gradual increase in intensity, duration and frequency of uterine contraction. The relaxation phase becomes less and less, ultimately a state of tonic contraction develops. Retraction, however, continues. The lower segment elongates and becomes progressively thinner to accommodate the fetus driven from the upper segment. *A circular groove encircling the uterus is formed between the active segment and the distended lower segment, called pathological retraction ring (Bandl's ring).* Due to pronounced retraction, there is fetal jeopardy or even death.

In primigravidae, further retraction ceases in response to obstruction and labour comes to a stand still a state of uterine exhaustion. Contractions may recommence after a brief period of rest with renewed vigour. *But in multiparae,* retraction continues with progressive circumferential dilatation and thinning of the lower segment. There is progressive rise of the Bandl's ring, moving nearer and nearer to the umbilicus and ultimately, the lower segment ruptures.

Clinical features

1. Patient is in agony from continuous pain and discomfort and becomes restless.
2. Features of exhaustion and ketoacidosis are evident.
3. Abdominal palpation reveals
   - Upper segment is hard and tender. Lower segment is distended and tender.
   - The pathological retraction ring is placed obliquely between the umbilicus and symphysis pubis and rises upwards in course of time.
   - Taut tender round ligaments may be felt on either side. This is because; the uterine attachments of the round ligaments have been raised by the shortening of the upper segment and distension of the lower segment.
   - Fetal parts may not be well defined.
   - FHS is usually absent
4. Internal examination reveals
   - Vagina is dry and hot and the discharge is offensive

- Cervix fully dilated.
- Membranes are absent
- Cause of obstructed labour is revealed.

Prevention

It is a preventable condition: The abnormality, either in the passage (bony or soft tissue) or in the passenger (malpresentation or malformation of the fetus) can be detected during antenatal or early intranatal period and delivery by caesarean section is done. Bandl's ring is rarely seen these days because of early detection and intervention of prolonged labour cases.

Treatment

- Rupture of uterus is to be excluded
- Internal version is contraindicated
- Correction of dehydration and keto-acidosis by infusion of Ringer's solution.
- Adequate pain relief
- Parenteral antibiotic is given (Ceftriaxone 1 gm IV)
- Caesarean delivery is done in majority of the cases. Rupture of uterus must be excluded before attempting destructive operation.

AMNIOTIC FLUID EMBOLISM (AFE)

AFE continues to be one of the most feared and devasting complications of pregnancy in which amniotic fluid, fetal cells, hair or other debris enters the mother's blood stream via the placenta and triggers an allergic reaction.

The disease spectrum ranges from a subclinical entity to one which is rapidly fatal. Most cases (80%) occur during labour, but it can occur either before labour or after delivery. About 25% of patients will die within one hour of onset.

The first careful description of this syndrome was Steiner and Lushbaugh in 1942.

Incidence

The incidence of this syndrome ranges from 1 in 8000 to 1 in 80,0000 pregnancies. Even today,

AFE is the leading cause of death during labour and the first few postpartum hours, and it remains a deadly and unpreventable obstetric emergency. Despite technological advances in critical care life support, the maternal mortality rate for AFE remains around 61%; a number of survivors have permanent hypoxia induced neurological damage.

WHAT CAUSES AFE?

It is mostly agreed that this condition results from amniotic fluid entering the uterine veins. AFE occurs when the barrier between amniotic fluid and maternal circulation is broken and, possibly under a pressure gradient, fluid abnormally enters the maternal venous system via the endocervical veins, the placental site (if placenta is separated), or a uterine trauma site. Why this entry into material circulation occurs in some women and not in others is not clearly understood.

Risk Factors

1. Older age
2. Multiparty
3. Intense uterine contractions, either physiological or drug induced
4. Abdominal trauma
5. Cesarean section
6. Uterine rupture
7. High cervical tear
8. Premature placental separation
9. Placental abruption
10. Intrauterine fetal demise or fetal distress.

Medical induction of labour nearly doubled the risk of overall, cases of amniotic-fluid embolism.

Clinical features

AFE usually occurs during labour but has been recorded during abortion, abdominal trauma, and amnioinfusion . Typically, a woman in the late stages of labour becomes acutely dyspneic, cyanotic with hypotension; she may experience

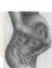

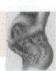

seizures quickly followed by cardiac arrest. Massive DIC–associated hemorrhage follows and then death. Most patients die within an hour of onset.

The initial signs and symptoms have a typically chronology, and the morbidity and morality of the manifestations steadily decreases with time. More than 80% of patients experience cardio respiratory arrest within the first few minutes. Approximately 50% of patients do not survive this onslaught of cardiopulmonary injury, but of those who do, 40 to 50% have coagulopathy and hemorrhage up to 4 hours later.

Diagnosis

The diagnosis of amniotic fluid embolism is always a clinical diagnosis and one of exclusion.

The postmortem diagnosis of an amniotic fluid embolism is made by demonstration of amniotic fluid debris in the pulmonary vasculature. The same findings when present in the blood vessels of the uterus and in particular the cervix also confirm the diagnosis in survivors. The diagnosis can also be made by cytological examination of blood from central venous of pulmonary catheterization. Measurement of maternal plasma zinc coproporphyrin, which is a component of meconium.

The second manifestation includes negative inotropism and left ventricular failure resulting in increasing pulmonary edema and hypotension quickly leading to shock. The third manifestation is a neurological response to the respiratory and hemodynamic injury, which may include seizures, confusion or coma.

About 40 to 50% of patients who survive to this point have severe coagulopathy, usually disseminated intravascular coagulation, which results in uncontrollable uterine bleeding along with bleeding from puncture sites such as insertion sites for intravenous and epidural catheters. This components of amniotic fluid, most notably thromboplastin, which initiate the extrinsic fluid, most notably thromboplastin, which initiate the extrinsic pathway of the clotting cascade and results in excessive fibriolytic activity.

Pathophysiology

The pathophysiology of AFE is poorly understood. When amniotic fluid and fetal cells enter the maternal circulation it possibly triggers an anaphylactic reaction to fetal antigens.

Amniotic fluid and debris enter the maternal circulation; this may trigger a massive anaphylactic reaction, activation of the complement cascade, or both. Progression usually occurs in 2 phases.

First phase: The patient experiences acute shortness of breath and hypertension. This rapidly progresses to cardiopulmonary arrest as the chambers of the heart fail to dilate and there is a reduction of oxygen to the heart and lungs. Not long after this stage the patient will lapse into a coma.

Second phase: Although many women do not survive beyond the first stage, about 40% of the initial survivors will pass onto the second phase. This is known as the hemorrhagic phase and may be accompanied by severe shivering, coughing, vomiting and the sensation of a bad taste in the mouth. This is also accompanied by excessive bleeding as the blood loses its ability to clot. As hypoxia is progressive, there is also fetal distress present.

Management

Once the signs and symptoms are recognized and a presumptive diagnosis is made, supportive measures should be implemented promptly. The treatment at best is only supportive.

Oxygenation

The fetus is very vulnerable to maternal hypoxia, which is initially profound in AFE. Therefore, the first priority is resuscitation of the mother and administration of oxygen by any means available at concentrations of 100%.

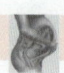

A more aggressive approach includes securing an airway through endotracheal intubation, providing mechanical ventilation for the patient with a high inspired fraction of oxygen (>60%), and the addition of positive end-expiratory pressure. The goal of oxygen therapy is to maintain arterial PaO_2 higher than 60 mm Hg and arterial oxygen saturation at 90% or higher.

Circulation

Maintaining cardiac output and blood pressure involves several simultaneous interventions. The Gel and Hankins recommend positioning the patient flat or in a slight Trendelenburg position to improve the venous blood return and perfusion of the central nervous system. Supportive measures include the initiation of fluid therapy, administration of pharmacological agents and electrocardiographic monitoring to detect and treat arrhythmias. Placement of pulmonary artery catheter is highly recommended for monitoring cardiac output, central venous pressure, and pulmonary artery pressures. In addition, pulmonary artery catheters provide direct access for blood samples to be sent for cytological analysis for amniotic fluid and fetal debris.

Volume replacement with isotonic crystalloid solution is a first-line therapy for maintaining blood pressure. Fluid therapy should be based on the findings of central venous monitoring.

Fetal management

The fetus is continuously monitored throughout. In some instances, and of course, most favorable for the fetus. AFE does not occur until after delivery. When AFE occurs before or during deliver, however, the fetus is in grave danger from the onset because of the maternal cardiopulmonary crisis. In addition to concern for fetal well-being, delivery of the fetus increases the chances for a good outcome for the mother because the weight of the gravid uterus on the interior vena cava impedes blood return to the heart and decreases systemic blood pressure.

Therefore, as soon as the mother's condition is stabilized, delivery of he viable infant should be expedited. If resuscitation of the mother is futile, an emergency bedside cesarean delivery may be necessary to save the infant.

Cardiopulmonary resuscitation (CPR) is initiated if the patient goes ino cardiac arrest. If she does not respond to resuscitation, a perimortem cesarean delivery is performed.

Coagulopathy and control of haemorrhage

If coagulopathy develops, it is treated with FFP (fresh frozen plasma). Platelets are transfused for platlet counts less than 20,000/ml. Administration of blood transfusions and blood components is considered the first line of treatment for correcting coagulopathy associated with AFE. Blood products include packed red blood cells, fresh frozen plasma, platelets and cryoprecipiate to maintain organ perfusion and urinary output until bleeding due to disseminated intravascular coagulation resolves.

BLOOD COAGULATION DISORDERS

DISORDERS OF BLOOD COAGULATION AND FIBRINOLYSIS IN OBSTETRICS

Physiology of blood coagulation

The bleeding from the injured vessels is controlled by haemostasis, formation of a clot and fibrinolysis (dissolution of clot). Haemostasis has four components:

1. Vascular component—vasoconstriction of the injured vessel.
2. Platelets aggregate at the mouth of the injured vessel.
3. Formation of a fibrin plug (blood coagulation) reinforcing the platelet plug.
4. Fibrinolysis (proteolysis) removing fibrin in the process of healing to maintain fluidity of blood.

Blood coagulation (mechanism)

The following mechanism is currently agreed.

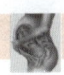

Prothrombin (factor II), a protein in plasma is an inert precursor of thrombin (glycoprotein, proteolytic enzyme). Thrombin is elaborated from prothrombin (present in plasma, 20–30 mg%) in the following mechanism.

1. *Intrinsic mechanism:* Factor XII is activated by contact with the damaged vessel to form activated factor X through the series of reactions involving factors XI, IX, platelet lipoprotein (platelet factor 3) and factor VIII.

2. *Extrinsic mechanism:* Damaged tissue at the injured vessel liberates tissue thrombo-plastin (tissue factor, factor III). This reacting with factor VII and calcium ion (factor IV) also activates factor X.

3. *Common pathway mechanism:* The activated factor X (derived from intrinsic and extrinsic pathways) being accelerated by factor V, platelet factor 3 and calcium ion converts prothrombin to thrombin. The latter converts soluble fibrinogen (factor I) into insoluble polymer fibrin strands. Factor XIII, fibrin stabilizing factor makes the fibrin strands more firm.

FIBRINOLYSIS

Fibrinolytic enzyme system operates to dissolve fibrin in the following steps (Fig. 11.6).

Plasminogen (a plasma globulin) is activated by activators present in plasma and tissues →

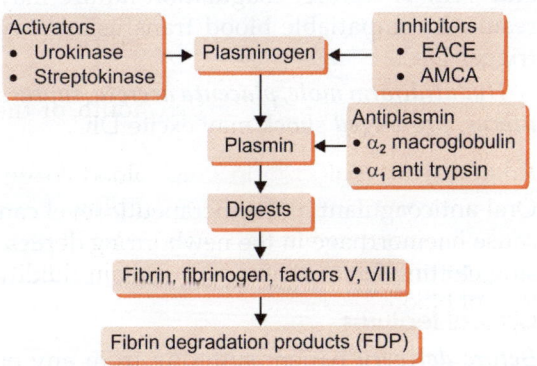

Fig. 11.6: Scheme showing plasma fibrinolytic system

Plasmin (a proteolytic enzyme) →digests fibrin →soluble products (fibrin degradation products). Plasmin digests both fibrin and fibrinogen. Plasminogen activators are set to action at the site of coagulation. Urokinase is a naturally occurring plasminogen activator enzyme which is isolated in urine. Plasminogen inhibitors inhibit fibrinolysis in the circulation. Blood coagulation and fibrinolysis act together to maintain haemostasis, fluidity of blood and an intact patent vascular tree.

EFFECT OF PREGNANCY ON BLOOD COAGULATION AND FIBRINOLYSIS SYSTEMS

Blood coagulation system

Fibrinogen level increases throughout pregnancy and labour from 250 mg% (prepregnancy level) to 400 mg%. Factors Vll, VIII, IX and X are also increased. These result in a state of hypercoagulability in late pregnancy and labour. Fibrin deposition occurs in the placental villi, placental bed, spiral arterial wall and at the placental bed on separation of placenta.

Fibrinolysis system

Plasma fibrinolytic activity decreases markedly during pregnancy, remain depressed in labour but returns to normal within an hour of delivery.

The placenta contains fibrinolytic inhibitors. There is no consistent increase in fibrinogen degradation products in plasma during pregnancy.

Disseminated intravascular coagulation (DIC) coagulation failure in obstetrics

Coagulation failure in obstetrics results from widespread intravascular coagulation →blood coagulation factors are used up →bleeding occurs from various sources. Plasma fibrinolytic activity is enhanced →digests fibrinogen → further bleeding. In acute DIC sudden purpura, bleeding from gastrointestinal tract, urinary and genital tract, operative site occur. Blood loss, hypovolaemic shock and fibrin deposition in the renal microcirculation may lead to renal cortical necrosis and acute renal failure. In chronic DIC, there can be thrombotic and haemorrhagic manifestation. Some patients in chronic DIC are clinically silent.

ETIOLOGY

Abruptio placentae or concealed accidental haemorrhage

This is number one cause of coagulation failure in obstetrics which operates in the following way:

1. Utilisation of fibrinogen and other clotting factors (factors V, VIII, platelets) for the massive retroplacental clot formation.
2. Liberation of tissue thromboplastin from damaged placenta and decidua into the circulation producing disseminated intravascular coagulation (DIC).
3. Secondary activation of the fibrinolytic enzyme system which can also digest fibrinogen. Fibrinogen-fibrin degradation products also act as anticoagulant. As a result, abruptio placentae may develop *acute haemorrhagic state* and becomes associated with prolonged coagulation time, lowered fibrinogen level and platelet count, high fibrinogen-fibrin degradation products. About 5% *abruptio placentae* cause coagulation failure and haemorrhagic state.

Intrauterine foetal death and missed abortion (beyond 20 weeks). This is the second common cause. This causes DIC due to thromboplastin absorption from the placenta and decidua. This may lead to haemorrhagic state due to prolonged coagulation time, lowered fibrinogen level and platelet count, high fibrinogen-fibrin degradation products.

Amniotic fluid embolism

This results in DIC leading to coagulation failure.

Septic abortion and intrauterine infection

Like Schwartzman reaction, DIC is caused by the bacterial endotoxin.

Caesarean section

This can rarely develop coagulation defect following uncomplicated caesarean section by either through entry into the circulation of the thromboplastin from the placenta and decidua or release of plasminogen activator from the uterus setting up fibrinolysis.

Pre-eclampsia and eclampsia

The syndrome can set up DIC and coagulation defect. The intravascular coagulation is manifested by fibrin deposits at the glomeruli, placental bed vessels and hepatic fibrin thrombi.

Hypertonic saline abortion

Hypertonic saline can cause placental damage and thromboplastin absorption leading to DIC and coagulation failure.

Dextran infusion

In infusion of low molecular weight dextran 40 for more than two pints, coagulation failure may develop as dextran can inactivate fibrinogen compound. This can also inhibit platelet adhesiveness.

Massive banked blood transfusion

Banked blood is deficient in platelets, factor V and VIII. Therefore, coagulation failure may result. Incompatiable blood transfusion may trigger DIC.

Hydatidiform mole, placenta accreta, rupture uterus, prolonged shock may excite DIC.

Anticoagulants

Oral anticoagulant in the therapeutic level can cause haemorrhage in the newborn by depressing clotting factors.

Clinical features

Before delivery patient suffering from any of the conditions as mentioned in aetiology may

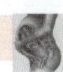

develop acute haemorrhagic states, viz., subcutaneous bruises, bleeding gums, haematuria, gastrointestinal haemorrhage, bleeding from needle pricks.

After delivery: Defective blood coagulation may lead to severe postpartum haemorrhage of nonclotted blood from the genital tract or from operation site although uterus appears contracted and firm. Patient becomes shocked.

TESTS FOR COAGULATION FAILURE

Bed-side tests

1. *Clot observation tests:* Venous blood (5 ml) is collected in dry test tube and is left to stand at 37°C. Normally, clot forms by 10 minutes, clot retracts and remains firm at the end of one hour. If the clot fails to form by 10 minutes, fibrinogen deficiency is taken; when clot fails to form by 30 minutes, fibrinogen level is probably less than 100 mg%. In others after 30 minutes, formed clot is fragmented when test tube is gently shaken. This can be due to fibrinogen deficiency or presence of fibrinolysins.
2. *Circulating fibrinolysin test:* 5 ml freshly drawn patient's blood is added to a similar amount of dotted normal blood. The presence of fibrinolysin is suggested if lysis occurs within one hour.

Laboratory tests

Prothrombin time: This gives measure of prothrombin concentration in plasma. This is prolonged over normal 10–14 seconds in coagulation failure.

Plasma fibrinogen is estimated by the laboratory assay. A lowered value below 100 mg% is obtained in coagulation defect.

Platelets are counted. A lowered value below 70,000/cu mm is obtained in coagulation defect.

Fibrenogen: Fibrin degradation products can be estimated by using latex agglutination test and staphylococcus clumping test. Value around 150 ug/ml is significant in fibrinolysis.

TREATMENT

Prevention

1. In abruptio placentae early induction by low rupture of membranes and early delivery are considered steps to prevent coagulation failure.
2. The conditions prone to develop coagulation failure are kept under observation and are treated to prevent coagulation failure.
3. Dextran 40 is used in a restricted way up to 1 litre.

Curative

Correction of coagulation failure

1. Best treatment of coagulation failure is by adequate fresh blood transfusion which provides all the clotting factors—fibrinogen, platelets, other clotting factors; one pint of fresh blood raises fibrinogen level by 25 mg%.
2. Fresh plasma and platelet rich plasma are also transfused. One pint plasma provide about 1 gm fibrinogen.
3. Cryoprecipitate bags having 150 mg fibrinogen per bag collected from a few donors can be also infused with much less risk of hepatitis.

Correction of fibrinolysis

On correction of deficiency of fibrinogen and other clotting factors, if the patient further bleeds, excess fibrinolytic activity is suspected for the cause of bleeding. In this situation the fibrinogen-fibrin degradation products show elevated level.

For bleeding due to excess fibrinolysis, inhibitors—*epsilon aminocaproicacid* (EACA), a synthetic amino acid is given IV 4 gm (10 ml caprostat–life pharmaceuticals) is infused mixed with 5% dextrose in first 30 minutes and then 1 gm/hour for next 12 hours.

IDIOPATHIC THROMBOCYTOPENIC PURPURA IN PREGNANCY

In this condition there is failure of haemostasis due to platelet deficiency. The bleeding time is prolonged. Platelet count is lowered but coagulation time is normal. Bleeding episodes as petechiae and bruising, nose and gum bleeding, melena, haematuria are clinical manifestations. Chronic idiopathic thrombocytopenic purpuric women may become pregnant. Regular oral steroid administration in pregnant mother to maintain remission of chronic ITP may be responsible for big babies which may cause difficult labour.

Antepartum and postpartum haemorrhages are not infrequent in such cases. In case of brisk haemorrhage in thrombocytopenic state, it is imperative to give fresh whole blood transfusion and/or platelet rich fresh plasma.

Effect on newborn

Newborn delivered of chronic ITP mother may suffer from neonatal thrombocytopenia and purpura of varying degree due to entry of platelet antibody from maternal to foetal circulation. Fortunately, the purpuric episode is mild and short lasting for 1–2 weeks. This needs treatment with steroids.

FOETAL DISTRESS

Definition

This signifies foetal asphyxia (foetal hypoxia and metabolic acidosis).

Causes

1. Late pregnancy—high-risk pregnancy (PIH, chronic hypertension, APH, IUGR, preterm labour)
2. During labour: Normal labour rarely
   - High-risk labour—on high-risk pregnancies, prolonged labour, CPD, cord complications.

DIAGNOSIS

I. Clinical foetal distress

1. By Intermittent auscultation of foetal heart rate persistent tachycardia above 160/min.,

persistent bradycardia below 120/min., Irregular PHR, Late deceleration—FH bradycardia starts at peak of contraction but lasts for 30–60 seconds—returns to normal.
2. Poor or no foetal movement for 6 hours in late pregnancy as reported by mother.
3. Passage of black meconium obtained by amniotic tap in late pregnancy.
4. Passage of green meconium in labour along with FHR abnormality.
5. Increasing caput succedeneum.

Diagnosis on clinical foetal distress is at times unnecessarily done. Every case must be evaluated by experienced obstetrician.

II. Continuous electronic FHR monitoring

By cardiotocography in late pregnancy (Non-stress testing - NST) and in labour (external and internal foetal heart cardiotocographic monitoring)—various FHR changes are obtained as curves on strip of paper in foetal distress (Fig. 11.7).

Effect of foetal distress

1. Low apgar scored baby below 3 at 5 min. is delivered
2. Neurological sequelae as seizures as a late complication.

Management

1. To stop oxytocin drip
2. To change maternal position to lateral from supine to relieve cord and aortocaval compression.
3. To administer oxygen to mother to improve foetal oxygenation.
4. To correct hypotension and acidosis by 5% dextrose and Ringer's lactate infusion.
5. Prompt delivery by caesarean section or safe vaginal delivery.
6. With meconium, baby's mouth and throat are sucked, laryngoscope is passed and tracheal suction is done. Intratracheal intubation and ventilation become necessary.

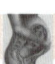

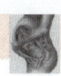

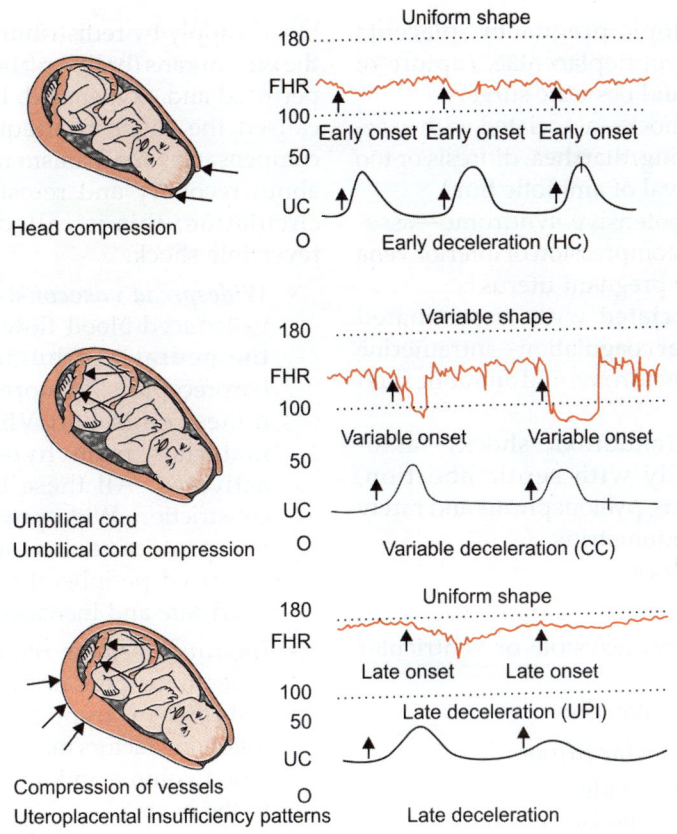

Fig. 11.7: Fetal heart rate, stress, showing early deceleration, variable deceleration and late deceleration

SHOCK IN OBSTETRICS

Definition

Shock is defined as a state of circulatory inadequacy with poor tissue perfusion resulting in generalized cellular hypoxia.

PRIMARY OR INITIAL SHOCK

It is a transient and usually a benign vasovagal attack resulting from sudden reduction of venous return to the heart caused by neurogenic vasodilatation and consequent peripheral pooling of blood. It can occur immediately following trauma, severe pain or emotional over-reaction such as due to fear, sorrow or surprise. Clinically, the patient generally develops unconsciousness, weakness, sinking sensation, pale and clammy limbs, weak and rapid pulse, and low blood pressure. The attack usually lasts for a few seconds or minutes.

SECONDARY OR TRUE SHOCK

This is the form of shock which occurs due to haemodynamic derangements with hypoperfusion of the cells. This type of shock is the true shock which is commonly referred to as 'shock'.

Classification of shock

1. **Hypovolaemic shock**
   - Haemorrhagic shock—Associated with postpartum or postabortal haemo-

 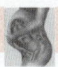

rrhage, ectopic pregnancy, placenta praevia, abruptioplacentae, rupture of the uterus and obstetric surgery.

- Fluid loss shock—associated with excessive vomiting, diarrhea, diuresis or too rapid removal of amniotic fluid.
- Supine hypotensive syndrome—associated with compression of inferior vena cava by the pregnant uterus.
- Shock associated with disseminated intravascular coagulation—intrauterine dead fetus syndrome and amniotic fluid embolism.

2. Septic shock (endotoxic shock)—associated typically with septic abortion, chorioamnionitis, pyelonephritis and rarely postpartum endometritis.
3. Cardiogenic shock

Failure of left ventricular ejection
- Cardiac arrest (asystole or ventricular fibrillation)
- Myocardial infarction

Failure of left ventricular filling
- Cardiac tamponade
- Pulmonary embolism

4. Neurogenic shock
- Chemical injury: Associated with aspiration of gastrointestinal contents during general anaesthesia specially in caesarean section *(Mendelson's syndrome)*
- Drug-induced: Associated with spinal anaesthesia.

Stages of shock

Deterioration of the circulation in shock is a progressive phenomenon and can be divided arbitrarily into 3 stages:
1. Compensated (reversible) shock
2. Progressive decompensated shock
3. Decompensated (irreversible) shock

COMPENSATED (REVERSIBLE) SHOCK

In the early stage of shock, an attempt is made to maintain adequate cerebral and coronary blood supply by redistribution of blood so that the vital organs (brain and heart) are adequately perfused and oxygenated. If the condition that caused the shock is adequately treated, the compensatory mechanism may be able to bring about recovery and re-establish the normal circulation; this is called compensated or reversible shock.

- *Widespread vasoconstriction:* In response to reduced blood flow and tissue anoxia, the neural and humoral factors (e.g., baroreceptors, hemoreceptors, catecholamines, renin and VEM or vasoexcitor materials from hypoxic kidney) are activated. All these bring about vasoconstriction. Widespread vasoconstriction is a protective mechanism as it causes increased peripheral resistance, increased heart rate and increased blood pressure.

- *Improved venous return to the heart:* In order to compensate the actual loss of blood volume in hypoglycemic shock the following factors may assist in restoring the blood volume and improve venous return to the heart.
  - Release of aldosterone from hypoxic kidney.
  - Release of ADH due to decreased effective circulating blood volume.
  - Reduced glomerular filtration rate (GFR) due to arteriolar constriction.
  - Shifting of tissue fluids into the plasma due to lowered capillary hydrostatic pressure (hypotension).

PROGRESSIVE DECOMPENSATED SHOCK

This is a stage when the patient suffers from some other stress or risk factors (e.g., pre-existing cardiovascular and lung disease) besides persistence of the shock so that there is progressive deterioration. The effects of progressive decompensated shock include the following:

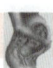

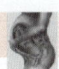

- Pulmonary hypoperfusion with resultant tachypnoea and adult respiratory distress syndrome.
- Tissue anoxia causing anaerobic glycolysis resulting in metabolic lactic acidosis.
- Anoxia of liver causing reduced clearance of lactate from it leading to acidosis.

DECOMPENSATED (IRREVERSIBLE) SHOCK

When the shock is so severe that inspite of compensatory mechanism and despite therapy and control of etiologic agent, which caused shock, no recovery takes place, it is called decompensated or irreversible shock. Its effects include the following:

- Progressive fall in the blood pressure due to deterioration in cardiac output attributed to release of myocardial depressant factor (MDF).
- Severe metabolic acidosis due to anaerobic glycolysis.
- Respiratory distress due to pulmonary edema, tachypnoea and adult respiratory distress syndrome (ARDS).
- Ischaemic cell death of brain, heart and kidneys due to reduced blood supply to these organs resulting in coma, worsened heart function and progressive renal failure.

GENERAL CHANGES IN SHOCK (WITH SPECIAL REFERENCE TO HYPOVOLAEMIC SHOCK)

There are four phases of changes. The first two phases reversible; the third one probably correctable and the fourth is irreversible.

- *First phase:* Sympathetic impulses and the level of circulating catecholamines increase in response to hypovolaemia, cardiogenic or neurogenic stimulus. Stretch receptors monitoring blood pressure in the carotid sinus and aortic arch supply information to the vasomotor centre via the ninth and tenth cranial nerves. The vasomotor centre responds by sending efferent impulses through the sympathetic nervous system.
- *Second phase:* As a result of excessive sympathetic stimulus, there is constriction of the pre and post-capillary sphincters, resulting in inadequate venous return leading to diminished cardiac output, clinical manifestations of which are hypotension and tachycardia.

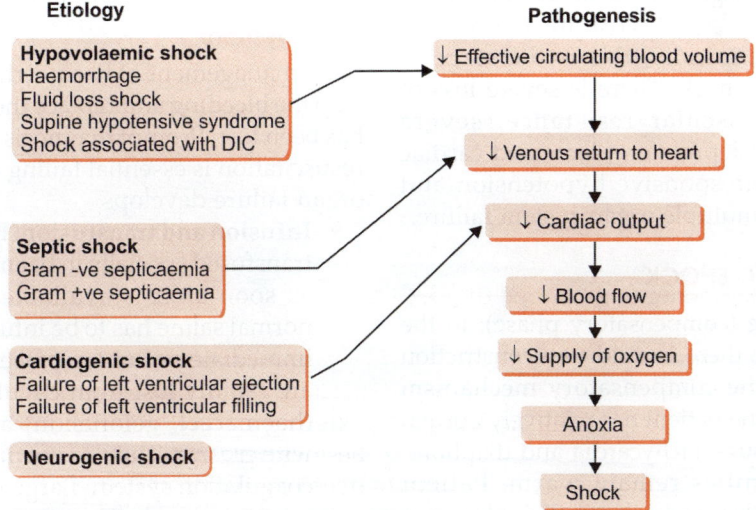

Fig. 11.8: Etiology (left) and pathogenesis (right) of shock

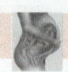

These mechanism attempt to correct hypo-volaemia, improve cardiac output and the perfusion of vital organs. At this stage, transfusion and control of hemorrhages are usually effective in restoring the normal circulatory balance and tissue perfusion.

On the other hand, if bleeding continues or treatment is delayed, the changes at microcirculatory unit will continue to persist and will pass on to the third and fourth phases of shock.

- **Third phase:** Prolonged anoxia of the tissues will lead to excessive production of lactic acid (acidosis). Lactic acid and anoxia causes relaxation of the precapillary sphincters but not the post-capillary sphincters. In addition, thromboxane A_2 leukotrienes (endogenous mediators) cause damage to the endothelial cells of the capillaries of the microcirculatory bed. These lead to formation of thrombus within the capillaries.
- **Fourth phase:** Consequent to persistent constriction of the post-capillary sphincter, blood remains stagnant within the capillary bed. Fluid from the capillaries leaks into the tissue spaces due to increased permeability. All fluids administered intravenously will go into the tissue spaces and circulatory blood volume cannot be restored. Clinically, this is the stage of irreversible shock. There is severe loss of systemic vascular resistance, severe myocardial depression (decreased cardiac output), unresponsive hypotension and ultimately multiple organ system failure.

HAEMORRHAGIC SHOCK

- **Early phase** (compensatory phase): In the early phase there is mild vasoconstriction and with the compensatory mechanism operating, the patient has relatively normal blood pressure, tachycardia and diaphoresis. Extremities remain warm. Patient appears restless and anxious. *This phase can be easily managed by volume replacement.*

- **Intermediate phase** *(reversible phase):* If the early phase remains untreated, the patient passes into the state of hypotension. Patient progressively becomes pale; tachycardia persists and due to intense vasoconstriction, the periphery becomes cold and there may be sweating. Due to diversion of blood to vital organs, the patient remains conscious and the urine output is within normal limits. *Still with adequate management, the shock state can be reversed.*
- **Late stage (irreversible):** Hypotension continues and cannot be reversed by fluid replacement because of stagnation of blood at the microvascular level. Extremities become cold and clammy because of vasoconstriction due to sympathetic stimulation. For the same reason, colour of the skin becomes ashen grey. Metabolic acidosis, coagulopathy and thrombocytopenia are associated. Practically, imperceptible low volume pulse, oliguria, mental confusion (multiple organ failure) are the combined results of circulatory failure and anaerobic metabolism. Treatment of any kind is practically useless in this phase and mortality varies between 3 and 100%.

Management

Basic management of haemorrhagic shock is to stop the bleeding and replace the volume which has been lost. Prompt diagnosis and immediate resuscitation is essential failing which multiple organ failure develops.

- **Infusion and transfusion:** Blood should be transfused specially in haemorrhagic shock as soon as it is available. Crystalloids: normal saline has to be infused initially for immediate volume replacement. But they are rapidly lost from circulation. Colloids (haemaccel, gelofusion) are iso-osmotic with plasma. They do not interfere with the coagulation system. Large volumes can be administered. They promote osmotic diuresis.

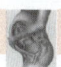

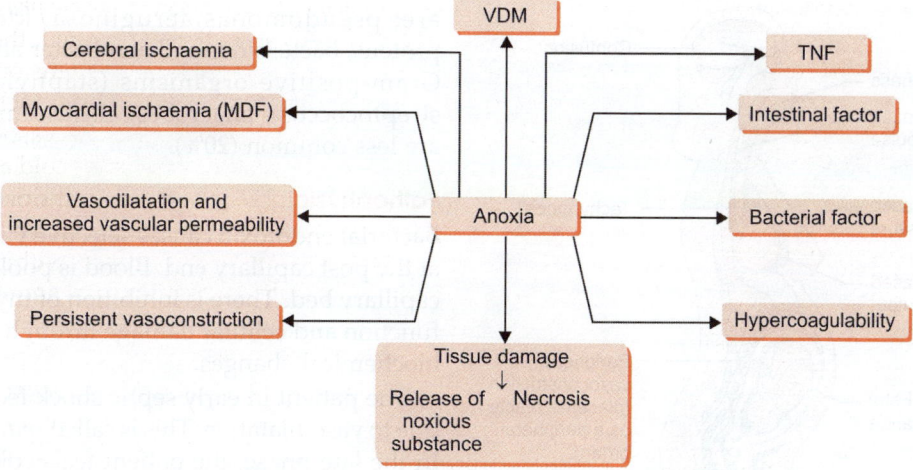

Fig. 11.9: Mechanisms involved in irreversibilty of shock with central role of anoxia

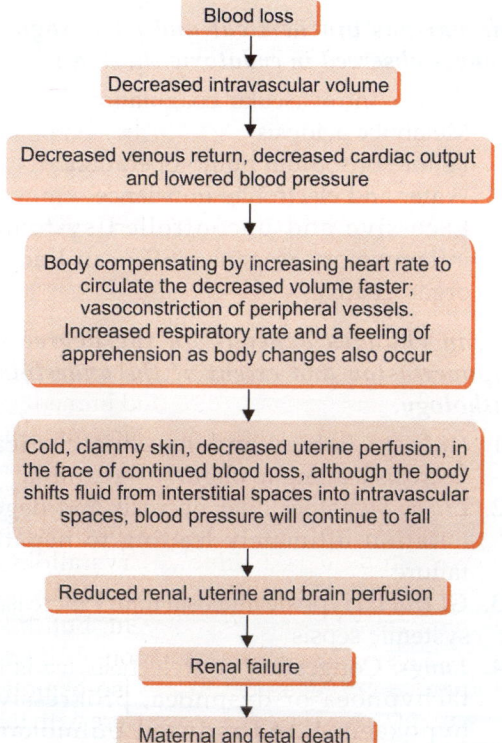

Fig. 11.10: The process of shock due to blood loss (hypovolaemic)

- **Maintenance of cardiac efficiency:** When a large volume of fluid or blood is to be administered, the cardiac competence or efficiency should be ascertained—otherwise there is a risk of overloading the circulation and cardiac failure. Haemodynamic monitoring should be aimed to maintain systolic BP > 90 mm Hg.

- **Administration of oxygen to avoid metabolic acidosis:** In the initial phase, administration of oxygen by face mask at a rate of 6–8 litres per minute is enough but in the late phases, ventilation by endotracheal intubation may be necessary.

- **Pharmacologic agents:** Use of vasopressor drugs should be kept to a minimum.

- **Control of haemorrhage:** Specific surgical and medical for control of haemorrhage should start along with the general management of shock.

- **Monitoring:** Clinical parameter like skin temperature, visible peripheral veins can be helpful to assess the degree of tissue perfusion. Urine output (> 30 ml/hr) is useful guide. Arterial blood pressure is a poor indicator to assess tissue perfusion.

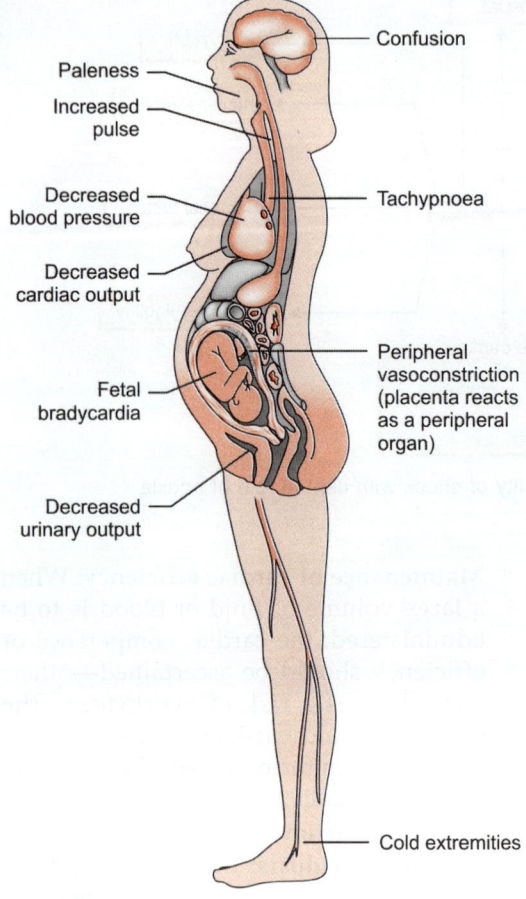

- Confusion
- Paleness
- Increased pulse
- Decreased blood pressure
- Tachypnoea
- Decreased cardiac output
- Peripheral vasoconstriction (placenta reacts as a peripheral organ)
- Fetal bradycardia
- Decreased urinary output
- Cold extremities

Fig. 11.11: Signs of hypovolemic shock

In critically ill patient, however, measurement of central venous pressure (CVP), to assess the adequacy of patients circulating volume and the contractile state of the cardium, is essential. Pulse oximeter and blood gas analysis are useful to assess tissue perfusion.

ENDOTOXIC SHOCK

Changes in endotoxic shock usually follows infection with Gram-negative organism (75–80%). The commonest organism involved is *Escherichia coli* (50%). Other organisms occasionally responsible for endotoxic shock are: pseudomonas aeruginosa, klebsiella, proteus, bacteroides and aerobacter aerogenes. Gram-positive organisms (staphylococcus, streptococcus), anaerobes, clostridium group are less common (20%).

Pathophysiology of endotoxic shock

Bacterial endotoxin causes selective vasospasm at the post capillary end. Blood is pooled in the capillary bed. There is inhibition of myocardial function and cellular damage through complex biochemical changes.

The patient in early septic shock feels warm due to vasodilatation. This is called *warm shock.* In the late phase, the patient feels cold due to vasoconstriction (sympathetic squeeze). This is called *cold shock* or *late shock.* Patient's skin becomes cold, clammy and ashen grey.

The various biochemical and pathological changes observed in endotoxic shock are

1. Diffuse intravascular coagulation
2. Metabolic acidosis
3. Failure of sodium pump operation
4. Water and electrolyte imbalance
5. Excessive and uncontrolled systemic inflammatory response (SIR) can lead to organ changes.

Organ changes depends on the degree of hypoperfusion and extent of the underlying pathology.

1. *Kidney:* Patchy and massive cortical necrosis leading to oliguria and anuria
2. *Liver:* Hepatocellular necrosis and degeneration ultimately leading to hepatic failure
3. *GI tract:* Hypoxic mucosal injury increases systemic sepsis
4. *Lungs:* Congestion or atelectasis leads to tachypnoea or dyspnoea, progressive hypoxaemia and reduced pulmonary compliance. ARDS results from increased capillary permeability and thickening of the alveolar capillary membranes.

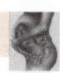

Table 11.2: Signs and symptoms of hypovolaemic shock

Assessment	Significance
Increased pulse rate	Heart attempting to circulate decreased blood volume
Decreased blood pressure	Less peripheral resistance because of decreased blood volume
Increased respiratory rate	Increased gas exchange to better oxygenate decreased red blood cell volume
Cold, clammy skin	Vasoconstriction occurs to maintain blood volume in central body core
Decreased urine output	Inadequate blood is entering kidney due to decreased blood volume
Dizziness or decreased level of consciousness	Inadequate blood is reaching cerebrum due to decreased blood volume
Decreased CVP	Decreased blood is returning to heart due to reduced blood volume

5. *Heart:* Cardiac output decreases depending on the degree of hypotension, hypoperfusion and vasoconstriction. Myocardial ischaemia → cardiac dysfunction → dysrrhythmias →cardiac failure →left ventricular end diastolic pressure (LVEDP) →pulmonary oedema →tissue hypoxia.

6. Ultimately multiple organ failure develops.

In the initial phase of endotoxic shock, because of precapillary dilatation and diversion of blood through metarteriolar shunt, the patient remains alert, there is marked flushing of the face and the skin feels warm. There are temperature change, > 38°C or < 36°C, bounding pulse, heart rate > 100 beats. Min, respiratory rate > 20/min, WBC > 12000/ml^3.

When, however, the state of shock persists, there is intense constriction of sphincters at either end of the capillary bed. The patient becomes pale and there is profuse sweating. Extremities are cold and clammy. Urine output is markedly reduced.

If the shock condition dose not improve, the patient passes clinically to the stage of *irreversible shock*. She remains cold and clammy with ashen grey cyanotic appearance. Severe sepsis is associated with hypotension (< 90 mm Hg systolic), organ hypoperfusion and dysfunction →lactic acidosis →oliguria, renal failure, ARDS, cardiac failure → multiple organ dysfunction syndrome.

Principles of management

Management of endotoxic shock can be formulated only on the basis of the pathological changes produced by endotoxaemia.

This includes administration of antibiotics, intravenous fluids treatment of intravascular coagulation and toxic myocarditis, administration of oxygen and elimination of the source of infection.

- *Antibiotics:* Endotoxic shock is most commonly due to Gram-negative organism, so proper antibiotics should be administered in adequate doses.

- *Intravenous fluid and electrolytes:* Septic shock associated with haemorrhagic hypotension should be treated by liberal infusion and blood transfusion. The amount of fluid to be administered can be precisely assessed by recording the central venous pressure. Oliguria with high specific gravity is an indication of liberal fluid administration, whereas a low specific gravity indicates fluid restriction. Impairment of renal function contraindicates administration of electrolytes. Estimation of blood electrolytes (Na, K, bicarbonate) is a helpful guide.

- *Correction of acidosis:* Acidosis and hypoxaemia depress myocardial contractility. Bicarbonate should be administered to correct persistent metabolic acidosis (pH < 7.2) only.

- *Maintenance of blood pressure*
  - *Inotropic agents:* In a critically ill patient when there is hypotension (MAP < 60 mm Hg) and impaired perfusion of vital organs despite adequate volume replacement, inotropes should be used. Adrenaline, noradrenaline, dopamine and dobutamine have both inotropic and vasoconstrictive effects. Dopamine is still the drug of choice.
  - *Vasodilator therapy:* In selected cases, (MAP > 70 mm Hg) after load reduction may improve stroke volume and reduce ventricular wall tension. Sodium nitroprusside and nitroglycerin could be used for that purpose.
  - *Diuretic therapy:* To reduce fluid over load (pre load) and pulmonary oedema, diuretics should be used. Frusemide is the drug of choice.
- *Corticosteroids:* The role of steroid is restricted to specific condition only. The dose recommended in septic shock is 50 mg of hydrocortisone per kg body weight. The advantages claimed are:
  - To exert an anti-endotoxin effect on the peripheral circulation
  - Stabilizes lysosomal membrane
  - To counteract anaerobic oxidative mechanism
  - To improve the regional blood flow (microcirculation) and thereby reverse the metabolic acidosis
- *Treatment of diffuse intravascular coagulation:* When there is low fibrinogen level, reduced platelet count and increased fibrin degradation products heparin therapy should be considered. Alternatively fresh-frozen plasma or whole blood transfusion could be done.
- *Elimination of source of infection:* Hysterectomy has been advocated in unresponsive endotoxic shock following septic abortion or puerperal sepsis.

- *H₂-blockers:* Ranitidine IV is given to prevent stress-induced bleeding and ulceration of the gastric mucosa.
- *Nutritional support:* Oral, or parenteral nutrition to provide 20–30 kcal kg/day with fat and carbohydrate (nonprotein) is optimum.

NEUROGENIC SHOCK

The basic pathological factors in both haemorrhagic and neurogenic shock are more or less the same except for the fact that haemorrhagic shock is hypovolaemic and neurogenic shock, initially is normovolaemic, though this becomes hypovolaemic in the later phase due to pooling and stagnation of blood in the microvascular capillaries.

The compensatory phase, in neurogenic shock, however is very transient. In the reversible phase, unlike hypovolaemic shock, pallor is absent; on the contrary, the face may be flushed. Moreover, neurogenic shock does not show expected response to volume replacement. Temperature remains normal or subnormal.

Management

- **Fluid replacement:** This is essential because a large volume of fluid or blood is trapped in the capillary bed either due to vasoconstriction or vasodilatation. The amount of fluid to be infused will depend on the CVP urinary output and specific gravity of urine.
- *Vasoactive drugs and corticosteroids:* Vasoactive drugs like phenylephrine may be used. Corticosteroids however is used in selected cases.
- *Correction of acidosis and ventilation:* The line of management is same as in endotoxic or haemorrhagic shock.
- *Elimination and correction of source of neurogenic stimulus:* (Like inversion of uterus, myocardial infarction and pulmonary embolism)—along with treatment of

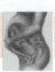

shock, these basic etiological factors for neurogenic shock should receive priority attention.

The female pelvis may be altered in size and shape by errors of development by diseases of the pelvic bones and joints, by deformities of the spinal column and lower extremities or because of accident.

Definition

Obstetric definition which states that alteration in the size and/or shape of the pelvis of sufficient degree so as to alter the normal mechanism of labour in an average size baby.

Common causes of contracted pelvis

1. Nutritional and environmental defects
   • Minor variation: common
   • Major: Rachitic and osteomalacic—rare
2. Diseases or injuries affecting the bones of the *pelvis*—fracture, tumours, tubercular arthritis; *spine*—kyphosis, scoliosis, spondylolisthesis, coccygeal deformity; *lower limbs*—poliomyelitis, hip joint disease.
3. Development defects—Naegele's pelvis, Robert's pelvis; high or low assimilation pelvis

RACHITIC FLAT PELVIS (Fig. 11.12)

Rickets is predominantly a disease of early childhood when the bones remain soft and unossified. At this time if the child lies or sits in bed, changes occur in the soft pelvis due to weight bearing. The classic changes in the pelvic bones are given below:

Inlet: Sacral promontory is pushed downwards and forwards producing a "reniform" shape of the inlet with marked shortening of the anteroposterior diameter without affecting the transverse diameter, which is often increased.

Cavity: Sacrum is flat and tilted backwards. There may be sharp angulation at the sacrococcygeal joint.

Outlet: Body weight transmitted through the ischium in sitting position results in widening of the transverse diameter of the outlet and the pubic arch.

OSTEOMALACIC PELVIS (Fig. 11.13)

The deformity is caused by softening of the pubic bones due to calcium and vitamin D deficiency and lack of exposure to sunrays.

• The promontory is pushed downwards and forwards.
• Approximation of the two ischial tuberosities and marked narrowing of the pubic arch occurs. Sacrum is markedly shortened. Coccyx is pushed forward.

Vaginal delivery is unlikely and if left uncared, may lead to obstructed labour.

ASYMMETRICAL OR OBLIQUELY CONTRACTED PELVIS

It is seen in

1. Naegele's pelvis

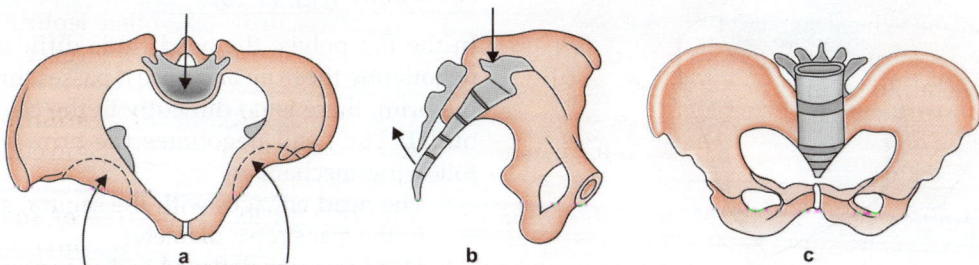

Fig. 11.12: Rachitic pelvis. **a.** Effect of walking, **b.** Effect on lying down position, **c.** Reniform shape of the inlet

 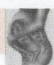

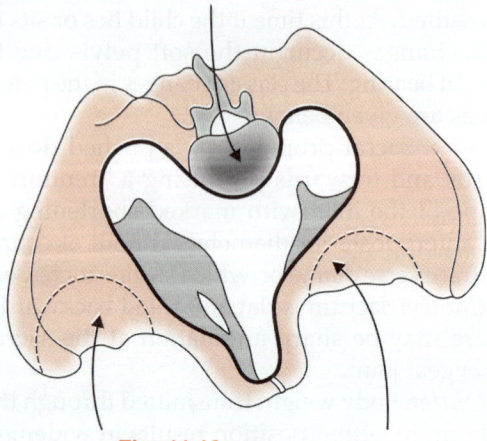

Fig. 11.13: Osteomalacic

2. Scoliotic pelvis
3. Due to disease affecting one hip or sacro-iliac joint
4. Tumours or fracture affecting one side of the pelvic bones during growing age

Naegele's pelvis (Fig. 11.14): This type of pelvis is extremely rare. It is produced due to arrested development of one ala of the sacrum. It may be:

• Congenital
• Acquired: The pelvis is obliquely contracted at all levels but more marked in the outlet. Iliopectineal line on the affected side is almost straight. Method of delivery is by caesarean section.

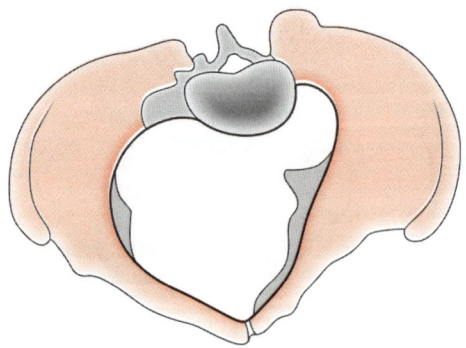

Fig. 11.14: Naegele's pelvis

Scoliosis involving only the lumbar region will cause deformity of the pelvis (Fig. 11.15). The acetabulum is pushed inwards on the weight bearing side. Oblique asymmetry of the pelvis results in contraction of one of the oblique diameters.

Robert's pelvis: Ala of both the sides are absent and the sacrum is fused with the innominate bones.

Kyphotic pelvis: The sacrum is tilted backwards in the upper part and forwards in the lower part. It is narrow and straight. The antero-posterior diameter of inlet is increased but is diminished at the outlet. Sub-pubic angle is narrow. Thus the feature is an extreme funnelling of the pelvis.

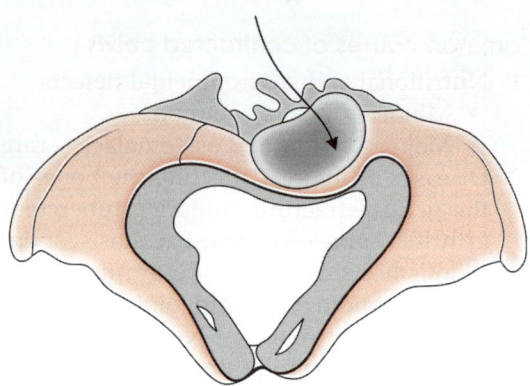

Fig. 11.15: Scoliotic pelvis

MECHANISM OF LABOUR IN CONTRACTED PELVIS WITH VERTEX PRESENTATION

FLAT PELVIS (Fig. 11.16)

In the flat pelvis, the head finds difficulty in negotiating the brim and once it passes through the brim, there is no difficulty in the cavity or outlet. The head negotiates the brim by the following mechanism:

• The head engages with the sagittal suture in the transverse diameter.
• Head remains deflexed and engagement is delayed.

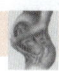

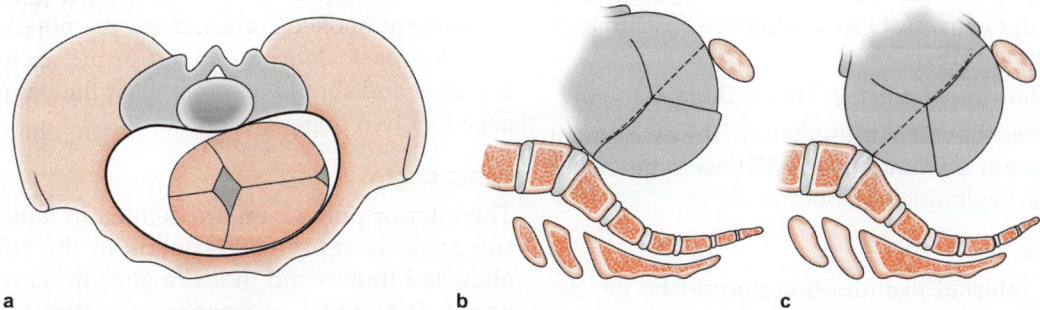

Fig. 11.16: Mechanism of labour in flat pelvis. **a.** Lateralisation of occiput to the sacral bay, **b.** and **c.** Engagement of the head by exaggerated parietal presentation

- If the anteroposterior diameter is too short, the occiput is mobilised to the same side, to occupy the sacral bay. The biparietal diameter is thus placed in the sacro-cotyloid diameter (9.5 cm or 3 ¼") and the narrow bitemporal diameter is placed in the narrow conjugate. If lateral mobilisation is not possible, there is a chance of extension of the head leading to brow or face presentation.
- Engagement occurs by exaggerated parietal presentation so that the supersubparietal diameter (8.5 cm) instead of the biparietal diameter (95 cm) passes through the pelvic brim.
- Moulding may be extreme and often there is an indentation or even a fracture of one parietal bone. However, the caput that forms is not big.
- Once the head negotiates the brim, there is no difficulty in the cavity and outlet and normal mechanism follows.

DIAGNOSIS OF CONTRACTED PELVIS

Past history
- *Medical:* Past history of fracture, rickets, osteomalacia, tuberculosis of the pelvic joints or spines, poliomyelitis is to be enquired.
- *Obstetrical:* A history of prolonged and a tedious labour followed by either sponta-neous or difficult instrumental delivery is suggestive of pelvic contraction. Difficult vaginal delivery ending in stillborn or early neonatal death or late neurological stig-mata following a difficult labour without any other aetiological factor points towards contracted pelvis. Weight of the baby, evidences of maternal injuries such is complete perineal tear, vesicovaginal or rectovaginal fistula, if available, are of useful guide.

Physical examination
- *Stature:* A small woman of less than 5 ft is likely to have a small pelvis.
- *Stigma:* Deformities (congenital or acqui-red) of pelvic bones, hip joint, spine.

Abdominal examination
- *Inspection:* Pendulous abdomen specially in primigravidae, is suspicious of inlet contraction.
- *Obstetrical:* In primigravidae, usually there is engagement of the head before the onset of labour. Presence of malpresen-tation in primigravidae, gives rise to a suspicion of pelvic contraction.

Assessment of the pelvis (pelvimetry)
Assessment of the pelvis can be done by bima-nual examination: clinical pelvimetry or by

imaging studies—radio-pelvimetry, computed tomography (CT) and magnetic resonance imaging (MRI)

Clinical pelvimetry: This is done manually.

Time: In vertex presentation, the assessment is done at any time beyond 37th week but better at the beginning of labour.

Steps

The internal examination should be gentle, thorough, methodical and purposeful (Fig. 11.17).

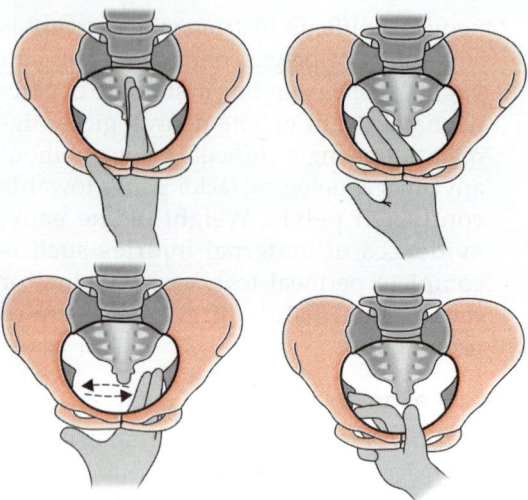

Fig. 11.17: Clinical assessment of the pelvis

Sacrum: The sacrum is smooth, well curved and usually inaccessible beyond lower three pieces.

Sacrosciatic notch: The configuration of the notch denotes the capacity of the posterior segment of the pelvis and the side walls of the lower pelvis.

Ischial spines: Spines are usually smooth and difficult to palpate.

Iliopectineal lines: To note for any breaking suggestive of narrow forepelvis.

Posterior surface of the symphysis pubis: It normally forms a smooth rounded curve.

Sacrococcygeal joint: Its mobility and presence of hooked coccus, if any are noted.

Pubic arch: Normally, the pubic arch is rounded and should accommodate the palmar aspect of two fingers.

Pubic angle

The inferior pubic rami are defined in female, the angle roughly corresponds to the fully abducted thumb and index fingers. In narrow angle, it roughly corresponds to the fully abducted middle and index fingers.

Transverse diameter of the outlet: It is measured by placing the knuckles of the first interphalangeal joints or knuckles of the clinched fist between the ischial tuberosities (Fig. 11.18).

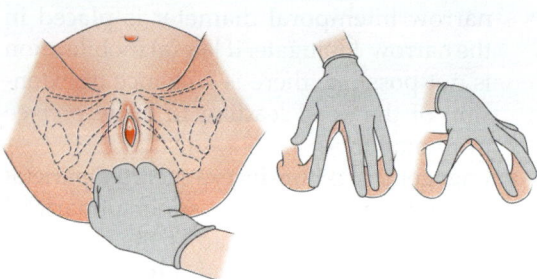

Fig. 11.18: Measurement of transverse diameter of the outlet and sub-pubic angle

Anteroposterior diameter of the outlet: The distance between the inferior margin of the symphysis pubis and the skin over the sacrococcygeal joint can be measured with the method employed for diagonal conjugate.

X-ray pelvimetry is of limited value in the diagnosis of pelvic contraction or cephalopelvic disproportion.

DISPROPORTION

The disparity in the relation between the head and the pelvis is called cephalopelvic disproportion. Disproportion may be either due to an average size baby with a small pelvis or due to a big baby with normal size pelvis (hydrocephalus) or due to a combination of both the factors.

Diagnosis of cephalopelvic disproportion at the brim

The presence and degree of cephalopelvic disproportion at the brim can be ascertained by the following:

- *Clinical*—abdominal method
- *Imaging pelvimetry*
- *Cephalometry*
- Ultrasound
- Magnetic resonance imaging (MRI)
- X-ray

Clinical

In multigravidae, a previous history of spontaneous delivery of an average size baby, reasonably rules out contracted pelvis. But in a primigravida with non-engagement of the head even at labour, one should rule out disproportion.

Abdominal method

The patient is placed in dorsal position with the thighs slightly flexed and separated. The head is grasped by the left hand. Two fingers (index and middle) of the right hand are placed above the symphysis pubis keeping the inner surface of the fingers in line with the anterior surface of the symphysis pubis to note the degree of overlapping, if any, when the head is pushed downwards and backwards.

Inferences

- The head can be pushed down in the pelvis without overlapping of the parietal bone on the symphysis pubis—no disproportion.
- Head can be pushed down a little but there is slight overlapping of the parietal bone evidenced by touch on the under surface of the fingers (overlapping by 0.5 cm or ¼" which is the thickness of the symphysis pubis)—moderate disproportion.

- Head cannot be pushed and instead the parietal bone overhangs the symphysis pubis displacing the fingers—severe disproportion.

X-ray pelvimetry: It is helpful in assessing cephalopelvic proportion in all planes of the pelvis—inlet, midpelvic and outlet.

Magnetic resonance imaging (MRI): It is useful to assess the fetal size, fetal head volume and pelvic soft tissues which are also important for successful vaginal delivery.

Degree of disproportion and contracted pelvis: Based on the clinical and supplemented by imaging pelvimetry, the following degrees of disproportion at the brim are evaluated.

- *Severe disproportion:* Where obstetric conjugate is < 7.5 cm (3").
- *Border line:* Where obstetric conjugate is between 9.5 and 10 cm. When both the anteroposterior diameter (< 10 cm) and the transverse diameter (< 12 cm) of the inlet are reduced the risk of dystocia is high than when only one diameter is contracted.

EFFECTS OF CONTRACTED PELVIS ON PREGNANCY AND LABOUR

Pregnancy

The general course of pregnancy is not much affected. However, the following may occur:

1. There is more chance of incarceration of the retroverted gravid uterus in flat pelvis.
2. Abdomen becomes pendulous specially in multigravida with lax abdominal wall.
3. Malpresentation are increased 3–4 times and so also increased frequency of unstable lie.

Labour

1. There is increased incidence of early rupture of the membranes.
2. Incidence of cord prolapse is increased.
3. Cervical dilatation is slowed.
4. There is increased tendency of prolonged labour and in neglected cases, obstructed

labour with features of exhaustion, dehydration, ketoacidosis and sepsis.

5. There is increased incidence of operative interference, shock, postpartum haemorrhage and sepsis.

Maternal injuries: The injuries of the genital tract may occur spontaneously or following operative delivery.

Fetal hazards: Fetal risks are due to trauma and asphyxia.

MANAGEMENT OF CONTRACTED PELVIS (INLET CONTRACTION)

Minor degrees of inlet contraction does not give rise to any problem and the cases are left to have a spontaneous vaginal delivery at term. The moderate and the severe degrees are to be dealt by any one of the following:

- Preterm induction of labour
- Elective caesarean section at term
- Trial labour

Preterm induction of labour: Preterm induction is limited only to moderate degrees of pelvic contraction. However, in selected multigravidae, with previous history of difficult vaginal delivery of an average size baby, the method may be employed 2–3 weeks prior to due date.

Elective caesarean section at term: Elective caesarean section at term is indicated in:

1. Major degree of inlet contraction.
2. Moderate degree of inlet contraction associated with outlet contraction or complicating factors like elderly primigravida, malpresentation, post caesarean pregnancy, etc.

TRIAL LABOUR

Definition

It is the conduction of spontaneous labour in a moderate degree of cephalopelvic disproportion portion, in an institution under supervision with watchful expectancy, hoping for a vaginal delivery.

Aims

A trial labour aims at avoiding an unnecessary caesarean section and at delivering a healthy baby.

Contraindications

- Associated midpelvic and outlet contraction
- Presence of complicating factors like elderly primigravida, malpresentation, postmaturity, post caesarean pregnancy, pre-eclampsia, medical disorders like heart disease, diabetes, tuberculosis etc.
- Where facilities for caesarean section is not available.

Conduction of trial labour

The management of a trial labour requires careful supervision and consideration. The following guidelines are prescribed.

- The labour should ideally be spontaneous in onset. But in those cases where the labour fails to start even at due date, induction of labour may be contemplated.
- Oral feeding remains suspended and hydration is maintained by intravenous drip. Adequate analgesic is administered.
- The progress of the labour is meticulously observed.
- Progressive dilatation of the cervix
- *If there is failure to progress* due to inadequate uterine contraction, augmentation of labour in carefully selected cases may be done by amniotomy along with oxytocin infusion. On no account should the procedure be employed before the cervix is at least 3 cm (2 fingers) dilated.
- *To watch* carefully the maternal and fetal conditions.
- *After the membranes rupture*, pelvic examination is to be done
- To exclude cord prolapse
- To note the colour of liquor
- To assess the pelvis once more

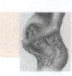
- To note the condition of the cervix including pressure of the presenting part on the cervix and the rate of descent of the head.

How long the trial to be continued?

So long as the progress is satisfactory and the maternal and fetal condition remain good, trial may be continued safely. However, if any omnious features appear, trial is to be terminated. Inspite of adequate uterine contractions if there is arrest of descent or dilatation of the cervix for a reasonable period (3–4 hours) in the active phase, labour is terminated by caesarean section.

Advantages of trial labour

- It eliminates unnecessary caesarean section
- It eliminates injudicious use of premature induction of labour.
- A successful trail ensures the woman a good future obstetrics

Disadvantages of trial labour

- Increased perineal morbidity or mortality due to asphyxia or intracranial haemorrhage when the trial is prolonged and/or ends in difficult delivery.
- Increased maternal morbidity due to the effects of prolonged labour and/or operative delivery.

RUPTURE OF THE UTERUS

Rupture of the uterus is the most serious accident than can complicate labour. It may also occur in pregnancy, though much less frequently. In either case the rupture may be spontaneous or traumatic.

Definition

Dissolution in the continuity of the uterine wall any time beyond 28 weeks of pregnancy is called rupture of the uterus.

Incidence

The incidence of uterine rupture probably depends on the standards of obstetric care and varies from 1:500 to 1:4000. The majority of rupture uterus occur in multipara.

Etiology

The causes of rupture of the uterus are broadly divided into:

- Spontaneous
- Scar rupture
- Iatrogenic

SPONTANEOUS

During pregnancy

It is indeed rare for an apparently uninjured uterus to give way during pregnancy. The causes are:

1. Previous damage, and thereby weakening of the uterine walls following dilatation and curettage operation or manual removal of placenta.
2. Grand multiparae
3. Congenital malformation of the uterus of bicornuate variety is a rare possibility.
4. In Couvelaire uterus

Spontaneous rupture during pregnancy is usually complete, involves the upper segment and usually occurs in later months of pregnancy.

During labour

Due to

1. *Obstructive rupture:* This is the end result of an obstructed labour. The rupture involves the lower segment and usually extends through one lateral side of the uterus to the upper segment.
2. *Non-obstructive rupture:* Grand multiparae are usually affected and rupture usually occurs in early labour. The rupture usually involves the fundal area and is complete.

SCAR RUPTURE

In about 2% of women who become pregnant again following a classical caesarean section, the scar may give way during the pregnancy or labour and in about half of these cases before the onset of labour. Therefore, any woman with such a scar is kept under observation during the later months of pregnancy. Rupture of the uterine scar after lower segment caesarean section is much rarer (0.4% or less).

A classical scar may rupture more frequently in a subsequent pregnancy. The classical scar is more vulnerable because of the following reasons:

- The involuting uterus keeps contracting during puerperium causing defective healing
- Difficulty in approximating the edges of the wound and catgut sutures are prematurely digested
- Placenta may be situated over the existing scar
- Incomplete haemostasis and infection during healing
- Inversion of endometrium or the serosa into the scar during repair
- Placenta implanted over the scar
- Several previous caesarean sections
- Rupture is less likely if previous caesarean section was done in labour as opposed to an elective section
- Fetal factors: Overdistension of the uterus by a large baby or multiple pregnancy may initiate rupture.

IATROGENIC OR TRAUMATIC

During pregnancy

1. Injudicious administration of oxytocin
2. Use of prostaglandins for the induction of abortion or labour
3. Forcible external version specially under general anaesthesia
4. Fall or blow on the abdomen

During labour

1. Internal podalic version
2. Destructive operation

3. Manual removal of placenta
4. Application of forceps or breech extraction through incompletely dilated cervix
5. Injudicious administration of oxytocin for augmentation of labour.

Pathology

The uterine rupture may be:

- Incomplete
- Complete

Rupture of the uterus is said to be complete when all the coats including the peritoneum are torn, and incomplete when this is not the case. Rupture of the lateral wall of the uterus, which in pregnancy is uncovered by peritoneum, may include the whole thickness of the muscular wall and still be incomplete, as it only opens up the broad ligament, but does not tear the peritoneum. Incomplete rupture is sometimes seen in well-marked cases of overdistension and haemorrhagic disruption of the uterine wall (Couvelaire uterus from concealed accidental haemorrhage).

Spontaneous rupture is more often complete than incomplete and traumatic rupture is more often incomplete than complete.

In the majority of cases, rupture begins in the lower uterine segment as this part of the uterine wall is thinnest and is most liable to overdistension. The rupture may be confined to the lower segment, or may extend upwards into the uterine body, even to the fundus, or downwards into the vaginal fornices. Tears of the anterior wall occasionally extend into the bladder. Sometimes rupture causes laceration of a large branch of the uterine or vaginal artery, or of large uterine veins causing serious haemorrhage.

Complete rupture is usually followed by the escape of the uterine contents (fetus or placenta, or both) into the peritoneal cavity. The empty uterus then retracts firmly and severe haemorrhage will not occur, unless large vessels have been torn. The fetus generally dies because of

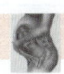

the effect of uterine retraction upon the utero-placental circulation.

When the rupture is small or incomplete the fetus remains in the uterine cavity and sometimes only a part of the fetus, the head or a limb escapes through the rent, the rest being retained in the uterus.

Diagnosis

The symptoms in ruptured uterus are not always characteristic, although they may arouse the suspicion that rupture has occurred.

Rupture during pregnancy

Typically

- Acute abdominal pain with features of shock and intra-abdominal haemorrhage
- Contracted uterus as seen after the third stage of labour
- Easily palpable fetus
- Absent fetal heart

Atypically

- Incomplete rupture producing localized abdominal pain and tenderness.
- Frank signs of haemorrhage and shock develop slowly.

The differential diagnosis is with accidental haemorrhage and other causes of acute abdomen in late pregnancy.

Rupture in labour

The attendant symptoms are influenced mainly by the rapidity with which the laceration is produced, and the amount of haemorrhage, which accompanies it.

- Premonitory symptoms are those of a long and difficult labour, tonic contraction and over stretching of the lower uterine segment.
- Sudden acute pain in the lower abdomen and previous labour pains appear to stop altogether.
- Signs of internal haemorrhage
- Abdominal palpation: Fetal parts are easily palpable through abdominal wall, together with hard -retracted fundus. This feature is characteristic of complete rupture.
- Vaginal examination
- Reveals haemorrhage through the cervical os
- Recession of the presenting part incomplete rupture
- Hematuria may be present
- Cervix hangs like a curtain

Sometimes, the suspicion of rupture does not arise until after the delivery of the patient either with or without artificial aid. The bad general condition of the patient then attracts attention. Considerable external bleeding occurs although the placenta has been expelled and the uterus is firmly retracted. Rupture is not suspected for several hours if there is gradual development of the symptoms.

The symptoms vary greatly, from severe pain and shock, and evidence of profuse intra-peritoneal haemorrhage, to just discomfort and very slight general disturbance. A thin and fibrous caesarean section scar may yield quietly and the fetus be gradually extruded into the peritoneal cavity. However, in the majority of cases the symptoms are severe. Because of the variation in symptoms the diagnosis may be difficult. The main symptoms of rupture of the uterus or the sudden and rapid development of symptoms of shock in a case in which the labour has been prolonged, or artificial delivery has been accomplished with difficulty. There is vaginal bleeding and, though delivery has taken place, the pain suddenly cease.

Due to intrauterine manipulations or extraction of the head by forceps through an imperfectly dilated cervix, the rupture starts in the cervix or lower uterine segment. It then runs up into the body, opening of the broad ligament. The majority of such cases are therefore cases of incomplete rupture.

Incomplete rupture through the anterior or lateral wall or the lower uterine segment may result in the formation of an extensive haema-

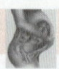

toma under the loose visceral peritoneum. Such a haematoma can sometimes be palpated as a diffuse, fluctuant, sometimes crepitant, swelling over the anterior or anterolateral aspect of the lower segment.

PROPHYLAXIS

The following guidelines are helpful to prevent or to detect at the earliest the tragic occurrence of rupture uterus.
- The at-risk mothers likely to rupture should have mandatory hospital delivery.

These are:
- Contracted pelvis
- Previous history of caesarean section, hysterotomy or myomectomy
- Uncorrected transverse lie
- Multiparity with pendulous abdomen
- Grand multiparity
- Known case of hydrocephalus
- General anaesthesia should not be used to give undue force in external version.
- Undue delay in the progress of labour in a multipara with previous uneventful delivery should be viewed with concern and the cause should be sought for.
- Judicious selection of cases with previous history of caesarean sections for vaginal delivery
- Judicious selection of cases and careful watch are mandatory during oxytocin infusion.
- There is hardly any place of internal podalic version in singleton features in present day obstetrics.
- Attempted forceps delivery or breech extraction through incompletely dilated cervix should be avoided.
- Destructive vaginal operations should be performed by skilled personnel
- Manual removal in morbid adherent placenta should be done by a senior person.

Treatment

Resuscitation and laparotomy

Depending upon the state of the clinical condition, either resuscitation is to be done followed by laparotomy or in acute conditions, resuscitation and laparotomy are to be done simultaneously.

LAPAROTOMY

Any of the three procedures may be adopted following laparotomy.
- *Hysterectomy*: In most cases of rupture uterus other than a rupture caesarean scar, the edges are ragged and irregular. Suturing is less feasible. The bleeding can be controlled and the risk of sepsis decreased by hysterectomy. Total hysterectomy is technically more difficult.

  If the patient is in poor general condition, speed is essential. Subtotal hysterectomy can be done more easily. Amputation is completed at the site of the rupture.
- *Repair:* This is mostly applicable to a scar rupture where the margins are clean.
- *Repair and sterilization:* This is mostly done in patients with a clean cut scar rupture having desired number of children.

Prognosis

Prognosis depends upon the manner in which labour is managed prior to the accident, type of rupture, morbid pathological changes at the site of the rupture and the effective management. Lower segment scar rupture gives a comparatively better prognosis. But rupture following obstructed labour either spontaneous or due to instrumentation gives a maternal death rate of about 20% or more.

CERVICAL DYSTOCIA

Definition

Failure of the cervix to dilate within a reasonable time in spite of good regular uterine contractions.

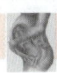

Varieties

- *Organic* (secondary dystocia) due to:
  a. Cervical stances as a sequel to previous amputation, cone biopsy, extensive cauterization or obstetric trauma
  b. Organic lesions as cervical myoma or carcinoma
  c. Post delivery
- *Functional* (primary dystocia):
  a. *Achalasia of the cervix:* In spite of the absence of any organic lesion and the well effacement of the cervix, the external os fails to dilate.
  b. *Rigid cervix:* This may be due to lack of softening of the cervix during pregnancy or cervical spasm resulted from overactive sympathetic tone.
  c. *Conglutination of the external os:* The sticking together of the lips of the cervix.

Complications

Annular detachment of the cervix: surprisingly the bleeding from the cervix is minimal because of fibrosis and avascular pressure necrosis leading to thrombosis of the vessels before detachment.

- Rupture uterus
- Postpartum haemorrhage: particularly if cervical laceration extends upwards tearing the main uterine vessels
- The constant and prolonged pressure on the cervix leads to anoxia and devitalization of the tissue, which eventually separates and comes away as a ring.
- In some cases the cervix becomes well effaced and the external os very thin, but dilatation does not take place.

Management

- **Organic dystocia**
- Caesarean section is the management of choice
- **Functional dystocia**
- Pethidine and antispasmodics: may be effective

- Caesarean section: if medical treatment fails or foetal distress developed

DISSEMINATED INTRAVASCULAR COAGULATION (DIC) IN OBSTETRICS

The first description of DIC comes from the lecture delivered by Walter H. Seegers in April of 1950. Disseminated intravascular coagulation is always a secondary hemostatic disorder, that is initiated by a underlying disease. Disseminated intravascular coagulation (DIC) is an acquired syndrome. Normally the coagulation system is activated and regulated in a confined site of injury resulting in clot formation and reabsorption of the clot. This disorder occurs when body's clotting mechanisms are activated inappropriately.

DEFINITION OF DIC (MINIMAL ACCEPTABLE CRITERIA)

A systematic thrombohemorrhagic disorder seen in association with well defined clinical situations and laboratory evidence of:

1. Procoagulant activation
2. Fibrinolytic activation
3. Inhibitor consumption and
4. Biochemical evidence of end-organ damage or failure.

Predisposing factors of DIC

About 50% of individuals with disseminated intravascular coagulation are patients with complications from pregnancy. Widespread infection and truma are responsible for the majority of the remaining cases.

Causes of DIC

There are many causes of disseminated intravascular coagulation. These can be classified as acute or chronic. The disorder may be the result of single or multiple conditions.

Other Causes of DIC

- Amniotic fluid embolism

 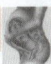

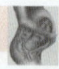

- Placental abruption
- Pre-eclampsia
- Eclampsia
- HELLP syndrome
- Retained fetus syndrome
- Abortion
- Hydatidiform mole
- Amniocentesis
- Cesarean section
- Placenta accreta
- Ruptured uterus
- Retained placenta
- Gynecologic malignancy
- Ovarian
- Utrine and breast cancer.
- Infections bacterial (e.g. Gram-negative infection, meningococcal infection)
- Viral (HIV, cytomegalovirus, varicella)
- Fungal (histoplasma)
- Parasitic (malaria)
- Tissue trauma such as burns, accidents, surgery or shock
- Acute liver failure
- Incompatible blood transfusion or massive blood transfusion (more than the total circulatory volume
- Venomous snake bites (e.g. saw-scaled vipers)
- Maligant disease (e.g. acute myelocytic leukemias)

Pathophysiology

DIC occurs when monocytes and endothelial cells are activated or injured by toxic substances elaborated in the course of certain diseases.

The response of monocytes and endothelial cells to injury is to generate tissue factor on the cell surface, overactivating the coagulation cascade which results in excessive generation of thrombin which depletes clotting factors and platelets and activates the fibrinolytic system.

As the clotting factors and platelets are consumed, there are less clotting factors available to be used at real sites of bleeding and excessive bleeding occurs.

Clinical presentation

DIC has a varied clinical presentation. Chronic DIC is infrequently seen in obstetrics and gynecology thus it is briefly outlined below:

CHRONIC DIC

In the chronic DIC clinical findings are:
- Signs of deep venous or arterial thrombosis or embolism
- Superficial venous thrombosis, especially without varicose veins
- Multiple thrombotic sites at the same time
- Serial thrombotic episodes.

ACUTE DIC

Obstetrical accidents are common events leading to disseminated intravascular coagulation. In acute DIC the onset of signs and symptoms, is typically acute and dramatic, classically characterized by dyspnea, hypoxemia, hypotension and cardiovascular collapse. Coagulopathy and hemorrahage are common and occur usually after the diagnosis is made.

In milder forms the presentation can be in the form of

- Ecchymoses of the skin, mucous membranes
- Visceral hemorrhage
- Ischemic tissue
- Multiple bleeding sites
- Hemodynamic shock disproportionate to bleeding.

Diagnosis of DIC

The diagnosis of DIC is mainly clinical. Full blood count (especially the platelet count), fibrin D-gradation products or D-dimer tests (markers of fibrinolysis), bleeding time and fibrinogen

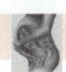

Table 11.3: Causes of DIC

DIC in obstetrics and gynecology	Other causes of DIC
Amniotic fluid embolism	Infections Bacterial (e.g. Gram-negative infection, meningococcal infection) Viral (HIV, cytomegalovirus, varicella) Fungal (histoplasma) Parasitic (malaria)
Placental abruption	Tissue trauma such as burns, accidents, surgery or shock Acute liver failure
	Incompatible blood transfusion or massive blood transfusion (more than the total circulatory volume
Pre-eclampsia	Venomous snake bites (e.g. saw-scaled vipers)
Eclampsia	
HELLP syndrome	
Retained fetus syndrome	Maligant disease (e.g. acute myelocytic leukemias)
Abortion	
Hydatidiform mole	
Amniocentesis	
Cesarean section	
Placenta accreta	
Ruptured uterus	
Retained placenta	
Gynecologic malignancy	
Ovarian, uterine and breast cancer	

levels. Decreased platelets, elevated FDPs or D-dimers, prolonged bleeding time and decreased fibrinogen are markers of DIC.

Differential diagnosis of DIC

- Air embolism
- Acute myocardial infarction
- Cardiomyopathy
- Anaphylaxis
- Aspiration pneumonitis should also be considered.

Treatment options for DIC syndrome

- Treat the underlying disease
- Avoid delay
- Treat vigorously (e.g. shock, sepsis, obstetrical problems)

Manage the DIC

Acute DIC

- Without bleeding or evidence of ischemia
- No treatment
- With bleeding
- Blood components as needed
- Fresh frozen plasma
- Cryoprecipitate
- Platelet transfusions
- With ischemia
- Anticoagulants
- Bleeding risk is corrected with blood products

Chronic DIC

- Without thromboembolism

- No specific therapy needed but prophy-lactic drugs (e.g. low-dose heparin, low-molecular-weight heparin)
- May be used for patients as high-risk of thrombosis with thromboembolism
- Heparin or low-molecular-weight heparin, trial of warfarin sodium.

Bick RL disseminated intravascular coagu-lation: A review of etiology pathophisiology, diagnosis and management: guidelines for care. Clin Appl Thrombosis/Homeostasis 2002; 8:1–31

HELLP SYNDROME

Incidence in pre-eclampsia ranges from 4–14%

Acronym of HELLP was first described in 1982 by Dr. Louis Winstein.

I Haemolysis

Hemolysis (H) elevated liver enzyme (EL) and low platelet count (LP) less than 1 lakh mm^3.

I Hemolysis: Red blood cells destruction as RBCs travel through constricted vessels causing anemia and changes in RBC morphology. Reduced O_2 carrying capacity.

Elevated bilirubin greater than 1.2 mg/dl and jaundice may also develop because of hemolysis of red blood cells.

II Elevated liver enzyme

Vasospasm decreases blood flow to the liver resulting in tissue ischemia and hemorrhagic necrosis.

Symptoms of hepatic damage include right upper quadrant or epigastric pain, nausea, vomiting and tenderness when liver is palpated.

Eventually, liver may rupture to cause sudden hypotension due to hemoperitoneum.

III Low platelets

Platelets aggregate at the site of damaged vas-cular endotheliun causing platelet consumption and thrombocytopenia.

Thrombocytopenia is considered as a platelet count less than 1 lakh mm^3.

S/S include bleeding gums, bruising, petechiae, bleeding from intravascular and from other sites.

Pathophysiology

I. Arteriolar vasospasm—damages the endo-thelial layer of small vessels—causing lesion
   a. These lesion allow formation of platelet aggregation and in turn a fibrin network.
   b. As RBCs are forced through the network under high pressure the cells are hemolysed.
II. Maternal hepatic damage results from microemboli in the liver
   a. Ischaemia and tissue damage results from the emboli
   b. Obstruction to the hepatic blood flow and fibrin deposits cause hepatic dis-tension
   c. Increasing intrahepatic pressure poten-tiates liver rupture (which is rare but often fatal).
III. Circulatory volume of platelets decreases as a result of an increase in consumption
   a. Circulatory platelet adhere to damaged endothelium
   b. As the platelets are consumed thrombo-cytopenia results.

Management

- Antiseizure prophylaxis with $MgSO_4$ is started/careful assessment of maternal and fetal status followed by delivery.
- Administration of corticosteroids improves perinatal and maternal outcome.
- Cesarean section is the common mode of delivery.
- Epidural anesthesia can be used safely if the platelet count is more than 1 lakh/mm^3
- Platelet transfusion should be given if the count is less than 50,000 mm^3.
- Patient should be managed in an ICU until there is improvement in platelet count, urine output, BP and liver enzymes.

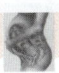

- Recurrence risk of "HELLP" syndrome is 3–10%
- Fresh frozen plasma may be needed if bleeding occurs and persists
- Delayed transfusion of packed RBCs is often necessary because of continued hemolysis.

POSTPARTUM HAEMORRHAGE

Postpartum haemorrhage is a life-threatening emergency with possible grave maternal outcome. According to WHO 5,29,000 women die annually due to the complications of pregnancy and childbirth.

Definition

- **Quantitative definition** is arbitrary and is related to the amount of blood loss in excess of 500 ml following the birth of the baby.
- **Clinical definition** states "any amount of bleeding from or into the genital tract following birth of the baby up to the end of puerperium which adversely affects the general condition of the patient evidenced by rise in pulse rate, and falling BP is called PPH.

Incidence

Incidence of PPH varies widely because lack of uniformity in definition and deficient data collection. Estimated incidence is 4–6% of all deliveries and the recurrence risk is 20–25%. PPH contributes to about 25% of all maternal deaths in India.

Types

Postpartum haemorrhage can be categorized as:

- Early or primary PPH
- Late or secondary PPH.

Primary PPH: is defined as blood loss from genital tract more than 500 ml in the first 24 hours of delivery (WHO).

Primary PPH has greater blood loss and morbidity and is more common.

Secondary PPH which occurs (24 hours to 6 wks) beyond 24 hours and within puerperium and also delayed or late PPH.

Primary PPH is divided into 2 types

Third stage haemorrhage: Where bleeding occurs before the expulsion of the placenta and

True PPH: Where bleeding occurs subsequent to the expulsion of placenta (majority).

Etiopathology

There are four primary causes of PPH.

The four Ts namely

- Tone (atonic uterus)
- Tissue (retained placenta)
- Trauma
- Thrombin (coagulation defects)

1. *Uterine atony:* Accounts for 90% of cases of PPH.

   The following are the conditions which often interfere with the retraction of the uterus as a whole and the placental site in particular.

   - Prolonged labour
   - Very rapid labour
   - Induced labour (use of high doses of oxytocin)
   - Over distended uterus
   - Large baby (wt. > 4 kg)
   - Multiple pregnancies
   - Hydramnios
   - Maternal factors
     - Increase age > 35 years
     - Increase parity
     - Obesity
     - Jaundice, hypertension
     - Fibroid uterus
   - Caesarean delivery
   - Chorioamnionitis
   - Previous history of PPH
   - Uterine inversion
   - Mismanaged III stage of labour

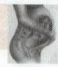

- Too rapid delivery
- Premature attempt to expel the placenta
- Pulling the cord
- Bladder not being evacuated
- Concealed bleeding

2. **Placenta related conditions**
   - Retained placenta
   - Succenturiate placenta
   - Placenta praevia
   - Morbid adhesions of the placenta

3. **Injury to the genital tract**
   - Extension of episiotomy
   - Paraurethral, vulval and vaginal tears
   - Cervical tears
   - Uterine rupture
   - Vulval and vaginal haematoma
   - Broad ligament haematoma
   - Retroperitoneal haemotoma

4. **Coagulation defects**
   - Abruptio placentae
   - Pre-eclampsia and HELLP syndrome
   - Amniotic fluid embolism
   - Sepsis
   - Intrauterine fetal death
   - Massive blood transfusion
   - Saline induced II trimester abortion.
   - Anticoagulant therapy
   - Idiopathic thrombocytopenic purpura
   - Liver disease

5. **Anemia**
   - Malnutrition/not taking iron supplements
   - Thalassaemia

PREDISPOSING FACTORS

Uterine atony and the possibility of immediate PPH in essentially normal women usually can be anticipated prior to delivery. The following conditions should alert the midwife to the potential of immediate PPH due to uterine atony.

- Over distended uterus
- Oxytocin induction or augmentation
- Rapid or precipitous labour and delivery
- Prolonged first and second stage of labour
- Grand multiparity
- History of uterine atony/PPH with previous childbearing.
- Use of uterine relaxing agents such as magnesium sulphate or terbutaline.

Clinical presentation

Clinical features depend on the antenatal haemoglobin levels and amount of bleeding leading to hypovolemia and acute anemia.

Diagnosis

In majority of cases profuse bleeding at the time of caesarean or after vaginal delivery makes. The diagnosis of PPH obvious. However, visual estimation of the amount of blood loss is always grossly inaccurate. Following methods have been proposed for estimation of blood loss at delivery.

- Collection of blood into bedpan or plastic bags
- A plastic calibrated drape and receptacle has been used to collect the blood.
- Weighing the sponges soaked in blood during C.S. and calculating the change in weight of the dry and soaked sponges.

Management

Principles of management is to ascertain the cause of bleeding and initiate prompt measures to control it. Interval between delivery, diagnosis of PPH and start of resuscitation with appropriate medical or surgical measures is an important prognostic factor for subsequent maternal morbidity and mortality associated with PPH.

Resuscitation

- It is important to work as a team, call for helps, summon senior obstetrician and anesthetist and enough staff. Alert blood bank and operation theatre of the emergency.
- Perform a quick but thorough physical examination
- Raise the foot end of the patient.
- Administer oxygen by mask.

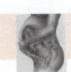

Table 11.4		
	Etiology process	**Clinical risk factors**
Abnormalities of Uterine **(tone)**	Overdistended uterus	Polyhydramnios multiple gestation contraction macrosoma
	Uterine muscle exhaustion	Rapid labour, prolonged labour, high parity
	Intra-amniotic infection	Fever, prolonged ROM
	Functional/Anatomic distortion of the uterus	Fibroid uterus, placenta previa Uterine anomalies
Retained products of conception **(tissue)**	Retained products Abnormal placenta Retained cotyledon or succinturiate lobe Retained blood clots	Incomplete placenta at delivery Previous uterine surgery High parity Abnormal placenta on ultrasonography Atonic uterus
Genital tract trauma **(trauma)**	Lacerations of the cervix, vagina or perineum Extensions, lacerations at C.S. Uterine rupture Uterine inversion	Precipitous delivery, operative delivery Malposition, deep engagement Previous uterine surgery High parity, fundal placenta
Abnormalities of coagulation **(thrombin)**	Pre-existing states hemophilia A Von Willebrand's disease Acquired in pregnancy Idiopathic thrombocytopenic purpura Thrombocytopenia with pre-eclampsia DIC pre-eclampsia dead fetus in utero Severe infection, abruption Amniotic fluid, embolus	H/o hereditary coagulation H/o liver diseases
	Therapeutic anticoagulation	H/o blood clot

- Secure intravenous access with at least 2 large bore IV cannula.
- Collect adequate sample, about 20 ml for blood grouping, cross-matching and complete blood counts, if necessary for coagulation profile.
- Arrange for at least 4–6 units of blood in severe bleeding and also for fresh frozen plasma and cryoprecipitate if coagulopathy is suspected.
- Start fluid replacement with rapid infusion of cystalloids like normal saline 0.9% or Ringer lactate solution to restore blood pressure. 5% dextrose solution is hypotonic and is not helpful for acute volume expansion. Colloids like albumin or Hartman's solutions may be used if there is delay in obtaining blood. Blood or blood component therapy should be initiated as soon as available.
- Self-retaining catheter should be inserted as full bladder interferes with contraction of uterus.
- Monitor vital signs, urine output, bleeding PV and fundal height. In severe bleeding monitoring by ECG, CVP line pulse oxymetry is necessary.

Prevention of PPH

I. Clinician should assess each woman's risk for PPH and make appropriate arrangements for her care.

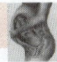

Table 11.5: Clinical presentation

	Mild bleeding	Moderate bleeding	Severe bleeding
Symptoms	Minimal	Fatigue Palpitations Restlessness	Drowsiness Disorientation Air hunger Fainting
Signs	Tachycardia pulse 100/ml	Pallor Tachycardia (110–120/ml) Low BP (postural hypotension)	Severe hypotension Tachypnoea Shock Anuria

Table 11.6: Clinical findings in PPH (Degrees of shock)

	Compensation	Mild	Moderate	Severe
Blood loss	500–1000 ml 10–15%	1000–1500 ml 15–25%	1500–2000 ml 25–35%	2000–3000 ml 35–45%
Blood pressure change (systolic)	None	Slight fall (80–100 mm Hg)	Marked fall (70–80 mm Hg)	Profound fall (50–70 mm Hg)
Symptoms and signs	Palpitations, dizziness and tachycardia	Weakness, sweating and tachycardia	Restlessness Pallor Oliguria	Collapse Air hunger Anuria

Uterotonic drugs

Routine oxytocin administration in 3rd stage of labour can reduce the risk of PPH by more than 40%. Administration of oxytocin is most beneficial in prevention of PPH and has not been demonstrated to increase the risk of retained placenta or the duration of the third stage of labour. Management of the 3rd stage of labour should therefore include the administration of oxytocin after the delivery of the anterior shoulder.

Effective protocols include 10 units IM, five units by IV push or 10–20 units per litre IV drip run at 100 to 150 cc/hr.

II. **Routine prophylactic oxytocin after delivery of the shoulder reduces the risk of PPH.**

III. **Third stage care should also include early cord clamping controlled cord traction with uterine palpation and inspection of** both the placenta and the lower genital tract.

Management of established PPH

Early recognition of PPH is a very important factor in management. One should routinely observe women after delivery for signs of excessive bleeding.

A stepwise approach to the management of Post partum haemorrhage.

Step 1: Initial assessment and treatment

- Resuscitation
  - Large bolus IV
  - Oxygen by mask
  - Monitor BP, P, R
  - Urine output
  - Catheter
  - O_2 saturation
- Assess etiology

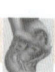

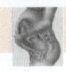

- Explore uterus (tone tissue)
- Explore lower genital tract (trauma)
- Review history (thrombin)
- observe clots
- Laboratory tests
  - CBC
  - Coagulation screen
  - Group and cross-matching

Step II: Directed therapy

- Tone
  - Massage
  - Compress
  - Drugs
- Tissue
  - Manual removal
  - Curettage
- Trauma
  - Correct inversion
  - Repair laceration
  - Identify rupture
- Thrombin
  - Reverse
  - Anticoagulation
  - Replace factors

Step III: Intractable PPH

- Get help
  - Obstetrician/surgeon
  - Anaesthesiologists
  - Lab and ICU
- Local control
  - Manual compression
  - Pack uterus
  - Vasopressin
  - embolization
- BP and coagulation
  - Crystalloid
  - Blood products

Step IV Surgery

- Repair laceration
- Ligate vessels
  - Uterines
  - Internal iliac artery

- Ovarians
- Hysterectomy

Step V: Post-hysterectomy bleeding

- Abdominal packing
- Angiographic embolization

IV **Initial treatment of PPH** includes early recognition followed by prompt attention to the resuscitation and a simultaneous search for the cause of bleeding. Baseline laboratory tests should be ordered.

V **The second step in the management of PPH** involves attention to the specific cause; proceed with massage, compression and medications for atony, evacuation of the uterus for retained blood clots and products of conception, physical repair of any trauma and reversal of coagulation defects.

VI **For the small proportion of women** not responding to the initial management steps a multidisciplinary team should be assembled including a second obstetrician or surgeon, anesthesiologist and the associated staff from the operating room, blood bank and intensive care unit. If invasive radiology services are available consideration may be given to angiographic embolization. While such arrangements are being made, blood loss should be minimized by compression, packing and or vasopressin. Fluid and blood component therapy must be continued to maintain haemodynamic and coagulation status.

Surgical approach (internal iliac artery ligation)

It involves identifying the bifurcation of the common iliac artery where ureter crosses it. A 5.8 cm incision is made in the peritoneum lateral and parallel to the line of the uterus. With the peritoneum open the ureter is then retracted medically and the artery is ligated 2.5 cm distal to the bifurcation of internal and external iliacs.

A right-angled clamp is passed gently behind the artery and appropriate nonabsorbable suture material is fed around the artery and two free ligatures tied 1.5 to 2 cm apart. External iliac artery and femoral pulse must be identified before and after tying the ligatures.

VII **The approach to interactable PPH** will be individualized depending on the clinical situation and the skills and the technology available. Continued monitoring and fluid and blood component replacement and use of all available expertise are essential.

VIII **Uterine vessel ligation**: Waters first described this procedure in 1952 and others have subsequently reported success rates of 80–90%. In this technique the uterine artery is ligated at the level where it runs along the uterine border beside the upper part of the lower uterine segment. Uterine vessel ligation may be effective in controlling PPH. Internal iliac artery ligation has been reported for use in PPH however its effectiveness is not yet proven. This procedure requires more extensive surgical skills and the situation may deteriorate if the iliac veins are injured

B-Lynch surgical technique for the control of massive PPH

Technique

1. The patient should be under general anaesthesia, is catheterized and placed in Lloyd-Davies position.
2. The Abdomen is opened or if the patient has had caesarean section following which she bleed, the same incision is reopened.
3. The uterine cavity is evacuated, examined and swabbed out.
4. The uterus is rechecked to identify any bleeding point. If the bleeding is diffused bimanual compression is first tried to assess the potential chance of success of the B-Lynch suturing technique. The vagina is swabbed out to confirm adequate control of bleeding.

Table 11.7: Drug therapy for PPH

Drug	Dose	Side effects	Contraindications
Oxytocin	10 units IM/ml 5 units IV bolus 10 to 20 units/litre	Usually none painful contractions nausea, vomiting (water intoxication)	Hypersensitivity to drug
Methylergonovine maleate	0.25 mg IM/0.125 mg IV repeat every 5 mins as needed maximum 5 doses	Peripheral vasospasm Hypertension Nausea, vomiting	Hypertension Hypersensitivity to drug
Carboprost (15-methyl PGF$_{2\alpha}$)	0.25 IM/ml repeat every 15 mins as needed maximum 8 doses	Flushing, diarrhea, nausea, vomiting bronchospasm, flushing, restlessness, Oxygen desaturation	Active cardiac Renal or Hepatic disease Hypersensitivity to drug
Vasopressin	20 units diluted in 100 ml normal saline = (0.2 units/ml) inject 1 ml at bleeding site avoid intravascular injection	Acute hypertension Bronchospasm, nausea vomiting, abdominal cramps angina, headache vertigo, death with intravascular injection	Coronary artery disease Hypersensitivity to drug

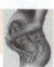

5. If bleeding is controlled , a 70 mm round body hand needle on which a No. 2 chromic catgut suture is mounted and is used to puncture the uterus 3 cm from the right lower edge of the uterine incision and 3 cm from the right lateral border.

6. The mounted No. 2 chromic catgut is threaded through the uterine cavity to emerge at the upper incision margin 3 cm above and 4 cm from the lateral border.

7. The chromic catgut now visible is passed over to compress the uterine fundus approximately 3 to 4 cm from the right cornual border.

8. The chromic catgut is pulled under moderate tension assisted by manual compression. The length of the catgut is passed back posteriorly through the same surface making as for the right side, the suture lying horizontally.

9. The two lengths of the catgut are pulled by the bimanual compression to minimize stroma and to achieve compression. During such compression the vagina is checked that the bleeding is controlled.

10. The lower transverse uterine incision is closed in a normal way in two layers with or without closure of the lower uterine segment peritoneum.

Emergency peripartum hysterectomy

Emergency peripartum hysterectomy is the most common treatment modality when massive postpartum haemorrhage requires surgical intervention.

Each year thousands of women die from PPH around the world. The prevention and management of postpartum haemorrhage are therefore very important aspects of maternity care. Clinicians should identify risk factors, take steps to prevent PPH and learn and employ as many of the above said management techniques.

Placenta accrete is defined as the abnormal adherence, either in whole or in part, of the afterbirth to the underlying uterine wall. The placental villi adhere into, or penetrate through the myometrium.

Pathology

Normally the decidua basalis lies between the myometrium and the placenta. The plane of cleavage for placental separations is in the spongy layer of the decidua basalis. In placenta accreta the decidua basalis is partially or completely absent, so that the placenta is attached directly to the myometrium. The villi may remain superficial to the uterine muscle or may penetrate it deeply. This condition is caused by a defect in the decidua rather than by any abnormal invasive properties of the trophoblast.

In the superficial area of the myometrium a large number of venous channels develop just beneath the placenta. Rupture of these sinuses by forceful extractions of the placenta is the source of the profuse hemorrhage that occurs.

Classification

1. By extent
   - *Complete:* The whole placenta is adherent to the myometrium

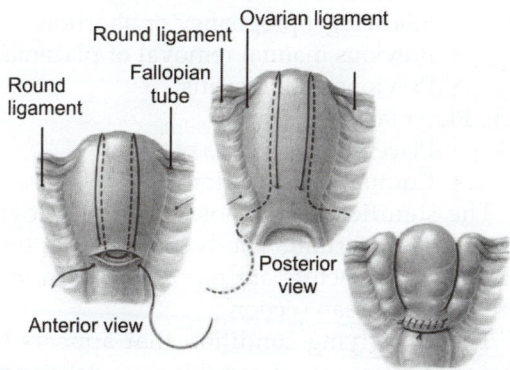

Fig. 11.19: B-Lynch surgical technique

 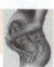

- Partial: one or more cotyledons or part of a cotyledon is adherent
2. By depth
  - *Accreta:* The placenta is adherent to the myometrium. There is no line of cleavage.
  - *Increta:* the villi penetrate the uterine muscle but not its full thickness.
  - *Precreta:* the villi penetrate the wall of the uterus and perforate the serosa. Intraperitoneal bleeding occurs frequently. Occasionally the uterus is ruptured. The villi may grow into the cavity of the bladder and cause gross hematuria.

Incidence

The true incidence is impossible to determine. The reported range varies from 1:540 to 1:93,000 deliveries.

Etiology

1. Maternal factors
   - Other gravidas
   - Multiparity. Placenta accreta is rare in primigravidas.
2. Uterine factors
   - Previous cesarean section. Often the placenta is implanted over the uterine scar.
   - Previous uterine surgery
   - Previous uterine curettage. Mainly following a pregnancy or abortion.
   - Previous manual removal of placenta.
   - Previous endometritis.
3. Placental factors
   - Placenta previa
   - Cornual implantation

The significance of most of the etiologic factors is uncertain. The two most frequent predisposing factors are placenta previa and previous cesarean section.

The underlying condition that appears to common to all casual conditions is deficiency of the endometrium and the decidua.

1. The decidua overlying the scar of a previous cesarean section is often deficient.
2. In women who have placenta previa the decidua of the lower uterine segment is relatively poorly developed.
3. The decidua of the uterine cornu is usually hypoplastic.
4. With increasing age and parity there is, in many women, a progressive inadequacy of decidua.
5. Previous curettage or manual removal of placenta is probably not an etiological but an indication that an abnormal adherence to the placenta was the reason for the precedure's being necessary.

CLINICAL PICTURE

Pregnancy

1. Most patients have a normal pregnancy
2. The incidence of antepartum bleeding is increased, but this is usually associated with placenta previa.
3. Premature labour occurs but only when precipitated by bleeding
4. Rarely rupture of the uterus takes place.

Labour: first and second page

These are normal in almost all cases

Third stage of labour

1. Retained placenta: this is the main and presenting feature.
2. Postpartum hemorrhage: The amount of bleeding depends on the degree of placental attachment. In complete placenta accreta there is no bleeding. In the partial variety bleeding takes place from the uterine vessels underlying the detached area, while the adherent portion prevents the uterus from retracting properly. Often the bleeding is precipitated by the obstetrician as he attempts manual removal of the placenta. In a recent report of 22 cases the average loss of blood was 3826 ml and

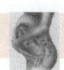

the mean amount of blood transfused was 8 units.

3. Uterine inversion: a rare but serious complication, is uterine inversion. This may occur spontaneously but is more often the result of attempts to remove the placenta.

4. *Rupture of the uterus:* This may occur during too vigorous attempts to extract the afterbirth.

Diagnosis

The gross diagnosis is provisional and is made in two ways:

1. *Direct intrauterine palpation:* No line of cleavage can be found between the placenta and uterus. The examining fingers slide over the fetal side of the placenta.

2. Study of the uterus and placenta following hysterectomy.

Microscopic examination established the diagnosis by demonstrating chorionic villi in the myometrium.

The different diagnosis includes

1. Retained incarcerated placenta
2. Adherent placenta where there is a line of cleavage
3. Retained placental fragments
4. Subinvolution of the placental site
5. Choriocarcinoma.

Management

The safest treatment is hysterectomy. Since this puts an end to child bearing, a conservative method of therapy has evolved based on the availability of blood and antibiotics. When placenta accreta is suspected, the following plan of management is useful.

Diagnosis and preliminary treatment

1. An intravenous infusion is started with a wide-bore needle.
2. Blood is cross-matched.
3. Expert anesthesia should be available.
4. The operating room must be ready for an emergency.

5. Intrauterine exploration is performed to see whether placenta accreta is present and if so whether it is complete or partial.

6. In making the diagnosis an attempt is made to remove the placenta. In most instances placenta accreta is not present. Overzealous attempts to extract the placenta must be avoided since the uterus can be ruptured.

Indication for hysterectomy

1. Further pregnancy is not desired
2. Uncontrolled hemorrhage
3. Failure of conservative management
4. Intrauterine suppuration
5. Placenta previa accreta

Conservative management (total placenta accreta)

1. There is no bleeding unless attempts are made to remove the placenta.
2. The cord is cut short and the blood drained from the placenta
3. The placenta is left in the uterus
4. Broad-spectrum antibiotics are given
5. The placenta becomes organised and partially absorbed, and the superficial portion sloughs off.
6. In some cases suppuration takes place and generalized infection may set in.

Conservative management (partial placenta accreta)

1. All separated placenta is removed manually. The part of the placenta that is abnormally attached is left.
2. An intravenous oxytocin infusion is maintained for 48 hours.
3. The patient is observed carefully and constantly.
4. Broad-spectrum antibiotics are given.
5. If there is no bleeding after 48 hours, the first stage of conservative management has been successful.

Vasa previa: Vasa previa occurs when the fetal blood vessels travel across the fetal membranes without any support from the umbilical cord and placental tissue. The blood vessels travel down across the lower part of the uterus right between the unborn child and the cervical opening. Vasa previa has a very high fetal mortality rate due to a number of reasons. The vessels can become pinched when compressed between the baby and the birth canal, or the vessels can actually tear and rupture.

Types of vasa previa: Multi-lobed placenta and velamentous insertion of the umbilical cord. Velamentous insertion occurs when the blood vessels traverse across the amniotic membranes finally meeting an umbilical cord.

Multi-lobed placenta vasa previa can cause harm to the mother, her child or birth. Symptoms of this disorder include bleeding during the first trimester of pregnancy and postpartum hemorrhaging when one lobe fails to separate upon birth. Risk factors for this type of vasa previa include smoking during pregnancy, pregnancy when the mother is over thirty-four, vomiting during the first trimester and diabetes.

VELAMENTOUS INSERTION OF THE UMBILICAL CORD

Normally, the veins of the baby run from the middle of the placenta via the umbilical cord to the baby. Velamentous insertion means that the veins, unprotected by Wharton's jelly, traverse the membranes before they come together into the umbilical cord.

The umbilical cord inserts on the placental mass in about 99% of cases. The insertion site may vary from the center of the fetal surface to the border of the placenta. The term velamen-

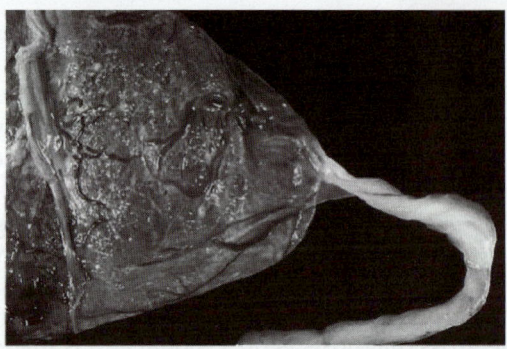

Fig. 11.20: Velamentous insertion of the umbilical cord

tous insertion is used to describe the condition in which the umbilical cord inserts on the chorioamniotic membranes rather than on the placental mass.

Therefore, a variable segment of the umbilical vessels runs between the amnion and the chorion, loosing the protection of the Wharton's jelly.

The incidence of this condition is about 1.1% in singleton pregnancies and 8.7% in twin gestations.

The most significant clinical problem arising from a velamentous insertion of the umbilical cord is vasa previa, a dangerous condition in which the velamentous umbilical vessels traverse the fetal membranes in the lower utrine segment below the presenting part. These unprotected vessels may rupture at any time during pregnancy, causing fetal exsanguination and death. Although spontaneous rupture has been reported before labour and with or without intact membranes, this accident occurs most often during amniotomy.

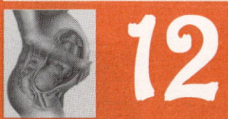

12

Obstetric Interventions and Operations

OUTLINE

- D and E
- Hysterotomy
- Version
- Episiotomy
- Forceps
- Ventouse
- Caesarean section
- Destructive operations in the fetus

Introduction

Obstetric operations are surgical procedures and as such irrespective of the nature of operation, asepsis and antiseptic precautions are to be taken.

The following preliminaries are to be followed with a few additions or alterations as and when required. These are:

1. *Anaesthesia:* Either general or local is used. In some cases, the operation may be performed with intravenous diazepam sedation.
2. *The patient is to be placed* in lithotomy position.
3. *Full surgical asepsis* is to be taken.
   a. Surgeon should wear sterile mask, gown and gloves.
   b. Vulva and vagina are to be swabbed with antiseptic solution.
   c. The perineum is to be draped by sterile towel and the legs with leggings.

4. *To empty the bladder:* If the patient is ambulant, she is asked to empty the bladder before she is placed on the table; otherwise catheterization is to be done.
5. *Vaginal examination* is done.

DILATATION AND EVACUATION

The operation consists of dilatation of the cervix and evacuation of the products of conception from the uterine cavity. The operation may be performed:

- *One stage:* Dilatation of the cervix and evacuation of the uterus are done in the same sitting.
- *Two stage*
  a. First phase includes slow dilatation of the cervix.
  b. Second phase includes rapid dilatation of the cervix and evacuation.

ONE STAGE OPERATION

Indications

1. Incomplete abortion (commonest)
2. Inevitable abortion
3. Medical termination of pregnancy (6–8 weeks)
4. Hydatidiform mole in the process of expulsion.

Procedures

Preliminaries: The steps to be followed are those mentioned earlier. The patient is put under general anaesthesia. Internal examination is done to note the size and position of the uterus and state of dilatation of the cervix.

Steps (incomplete abortion)

1. If the cervix is not sufficiently dilated to admit the index finger it should be dilated.
2. Posterior vaginal speculum is introduced and an assistant is asked to hold it. The anterior lip of the cervix is grasped by an Allis forceps to steady the cervix. The uterine sound is introduced to note the length of the uterine cavity and the position of the uterus.
3. The cervix is dilated up to the desired extent by the graduated metal dilators.
4. The products are removed by ovum forceps. The uterine cavity is finally curetted gently by a flushing (blunt) curette. Injection methergin 0.2 mg is to be administered intravenously.
5. The speculum and the Allis forceps are to be removed. The uterus is to be massaged bimanually with the help of the external hand and the internal fingers, placed inside the vagina.
6. After being satisfied that the uterus is remaining firm and the bleeding is minimal, the vagina and perineum are toileted; a sterile vulval pad is placed and the patient is sent back to her bed.

Post abortion care

- Emergency treatment of complications of any abortion spontaneous or induced
- Family planning counselling and referral services
- Linkages to other reproductive health services.

Medical termination of pregnancy in one stage: The procedure is similar to that followed in second phase of two stage operation. To prevent damage to the cervix during rapid dilatation, a two stage operation is, however, preferred in such cases.

TWO STAGE OPERATION

Indications

1. Induction of 1st trimester abortion (commonest)
2. Missed abortion (uterus 8–10 weeks)
3. Hydatidiform mole with unfavourable cervix (long, firm and closed os).

Procedures

1. First phase

It consists of introduction of laminaria tent into the cervical canal to affect its slow dilatation. The same may be effective by intravaginal prostaglandin E_2 gel 2 mg or pessary 3 mg into the posterior fornix at least 12 hours beforehand.

Steps of introduction of tents

The preliminaries to be followed are those mentioned earlier.

1. The patient should empty her bladder beforehand
2. No anaesthesia is required.
3. The appropriate size and number of the tent required are selected. The threads attached to one end are tied to the roller gauze.

Steps

1. Internal examination is done to note the size and position of the uterus and state of the cervix.
2. Posterior vaginal speculum is introduced and an assistant is asked to hold it. The anterior lip of the cervix is grasped by an Allis forceps to steady the cervix.
3. The cervical canal may have to be dilated especially in primigravidae by one or two smaller metal dilators (Hawkin Ambler– size 3/6 or 4/7) to facilitate the introduction of the tents.
4. The tents are introduced one after the other, holding it by tent introducing forceps. The tents should be introduced for at least 4 cm (1½") so that the tips are placed beyond the

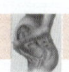

internal os. The tents can also be introduced manually.

5. The roller gauze is used to pack the upper vagina so as to prevent the displacement of the tents.

6. The patient is returned and preferably confined to her bed.

7. Prophylactic antibiotic is usually administered.

2. Second phase

It consists of further dilatation of the cervix by graduated metal dilators followed by evacuation of the uterus.

Procedures

- The patient is brought back to the operation theatre usually after 12 hours. The patient should empty her bladder beforehand.
- *Preliminaries:* The steps to be followed are those previously mentioned. The operation may be conducted under intravenous diazepam sedation, local paracervical block or under general anaesthesia.

Steps (MTP— 8 weeks)

1. The posterior vaginal speculum is introduced after removing the roller gauze. The tents are removed with the help of sponge holding forceps. The vagina and the cervix are swabbed with antiseptic solution. The posterior vaginal speculum is removed.

2. Vaginal examination is done to note once more the size of the uterus/position of the uterus and state of dilatation of the cervix.

3. Posterior vaginal speculum is reintroduced and is to be held by an assistant. The anterior lip of the cervix is to be grasped by the Allis forceps to steady the cervix. The uterine sound is to be introduced into the uterine cavity to ascertain the length of the cavity and position of the uterus.

4. The cervix is dilated with the graduated metal dilators up to the desired extent

(10/13 to 12/15) to facilitate introduction of the ovum forceps.

5. The products are removed by introducing the ovum forceps. Intravenous methergin 0.2 mg is to be given during this stage to minimize blood loss. Firm and well contracted uterus facilitates curettage.

6. The uterine cavity is thoroughly curetted by a flushing curette.

7. The posterior vaginal speculum and the Allis forceps are removed. The uterus is massaged bimanually and after being satisfied that the uterus is empty, the patient is sent to her bed after placing a sterile vulval pad.

8. Intramuscular methergin 0.2 mg may be repeated, and prophylactic antibiotic may be prescribed.

DANGERS OF D AND E OPERATION

Immediate

1. Excessive haemorrhage may be due to:
   a. Incomplete evacuation
   b. Atonic uterus
2. Injury
   a. Cervical lacerations of varying degree which may lead to formation of a broad ligament haematoma
   b. Uterine perforation
3. Shock may be due to:
   a. Uterine perforation
   b. Excessive blood loss
   c. Anaesthetic complications
4. Increased morbidity

Late

1. Pelvic inflammation
2. Infertility
3. Cervical incompetence
4. Uterine synechiae

Suction evacuation

It is a procedure in which the products of conception are sucked out from the uterus with the help of a cannula fitted to a suction apparatus.

Indications

1. Medical termination of pregnancy during first trimester (commonest)
2. Inevitable abortion.
3. Recent incomplete abortion
4. Hydatidiform mole.

Procedures

Preliminaries: General anaesthesia is usually not needed. If the patient is apprehensive, intravenous diazepam 5–10 mg supplemented by paracervical block is quite effective. The patient is put on the table after she empties her bladder.

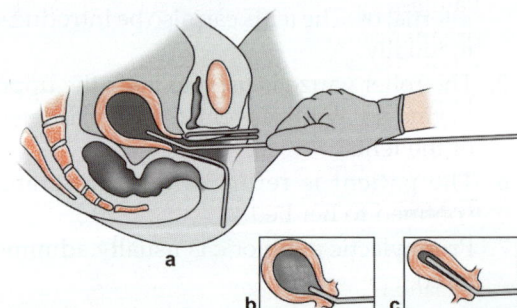

Fig. 12.1: Suction evacuation. **a.** Suction cannula attached to the pump is introduced into the uterine cavity, **b.** Size of the uterine cavity prior to aspiration, **c.** Reduction of uterine cavity following aspiration

Steps (Fig. 12.1)

1. Vaginal examination is done to note the size and position of the uterus and to note the state of cervix.
2. Posterior vaginal speculum is introduced and an assistant is asked to hold it.
3. The anterior lip of the cervix is to be grasped by an Allis forceps. A uterine sound is to be introduced to note the length of the uterine cavity and position of the uterus.
4. The cervix may have to be dilated with smaller size graduated metal dilators up to one size less than that of the suction cannula.
5. Intravenous methergin 0.2 mg is administered.
6. The appropriate suction cannula is fitted to the suction apparatus by a thick rubber or plastic tubing. The cannula is then introduced into the uterus, the tip is to be placed in the middle of the uterine cavity.
7. The pressure of the suction is raised to 400–600 mm Hg. The cannula is moved up and down and rotated within the uterine cavity with the pressure on.
8. The vacuum should be broken before withdrawing the cannula down through the cervical canal to prevent injury to the internal os.
9. It is better to curette the uterine cavity by a small flushing curette at the end of suction and the cannula is reintroduced to suck out any remnants.
10. After being satisfied that the uterus is remaining firm, and there is minimal vaginal bleeding, the patient is brought down from the table after placing a sterile vulval pad.

Complications

Similar complications as mentioned in D and E operation may occur. Use of a plastic cannula can minimize uterine perforation. Blood loss and incomplete evacuation are less likely with pregnancy of 8 weeks or less.

HYSTEROTOMY

Hysterotomy is an operative procedure extracting the products of conception out of the womb before 28th week by cutting through the anterior wall of the uterus. The operation is usually done through the abdominal route but can also be done vaginally.

Indications

- Medical termination of pregnancy (mid-trimester)
- Evacuation of a molar pregnancy

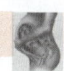

- Painless vaginal bleeding in midtrimester pregnancy with cervix remaining unfavourable. The bleeding is mostly due to low lying placenta.

Complications

- Immediate
- Remote

Immediate

- Uterine bleeding
- Peritonitis
- Intestinal obstruction
- Anaesthetic hazards. All these lead to increased morbidity and an occasional death.

Remote

- Menstrual abnormality—menorrhagia or irregular periods
- Scar endometriosis (1%)
- Scar rupture in subsequent pregnancy. While concurrent sterilization eliminates the hazards, but those left exposed to future pregnancy become a growing concern.

VERSION

Definition

It is a manipulative procedure designed to change the lie or to bring the comparatively favourable pole to the lower pole of the uterus.

Types

According to the methods employed, the following are the types:

- External
- Internal
- Bipolar

External: The manoeuvre is done solely by external manipulation.

Internal: The conversion is done principally by one hand introducing into the uterus and the other hand on the abdomen.

Bipolar (Braxton-Hicks): The conversion is done introducing one or two fingers through the cervix and the other hand on the abdomen.

In fact, all the manoeuvres are bipolar in the sense that both the poles of the fetus are to be manipulated to bring about conversion. *When the cephalic pole is brought down to the lower pole of the uterus, it is called cephalic version and when the podalic pole is brought down, it is called podalic version.*

EXTERNAL CEPHALIC VERSION

External cephalic version is done to bring the favourable cephalic pole in the lower pole of the uterus.

Indications

- Breech presentation
- Transverse lie

Selection of time, contraindication, difficulties and complications have already been described.

Procedures

In breech presentation

The manoeuvre is carried out after 35 weeks in the labour—delivery complex. *Any one of the following tocolytic drugs, if required, can be administered* by intravenous infusion. The maternal heart rate and blood pressure are measured every 5 minutes. A reactive NST should precede the manoeuvre.

Drugs: Terbutaline—0.25 mg SC or Isoxsuprine 50–100 µg/min IV could be used.

Preliminaries: The patient is asked to empty her bladder. She is to lie on her back with the shoulders slightly raised and the thighs slightly flexed. Abdomen is fully exposed. The obstetrician is to stand on the right side. The presentation, position of the back and limbs are checked and FHR is auscultated. Some use dusting powder on the abdomen to facilitate the hands to slide over the skin surface readily. The manipulation should be temporarily stopped during Braxton-Hicks contraction, and to be withheld, if the patient is in pain.

 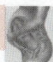

ACTUAL STEPS (Fig. 12.2)

Forward somersault movement

- *Step I:* The breech is mobilized using both hands to one iliac fossa towards which the back of the foetus lies. The podalic pole is grasped by the right hand in a manner like that of Pawlik's grip while the head is grasped by the left hand. If the breech is

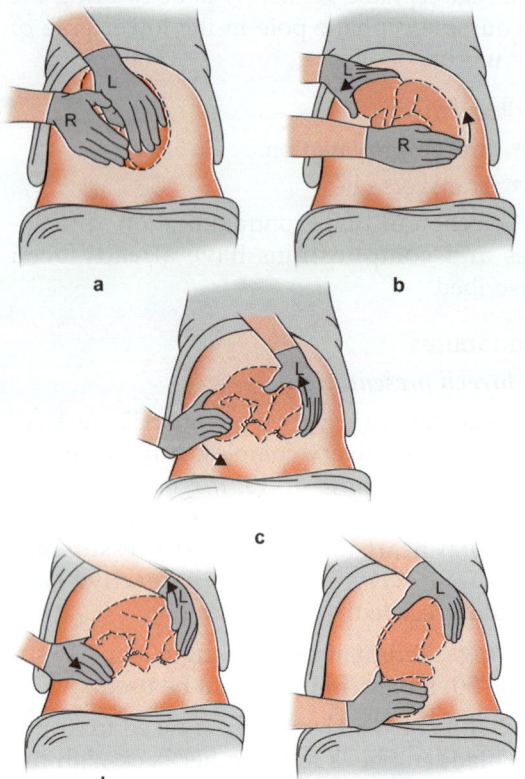

Fig. 12.2: Steps of external cephalic version. **a.** Mobilisation of the podalic pole to the iliac fossa towards which the back lies using both hands, **b.** Rotation of the trunk holding the poles both hands and maintaining flexion of the trunk, **c.** Change of hands to prevent crossing after the lie becomes transverse, **d.** Further mobilisation of the cephalic pole to bring it to the lower pole of the uterus, **e.** The lie becomes longitudinal with the cephalic pole being brought to the lower pole of the uterus.

engaged, it should be lifted up using both the hands. Rarely, the gloved fingers of an assistant may have to be introduced inside the vagina to push up the breech.

- *Step II:* The pressure is now exerted to the head and the breech in the opposite directions to keep the trunk well flexed which facilitates version. The pressure should be intermittent to push the head down towards the pelvis and the breech towards the fundus until the lie becomes transverse. The FHR is once more to be checked.

- *Step III:* The hand is now changed one after the other to hold the fetal poles to prevent crossing of the hand. The intermittent pressure is exerted till the head is brought to the lower pole of the uterus. As far as possible, the fetus should be allowed to turn by its own limb movements.

- *Step IV:* An attempt is made to push the head down to the brim. This may be difficult when the version is attempted in earlier period of gestation.

If the forward somersault technique fails, one may try hopefully the backward somersault technique.

A reactive NST should be obtained after completing the procedure: There may be undue bradycardia due to head compression which is expected to settle down by 10 minutes. If, however, fetal bradycardia persists, the possibility of cord entanglement should be kept in mind and in such cases reversion may have to be considered. *The patient is to be observed for about 30 minutes.*

1. To allow the FHR to settle down to normal.
2. To note for any vaginal bleeding or evidence of premature rupture of the membranes.

Instructions

1. The patient is advised to come on the next day to check the corrected position.

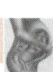

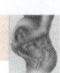

2. To report to the physician even earlier if there is vaginal bleeding or escape of liquor amnii or labour starts.

3. **Rh negative nonimmunized women must be protected** by intramuscular administration of 100 µg anti-D gamma globulin.

INTERNAL VERSION

Internal version is always a podalic version and is almost always completed with the extraction of the fetus.

Indications

Its only indication being the transverse lie in case of the second baby of twins.

However, it may be employed in singleton pregnancy to expedite delivery in adverse conditions where the caesarean section facilities are lacking. Such conditions are:

1. Transverse lie with cervix fully dilated
2. Cord prolapse with cervix fully dilated with transverse lie or head high up and the baby is alive.

Conditions to be fulfilled

The following conditions are to be fulfilled prior to internal version:

1. The cervix must be fully dilated.
2. Liquor amnii must be adequate for intrauterine fetal manipulation.
3. Fetus must be living.

Contraindications

It must not be attempted in neglected obstructed labour even if the baby is living.

Procedures

Preliminaries: The steps are to be followed as mentioned earlier. Patient should be deeply anaesthetized to make the uterus relaxed.

Actual steps

Step I: Introduction of the head

If the podalic pole of the fetus is on the left side of the mother, the right hand is to be introduced

and vice versa. The hand is to be introduced in a cone shaped manner. It is then pushed up into the uterine cavity keeping the back of the hand against the uterine wall until the hand reaches the podalic pole. If a hand is prolapsed outside, it is smeared with antiseptic solution and replaced inside the uterus.

Step II: The hand is to pass up to the breech and then along the thigh until a foot is grasped. During this procedure, the podalic pole may be made accessible by the external hand depressing the podalic pole. The identification of the foot is done by palpation of the heel. It is preferable to bring down the anterior or lower leg first but is not disadvantageous to grasp the first foot which one encounters.

Step III: While the leg is brought down by a steady traction, the cephalic pole is pushed up using the external hand.

Step IV: After one leg is brought down, there is no difficulty to deliver the other leg. The delivery is usually completed with breech extraction.

Step V: Routine exploration of the uterovaginal canal to exclude rupture of the uterus or any other injury.

Hazards

Maternal risk includes placental abruption, rupture of the uterus and increased morbidity. The fetal risk includes asphyxia cord accident and intracranial haemorrhage apart from all hazards of breech delivery leading to a high perinatal mortality of about 50%.

EPISIOTOMY

Episiotomy is a surgical incision of the perineum that is made both to prevent tearing of the perineum and to release pressure on the fetal head with birth. The advantage of an episiotomy is that it substitutes a clean cut for a ragged tear.

Definition

A surgically planned incision on the perineum and the posterior vaginal wall during the second stage of labour is called episiotomy (perineo-tomy).

Objectives

- **To enlarge** the vaginal introitus so as to facilitate easy and safe delivery of the fetus - spontaneous or manipulative.
- **To minimise** overstretching and rupture of the perineal muscles and fascia; to reduce the stress and strain on the fetal head.

Indications

- *Anticipating perineal tear*
  1. This is widely indicated in primigravidae as an elective procedure.
  2. Other indications are face to pubis or face delivery, big baby, narrow pubic arch.
- *Inelastic perineum*
  1. Elderly primigravida
  2. Old perineal scar of episiotomy or perineorrhaphy.
- *Manipulative delivery:* This is needed to get more space for operative or manipulative delivery such as forceps, breech or internal version especially in primigravidae.
- *To cut short the second stage:* In heart disease, severe pre-eclampsia or eclampsia, post caesarean cases, postmaturity, etc.
- *Fetal interest*
  1. Fetal distress
  2. Premature baby—to minimise compression of the soft and pliable skull bones thereby preventing intracranial damages.
  3. Breech delivery—to minimise compression of the after coming head and to facilitate manipulation, if required.

Common indications

1. Threatened perineal injury in primigravidae
2. Rigid perineum
3. Forceps, breech, occipitoposterior or face delivery.

Timing of the episiotomy: Bulging thinned perineum during contraction just prior to crowning is the ideal time.

Types

The following are the various types of episiotomy:
- Mediolateral
- Median
- Lateral
- 'J' shaped

Mediolateral: The incision is made downwards and outwards from the midpoint of the fourchette either to the right or left. It is directed diagonally in a straight line which runs about 2.5 cm away from the anus.

Median: The incision commences from the centre of the fourchette and extends posteriorly along the midline for about 2.5 cm.

Lateral: The incision starts from about 1 cm away from the centre of the fourchette and extends laterally.

'J' shaped: The incision begins in the centre of the fourchette and is directed posteriorly along the midline for about 1.5 cm and then directed downwards and outwards along 5 or 7 O'clock position to avoid the anal sphincter.

STEPS OF MEDIOLATERAL EPISIOTOMY

Structures cut

1. Posterior vaginal wall
2. Superficial and deep transverse perineal muscles, bulbospongiosus and part of levator ani.
3. Fascia covering those muscles
4. Transverse perineal branches of pudendal vessels and nerves
5. Subcutaneous tissue and skin.

Repair

Timing of repair: The repair is done soon after the expulsion of placenta. If repair is done prior to that, disruption of the wound is inevitable, if subsequent manual removal or exploration of the genital tract is needed. Oozing during this period should be controlled by pressure with a sterile gauze swab and bleeding by the artery forceps. Early repair prevents sepsis and

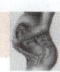

eliminates the patient's prolonged apprehension of 'stitches'.

Preliminaries: The patient is placed in lithotomy position. A good light source from behind is needed. The perineum including the wounded area is cleansed with antiseptic solution. Blood clots are removed from the vagina and the wounded area. The patient is draped properly and repair should be done under strict aseptic precautions. If the repair field is obscured by oozing of blood from above, a vaginal pack may be inserted and is placed high up. Do not forget to remove the pack after the repair is completed.

Repair: The repair is done in three layers. The principles to be followed are:

1. Perfect haemostasis
2. To obliterate the dead space
3. Suture without tension

The repair is to be done in the following order

1. Vaginal mucosa and submucosal tissues
2. Perineal muscles
3. Skin and subcutaneous tissues.

POSTOPERATIVE CARE

Dressing: The wound is to be dressed each time following urination and defaecation to keep the area clean and dry. The dressing is done by swabbing with cotton swabs soaked in antiseptic solution followed by application of antiseptic powder or ointment (Furacin or Neosporin). The state of healing is attested by observing for redness, edema, ecchymosis, discharge and approximation (REEDA scale)

Comfort: To relieve pain in the area, application of heat or cold, sitz bath may be used. Analgesic drugs (aspirin) may be given as and when required.

Ambulance: The patient is allowed to move out of the bed after 24 hours.

Complications

- Immediate
- Remote

Immediate

1. **Extension of the incision** to involve the rectum.
2. **Vulval haematoma**
3. **Infection:** The clinical features are:
   - Throbbing pain on the perineum
   - Rise in temperature
   - The wounded area looks moist, red and swollen
   - Offensive discharge comes out through the wounded margins.

Treatment

- To facilitate drainage of pus by cutting one or two stitches
- Local dressing with antiseptic powder or ointment
- Magnesium sulphate compression or application of infrared heat to the area to reduce oedema and pain
- Systemic antibiotic.

4. *Wound dehiscence:* Infection is the principal cause of wound disruption or non-union. The wound should be dressed daily until the local infection subsides and healthy granulation tissue forms in the margins. Secondary sutures are given under local anaesthesia using cutting needle and nylon.

Remote

1. **Dyspareunia:** This is due to a narrow vaginal introitus which may result from faulty technique of repair or due to painful perineal scar.
2. **Chance of perineal lacerations** in subsequent labour, if not managed properly.

FORCEPS

Obstetric forceps is a pair of instruments specially designed to assist extraction of the head and thereby accomplishing delivery of the fetus.

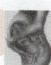

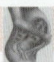

Varieties of obstetric forceps

Ever since either Peter I or Peter II of the Chamberlain family invented the forceps around AD 1600, many designs were invented or modified. But only three varieties are commonly used in present day obstetric practice.

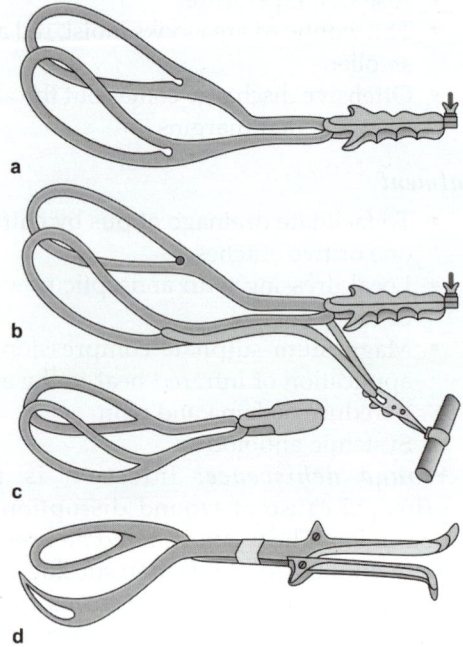

Fig. 12.3: Different types of obstetric forceps currently used. **a.** Long curved with axis traction device, **b.** The same with attached axis traction device, **c.** Wrigley's, **d.** Kielland's

These are

- *Long curved forceps with or without axis traction device*
- Short curved forceps
- *Kielland's forceps*

The basic construction of these forceps is the same in that each consists of two halves (blades) articulated by a lock.

LONG CURVED OBSTETRIC FORCEPS

Long curved obstetric forceps is relatively heavy and is about 37 cm (15") long.

Measurements: Length is 37 cm, distance in between the tips is 2.5 cm and widest diameter between the blades is 9 cm.

Blades

There are two blades and *are named right or left in relation to maternal pelvis in which they lie when applied. Each blade consists of the following parts:*

1. Blade
2. Shank
3. Lock
4. Handle with or without screw

Blade: The blade is fenestrated to facilitate a good grip of the fetal head. There is usually a slot in the lower part of the fenestrum of the blades to allow the upper end of the axis traction rod to be fitted.

The blade has got two curves

- *Pelvic curve:* The curve on the edge is to fit more or less the curve on the axis of the birth canal
- *Cephalic curve:* It is the curve on the flat surface which when articulated grasps the fetal head without compression.

Shank: It is the part between the blade and the lock. It increases the length of the instrument and thereby, facilitates locking of the blades outside the vulva.

Lock: The common method of articulation consists of a socket system located on the shank at its junction with the handle.

Handle: The handles are opposed when the blades are articulated. There is a finger guard on which a finger can be placed during traction.

A screw may be attached usually at the end (or at the base) of one blade (commonly left). It helps to keep the blades in the position.

Axis traction device

It can be applied with advantage in mid forceps operation, especially following manual rotation of the head. It provides traction in the correct

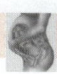

axis of the pelvic curve and as such, less force is necessary to deliver the head.

It consists of

1. Traction rods (two-right and left)
2. Traction handle

SHORT CURVED OBSTETRIC FORCEPS

The instrument is lighter, about a third of the weight of an ordinary long curved forceps. *The instrument is short which is due to reduction in the length of the shanks and handles.* It has a marked cephalic curve with a slight pelvic curve.

KIELLAND'S FORCEPS

It is a long straight (very slight pelvic curve) obstetric forceps without any axis traction device.

Indications of forceps operation

- *Delay in the second stage:* The forceps operation is commonly indicated for delay in the second stage of labour due to uterine inertia.
- *Fetal indications*
  1. Appearance of fetal distress in the second stage when prospect of vaginal delivery is safe.
  2. Cord prolapse
  3. Aftercoming head of breech
  4. Low birth weight baby
  5. Postmaturity
- *Maternal indications*
  1. Maternal distress
  2. Preeclampsia
  3. Post-caesarean pregnancy
  4. Heart disease

Conditions to be fulfilled prior to forceps operation

The following criteria are to be fulfilled prior to forceps applications:

- *Presentation and positions must be a suitable one* so as to apply the blades correctly to the sides of the head. Vertex, anterior face and aftercoming head are the ideal presentations.
- *The cervix must be fully dilated and effaced.*
- *Membranes must be ruptured.*
- *The head must be engaged* with no parts of the head palpable abdominally.
- *There should not be undue obstruction,* bony or otherwise at or below the station of the head.
- *Baby should be living.*
- *Uterus should be preferably contracting and relaxing* as a safeguard to postpartum haemorrhage.
- *The bladder must be emptied.*

Success of the operation depends on

1. Meticulous observation on the principles as laid down prior to forceps application.
2. Pre-application maternal and fetal health status.
3. Competence of the surgeon
4. Amenities available.

Types of forceps operation

The operations are classified according to the station of the fetal head at which the forceps are applied (Fig. 12.4).

- *High forceps operation* refers the application of the forceps in a fetal head where

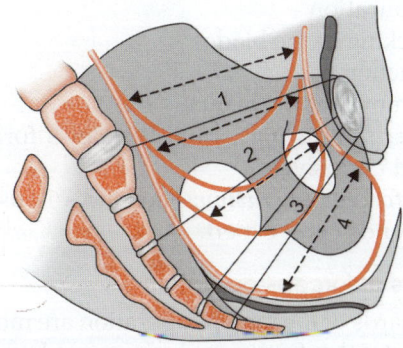

Fig. 12.4: Different types of forceps operation. 1. High forceps, 2. and 3. Mid forceps, 4. Low forceps

the biparietal diameter has not yet passed the plane of the pelvic inlet (non-engaged head). This type of forceps operation has long been abandoned in preference to caesarean section.

- *Mid forceps operation* refers to the application of the forceps where the biparietal diameter has passed the plane of the inlet but has not passed the level of ischial spines. It may be described with two sub varieties:
- *High mid:* Biparietal diameters has passed the plane of inlet but remains above the level of ischial spines.
- *Low mid:* Biparietal diameters has passed the plane of the inlet and lies at the level of ischial spines. So, the lower pole lies below the level of ischial spine.
- *Low forceps operation* refers to the application of the forceps where the biparietal diameter has passed the level of ischial spines.
- *Outlet forceps:* It is a variety of low forceps operation, where the forceps are applied on the fetal head lying on the perineum and is visible at the introitus in between contractions.

Thus, while all outlet forceps are low forceps but not all low forceps are outlet forceps operation.

Steps of low forceps operation

- Identification of the blades and their application
- Locking of the blades
- Traction
- Removal of the blades

Outlet forceps operation: Wrigley's forceps are used exclusively.

Mid forceps operation: Kielland's is useful in the hands of an expert.

Dangers of forceps operation

The hazards of the forceps operation are mostly related to the faulty technique and to the indication for which the forceps are applied rather than the instrument. *The hazards are grouped into*

- Maternal
- Fetal

Maternal

- Immediate
- Remote

Immediate: **The immediate complications are:**

- *Injury*
  - Extension of the episiotomy externally even to involve the rectum or its upward extension up to the vault of vagina
  - Vaginal lacerations
  - Cervical tear especially when applied through an incompletely dilated cervix
- *Postpartum haemorrhage:* due to
  - Trauma
  - Atonic uterus due to prolonged labour or effect of anaesthesia
- *Shock:* due to
  - Blood loss
  - Prolonged labour and dehydration
- *Sepsis:* due to improper asepsis and devitalisation of the local tissues
- *Anaesthetic hazards*

Remote

- *Chronic low backache:* Due to tension imposed on the softened ligaments guarding the lumbosacral or sacroiliac joints during lithotomy position.
- *Genital prolapse or stress incontinence:* This may occur specially when the head is dragged down through incompletely dilated cervix or in unrotated position or due to faulty repair of perineal lacerations.

Fetal

- Immediate
- Remote

Immediate

- Asphyxia due to intracranial stress out of prolonged compression

- *Rooting:* Touching or stroking the cheek along the side of mouth causes infant to turn head toward that side and begin to suck; should disappear at about 3–4 months, but may persist for up to 12 months.
- *Extrusion:* When tongue is touched or depressed, infant responds by forcing it outward; disappears by age of 4 months.

Extremities

- *Grasp:* Touching palms of hands or soles of feet near base of digits causes flexion of hands and toes. Palmar grasp lessens after age of 3 months, to be replaced by voluntary movement; plantar grasp lessens by 8 months of age.
- *Babinski:* Stroking outer sole of foot upward from head and across ball of foot causes toes to hyperextend and hallux to dorsiflex; disappears after age of 1 year.

Nursing diagnoses

- Airway clearance, ineffective, related to mucus obstruction
- Hypothermia related to body heat loss
- Risk for infection, related to newborn's susceptibility to pathogens
- Urinary elimination, altered, related to circumcision.

Mass

- *Moro:* Sudden jarring or change in equilibrium causes sudden extension and abduction of extremities and fanning of fingers, with index finger and thumb forming a C shape, followed by flexion and adduction of extremities, legs may weakly flex; infant may cry; disappears after age of 3–4 months usually strongest during first 2 months.
- *Startle:* A sudden loud noise causes abduction of the arms with flexion of elbows, hands remain clenched; disappears by age of 4 months.

- *Asymmetric tonic neck:* When infant's head is turned to one side, arm and leg extend on that side, and opposite arm and leg flex; disappears by age of 3–4 months, to be replaced by symmetric positioning of both sides of body.
- *Trunk incurvation:* Stroking infant's back alongside spine causes hips to move toward stimulated side; disappears by age of 4 weeks.

MINOR AILMENTS OF NEWBORN

Stuffy nose

It may lead to mouth breathing and excessive air swallowing which in turn may lead to abdominal distension and vomiting. The nostrils may be cleansed with cotton wool soaked in normal saline.

Sticky eyes

It may be due to a chemical irritant or bacterial conjunctivitis due to *Staphylococcus.* Use of erythromycin (0.5%) ointment every 6 hours for 7–10 days cures the condition.

Skin rash

- *The common form of skin rash is blotchy erythematous* located on the trunk, limbs and face. They disappear within a day or two. Pustules are rare. No treatment is required.
- *Napkin rash (ammonia dermatitis):* It is more common in artificially fed babies. It can be prevented by frequent care and attention to the napkin area along with immediate changes of the napkins after each soiling.
- *Perianal dermatitis:* It is situated around the anal opening. It is due to the alkalinity of the stool and is met in artificially fed babies. Use of lactose, instead of glucose, cures the state.
- *Thrush:* It produces a rash in the napkin area. The buttocks and the inner side of the thighs are also affected. Treatment with

1% gentian violet solution or nystatin suspension (100,000 units/ml), applied to each side of the mouth with a cotton-tipped swab 3–4 times a day is effective.

Congenital phimosis

Pinpoint prepuce which makes the baby cry during act of micturition, requires dilatation by mosquito forceps.

Genital crisis

Mastitis neonatorum, hydrocele of the newborn developed in the neonatal period, or vaginal bleeding during first week require no treatment apart from assurance to the mother.

Physiological jaundice

This is observed in 60% of the term and 80% of preterm neonates.

Constipation

It is commonly met in artificially fed babies. Correction of the diet and extra water is usually effective. If it fails, milk of magnesia 4 ml by mouth is effective. Insertion of a catheter or a suppository into the rectum is to be avoided.

PRETERM BABY

DEFINITION

Preterm baby weighs less than 2.5 kg at birth and is less than 259 completed days, born before 37 completed weeks of gestation calculating from the first day of last menstrual period and is arbitrarily defined as preterm baby. Babies born before 37 completed weeks usually weigh 2500 gm or less.

INCIDENCE

Preterm baby constitutes two-thirds of low birth weight babies. The incidence of low birth weight baby is about 30–40% in the developing countries, as such the incidence of preterm baby is about 20–25%. In affluent societies and in the developed countries, the incidence of the former is less than 10%.

FEATURES OF PRETERM BABY

Physical

1. **Birth weight less than 2.5 kg**
2. Birth length (crownheel) less than 47 cm.
3. **Head, trunk,** head circumference is less than 33 cm, *3 cm bigger than chest circumference*. Abdomen is protruberant. Subcutaneous fat is poor, baby looks red. *Vernix is abundant*. It begins to disappear after 36 weeks till it clears at 41 weeks. Lanugo hair is present especially on back and limbs. Skull bones are soft and sutures are widely separate.
4. **Eyes:** Eye lids fuse during third month of foetal life and do not reopen till 28–30 weeks. Thus eyes are more closed.
5. **Genitals:** In male, *testes may remain undescended,* scrotum poorly developed. In female, *labia majora are poorly developed,* do not cover labia minora.

Functional

1. **Central nervous system:** *Immaturity of CNS* → inactive and lethargy → cry is weak and feeble. Suckling and swallowing reflexes are poorly developed until 34 week.
2. **Respiratory system:** Ribs are very soft → *inspiratory insuction due to negative intrathoracic pressure.* Deficiency of pulmonary surfactant in pulmonary alveoli hampers alveolar expansion. Resuscitation difficulties → often *hyaline membrane disease.*
3. **Cardiovascular system:** Before 34 weeks ductus arteriosus remains patent in one-third.
4. **Gastrointestinal system:** Poor suckling and swallowing → poor self feeding. *Regurgitation and aspiration* are common, because of incoordinated sucking, swallow-

Table 14.1: Determination of gestational age by physical criteria

Criteria	36 weeks or less	37 to 38 weeks	39 weeks or more
Sole creases	Only anterior 1/3 transverse crease	Occasional creases anterior 2/3	Sole covered with creases
Breast nodule diameter	2 mm	4 mm	7 mm
Scalp hair	Fine and fuzzy	Fine and fuzzy	Coarse and silky
Ear lobe	Pliable, no cartilage	Some cartilage	Stiffened by thick cartilage
Genitalia	Small scrotum, few rugae, prominent labia minora	Intermediate	Full scrotum, full rugae, labia majora prominent

ing small capacity of stomach and poor cough reflex.

Immaturity of glucuronyl transferase system in liver→hyperbilirubinaemia. Hypoglycaemia develops due to poor hepatic glycogen store, delayed feeding, birth asphyxia and respiratory distress syndrome.

5. **Hypothermia** occurs when axillary temperature drops below 36.5°C (97.7°F). Preterm baby is prone to hypothermia.

6. **Infection:** Low level of IgG and inefficient cellular immunity make infection prone.

7. **Renal function:** Blood urea nitrogen is high due to poor glomerular filtration rate.

8. Biochemical disturbances are *hypoglycaemia, hypocalcaemia, hypoprotenaemia, hypoxia and acidosis.*

9. *Nutrition handicaps:* Baby develops anaemia by 6–8 weeks due to poor iron store.

Complications

- *Asphyxia:* The babies are likely to be asphyxiated because of anatomical and functional immaturity.
- *Hypothermia:* A low birth weight baby has reduced subcutaneous as well as brown fat.
- *Pulmonary syndrome:* This includes:
  - Pulmonary oedema
  - Intra-alveolar haemorrhage
  - Idiopathic respiratory distress syndrome (RDS). The first two are the effects of

hypoxia; RDS is one of the major causes of death.

- *Cerebral haemorrhage:* The causes are:
  - Soft skull bones allow dangerous degree of moulding leading to subdural or subarachnoid haemorrhage.
  - Fragile subependymal capillaries cannot withstand minor degree of hypoxia leading to intraventricular haemorrhage.
  - Associated hypoprothrombinemia.
- *Fetal shock:* Apart from the shock sustained during delivery, it may appear following improper resuscitative manipulation during the first day or second.
- *Heart failure:* It may be precipitated by asphyxia with rapid development of pulmonary oedema which in turn impairs pulmonary aeration and aggravates pulmonary oedema.
- *Oliguria, anuria:* As the immature kidneys are unable to handle water, solute and acid loads.
- *Infection:* Both the humoral and cellular immune response is poor. The common types of infection are bronchopneumonia, meningitis and gastroenteritis.
- *Jaundice:* Because of hepatic insufficiency, the bilirubin produced by the excessive haemolysis cannot be conjugated adequately for excretion as bile, leading to rise in unconjugated bilirubin which is

responsible for exaggerated physiological jaundice.

- *Dehydration and acidaemia* occur due to immature renal function may occure abruptly.
- *Anaemia:* Lack of stored iron, hypofunction of the bone marrow and excessive haemolysis all contribute to anaemia.
- Retinopathy of prematurity is a multifactorial disorder of the retina caused by abnormal neovascularisation. It is an important cause of blindness for the children under 6 years. The cause is mostly related to the liberal administration of high concentration of oxygen above 40% for a prolonged period (1–2 days) following birth.

Prognosis

The chance of survival is directly related to the birth weight. A baby weighing more than 1500 gm is most likely (95%) to survive. With intensive neonatal care the survival rate of the baby weighing 751–1000 gm is to the extent of 80%.

Management

- Prevention of prematurity
- Management of preterm labour
- Care of preterm baby afterbirth

The prevention of prematurity and the management of preterm labour (refer pg. 278).

CARE OF THE PRETERM NEONATE

Immediate management following birth

- The cord is to be clamped quickly to prevent hypervolaemia and development of hyperbilirubinemia.
- The cord length is kept long (about 10–12 cm) in case exchange transfusion is required.
- The air passage should be cleared of mucus promptly and gently using a mucus sucker.
- Adequate oxygenation through mask or nasal catheter in concentration not exceeding 35%.

- The baby should be wrapped including head in a sterile warm towel (normal temperature 36.5°–37.5°C).
- Aqueous solution of vitamin K 1 mg is to be injected intramuscularly to prevent haemorrhagic manifestations.

Intensive care protocol

Those requiring "special care" are judged by:
1. Inability to suckle the breast and to swallow
2. Incapacity to regulate the temperature within limited range from 96°–99°F (35.6°–37.2°C)
3. Inability to control the cardiorespiratory function without cyanotic attacks.

The principles that are to be taken for the babies requiring special care are

- To maintain a relatively stable thermoneutral condition. Keep delivery room warm, dry and then wrap the baby with a warm towel, keep the baby with mother skin to skin contact.
- Adequate humidification to counterbalance increased insensible water loss.
- Oxygen therapy and adequate ventilation
- To prevent infection
- To maintain nutrition and adequate nursing care

To maintain body temperature: As the premature babies are extremely thermolabile, they can easily develop hyperpyrexia or hypothermia. The rectal temperature should be between 96° and 99°F (35.6°–37.2°C).

The smaller babies are best placed in the incubator where temperature and humidity can be better stabilized. The skin temperature should be maintained at 36°–37°C with surrounding humidity at least 50%.

Respiratory support: To tide over the initial cyanotic phase, measures are taken to clear the air passage and to administer oxygen. The baby is placed in the incubator with oxygen running alternatively. Baby's head is kept in an oxygen head box for prolonged oxygen therapy. Some

of the neonates may initially require endo-tracheal intubation and mechanical ventilation. Ventilatory status is monitored by blood gas sampling at regular intervals. Continuous oxygen monitoring is done by pulse oximeter. Desirable level of arterial blood gas values should be (i) PaO_2 55–56 mm Hg, (ii) $PaCO_2$ 35–45 mm Hg and (iii) PH 7.35–7.45 and pulse oximeter reading should be 90–92% oxygen saturation.

Infection: The main sites of infection are respiratory tract, gastrointestinal tract, skin and the umbilicus.

Prophylactic antibiotic therapy is to be given when the babies are born following premature rupture of the membranes. The common antibiotics used are Ampicillin 100 mg/kg per day Amikacin 10 mg/kg per day to be given intramuscularly in two divided doses for 5–7 days.

Nutrition: Preterm infants are often unable to suck and swallow. Enteral feeding may be possible depending on gestation age and vigour. Babies may require gavage feeding or parenteral nutrition. Human milk is the first choice of nutrition for all low birth weight babies.

Commencement: Early feeding between 1 and 2 hours of birth is now widely recommended. It eliminates hypoglycaemia, lowers serum bilirubin and neurological sequelae.

Intervals: Depending upon the birth weight, the interval of feeding ranges from hourly in extreme prematurity to 3 hourly feeds in babies born after 36 weeks.

Methods: The methods used depend on the size and vigour of the infant and his ability to suck and swallow. Thus, while a comparatively bigger baby with vigour can be put to the breast right from the beginning, the smaller one should be fed by any of the following methods:

- Tube (gavage)
- Pipette, dropper, katori and spoon
- Bottle
- Intravenous

Fluid requirement varies from 60–80 ml/kg/day of 10% dextrose water on first day and to increase by 15 ml/kg/day. Amount should be more, if phototherapy is used. Monitoring of fluid is done by measuring body weight, urine output, its specific gravity and serum sodium.

Position: The baby, when fed in a cot, should be placed on one side with the head raised a little to prevent regurgitation.

Adequate nursing care: The most important single factor is high standard of nursing and one trained nurse can adequately take care of two or three infants.

1. The temperature should be taken twice daily and the baby should be weighed daily to know whether over or undehydrated.
2. Constant supervision especially during the crucial first 48 hours, is imperative.
3. Mother should be allowed to keep her baby in the nursery.
4. Mother is taught for the general care of the baby and manual expression of breast milk by pressing over the areola and the nipple.

Favourable signs of progress

The following are the favorable signs

1. The colour of the skin remains pink all the time.
2. Smooth and regular breathing.
3. Increasing vigour evidenced by:
   1. Movement of the limbs
   2. Cry
4. Progressive gain in weight. Baby looses 1–2% weight everyday for the first 5–7 days. Thereafter baby gains 1–1.5% of birth weight daily. Baby regains birth weight by 10–14 days.

When to discharge?

The premature babies are discharged

1. When they attain sufficient weight
2. Attain good vigour
3. Able to suckle the breast successfully

KANGAROO CARE FOR PRETERM INFANTS

Kangaroo care consists of placing a diaper clad premature baby in an upright position on a parent's bare chest-tummy to tummy, in between the breasts. The baby's head is turned so that the ear is above the parent's heart. Due to lack of power and reliable equipment, Kangaroo care was found to be an inexpensive and very beneficial experience to premature babies.

The most common factor associated with neonatal death is prematurity. The preterm infants, regardless of birth weight, are those delivered before 37 weeks from the first day of the last menstrual period. Prematurity and low birth weight usually occur together, both carrying a high rate of morbidity and mortality, unless optimal care is given to maintain life. The preterm infants require a great deal of special attention which needs intensive care nursery and it is very expensive.

Meaning

- Kangaroo care is a form of skin-to-skin contact between a parent and their preterm baby.
- The baby wearing only a diaper, is held in an upright position against the parent's bare chest.
- Baby is held this way for 20 minutes to 4 hours a day.
- This is called Kangaroo care because a baby is snuggled against its mother.

History

Kangaroo care first began in South America due to a lack of baby equipment and increased risk of infection in the hospital. Preterm babies were sent home being carried between their mothers breast in an upright position and fed only mothers milk.

Kangaroo care has proven to be successful in poor developed countries.

Kangaroo care soon spread to countries in Europe and is becoming widespread throughout United States. It was first implemented by Dr. Martinez and Rey in Bogatta Columbia in 1979.

Indications

- To bring about the closer physical contact between the infant and family.
- To increased parent-infant bonding.
- To offer more parent-child activities to families separated by infant hospitalization.
- To improve the general well-being of the infant.
- To improve and prolong breastfeeding.

Type of Kangaroo care

Five categories of Kangaroo care have been identified, based on how long after the infant's birth intervention are given:

- *Late Kangaroo care:* Usually it is begun several days or weeks after birth when the infant has become physiologically stable.
- *Intermediate Kangaroo care:* Begins within the first week of life while the infant is still unable or may still be on a ventilator.
- *Early Kangaroo care:* It is initiated in the first days or hours of life in the infant who can be stabilised in a warmed incubator with IV fluids and oxygen, if necessary.
- *Very early Kangaroo care:* It is initiated in the first hour of life in the delivery or recovery room.
- *Birth Kangaroo care:* It refers to placing the infant skin-to-skin on the mother's abdomen in the first minute after delivery.

General instructions

- Wear front open shirt
- Mother's arms and chest must be free of rashes or sores.
- Avoid using strong smelling perfumes.
- Kangaroo care begins when the baby is physically stable and can tolerate activities.
- When mother feels well enough to hold her baby.
- Kangaroo care should be practised at least for half to one hour.

Procedure

- Set up plans for Kangaroo care
- The baby should wear only a diaper
- Place the mother in a comfortable position.
- Provide privacy
- Check the vital signs of the baby
- Hold the baby in an upright position against the parent's bare chest.
- The baby is held in this way for 20 minutes to 3 hours a day.
- Monitor the baby during Kangaroo care.
- After Kangaroo care place the baby back to the cradle.

Benefits

To the baby

- Regulates temperature
- Increased parent infant bonding
- Comfort from hearing parent's heartbeat
- Early breastfeeding
- Early discharge
- Promotes deep sleep
- Decreased breathing pauses and apnoea
- Increased oxygen level
- Decreased number of slow heart rate spells.

To the parents

- Increased parent-infant bonding
- Increased breast milk supply
- Earlier breastfeeding
- Continuous breastfeeding for longer periods of time
- Increased readiness for discharge
- Increased confidence in ability to care the baby
- Increased sense of control
- Increased ability to cope with the stress and emotions of having a high-risk infant.

Risks of Kangaroo care

To the parents

Feeling too warm or sweating

To the baby

- Potential for displacement of intravenous canula
- Potential for displacement of endotracheal tube

Disadvantages

For the baby

Limited to stable weight gain for infants who are fed with specific hospital guidelines.

For the parents

- Time consuming
- Require intense commitment

Kangaroo care is a method of care that uses skin to skin contact of infant to parent. The baby is placed between mother's breasts for many days at a stretch, maintaining an upright posture at an angle of 60 degree during sleep. The skin warms and calms the infant and promotes bonding. Thus Kangaroo care is best for the preterm babies.

INTRAUTERINE GROWTH RESTRICTION (IUGR)

Definition

Intrauterine growth restriction is said to be present in those babies whose birth weight is below the tenth percentile of the average for the gestational age. Growth restriction can occur in preterm, term or post-term babies.

Incidence

In developed countries, its overall incidence is about 2–8%. The incidence among the term babies is about 5% and that among the post term babies is about 15%.

Types

Based on the clinical evaluation and ultrasound examination the small fetuses are divided into:

1. Fetuses that are small and healthy. The birth weight is less than 10th percentile for their gestational age. They have normal ponderal index, normal subcutaneous fat and usually have uneventful neonatal course.
2. Fetuses where growth is restricted by pathological process (true IUGR). Depen-

Table 14.2: Features of symmetrical and asymmetrical IUGR fetuses

Symmetrical	Asymmetrical
Uniformly small	Head larger than abdomen
Ponderal index (birth weight/crown-heel length^3)—normal	Low
HC : AC and	Elevated
FL : AC ratios—normal	
Etiology: Genetic disease or infection—(intrinsic to fetus)	Chronic placental insufficiency—(extrinsic to fetus)
Total cell number—less	Normal
Cell size—normal	Smaller
Neonatal course—complicated with poor prognosis	Usually uncomplicated having good prognosis

ding upon the relative size of their head, abdomen and femur, the fetuses are subdivided into (Table 14.2):

- Symmetrical or Type I
- Asymmetrical or Type II

Symmetrical (20%): The fetus is affected by the noxious effect very early in the phase of cellular hyperplasia. The total cell number is less. This form of growth retardation is most often caused by structural or chromosomal abnormalities or congenital infection (TORCH). The pathologic process is intrinsic to the fetus and involves all the organs including the head.

Asymmetrical (80%): The fetus is affected in later months during the phase of cellular hypertrophy. The total cell number remains the same but size is smaller than normal. The pathologic processes that too often result in asymmetric growth retardation, are maternal diseases extrinsic to the fetus. These diseases alter the fetal size by reducing uteroplacental blood flow or by restricting the oxygen and nutrient transfer or by reducing the placental size.

Etiology

The causes of fetal restriction can be divided into four groups:

1. Maternal
2. Fetal
3. Placental
4. Unknown

Maternal

- **Constitutional:** Small women, maternal genetic and racial factor may be associated with small babies. These babies are not at increased risk.
- **Maternal nutrition before and during pregnancy:** Critical substrate requirement for fetal growth such as glucose, amino acids and oxygen are deficient during pregnancy. This is an important cause of IUGR in women with undernutrition.

Maternal diseases

Anaemia, hypertension, thrombophilia, heart disease, chronic renal disease, collagen vascular diseases are the important causes.

Toxins

Alcohol, smoking, cocaine, heroin, drugs.

Fetal

There is enough substrate in the maternal blood and also crosses the placenta but is not utilized by the fetus. The failure of nonutilization may be due to:

1. Structural anomalies either cardiovascular, renal or others

2. Chromosomal abnormality is associated with 8–12% of growth retarded infants.
3. Infection TORCH agents (toxoplasmosis, rubella, cytomegalovirus and herpes simplex) and malaria.
4. Multiple pregnancy: There is mechanical hindrance to growth and excessive fetal demand.

Placental

The causes include cases of poor uterine blood flow to the placental site for a long time. This leads to chronic placental insufficiency with inadequate substrate transfer. The placental pathology includes placenta praevia, abruption, circumvallate, infarction and mosaicism.

Unknown

The cause remains unknown in about 40 per cent.

Pathophysiology

Basic pathology in small for gestational age is due to reduced availability of nutrients in the mother or its reduced transfer by the placenta to the fetus. It may also be due to reduced ultilisation by the fetus. Brain cell size as well as cell numbers are reduced. Liver glycogen content is reduced. There is oligohydramnios as the renal and pulmonary contribution to amniotic fluid are diminished due to reduction in blood flow to these organs. The SGA fetus is at risk of intrauterine hypoxia and acidosis, which, if severe, may lead to intrauterine fetal death.

Diagnosis

Significant improvements have been made by clinical and biophysical methods in detecting growth restricted fetus.

Clinical

- Clinical palpation of the uterus for the fundal height, liquor volume and fetal mass may be used for screening.

- Symphysis fundal height (SFH) measurement in centimeters closely correlated with gestational age after 24 weeks. A lag of 4 cm or more suggests growth restriction.
- Maternal weight gain remains stationary or at times falling during the second half of pregnancy.
- Measurement of the abdominal girth showing stationary or falling values.

Biophysical

USG is extremely useful to diagnose the growth retardation.

Physical features at birth

- Weight deficit at birth is about 600 gm below the minimum in percentile standard.
- Length is unaffected.
- Head circumference is relatively larger than the body in asymmetric variety.
- Physical features show dry and wrinkled skin because of less subcutaneous fat, scaphoid abdomen, thin meconium stained vernix caseosa and thin umbilical cord. All these give the baby an "old man look". Pinna of ear has cartilaginous ridges. Planter creases are well defined (Fig. 14.1).
- The baby is alert, active and having normal cry. Eyes are open.
- Reflexes are normal including Moro-reflex.

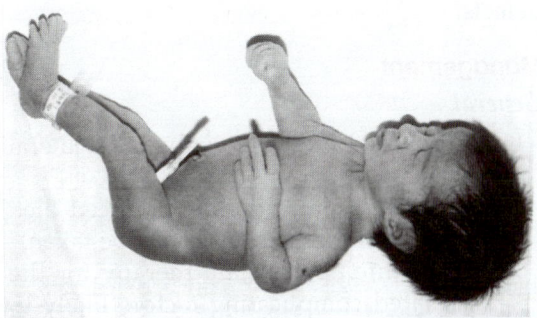

Fig. 14.1: Physical features (wrinkled skin, scaphoid abdomen) give the baby an "old man-look"

Complication
Fetal

- Antenatal: Chronic fetal distress, fetal death
- Intranatal: Hypoxia and acidosis

Afterbirth
Immediate

- Asphyxia (intrauterine and neonatal) and RDS
- Hypoglycaemia due to shortage of glycogen reserve in the liver as a result of chronic hypoxia
- Meconium aspiration syndrome
- Microcoagulation leading to DIC during first day of life
- Hypothermia
- Pulmonary haemorrhage
- Polycythaemia
- Necrotizing enterocolitis due to reduced intestinal blood flow
- Intraventricular haemorrhage (IVH).

Late

Symmetrical growth retarded baby is likely to grow slowly after birth. Whereas the asymmetrical one do tend to catch up growth in early infancy. The fetuses having retardation of growth evidenced before third trimester, are likely to have retarded neurologic and intellectual development infancy. The worst prognosis is for IUGR caused by congenital infection, congenital abnormalities and chromosomal defects.

Management
General

1. Adequate bed rest especially in left lateral position
2. To correct malnutrition by balanced diet: 300 extracalories per day are to be taken.
3. To institute appropriate therapy for the associated complicating factors likely to produce growth restriction
4. Avoidance of smoking and alcohol

5. Maternal hyperoxygenation (55%) for short term prolongation of pregnancy.
6. Low dose Aspirin (50 mg daily) may be helpful in very selected cases with history of recurrence.

PROBLEMS OF THE NEWBORN

ASPHYXIA NEONATORUM

Although the majority of infants gasp and establish respirations within 60 seconds of birth, some do not. This failure to initiate and sustain respiration at birth is known as *asphyxia* and *hypercapnia* which may or may not have been present before birth.

Birth asphyxia is clinically defined as failure to initiate and maintain spontaneous respiration following birth. Perinatal asphyxia is the more appropriate term. *Perinatal asphyxia* is the state of decreased oxygen delivery (hypoxia) to the fetus or neonate resulting in inadequate tissue perfusion (ischaemia). It is manifested by low Apgar score and metabolic acidosis. Often it is the continuation of antepartum or intra-partum event.

The basic requirements for initiation and maintenance of pulmonary respiration are:
1. Intact neurological and respiratory apparatus
2. Clear airway
3. Adequate alveolar area
4. Expanded alveoli with the presence of surfactant.
5. Sufficient pulmonary perfusion
6. Satisfactory lymphatic drainage
7. Oxygen diffusion and dissociation capacity
8. Carbonic anhydrase activity of blood.

Causes of perinatal asphyxia

90% of asphyxial event occur in the antepartum or intrapartum periods as a result of placental insufficiency. The rests are postnatal. Asphyxia can be classified broadly into the following groups:

A. Continuation of intrauterine hypoxia (placental insufficiency)

B. *Prenatal and intranatal medication to the mother*

C. *Birth trauma to the neonate*

D. *Postnatal factors*

Continuation of intrauterine hypoxia

- The placenta, as a respiratory organ of the fetus fails functionally either due to anatomical changes in the placenta or due to inadequacy or uteroplacental circulation. Premature placental separation, circumvallate placenta, hypertensive disorders in pregnancy, abnormal labour, cord compression, vascular anomalies in cord are some of the important causes.

- **Maternal hypoxic states:** The maternal disease such as anaemia, eclampsia, cyanotic, cardiovascular disorders, status asthmaticus, dehydration, hypotension are responsible for maternal and therefore to fetal and neonatal hypoxia.

BIRTH TRAUMA

Malpresentation such as breech, oblique lie, occipito-posterior often requires manipulative and operative vaginal delivery (forceps or ventouse). Prolonged second stage of labour in contracted pelvis, often cause asphyxia. Increased intracran ial tension → cerebral oedema and congestion → increased intracranial pressure → asphyxia.

Medications

Morphine, pethidine and anaesthetic agents depress the respiratory centres directly and the chance of development of asphyxia is increased.

Postnatal

Postnatal asphyxia is secondary to pulmonary, cardiovascular and neurological abnormalities of the neonate.

DEGREES OF ASPHYXIA (Table 14.3)

The length of time to which the fetus or neonate is subjected to hypoxia determines the outcome. It is considered that the human neonate responds to hypoxia in a similar manner to other young mammals. This involves an initial response of gasping respirations followed by a period of apnoea lasting 1–1½ minutes → primary apnoea, if not resolved by intervention techniques, is followed by a further episode of gasping respirations which accelerate while diminishing in depth until, approximately 8 minutes after birth, respirations cease completely → terminal apnoea. This suggest that it should be possible to determine the degree of asphyxia by assessment of the infant's condition at birth. The apgar score provides a guide to the severity of birth asphyxia though does not

Table 14.3: Degrees of birth asphyxia

Mild asphyxia	Severe asphyxia
Heart rate not severely depressed (60–80 bpm)	Slow feeble heart rate (less than 40 bpm)
Short delay in onset of respiration	No attempt to breathe
Good muscle tone	Poor muscle tone
Responsive to stimuli	Limp, unresponsive to stimuli
Deeply cyanosed (asphyxia livida)	Pale, gray (asphyxia pallida)
Apgar score 5–7	*Apgar score less than 5*
No significant deprivation of oxygen during labour	Oxygen lack has been prolonged before or after delivery, circulatory failure is present, baby is shocked

necessarily reflect the metabolic status of the infant. This presents a dilemma of the birth attendant who may be uncertain as to whether primary or secondary (terminal) apnoea is present at birth. It is advisable, therefore, to be prepared to undertake specific resuscitative measures for any infant who is asphyxiated at birth.

Clinical features

The clinical features depend upon the etiology, intensity and duration of oxygen lack, plasma carbon dioxide excess and subsequent acidosis. According to the intensity of clinical features they have been classified previously as asphyxia livida (stage of cyanosis) and asphyxia pallida (stage of shock).

Clinical sequences of birth asphyxia

Initial response is hyperpnea and hypertension → primary apnoea → gasping attempt to breathe → (if unresolved) → secondary apnoea → bradycardia and shock → diminished cerebral blood flow → cerebral haemorrhage → hypoxic ischaemic encephalopathy → (if severe) → either death or handicap (if the baby survives).

Management

Management of perinatal asphyxia can be divided into two. They are:

1. Prophylactic
2. Definitive

Prophylactic

1. Antenatal detection of high-risk patients.
2. Scrupulous fetal monitoring, particularly in high risk pregnancy group to ensure early detection of fetal distress and timely termination of pregnancy and/or labour.
3. Intrapartum use of electronic fetal monitoring and scalp blood pH assessment when indicated. Scalp blood pH < 7.0 is substantial evidence of prolonged intra-uterine asphyxia.
4. Judicious administration of anaesthetic agents and sedatives during labour.

Definitive

Apgar rating (Table 14.4)

Classically, the evaluation of the cardio-pulmonary status in the newborn has been assessed by Apgar rating at 1 and 5 minutes after birth. But it must be emphasized that in certain circumstances, it is inappropriate to delay resuscitative efforts until the 1 minute Apgar score is obtained. However, most infants, born with Apgar scores of 7–10 are essentially normal.

Babies with Apgar score 7–10: Pink, breathing regular, HR > 100)

Signs	Scoring		
	0	1	6
Respiratory effort	Absent	Slow, irregular	Good, crying
Heart rate	Absent	Slow (below 100)	Over 100
Muscle tone	Flaccid	Flexion of extremities	Active body movements
Reflex irritability	No response	Grimace	Cry
Colour	Blue, pale	Body pink, extremities blue	Complete pink

Table 14.4: Apgar scoring

- Total score =10
- Mild depression = 4–6
- No depression = 7–10
- Severe depression = 0–3

- The oropharynx and the nasopharynx are to be cleared off any mucus by suction.
- Oxygen is administered when required only.
- The condition reassessed at 5 minute and if found normal, the infant should be given to mother.

Babies with Apgar score 4–6: (Peripheral cyanosis, breathing irregular, HR > 100)

- Baby may follow primary apnoea.
- Place under a radiant heater, dry the baby.
- The baby is put flat or slight head down position with the face on one side to facilitate gravitational drainage of fluid from the respiratory passage.
- Immediate suction of the oropharynx and nasopharynx is done either by mucus sucker or by suction apparatus (mechanical or electrical) whichever is available.
- Stimulus to back and sole (gentle rubbing).
- Simultaneously oxygen (100%) is administered at a rate of 5 liters/min. by bag and mask at a pressure range of 25–30 cm H_2O.
- Intermittent positive pressure ventilation (IPPV) is given, if necessary.
- Support should be continued until respirations are spontaneous and the heart rate is > 100 bpm. Such an infant may be acidotic but it is corrected spontaneously after respiration is established.

In majority of cases, the baby takes independent respiration with these simple measures. The Apgar rating is done with 5 minutes and if found satisfactory, the baby is returned to the mother.

If the above measures fail (secondary apnoea), oral suction followed by tracheal intubation is done. The tracheal tube is connected to resuscitation bag through which oxygen is administered at the rate of 5–8 litres/minute. Intermittent positive pressure ventilation (IPPV) is maintained at the rate of 40–60 per minute. Gentle external cardiac massage is performed

if the heart rate is <60/min. When there is history of administration of a central depressant drug such as pethidine or morphine to the mother within 3 hours of delivery, suitable antidote, e.g. naloxone hydrochloride 100 μg/kg IM (single dose) may have to be repeated.

Babies with Apgar score below 4: (Central cyanosis, no breathing, HR < 100)

Tracheal intubation and intermittent positive pressure ventilation must be started immediately. In such circumstances, where arrangement for intermittent positive pressure ventilation cannot be made, gentle mouth to mouth respiration is life saving. For circulation to maintain, cardiac massage is given if after intubation and ventilation with 100% O_2 for 30 sec. the heart rate remains = 60 bpm.

Medication

Medication is needed if despite ventilation and cardiac massage improvement has not been observed.

Naloxone hydrochloride: Up to 400 μg (or approximately 100 μg per kg body weight) may be administered intravenously (through the umbilical vein) or intramuscularly to reverse the effect of maternal narcotic drugs. It must not be given until respiration is affected. Naloxone has the advantage of not having a respiratory depressant effect itself, therefore, no harm arises if it is given in the absence of narcotic analgesia. The dose can be repeated safely.

Sodium bicarbonate: 5 ml of 5% or 8.4% solution given intravenously assists in the correction of metabolic acidosis. It should be administered slowly, 1 ml per minute, in order to avoid rapid elevation of serum osmolality with the attendant risk of intracranial haemorrhage. It should not be given prior to ventilation being established.

Dextrose: 5 ml of 5% or 10% solution may be given intravenously to correct or prevent hypocalcemia.

Konakion (vitamin K): Up to 1 mg may be given intramuscularly to reduce the risks

associated with haemorrhage. Some centres give vitamin K orally.

Dexamethasone: 1–2 mg may be given intravenously or intramuscularly to minimise the risk of cerebral oedema if severe asphyxia is present.

EXTERNAL CARDIAC MASSAGE

If bradycardia persists or the heart rate is less than 40 beats per minute, external cardiac massage may be applied. This is achieved by placing the tips of the index and middle fingers of one hand over the middle of the sternum and depressing the chest with fingertip pressure only at a rate of 100–120 times per minute. (Excessive pressure over the lower end of the sternum may cause rib, lung or liver damage).

Complications

Immediate

- Cardiovascular—hypotension, cardiac failure.
- Renal—acute cortical necrosis, renal failure.
- Liver function—compromised.
- Gastrointestinal—ulcers and necrotizing enterocolitis.
- Lungs—persistent pulmonary hypertension.
- Brain—cerebral oedema, seizures.

Delayed

- Retarded mental and physical growth.
- Epilepsy: up to 30% in severe asphyxia.
- Minimal brain dysfunction.

BIRTH INJURIES

Birth injuries are defined as those sustained during labour and delivery. Birth injuries may be severe enough to cause neonatal deaths, stillbirths or number of morbidities (Table 14.5).

Predisposing factors

- Prolonged or obstructed labour
- Fetal macrosomia
- Cephalopelvic disproportion

- Abnormal presentation (breech)
- Instrumental delivery (forceps or ventouse)
- Difficult labour
- Shoulder dystocia
- Precipitate labour
- Manipulative delivery

INJURIES OF HEAD

Moulding of the baby's head varies according to the presentation, position and duration of labour. Damage may occur to the superficial tissues of the presenting part causing bruising or abrasion. When moulding is excessive cranial compression may take place and can lead to serious intracranial injury. A large caput succedaneum, not to be confused with cephalhaematoma, is often present in such cases.

Mothers can be very depressed by the appearance of a caput or cephalhaematoma. They need reassurance as these injuries are rarely harmful on their own, should disappear completely, and will not compromise the baby's development.

CEPHALHAEMATOMA (Fig. 14.2)

A cephalhaematoma is a swelling on the infant's skull, an effusion of blood under periosteum covering it, due to friction between the skull and pelvis. It occurs in cases of cephalopelvic disproportion and precipitate labour, when tearing of the periosteum from the bone causes bleeding.

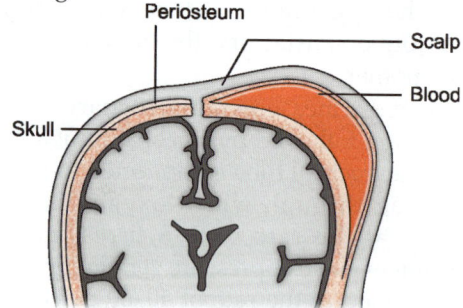

Fig. 14.2: Cephalhaematoma

Table 14.5: Birth injuries

Type of injury	Organ(s) affected
Soft tissue	Skin—Laceration, abrasions, fat necrosis
Nerve	Facial nerve, brachial plexus, spinal cord, phrenic nerve, Horners' syndrome
Eye	Haemorrhage—sub-conjunctiva, retina
Viscera	Rupture of liver, adrenal gland, spleen
Scalp	Laceration, abscess, haemorrhage
Dislocation	Hip, shoulder, cervical vertebrae
Skull	Cephalhaematoma, subgaleal haematoma, fractures
Intracranial	Haemorrhages—intraventricular, subdural, subarachnoid
Bones	Fractures—clavicle, humerus, femur

As the periosteum is adherent to the edges of the skull bones, the swelling is confined to one bone.

No treatment is necessary, the blood is absorbed and the swelling subsides. A ridge of bone may later be felt round the periphery of the swelling, due to the accumulation of osteoblasts.

- Appears after 12 hours
- Never crosses a suture
- Tends to grow larger
- Persists for weeks
- Is circumscribed, does not pit
- A double cephalhaematoma is usually bilateral (Fig. 14.3).

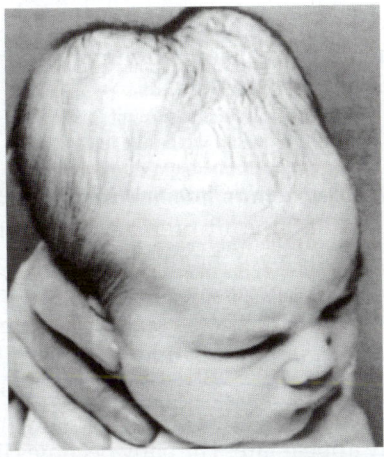

Fig. 14.3: Bilateral cephalhaematoma

SUBAPONEUROTIC HAEMORRHAGE (Fig. 14.4)

A subaponeurotic haemorrhage is occasionally seen following spontaneous delivery but more often is associated with vacuum extraction. Bleeding occurs below the epicranial aponeurosis. It can be confused with a caput succedaneum as the swelling extends across the suture lines. The infant must be observed for signs of hyperbilirubinaemia and anaemia. If the haemorrhage is severe, a blood transfusion may be necessary. Death due to massive haemorrhage is a possibility.

- It is present at birth
- Crosses suture lines
- Increases in size
- Resolves over 2–3 weeks
- Firm, fluctuant mass
- Can extend into subcutaneous tissue of neck and eyelids

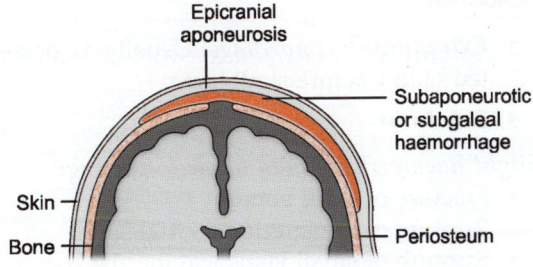

Fig. 14.4: Subaponeurotic haemorrhage

- Bruising may be apparent for days and sometimes weeks.

SCALP INJURIES

Minor injuries of the scalp such as abrasion in forceps delivery (tip of the blades), incised wound inflicted during caesarean section, episiotomy may be met with. On occasion, the incised wound may cause brisk haemorrhage and requires stitches. The wound should be dressed with an antiseptic solution like 2% mercurochrome.

FRACTURE SKULL

Fracture of the vault of the skull (frontal or anterior part of the parietal bone) may be of fissure or depressed type. Fractures are due to:

1. Effect of difficult forceps delivery in disproportion or due to wrong application of the forceps (blades not placed over the biparietal diameter).
2. Projected sacral promontory of the flat pelvis may produce depressed fracture even though the delivery is spontaneous.

The fracture may be associated with cephal-haematoma, extradural or subdural haemorr-hage or a haematoma or brain contusions.

INTRACRANIAL HAEMORRHAGE

Types

- Traumatic
- Anoxic

TRAUMATIC

- *Extradural haemorrhage:* Usually associated with fracture skull bone.

- **Subdural**

Slight haemorrhage may occur following:
- Fracture of skull bone
- Rupture of the inferior sagittal sinus
- Rupture of small veins leaving the cortex. The haemorrhage, so occurring, produces

haematoma which may remain stationary or increase in size. Neurological symptoms may appear acutely or may have insidious onset, like vomiting, irritability and failure to gain weight. Hydrocephalus and mental retardation may be a late sequelae.

Massive haemorrhage: massive subdural haemorrhage usually results from

- Tear of the tentorium cerebelli thereby opening up the straight sinus or rupture of the vein of Galen or its tributaries.
- Injury to the superior sagittal sinus.

Causes

1. Excessive moulding in deflexed vertex with gross disproportion.
2. Rapid compression of the head during delivery of the aftercoming head of breech or in precipitate labour.
3. Forcible forceps traction following wrong application of the blades.

Clinical features

The haemorrhage may be fatal and the baby is delivered stillborn or with severe respiratory depression having Apgar score 0–3. In lesser affection the baby recovers from the respiratory depression. Gradually, the features of cerebral irritation appear, such as, frequent high pitch cry, neck retraction, incoordinate ocular movements, convulsion, vomiting and bulging of the anterior fontanelle.

ANOXIC

- *Intraventricular haemorrhage (IVH):* It is more common in premature infants. The mechanism of haemorrhage is due to intense congestion of the fragile choroidal plexus due to anoxia leading to rupture.
- *Subarachnoid:* This may be due to tear of some tributary veins running from the brain to one of the sinuses. The symptoms may appear late. The baby becomes listless,

there is twitching of the extremities or inco-ordinated eye movements.

- *Intracerebral:* Small petechial haemorrhage may occur in the brain substance (paren-chyma) due to anoxia. It usually occurs in mature babies following prolonged labour. The features are, loss of weight, flaccid limbs or worried and anxious expression.

Prevention

Comprehensive antenatal and intranatal care is the key to success in the reduction of intracranial injuries.

- *To prevent or to detect at the earliest,* intra-uterine fetal asphyxia by intensive fetal monitoring, clinical and/or electronic, especially while conducting premature labour.
- *To avoid traumatic vaginal delivery* in preference to caesarean section. Difficult forceps should be avoided.
- *To extend the use of caesarean section* in breech more liberally. Gentleness is to be executed in vaginal breech delivery.
- *Administration of vitamin K 1 mg intra-muscularly* soon afterbirth in susceptible babies.

Investigations

1. Ultrasonography is used to detect intraven-tricular haemorrhage.
2. Doppler ultrasonography can detect any change in cerebral circulation.
3. CT scan is useful to detect cortical neuronal injury.
4. Magnetic resonance imaging (MRI) is used to evaluate any hypoxic ischaemic brain injury.

Treatment

- The baby should be nursed in quiet surro-undings.
- Incubator nursery is preferable to supply oxygen and to maintain the temperature and humidity.

- To maintain cleanliness of the air passage.
- To maintain normal range of $PaCO_2$ and to avoid hypoxemia.
- To restrict handling the baby, as such bathing, weighing and measuring should be withheld.
- Feeding by nasogastric tube is advisable. Fluid balance is to be maintained, if necessary, by parenteral route.
- To administer vitamin K 1 mg intramus-cularly to prevent further bleeding due to hypoprothrombinaemia.
- Prophylactic antibiotic is to be adminis-tered.
- Anticonvulsant: Any of the following may be useful:
  - Phenobarbitone—5–10 mg/kg/day in divided doses at 6 hourly intervals intramuscularly.
  - Phenytoin 10–15 mg/kg intravenously as loading dose at the rate of 0.5 mg/kg/min followed by maintenance dose of 5 mg/kg/day with cardiac monito-ring.
  - Diazepam 0.1 mg/kg intramuscularly thrice daily.
- Subdural haematoma
  - Subdural tap—aspiration of the blood through lateral angles of the anterior fontanelle may be required which may have to be repeated.
  - Surgical removal of the clot including the capsule may have to be done to prevent development of neurological sequelae.
  - Rarely subdural—peritoneal shunting may be needed. Neurosurgeon is consulted.

OTHER INJURIES

Skin and subcutaneous tissues

Bruises and lacerations on the face are usually caused by forceps blades. These are treated with application of 1% lotio mercurochrome. The scalp may be oedematous and bruised, if allowed to remain on the perineum for a long period. Buttocks in breech presentation, or eyelids, lips or nose in face presentation, similarly oedematous and congested.

Muscle injuries
Torticollis/WRY neck
Torticollis results from injury to the sterno-mastoid muscle during birth when either the muscle is torn or its blood supply is impaired. This may occur during delivery of the anterior shoulder in a vertex presentation or while rotating the shoulders during a breech delivery. It usually presents 1 or 2 weeks after birth as a small painless lump 2 cm or so in size, commonly on the left side of the neck. It is no longer thought to be a haematoma but it is probably a mixture of blood and fibrous tissue. The swelling will resolve over several weeks. Muscle-stretching exercises should be taught to parents to prevent shortening. Infants should sleep on the opposite side to the injury to increase passive stressing.

Nerve injuries
The most common are facial nerve and brachial plexus injuries.

Facial palsy
This is usually associated with forceps deliveries where the facial nerve has been compressed against the ramus of the mandible. There is unilateral facial weakness, the eyelid of the affected side remaining open while the mouth is drawn over to the normal side. Minimal feeding difficulties occur. No treatment is required. Occasionally methyl cellulose eye drops may be required, usually if the eyelids remain open. Spontaneous improvement should be seen in 7–10 days. Non-traumatic causes of facial palsy include nuclear agenesis and primary muscle disorders. Recovery is poor in the later cases.

Brachial palsy
These are caused by stretching or disruption of the nerves of the brachial plexus which is a group of nerves at the apex of the axilla, lying under the clavicle. Injuries can be caused by excessive lateral flexion of the head and neck in cases of shoulder dystocia or breech presentation. *There are three main types of injury:*

- *Erb's palsy:* This involves damage to upper roots of the brachial plexus. The baby's inwardly rotated arm lies limply by his side and he cannot flex his elbow or lift his arm, although there is movement of the arm and fingers. The half-closed hand is turned outwards (Waiter's tip position). In this 5th and 6th cervical nerve roots are involved. (Fig. 14.5).

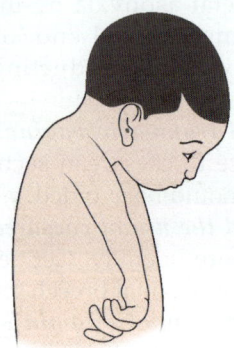

Fig. 14.5: Erb's palsy (Waiter's tip)

- *Klumpke's palsy:* Klumpke's palsy involves the lower arm, wrist and hand, with wrist drop and limp fingers caused by damage to spinal roots C8 and T1. The upper arm has normal movement.
- *Total brachial plexus palsy:* There is damage to all brachial plexus nerve roots with complete paralysis of the arm and hand, lack of sensation and circulatory problems.

These injuries require further investigation including X-rays of clavicle, arm, cervical spine and chest. Careful assessment of joints is particularly important. Treatment consists of resting the arm for 7–20 days followed by gentle physiotherapy to avoid contractures. Parents should be taught a full range of passive move-

ment, for shoulder, elbow and wrist. Complete spontaneous recovery is more common with Erb's than Klumpke's or total brachial plexus palsy but may take from several months up to 2 years. Follow-up is necessary.

Fractures
- *Skull bone* (discussed before)
- *Spines:* Fracture of the odontoid process or fracture dislocation of the fifth-sixth cervical vertebrae may occur due to acute bending of the spine while delivering the after-coming head. The result is instantaneous death of the baby due to compression on the medulla.
- **Long bones:** Bones commonly involved in fractures are the humerus, the clavicle and the femur. These occur in breech delivery. Fractures are usually of greenstick type but may be complete. Rapid union occurs with callus formation. Deformity is a rarity even when the bone ends are not in good alignment.

Treatments
Fracture femur and humerus are treated by splinting. X-ray studies are done. Closed reduction and casting are needed when bones are displaced. Limb motion is restricted. Healing with callus formation occurs over 2 to 4 weeks.

Dislocations
The common sites of dislocations of joints are shoulder, hip, jaw and fifth-sixth cervical vertebrae. Confirmation is done by radiology or ultrasonography and the help of an orthopaedic surgeon should be sought.

Visceral injuries
Liver, kidneys, adrenals or lungs are commonly injured mainly during breech delivery. The commonest result of the delivery is haemorrhage. Severe haemorrhage is fatal. In minor haemorrhage, the baby presents features of blood loss in addition to the disturbed function of the organ involved.

Treatment is directed
- To correct hypovolaemia and anaemia
- Specific management, surgical or otherwise, to tackle the injured viscera.

Prevention of injuries
Comprehensive antenatal and intranatal care is the key to success in the reduction of birth trauma and consequently in the reduction of perinatal mortality and neonatal morbidity.

ANTENATAL PERIOD

To screen out the at risk babies likely to be traumatised during vaginal delivery and to employ liberal use of elective caesarean section is important. Contracted pelvis and cephalo-pelvic disproportion or malpresentation like breech or transverse lie are included in the list.
- Normal
- Preterm labour
- Forceps
- Ventouse
- Breech

NORMAL DELIVERY

- *Continuous fetal monitoring,* if available, is able to detect early evidences of fetal distress; pH determination by fetal blood sampling can reveal any emergency, when the delivery has to be hastened before the baby becomes compromised. This can prevent traumatic cerebral anoxia.
- Episiotomy is to be done carefully after placing two fingers in between the head and the stressed perineum to prevent injury to the scalp.
- The neck should not be unduly stressed while delivering the shoulders to minimise injuries to the brachial plexus or sternomastoid.

Special care in preterm delivery
1. To prevent anoxia
2. To avoid strong sedative

3. Liberal episiotomy and use of forceps to minimise intracranial compression
4. To administer vitamin K 1 mg intramuscularly to prevent or minimise haemorrhage from the traumatised area.

Forceps delivery

Majority of the severe injuries are inflicted by injudicious applications of forceps.

- Difficult forceps are to be avoided in preference to the safer caesarean section.
- Never apply traction unless the application is a correct one (blades should be placed over the biparietal plane).
- *Ventouse delivery:* It is relatively less traumatic but it should be avoided in preterm babies.
- *Vaginal breech delivery:* Proper selection of cases and utmost care and gentleness are to be executed while conducting vaginal breech delivery.

JAUNDICE IN NEWBORN

Definition

Jaundice develops in newborn as yellow staining of skin and mucosa by the yellow pigment, bilirubin, when in excess of 2 mg per 100 ml of blood.

Physiology of bilirubin in newborn

Bilirubin formation

Newborn red cells breakdown at 90 days and are taken by

RE cells
↓
Noniron haeme → Bilirubin ← Tissue haeme
↓
Bilirubin transport through serum albumin (unconjugated bilirubin)

In foetus, this is transported via placenta to maternal circulation. Maternal unconjugated bilirubin, when high, goes to foetus.

Bilirubin conjugation and excretion

Hepatic cells conjugate unconjugated bilirubin with glucoronic acid and transferred as uridine diphosphoglucoronic acid with the help of hepatic enzyme, glucuronyl transferase.

Conjugated bilirubin (bilirubin glucuronide) is water soluble.

Excreted from hepatocytes to canalicular apparatus
↓
Biliary tree → intestine

Intestinal phase

Bilirubin glucuronide is converted to urobilinogen by intestinal bacteria one of urobilinogen (stercobilinogen) is oxidized to yellow pigment (stercobilin) → half excreted in stool
↓
Another half of urobilinogen absorbed → goes to liver to be excreted into bile again (enterohepatic circulation). Some urobilinogen is excreted as urinary urobilinogen.

Causes of jaundice in newborn

1. **Physiological jaundice** (appearing during 2–4th day of birth) due to hepatic immaturity is the commonest cause.
2. **Increased haemolysis:** Haemolytic diseases of newborn–Rh iso-immunization, ABO iso-immunization, other blood group immunization (appearing within 24 hours of birth).
3. **Jaundice in prematurity**

Other uncommon causes are: Deficiency of red cell enzyme glucose-6-phosphate dehydrogenase deficiency, haemoglobinopathies, hepatitis, portal pyaemia, galactosaemia and congenital obliteration of bile duct.

Uncommon causes are detailed as

1. *E. coli* septicaemia, huge cephalhematoma causing haemolysis
2. Haemoglobinopathies

3. Hereditary spherocytosis due to defect in red cell membranes.

4. *Iatrogenic:* Excess vitamin K administration of 5 mg may cause haemolysis. Sulphonamide and salicylates (aspirin) unbounds bilirubin from plasma albumin.

Defective conjugation

5. *Breast milk jaundice* develops in some babies, during 4–7th day, passing off by 7–10 weeks. This never causes kernicterus.

6. *Failure of conjugated bilirubin excretion.*

7. *Hepatitis:* Viral, *E. coli,* syphilis.

8. *Infective:* Portal pyaemia from infected umbilicus can cause jaundice towards end of the week.

9. *Metabolic:* Galactosaemia due to hereditary deficiency of hepatic enzyme converting galactose (derived from milk lactose) into glucose 1 phosphate. The latter accumulated leads to enlarged liver and jaundice during first few weeks of milk feeding. Lactose free milk is given in feeds.

10. *Congenital obliteration* of bile duct. Jaundice appears on second week. Stool is clay coloured, urine contains no urobilinogen. Early surgery can save neonate.

11. *Miscellaneous:* Hypothyroidism, infant of diabetic mother, Down's syndrome, with pyloric stenosis, intestinal obstruction.

PHYSIOLOGICAL JAUNDICE IN NEWBORN AND JAUNDICE IN PREMATURITY

This is unconjugated nonhaemolytic jaundice. Neonatal jaundice is physiological when it is been excreted into bile again (enterohepatic circulation) no other pathological cause is found.

Cause

1. Early breakdown of red cells due to short span of red cells.

2. Transient defect in conjugation of bilirubin due to immaturity of liver because of lower level of Y (ligandin) and Z (fatty acid binding) anion-binding protein.

3. Reduced conversion of bilirubin to urobilinogen by intestinal bacteria.

Time of onset

2nd–4th day afterbirth never within first 24 hours.

Duration

Mature, one week; premature 2 weeks. Serum bilirubin (mostly unconjugated) rises to 12 mg% in mature, 15 mg% in premature and then gradually falls.

Complications

Seldom kernicterus develops as in haemolytic jaundice in newborn.

Clinical feature

Baby becomes jaundiced, lethargic with disinclination to feeds. Stool becomes dark green and urine dark.

Treatment

In both mature and preterm infant, no initial treatment but more fluids are required.

Phototherapy (exposure to sunlight or blue light) is given to infant.

Phenobarbitone is administered 5 mg/kg/day to enhance bilirubin conjugation.

In premature, exchange transfusion may be rarely necessary.

HYPERBILIRUBINAEMIA

It means rise of unconjugated bilirubin above 10 mg/100 ml within first 24–28 hours of birth.

Causes are same as jaundice in newborn.

Clinical features

Jaundice appears at birth or soon after. The skin colour of jaundice due to unconjugated bilirubin is bright yellow or orange. Child becomes lethargic with disinclination to take feeds.

Complications

Kernicterus when bilirubin reaches 16–20 mg%.

Treatment of hyperbilirubinaemia

1. Neonate is referred to hospital care, with facilities of exchange transfusion.
2. Phototherapy is effectively given to jaundiced baby due to hyperbilirubinaemia (serum bilirubin above 10 mg%). This is also given to preterm baby for prevention of hyperbilirubinaemia.

Procedure

Phototherapy unit with fluorescent tubes are available. Naked infant is exposed under light source kept at a distance of 45 cm from skin. Eyes of baby are covered with shield to prevent retinal damage. Baby is turned every 2 hours and phototherapy is continued for 8 hours.

In rural India age old practice of exposure of infant in sunlight can also serve the purpose. Phototherapy is given daily till bilirubin comes down below 7 mg%. Serum bilirubin is regularly monitored.

Mechanism of action

1. Light at 420–460 nm. Wavelength causes photooxidation of bilirubin→water soluble product being excreted in bile, faeces and urine.
2. Promotes hepatic excretion of unconjugated bilirubin.

Complications

1. Loose green stool due to intestinal irritation.
2. Dehydration due to increased water loss (extra fluid is provided).
3. Phenobarbitone therapy is given as hepatic enzyme inducer for bilirubin conjugation in dosage of 5 mg/kg/day.
4. Exchange transfusion is effective treatment and is repeated within first week.

HYDROPS FOETALIS IS OEDEMATOUS STILLBORN BABY

A. **Immunized hydrops foetalis**—blood group immunization.
B. **Nonimmunized hydrops foetalis**—more common
   1. Twin pregnancy—twin transfusion
   2. Alpha thalassaemia
   3. Chromosomal—Down syndrome, Turner syndrome.
   4. Malformations
   5. Cardiac failure—congenital heart disease.

Diagnosis

Ultrasonography, foetal echocardiography, amniocentesis, foetal blood sampling for karyotyping, amniotic fluid bilirubin spectro-photometry are all employed.

Treatment as per cause

Prognosis

For immune hydrops prospect of survival is good. For non-immune hydrops, it is poor, only 10–20% survive.

ALIMENTARY DISORDERS

Diarrhoea

It is frequent passage of loose, watery stool which contains mucus and may be green due to unchanged bile.

Diarrhoea of infective origin contains pus cells. Breast fed babies are much less to develop diarrhoea than bottle fed babies.

Causes

1. *Gastroenteritis:* This µ caused by bacteria-certain strains of *E. coli, Salmonella shigella, Paradysentrica, Klebseilla, Staphylococcus aureus,* paracolon bacilli, group B haemolytic streptococci.
   Fungal agents like *Candida albicans* can cause diarrhoea. Virus like Rota, Echo and coxsackie can also cause diarrhoea.

2. *Parenteral infection:* Occasionally infection elsewhere in the body such as otitis media, infection of upper respiratory tract, pyelonephritis, septicaemia and meningitis may cause intestinal hypermotility and diarrhoea will result.

3. **Dietetic errors**
   - Underfeeding may cause the passage of small frequent green mucoid stools so called hunger stools.
   - Overfeeding is a rare condition but may cause the frequent passage of a large fairly loose stools without mucus.
   - *Milk sensitivity:* Occasionally cow's milk in a bottle fed baby with sensitivity will cause diarrhoea with frequent stools continuing mucus and streaks of blood. There is often perianal excoriation. Such a diarrhoea initially should be regarded as infective as a diagnosis of milk sensitivity can only be made by consistent relapse on re-exposure to cow's milk.
   - Protein, fat or carbohydrate intolerance. In artificially fed babies diarrhoea may be caused if the milk used contains too much protein, fat or carbohydrate. Excessive carbohydrate produces loose motion with soury smell. Besides, the child may be born with congenital lactose intolerance or may develop temporary lactose intolerance as a result of suffering from severe diarrhoea. Under this situation, baby should have soya bean milk instead of cow's milk.

Effects of diarrhoea

Dehydration, electrolyte imbalance and acidosis. Dehydration becomes mild, then becomes severe. Death comes in severe cases.

Management

1. *Isolation:* Especially if in a nursery, the baby having diarrhoea must be isolated from the others as infective diarrhoea is highly contagious.

2. *Stopping milk feeds:* Breastfed babies are allowed to continue breastfeeding unless in exceptional circumstance. All other milk foods must be stopped temporarily and feeds replaced by clear fluids such as 1/5 normal saline with 5% dextrose or half strength Hartmann's solution in 5% dextrose for 12 hours. This is followed by breastfeed or skimmed milk.

3. *Treatment of dehydration:* In mild dehydration, at home, oral rehydration therapy of home available fluid is given. In severe dehydration, such as depressed fontanelle, inelastic skin, dry tongue, thirst, oliguria, loss of weight, baby is transferred to neonatal care unit and intravenous therapy is necessary. In acute dehydration the only signs may be acute loss of weight and poor or absent peripheral pulse. Occasionally such children lie in a state of shock. The fluids used should be 5% dextrose in 1/5 normal saline or half strength Hartmann's solution. If there is any evidence of acidosis, 7.5% or 8.4% soda bicarbonate 1 to 3 mEq per kg of baby weight is given IV.

   The amount of fluid should be 120–180 ml per kg body weight; but if fluid loss is excessive this rate may have to be increased.

   In severe cases there should be electrolyte control with special care taken to watch for low sodium and potassium levels.

4. *Antibiotic therapy:* In the neonatal period inj. cefotaxime (Biotax) 50–100 mg/kg IV or IM 12 hourly and inj. gentamicin 5 mg/kg/day or inj. kanamycin 15 mg/kg/day in divided doses are the best antibiotics given for 5–7 days. Chloramphenicol may cause shock and hypothermia (gray-baby syndrome) and therefore is not used for newborn. A stool sent for culture must always be taken before antibiotic therapy is commenced.

PERSISTENT MILD DIARRHOEA

If all investigations are negative and the diarrhoea is persistent, improvement often follows without any treatment. This is often seen in breast fed baby and is physiological.

Prevention of diarrhoea

1. Meticulous attention to sterilization of feeding utensils and milk in the case of artificially fed babies.
2. Always washing the hands before feeding a child and also that of nipples before breastfeeding.
3. In nurseries immediate isolation of any child having diarrhoea and immediate taking of a stool swab for culture.
4. In a nursery if more than one cases of diarrhoea occur all the children should have stool swabs taken and source of infection is looked for.

VOMITING

Vomiting is common in the newborn period and sometimes occurs in abnormal baby. It may, however, be the first sign of serious disease and every baby who vomits must be examined carefully. Of extreme importance is the fact that the majority of children with bile stained vomit have an organic cause for the vomiting.

Causes

1. *Cerebral causes:* Birth trauma-vomiting is common in babies with intracranial haemorrhage. Meningitis can be a cause.
2. *Ingestion of blood and mucus*
3. *Underfeeding and aerophagy* can cause vomiting.
4. *Infections:* Gastroenteritis or infections outside the alimentary tract (pyelonephritis) may cause vomiting. In gastroenteritis the vomiting is usually followed by diarrhoea.
5. *Biochemical:* Uraemia in congenital renal abnormalities.

6. *Obstruction:* In high alimentary obstruction vomiting is early and there is little distension. In low alimentary obstruction vomiting is the late and accompanied by abdominal distension.

Treatment

This is really the treatment of underlying cause. Fluid loss has to be corrected and biochemical upset also corrected especially alkalosis. Early diagnosis of cases of obstruction is most important.

CONVULSIONS (SEIZURE) IN NEWBORN

It is twitching of limbs, generalised stiffness without clonic phase and sudden jerky movements. This is differentiated from jitteriness or course tremors.

Causes and diagnosis

Disturbance in cerebral tissue is the cause.

1. *Traumatic—trauma* causes oedema of brain and intracranial haemorrhage (subdural or subarachnoid). Convulsion develops at 2–7 days.
   Diagnosis: Bulged fontanelle, blood stained CSF, X-ray skull shows fracture CAT.
2. *Asphyxia* leads to cerebral oedema, scanty petechial cerebral haemorrhage and fits on first day. Some develop epilepsy later.
   Diagnosis is made from moderate to severe low Apgar score.
   Trauma and asphyxia lead to one fourth of neonatal convulsion.
3. *Metabolic*
   - Hypocalcaemia (10–20%) develops particularly in IUGR and preterm when blood calcium level is less than 7 mg%.
   - Hypomagnesemia can be associated with hypocalcaemia when blood magnesium level is 1.25 mg%. Isolated disorder occurs in congenital metabolic disorder.

- Hyperbilirubinaemia causes convulsion (kernicterus) with plasma unconjugated bilirubin over 20 mg% in full term and 16 mg% in preterm baby.
- Hypoglycaemia blood glucose less than 20 mg% causes convulsion in newborn particularly in preterm and small for date baby. Symptoms are hypotonia, apnoea, stupor, jitteriness and convulsion.

4. *Infections:* Neonatal septicaemia leads to meningitis and convulsion. Lumbar puncture and CSF examination are mandatory. Gram-negative coliform bacilli is the commonest bacteria, rarely staphylococcus is the bacteria. Blood culture comes positive.

Neonatal tetanus causes tonic spasm simulating convulsions.

5. *Developmental defect* of brain as in microcephaly, hydrocephalus agenesis of corpus callosum cause convulsion.

6. *Withdrawal syndrome:* If mother had barbiturates, heroin, morphine, alcohol during pregnancy infant develops withdrawal symptom (incessant cry, sweating) and convulsion.

7. *Cause unknown:* Convulsion may occur where no cause can be identified.

Treatment

1. Oral feeding is suspended if convulsion is recurrent. Intravenous line is set up.
2. Oxygen is given if there is cyanosis.
3. For hypoglycaemia, 25% dextrose 2–3 ml/kg body weight is given initially over 3 mins, then 10% dextrose 100 ml/kg/day as maintenance therapy. If blood glucose level remains low with above treatment, hydrocortisone 5 mg/kg every 12 hours is administered.
4. Sedation and anticonvulsants—as anticonvulsant, inj. diazepam 0.2 mg/kg is given IV phenytoin (Dilantin) 5–10 mg/kg IV in 5–10 mins is given for convulsion.

Maintenance dose is 4–7 mg/kg/day in divided two doses IV or orally. After control of convulsions, anticonvulsants are tapered off and given for 4–12 weeks depending on EEG status.

To relieve cerebral oedema, mannitol 20% 10 ml/kg is given over 30–60 min. Inj. dexamethasone 1 mg IV is given followed by 0.5 mg 6 hourly.

5. Other specific treatment. Appropriate antibiotic for meningitis, exchange transfusion for hyperbilirubinaemia, calcium gluconate 10% 5–10 ml slowly injected over 5–10 minutes for hypocalcaemia.

6. Monitoring of blood pressure, serum electrolytes, blood pH is done. EEG is done for prognosis.

Prognosis

About one-fourth neonates die. High rate of neurological sequelae follow asphyxia, birth injury, hypoglycaemia, meningitis.

HAEMORRHAGIC DISEASE IN NEWBORN

Definition

Spontaneous haemorrhage from various site especially in the alimentary tract in the newborn. This occurs commonly during the first week of life with an incidence up to 1%.

Cause

Low prothrombin level and deficiencies of vitamin dependant coagulation factors, II, VII, IX and X result in decreased prothrombin activity. Asphyxia, trauma, prematurity and

---

🔑 Box 14.1: Nursing diagnoses

- Airway clearance, ineffective, related to mucus obstruction.
- Hypothermia related to body heat loss.
- Risk for Infection, related to newborn's susceptibility to pathogens.
- Urinary elimination, altered, related to circumcision.

infection predispose the condition, perhaps due to damage to the capillaries. In some cases, disseminated intravascular coagulopathy (DIC) may develop.

Sites of haemorrhage

1. Alimentary tract haematemesis and melaena neonatorum–the commonest site
2. Lungs
3. Vagina
4. Umbilicus
5. Skin, nose, urinary tract (haematuria)
6. Intracranial haemorrhage.

Clinical features

Haemorrhage starts on second, third or fourth day; prematures become more prone to develop the condition. Blood in vomitus is bright red and it may be slight or copious. Likewise, stool may be tarry or frank blood is visible in the stool. In brisk haemorrhage, baby appears pale, collapsed and many die.

Treatment

Prophylaxis Inj. vitamin K 1 mg is given IM x 2 days to high-risk neonates.

Curative

1. The baby is placed in head down position turned to one side while there is haematemesis.
2. Unnecessary handling of the baby is avoided.
3. In affected babies, breastfeeding is temporarily suspended. Bottlefeeding is also stopped in artificially fed babies when there is haematemesis.
4. Fluids: In cases of blood-vomiting nothing by mouth is given. Compatible fresh blood transfusion or plasma (where blood is not available) becomes necessary in severe cases. Glucose is given IV.
5. Vitamin K: Inj. vitamin K, or vitamin K analogue 1 mg is given immediately and may have to be repeated next day. Higher dosage of water soluble vitamin K analogue is dangerous as it may cause jaundice and kernicterus.

Secondary anaemia: This is treated later on by giving iron suspension (2–4 mg elemental iron/kg).

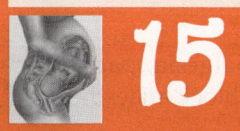

15

Pharmacology and Child Birth

OUTLINE

- Analgesics and antispasmodies in pregnancy
- Drugs used in pregnancy, labour and puerperium

ANALGESICS AND ANTISPASMODICS IN PREGNANCY AND LABOUR

GENERAL ACHES, PAIN AND DISCOMFORT

Analgesics and antispasmodics should be considered only after all serious causes of pain (like acute abdomen, urinary tract infection and venous thrombosis) have been excluded and simple drug measures like massage and hot water bag, etc. have been given a try.

The drugs commonly prescribed include paracetamol, soluble aspirin, ibuprofen, gels or creams for local application.

The commonly prescribed medicaments include the following

- *Paracetamol* 500 mg/1 tab b.d. or t.d.s. generally safe during pregnancy and lactation.
- *Soluble aspirin* one 350 mg (enteric coated) tablet b.d. after a meal. Risk of maternal or fetal bleeding on long term usage.
  Caution: Use with care in patients of gastric irritation and ulcer.
- *Ibuprofen* 200 mg tab, one tab b.d. when required, preferably on full stomach.
  Use with caution in patients with gastric irritation. There are a variety of nonsteroidal antiinflammatory drugs (NSAIDs) like ibuprofen, naproxen, indomethacin, etc. commonly used in practice.

Analgesics and antispasmodics for colics during pregnancy (other than uterine colic), *intestinal colics, biliary colic and ureteric colics.*

The drugs in common usage include hyoscine, dicyclomine, va; ethamate and drotaverine. These drugs should be prescribed after excluding obstruction and inflammation. The salient features of these drugs are as follows:

- *Hyoscine-N-butyl bromide (Buscopan):* This drug is a smooth muscle relaxant, and is prescribed in doses of 10 to 20 mg orally or parenterally.
- *Dicyclomine hydrochloride:* This is available as an injection of 20 mg, and also as an oral tablet of 20 mg in combination with dextropropoxyphene 65 mg and acetaminophen 400 mg (Spasmoproxyvon).
- *Valethamate (Epidosin, Valosin):* Available as oral tablet of 10 mg and as injectable of 8.0 mg. Useful for colics and to facilitate cervical dilatation during labour. It may be repeated at every 20 to 30 minutes if necessary. It often causes flushing, dryness of the mouth, difficulty in swallowing and tachycardia.
- *Drotaverine (Drotin):* Available as oral table of 40 mg b.d. or t.d.s. or injection of 40 mg in 2 ml ampoules. The dose may be repeated after 4 hours if required. It is useful in management of smooth muscle

spasms and also to assist cervical dilatation during labour.

ANALGESICS FOR PAIN RELIEF DURING LABOUR

Prescribed pethidine, promethazine hydrochloride, pentazocine, tramadol, ketamine, local and regional anaesthetic agents, and anaesthetic gases, all these drugs should be used only when the patient is in established labour and has entered the active phase of cervical dilatation.

- Pethidine is available as 100 mg in every 2 ml ampoules. This drug should be withheld if the patient is in advanced labour and likely to deliver within an hour. The drug crosses the placenta and can cause respiratory depression in the newborn. It can cause vomiting in labour. Nalorphine must be available for administration to the newborn suffering from drug-induced respiratory depression.
- *Promethazine HCl (Phenergan):* Available as 2 ml ampoule containing 25 mg/ml. This drug is an antihistamine which potentiates the action of pethidine or pentazocine. The combination helps to provide better relief at reduced doses, and thus reduces the chances of birth asphyxia.
- *Pentazocine (Penzyl, Fortwin, Pentawin, Dolowin):* This drug is available as 1 ml ampoule of 30 mg each. It is also an opioid analgesic and exerts mixed agonist and antagonist actions at the receptor level. It has a ceiling effect on respiratory depression *which can be countered with nalorphine.*
- *Tramadol (Contramal, Tramazac, Tramadol, Domadol):* This drug is available as 1 to 2 ml ampoules containing 50 mg/ml. It is advisable not to exceed the dose of 1 mg /kg body weight to minimize complications. This drug is a semisynthetic opiate derivative with a longer duration of action, effective analgesia and minimum depressive action on the fetal respiration.

- Lumbar epidural analgesia, paracervical block and pudendal block anaesthesia.

DRUGS USED IN PREGNANCY, LABOUR AND PUERPERIUM

ANTIEMETICS IN PREGNANCY

Antiemetics are prescribed for patients who do not respond well to conservative measures or who are admitted with excessive vomiting affecting their health status. Amongst the commonly used drugs are meclozine, cyclizine, promethazine and diphenhydramine as mentioned earlier. However, other drugs often prescribed include prochlorperazine (Emidoxyn, Stemetil), trifluoperazine (Trazine), doxylamine (Doxinate, Pymidoxin), pyridoxine HCl or vitamin B (Benadon, B-Long, Pyricontin) and metoclopramide (Perinorm, Maxeron, Reglan) to be used as a second line of treatment if the earlier treatments fail.

Antiemetic drugs to be avoided during pregnancy include domperidone, cisapride and ondansetron.

STEROIDS DURING PREGNANCY

Corticosteriods are prescribed for many different indications during pregnancy. They are administered through various routes—topical, inhalational, oral or parenteral preparations. These should be used with caution during pregnancy.

Common clinical indications

Amongst the common indications for the use of steroid drugs, the following are important:
- Severe bronchial asthma
- Autoimmune and collagen disorders—rheumatoid arthritis and systemic lupus erythematosus (SLE).
- Sometimes in recurrent pregnancy losses due to phospholipids antibodies.
- Threatened preterm labour prior to 34 weeks of gestation to prevent hyaline mem-

brane disease/respiratory distress synd-rome (HMD/RDS).

- Acute allergic emergencies and anaphy-laxis.
- Endotoxic and septic shock.
- Acute attack of ulcerative colitis.
- Herpes gestationis, impetigo herpetiformis gestationis.
- Immunosuppressant pregnant women with kidney transplant.
- Psoriasis
- Severe pruritus

SYSTEMIC STEROIDS IN CLINICAL USE

Hydrocortisone preparations (Efcorlin, Lycortin-S)

These contain hydrocortisone succinate 134 mg equivalent to 100 mg hydrocortisone (for parenteral/intramuscular/intravenous use). Hydrocortisone acetate is used only for topical use.

Prednisolone preparations

Prednisolone is more potent than hydrocor-tisone. It is available in many forms. For oral use, plain prednisolone table of 5.0 mg each (Deltacortril, Wysolone). Injectable prednisolone such as methylprednisolone acetate available as Depo-Medrol, and methylprednisolone sodium succinate (solu-Modrol) available as 8 ml (500 mg) vials and 16 ml (1.0 g) vials.

Betamethasone preparations (Betnelan, Betnesol)

It is more potent than prednisolone. For oral use, Betnelan or Betnesol tab. of 0.5 to 1.0 mg strength and also as injection Betnesol as 4.0 mg ampoules.

Dexamethasone preparations

It is a very potent glucocorticoid which causes marked suppression of the pituitary-adrenal axis. It is available as oral tab. by the name Decdan and Dexona, and as injectable from of the same name.

Contraindications and special precautions

Avoid using steroids or exercise caution when prescribing these drugs for the following:

Peptic ulcer, live virus immunization, systemic bacterial infection, diabetes mellitus, lactation, tuberculosis, hypertension, psy-chiatric states, osteoporosis, systemic fungal infection, chronic nephritis, herpes simplex, keratitis, etc.

DRUGS IN ASTHAMA (DURING PREGNANCY)

Asthma is a common clinical disorder encoun-tered during pregnancy. It is often aggravated during pregnancy. Allergic stimuli, weather changes, pollution and emotional stress may aggravate the condition.

Management of asthma during pregnancy
Mild disease

- *Salbutamol inhaler* (Asthalin, Salbutamol): The recommended dose is 1 to 2 puffs every 3 to 6 hours or as needed. Each puff is a metered dose providing 100 mg.
- *Beclomethasone inhaler* (Becloate, Becorde): The recommended dose is 2 to 4 puffs two to four times daily. Each puff provides 100 µg.

Moderate to severe disease

- Salbutamol inhaler as above
- Beclomethasone inhaler as above
- Sodium chromoglycate inhaler (Fintal, Cromal-5): This drug stabilizes the mast cell membrane.

Fintal inhaler provides 400 metered doses of 1.0 mg/dose. The dose recommended is 2 puffs four to eight times per day. Cromal-5 inhaler provides 112 metered doses of 5.0 µg/dose since the drug concentration is much higher, the recommended dose is ¼ the dose of Fintal.

- Aerocort inhaler provides combined drugs salbutamol 100 µg and veclomethasone 50 µg per puff. Combined puffs make patient compliance easy. For patients who do not

respond to inhaler drugs satisfactorily, the clinician must consider to prescribe deriphyllin additionally.

- Deriphyllin is a combination of etophylline + theophylline. It is available in four strengths: Deriphyllin-100 mg tab, deriphyllin—retard of 150, 300 and 450 mg strength. The dose is decided upon individual needs and response to therapy.

Drug management of an acute asthmatic attack during pregnancy

This is an acute emergency requiring hospitalization, intensive monitoring and treatment. The principles of treatment are as follows:

- Comfortable position—propped-up position makes patient comfortable.
- Oxygen inhalation
- Correction of dehydration and acidosis.

Bronchodilators aerosols—subcutaneous, intramuscular or intravenously. This is provided by Asthalin respirator solution 15 ml containing 5.0 mg/ml. This is given through a nebulizer. It takes 3 to 5 min to act, thereafter it may be discontinued. This may be followed up with injection salbutamol (Croysal 500 mg/ml) administered subcutaneously if necessary. The other bronchodilators used in clinical practice include aminophylline as 250 to 500 mg diluted in 20 to 50 ml of 5% dextrose slow intravenously. Avoid its use in patients already on theophylline. Alternatively injection deriphyllin may be given intravenously. Therapy should be monitored with blood gas analysis.

Other supportive measures

These include

- Antibiotics
- Steroids
- Antihistaminics
- Expectorants

For the asthmatic patient in labour, avoid use of pethidine for pain relief. Labour epidural analgesia is the method of choice for pain relief as also for anaesthesia in case a caesarean section becomes necessary. For stress prophylaxis, 100 mg hydrocortisone IV/8 hourly should be prescribed for any patient who has been on steroid therapy earlier. In the third stage of labour, avoid the use of injection methergin and $PGF_{2\alpha}$, as these may cause bronchospasm. Oxytocin is the drug of choice, failing which, PGE_2 may be used with care.

Antihypertensive drugs during pregnancy

The drugs commonly prescribed for the control of high blood pressure during pregnancy include the following: methyldopa, labetalol, propranolol and hydralazine. In case of sever pre-eclampsia, impending eclampsia or manifest eclampsia, drugs like magnesium sulphate and nifedipine have an important role to play to get the condition under rapid control (Table 15.1).

Low-dose aspirin is often prescribed from the 24th week of pregnancy to women who are considered to be prone to develop pre-eclampsia. Aspirin exerts anti-thromboxane effect and thus helps to prevent the hypertension-proteinuria syndrome. Nifedipine is a calcium channel blocker. It is prescribed orally in doses of 5 mg and 10 mg capsules, or sublingually when the clinical condition requires rapid lowering of the blood pressure. The patient must be carefully monitored by serial recording of the blood pressure.

Parenteral hydralazine administered in doses of 5 to 10 mg slow intravenously over 20 min helps to control the diastolic blood pressure between 90 to 100 mm Hg. It may be repeated after 20 min if necessary. It may be given in the form of an infusion of 50 mg hydralazine in 500 ml physiological saline or Ringer lactate solution at 40 to 60 drops per minute until the diastolic pressure is brought under control, followed by a maintenance dose.

In cases of threatened eclampsia requiring induction of labour or caesarean section immediately, continuous lumbar epidural anaesthesia would be recommended, as it lowers the blood pressure and accelerates the process of delivery.

Table 15.1: Antihypertensive drugs in pregnancy

Drug	Mode of action	Dose and remarks
Methyldopa	• Inhibition of vasoconstricting impulses from medulla oblongata • Inhibition of impulses from the hypothalamus	250–500 mg, three to four times daily
Propranolol	• Beta-adrenergic blockade	30–40 mg, four times daily
Hydralazine	• Decreased cardiac output acts directly on the muscle coat of the blood vessels and causes vasodilatation and lowered pressure	20–40 mg q.d.s. tachyphylaxis on prolonged usage
Labetalol	• It is both an alpha and beta-blocker.	100 mg/two to three times daily

In case, the above measures fail to control the blood pressure and the patient develops eclamptic convulsions or if the patient is admitted as an emergency case of eclampsia, the recommended treatment is as follows:

- *Initial dose:* 10 g of 50% solution of magnesium sulphate prepared in 20 ml, administered as 10 ml, deep IM on each buttock.
- *Subsequent doses:* 5 g of 50% magnesium sulphate administered deep IM every 4 hours on alternate buttocks.

Monitoring of treatment

Monitor the following parameters every hour, and just prior to giving the next top-up dose at half the rate.

- *Respiratory rate:* It should be more than 12/min.
- Patellar reflex present.
- *Urinary output:* This should be more than 25 ml/hour.

Close monitoring of the BP and pulse rate are mandatory. Parenteral hydralazine is not available in India.

The magnesium sulphate therapy must be continued for at least 24 hours after delivery.

Modes of action

- Impedes acetylcholine release
- Decreases the sensitivity of the motor end plate to acetylcholine.
- Exerts a central anticonvulsant effect

Antidote

To counter the excess effects of magnesium sulphate, the clinician should administer 10 ml of 10% calcium gluconate slow intravenously over a few minutes.

Presently, 'magnesium sulphate' is the treatment of choice in the management of eclampsia.

DIURETICS

The diuretics are used in the following conditions during pregnancy:

- Pregnancy induced hypertension with massive oedema
- Severe anaemia in pregnancy with heart failure
- Prior to blood transfusion in severe anaemia
- As an adjunct to certain antihypertensive drugs such as hydralazine or diazoxide.

Common preparation used

- Frusemide (loop diuretic): *Dose*—40 mg tab. daily following breakfast for 5 days a week. In acute conditions, the drug is administered parenterally in doses of 40–120 mg daily. *Mode of action*—It directly prevents reabsorption of sodium and potassium mainly from the loop of Henle.

Hazards

- *Maternal complications include:* weakness, fatigue, muscle cramps, hyperkalaemia

and postural hypotension. These can be corrected by potassium supplement during therapy.

- *Fetal*
  - In pre-eclampsia, its routine use should be restricted, as it is likely to cause further reduction of maternal plasma volume, which is already lowered. This may result in diminished placental perfusion leading to fetal compromise. Other hazards include thrombocytopenia and hyponatraemia.
  - *Hydrochlorthiazide (Esidrex): Dose*—25–50 mg tab. daily after breakfast for 5 days a week.
    Mode of action: The same mechanism as that of frusemide, but by acting on the proximal and distal convoluted tubules. Maternal and fetal hazards are the same as those of frusemide.
  - *Spironolactone (Aldactone):* The drug antagonizes aldosterone by competitive inhibition in the distal tubules thereby preventing the potassium excretion and decreasing the sodium reabsorption. *Dose:* initially 25 mg tab. may be raised to even 100 mg in divided doses. *Advantages:* There is no potassium loss. It has also some hypotensive action.

ANTICONVULSANTS

The commonly used drugs are given in Table 15.2.

TOCOLYTICS IN OBSTETRICS FOR THE NEXT 12 TO 48 HOURS, AT THE END OF WHICH THE THERAPY CAN BE SWITCHED OVER TO ORAL MEDICATION

Monitoring ritodrine infusion

Clinical parameters serially monitored include pulse rate, respiratory rate, blood pressure and auscultation of the lung bases to detect in time any tachycardia, hypotension and/or pulmonary oedema. The clinician should adjust the infusion rate so that the pulse rate does not exceed 120/ min, the systolic pressure does not drop below 90 mm Hg. and the lung bases are free of crepitations. It is mandatory to maintain a strict fluid intake-output chart to prevent fluid overload. Keep a watch on the electrolyte balance, and monitor fetal well-being with serial cardiotocography (CTG).

Oral ritodrine therapy: This should commence 30 to 60 min before discontinuing ritodrine infusion. The usual dose is 10 mg 4 to 8 hourly until clinical situation demands. Restrict its use in the third trimester only.

IM ritodrine therapy: This may be advised every 4 to 8 hours/for 12 to 24 hours after the uterine contractions cease.

Isoxsuprine HCl (Duvadilan, Perivalan)

Available as 10.0 mg tablet or as injection in 2.0 ml ampoules. Dosage schedule, 2 tablets orally after meals 4 to 8 hourly until uterine activity ceases. Thereafter reduce the dose to 1 tablet t.d.s. as long as clinically indicated.

It is administered intramuscularly, starting with a low dose of 5.0 mg, and gradually increasing the subsequent doses by 5.0 mg serially to 10–15–20 mg respectively, until contractions cease or side effects limit further increments of the drug. Once the end point of quiescence has been achieved switch over to oral medication.

Salbutamol (Asthalin, Bronkotab)

Oral Salbutamol tablets of 2.0 mg are available. These are prescribed in dose of ½ to 1 tablet or as injection 0.5 mg/ml in doses of 1 to 2 ml on admission followed by oral therapy. Monitor therapy as for any tocolytic agent.

Terbutaline (Bricanyl)

Available as injection containing 0.5 mg drug per ml in ampoules. The initial dose is ½ to 1.0 ml subcutaneously every 6 to 8 hourly. Once the contractions subside, therapy may be continued using ½ to 1 tablet every 8 hours until necessary.

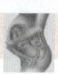

Table 15.2: Anticonvulsants

Drug	Mode of action	Dose and remarks
Diazepam	Central muscle relaxant and anti-convulsant	Initially 20–40 mg IV to be followed by an infusion containing 500 ml of dextrose with 40 mg of diazepam, the drip rate being 30 drops/minute or adjusted as per need.
Magnesium sulphate	It increases cerebral blood flow as established with Doppler studies. It reduces cerebral vasospatic ischaemia. Elevated concentration of circulatory magnesium decreases the acetylcholine release and reduces the motor end plate sensitivity to acetylcholine. It thereby reduces neuro-muscular irritability. It also decreases intracranial oedema and helps in diuresis. Its peripheral vasodilatation effect improves the uterine blood supply.	20 ml of 20% IV slowly in 3–4 minutes. To be followed immediately. IM 10 ml of 50% and is given 4 hourly till 24 hours postpartum. Repeat injections are given only if the knee jerks are present, urine output exceeds100 ml in previous 4 hours and the respiration is more than 10 per minute. The therapeutic level of serum magnesium is 4–7 mEq/L (not more than 20 gm should be given in 24 hrs).
Phenytoin	Centrally acting anticonvulsant	Eclampsia:10 mg /kg IV—at the rate not more than 50 mg /min followed 2 hours later by 5 mg /kg. Epilepsy: 300–400 mg daily orally in divided doses.
Phenobarbitone	Perhaps by inhibiting reticular activating system (RAS)	120–240 mg in divided doses.
Paraldehyde	Depresses the sensory area of the cortex, raises the threshold for convulsion. It is excreted mainly through the lungs and partly through kidneys.	2–10 ml deep IM into the gluteal region.

Table 15.3: Anticoagulants

Drug	Mode of action	Dose and remarks
Heparin	Inhibits action of thrombin, it also enhances the activity of anti thrombin III	5,000–10,000 IU. To be administered parenterally 2,500 IUSC every 24 hours
Warfarin	Interferes with synthesis of vit. K dependent factors (II,VII,IX, X)	10 mg orally daily for initial 2 days then 3–9 mg daily (taken at the same time each day depending upon the prothrombin time (INR)

Contraindications to tocolysis: These include cardiac disease, severe pre-eclampsia and eclampsia, intrauterine infection, intra-uterine fetal demise and antepartum haemo-rrhage. Use with great caution in cases of gestational diabetes.

OXYTOCICS IN OBSTETRICS

Definition

Oxytocics are the drugs of varying chemical nature that have the power to excite contrac-tions of the uterine muscles. Among a large

 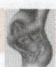

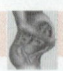

number of drugs belonging to this group, the following are the important ones and are extensively used in clinical practice:

- Oxytocin
- Ergot derivatives
- Prostaglandins

OXYTOCIN

Mode of action: Oxytocin is thought to bind to oestrogen dependent receptors on myometrial cell membranes. Bound intracellular calcium near the cell membrane is eventually mobilized from the sarcoplasmic reticulum to activate the contractile protein. Oxytocin is also thought to release prostaglandins from the deciduas. The uterine contractions are similar to the physiological pattern, i.e.causing fundal contraction with relaxation of the cervix.

Preparation used

1. Synthetic oxytocin (Syntocinon-Sandoz or Pitocin-Parke-Davis) is widely used. It has only got oxytocic effect without any vasopressor action. The Syntocinon is available in ampoules containing 51 U/ml; the Pitocin in 51 U/ml.
2. *Syntometrine (Sandoz):* A combination of syntocinon 5 units and ergometrine 0.5 mg.
3. *Desamino oxytocin:* It is not inactivated by oxytocinase and is 50–100% more effective than oxytocin. It is used as buccal tablets containing 501 U.
4. Oxytocin nasal solution contains 40 units/ml.

Indications

Oxytocin may be conveniently used in pregnancy, labour or puerperium. The indications are grouped as follows:

- Therapeutic
- Diagnostic

Therapeutic

- Pregnancy
- Labour
- Puerperium

Pregnancy

Early

- To accelerate abortion—inevitable or missed and to expedite expulsion of hydatidiform mole
- To stop bleeding following evacuation of the uterus
- Used as an adjunct to induction of abortion along with other abortifacient agents

Late

- To induce labour
- To facilitate cervical ripening for effective induction

Labour

- Augmentation of labour
- Uterine inertia
- In active management of third stage, it is used along with ergometrine (Syntometrine) during crowning of the head.
- Following expulsion of placenta as an alternative to ergometrine

Puerperium

To minimize blood loss and to control postpartum haemorrhage.

Diagnostic

- Oxytocin challenge test (OCT)
- Oxytocin sensitivity test (OST)

Contraindications

In later months of pregnancy

- Grand multipara
- Contracted pelvis
- Previous history of caesarean section or hysterotomy
- Malpresentation

During labour

- All the contraindications mentioned in pregnancy
- Obstructed labour
- Incoordinate uterine contraction

Any time
- Hypovolaemic state
- Cardiac disease

Dangers

The dangers are particularly noticed when the drug is administered late in pregnancy or during labour.
- Maternal
- Fetal

Maternal

Uterine rupture

The causes are

1. Wrong selection of cases
2. Injudicious administration of the amount of oxytocin
3. Improper supervision
4. Hypersensitivity of the uterus to oxytocin. These factors either singly or in combination produce violent uterine contractions leading to rupture. Intramuscular oxytocin must not be used while the fetus is inside the uterus. Sudden onset of violent contractions may be responsible for rupture and occasionally amniotic fluid embolism.

Hypotension

There is occasional fail of blood pressure following rapid intravenous administration of oxytocin. This is more likely in cases when the circulation is already compromised by hypovolaemia or a heart disease. As such, rapid intravenous administration is to be avoided.

Antidiuresis

The antidiuretic effect may be evident when the rate of infusion is raised to 40–50 milliunits per minute. One should take a cautious attitude even when the rate exceeds 20 mU/min. The dose should therefore be raised by increasing the strength of the oxytocin solution rather than the rate of infusion. Ringer lactate solution is preferable to customary 5 percent dextrose to prevent water intoxication.

Fetal

- Increased uterine tonus or tetanic contractions may produce asphyxia or even fetal death due to impairment of placental blood flow especially in a previously compromised foetus. Hence, a careful fetal monitoring is mandatory even when a low dose is administered.
- Increased incidence of neonatal jaundice following the use of oxytocin in labour is probably related more to prematurity and rarely to haemolysis due to vasopressin factor of oxytocin. Infusion of oxytocin in doses as high as 32 mU/min for a prolonged period during labour is often related.

Routes of administration

- Controlled intravenous infusion is the widely used method.
- Bolus IV or IM
- Intramuscular
- Buccal tablets or nasal spray—limited use on trial basis.

Methods of administration

- Controlled intravenous infusion
- Intramuscular

CONTROLLED INTRAVENOUS INFUSION

- For induction of labour
- Use in labour

For induction of labour

Principles

1. Because of erratic response of the uterus to a particular dose, the oxytocin should be started with a low dose but escalated quickly where there is no response. When the optimal response is achieved (uterine contraction sustained for about 45 seconds and numbering 3 contractions in 10 minutes), the administration of the particular concentration in mU/per minute is to be continued. This is called oxytocin titration technique.

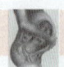

2. The objective of oxytocin administration is not only to initiate effective uterine contractions but also to maintain the normal pattern of uterine activity till delivery and at least 30–60 minutes beyond that.

Calculation of the infused dose: Now-a-days the infusion is expressed in terms of milliunits per minute. This can give an accurate idea about the exact amount administered per minute irrespective of the concentration of the solution.

Regulation of the drip

The drip is regulated by:
- Manually, counting the drops per minute commonly practised.
- Using electronic drop counter attached to the set.
- Cardiff oxytocin infusion pump which automatically controls the amount of fluid to be infused.

Convenient regime

Ordinarily, a multigravida uterus or the uterus which is already contracting is much more sensitive to oxytocin. In this respect, the primigravida uterus is less responsive because of wide variation in response, it is a sound practice to start with a low dose (4 mU/minute) and to escalate quickly if there is no response. The patient should preferably lie on one side or in semi-Fowler's position to minimize vena caval compression.

In majority of cases, a dose of less than 16 milliunits per minute (2 units in 500 ml Ringer's solution with drop rate of 60/minute) is enough to achieve the objective. Conditions where fluid overload is to be avoided infusion with high concentration and reduced drop rate is preferred. However, in an unresponsive state, higher doses may be required especially when induction is done in lesser weeks of gestation or in cases of intrauterine fetal death. The total dose required to initiate labour ranges from 600 to 12000 milliunits with an average of 4000 milliunits.

Use in labour

Oxytocin infusion is used during labour in uterine inertia or for augmentation of labour. The procedure consists of low rupture of the membranes followed by oxytocin infusion, if the liquor is found clear. One should assess the case carefully and feto pelvic disproportion should be ruled out. A low dose infusion is usually enough to stimulate the uterine contraction. An initial dose of 2 mU/minute may be stepped up to the usual maximum of 3–4 mU/minute to achieve the objective.

Observation

- The mother should never be left alone when the oxytocin infusion is running.
- Rate of flow of the infusion should be observed and properly adjusted especially when the drip is regulated by counting the drops per minute.
- Response to uterine contraction should be meticulously observed by noting the hardening of the uterus on abdominal palpation. In the absence of electronic gadgets, the number of uterine contraction in 10 minutes and the tonus of the uterus in between contractions (using finger tip palpation) should be noted.
- Fetal heart rate should be noted every 15 minutes interval. Continuous electronic fetal monitoring, if available, is undoubtedly ideal, especially for high-risk cases. Cardiotocographic equipment can record FHR and uterine contractions simultaneously.
- Maternal condition: Pulse rate is to be noted frequently and the blood pressure is to be checked hourly. The amount of urine should be noted when larger doses are administered (in excess of 20 mU minute). Any untoward symptoms like precordial

Table 15.4: Calculation of the dose delivered in milliunits (mU) and its correlation with drop rate per minute

Units of oxytocin mixed in 500 ml Ringer's solution (1 unit =1000 milliunits) (mU)	Drops per minute (15 drops = 1 ml)		
	15		30
	In terms of mU/minute		
1	2	4	8
2	4	8	16
8	16	32	64

Table 15.5: Showing the convenient regime

Dose of oxytocin	Solution used	Escalating drop rate at intervals of 15–30 min
To start with 1 unit	500 ml Ringer's solution	15–30–60
If no response—2 units	- do-	-do-
If still no response—8 units	- do-	-do-

pain or uneasiness should be detected promptly.

- Progress of labour: Progressive descent of the head and the rate of cervical dilatation are to be noted. The colour of the liquor is to be inspected periodically.

Indications of stopping the infusion

1. Nature of uterine contractions
   - Abnormal uterine contractions occurring frequently (every 2 minutes or less) or lasting more than 60 sec.
   - Increased tonus in between contractions.
2. Evidences of fetal distress
3. Appearance of untoward maternal symptoms

How to minimize the hazards?

- Judicious selection of cases (mentioned earlier)
- To administer a controlled intravenous infusion starting with a low dose.

- Meticulous supervision (vide supra) to note:
  1. Behaviour of the uterine contractions
  2. Maternal condition
  3. Fetal condition
- To stop the infusion at the earliest or IM after the birth of the baby as an alternative to ergometrine.

INTRAMUSCULAR

The preparation used is syntometrine
1. As a prophylaxis against haemorrhage, 1 amp is administered with the crowning of the head or immediately after the birth of the baby.
2. As a routine following delivery of the placenta.

Diagnostic

- Oxytocin challenge test
- Oxytocin sensitivity test

 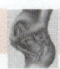

OXYTOCIN CHALLENGE TEST (OCT)

It is an invasive method of stress test to assess the fetal wellbeing in utero during pregnancy as suggested by alteration in FHR in response to uterine contractions.

Principles

The test is based on determination of the respiratory function of the fetoplacental unit during induced contractions when the blood flow through the unit is curtailed. The objective is to detect the degree of fetal compromise so that a suitable time can be selected to terminate the pregnancy.

Candidates for the test

The patients with medical-obstetrical problems related to uteroplacental compromises such as:

- Intrauterine growth retardation
- Postmaturity
- Hypertensive disorders of pregnancy
- Diabetes, are suitable candidates.

Contraindications

- Established compromised fetus
- Previous history of caesarean section
- Complications likely to produce preterm labour
- APH: Thus, its use is very much selective.

Procedure

The oxytocin infusion is started in the same manner as mentioned earlier. The initial rate of infusion is 1 mU/minute which is stepped up at intervals of 15 minutes until the effective uterine contractions are established (vide supra). The alteration of the FHR during contractions can be interpreted by electronic cardiotocographic equipment fitted to the patient's abdomen. Alternatively, clinical monitoring can effectively be performed using hand to palpate the hardening of the uterus during contraction and auscultation of FHR during contraction and for one minute thereafter. It takes at least 1–2 hours to perform the test.

Interpretation

Positive: Persistent late deceleration of the FHR—bradycardia develops after the contraction starts reaching its nadir after the peak of uterine contractions. The recovery of the baseline fetal heart rate does not occur until the contraction is over.

Negative: No delayed deceleration is observed even with 3 contractions in 10 minutes.

Suspicious: Inconsistent but definite decelerations do not persist with most uterine contractions.

Unsatisfactory: Due to poor quality of recording.

Hyperstimulation: Decelerations of FHR occur with uterine contractions lasting more than 90 seconds or occurring more frequently than every two minutes.

Importance

Negative test is of value but there is 50% chance of false positive result and as such positive test cases are subjected to other methods of evaluating the wellbeing of the fetus.

OXYTOCIN SENSITIVITY TEST (OST)

The test was devised by Nixon and Smith to assess the irritability of the uterus following the administration of oxytocin.

Procedure

0.01 units of oxytocin is injected intravenously at the end of a spontaneous uterine contraction. The injection is to be administered at one minute intervals until an induced contraction starts. This can be evidenced by hardening of the uterus on abdominal palpation.

Inference

If the contraction fails to start even after 4 injections, the uterus is unlikely to be responsive to induction. Prediction of maturity of the fetus using the test is not reliable.

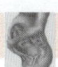

ERGOT DERIVATIVES

Out of many ergot derivatives, two are used extensively as oxytocics. These are:

- Ergometrine (ergonovine in USA)
- Methergin (methyl ergonovine in USA)

Mode of action

Ergometrine acts directly on the myometrium. It excites uterine contractions which come so frequently one after the other with increasing intensity that the uterus passes into a state of spasm without any relaxation in between.

Mode of administration

Ergometrine and methergin can be used parenterally or orally. As it produces tetanic uterine contractions, the preparation should only be used either in the late second stage of labour (after the delivery of the anterior shoulder) or following delivery of the baby.

It is highly effective in haemostasis to stop bleeding from uterine sinuses either following delivery or abortion.

Indications

- Therapeutic
- Prophylactic

Therapeutic

The indication of ergometrine or methergin is to stop the atonic uterine bleeding, following delivery, abortion or expulsion of hydatidiform mole.

Prophylactic

As a prophylaxis against excessive haemorrhage following delivery, it may be used after the delivery of the anterior shoulder (active management of third stage of labour). It minimizes the blood loss in the third stage to one-fifth of the normal and also shortens its duration. The same effect obtained if administered with crowning or following delivery of the baby.

Contraindications

The following are contraindication to its use:

Prophylactic

1. *Suspected plural pregnancy:* If given accidentally with the delivery of the first baby, the second one is likely to be compromised by the tetanic contraction of the uterus.
2. *Organic cardiac diseases:* It may cause sudden squeezing of blood of the uterine circulation into the general circulation causing overloading of the right heart and precipitating failure.
3. *Severe pre-eclampsia and eclampsia:* There may be sudden rise of blood pressure.
4. *Rh negative mother:* There is more chance of fetomaternal micro-transfusion.

Therapeutic

Heart disease or severe hypertensive disorders—because of its vasoconstrictive effect, it may cause transient hypertension especially when given intravenously. Oxytocin is a better substitute in such cases.

Hazards

1. Prolonged use may lead to gangrene of the toes due to its vasoconstrictive effect. Rarely, gangrene may occur even following short therapy.
2. Because of its vasoconstrictive action, it may precipitate rise of blood pressure especially in a hypertensive woman and even in a normotensive woman when given intravenously in the dose of 0.5 mg.
3. Prolonged use in puerperium may interfere with lactation by decreasing the concentration of prolactin.

Cautions

Ergometrine should not be used during pregnancy, first stage of labour, second stage prior to crowning of the head and in breech delivery prior to crowning.

PROSTAGLANDINS (PGS)

Use in obstetrics

- Induction of abortion (MTP and missed abortion)
- Termination of molar pregnancy
- Induction of labour
- Cervical ripening prior to induction of abortion or labour
- Acceleration of labour
- Management of atonic postpartum haemorrhage (refractory cases)
- Medical management of tubal ectopic pregnancy

Contraindications

Absolute

- Hypersensitivity of the compound
- Asthma
- Acute PID

Relative

- Hypertension
- Cardiovascular disease
- Renal disease
- Peptic ulcer

- Jaundice
- Uterine scar

OXYTOCIC EFFECT

Mechanism of action

Both PGE_2 and $PGF_{2\alpha}$ have got an oxytocic effect on the pregnant uterus when used in appropriate dose. The probable mechanism of action is change in myometrial cell membrane permeability and/or alteration of membrane-bound Ca^{++}. PGs also sensitise the myometrium to oxytocin. PGE_2 is at least 5 times more potent than $PGF_{2\alpha}$. $PGF_{2\alpha}$ acts predominantly on the myometrium, while PGE_2 acts mainly on the cervix due to its collagenolytic property.

Advantages

- It has got powerful oxytocic effect, irrespective of period of pregnancy. As such, it can be used independently especially in induction of abortion with success.
- In later months, where the preinduction score is low or in intrauterine death, it is more effective than oxytocin. Thus, it is a

Table 15.6: Composition of different ergot preparations

Preparations	Ampoules	Tablet
Ergometrine (ergonovine)	0.25 mg or 0.5 mg	0.5–1 mg
Methergin (methylergonovine)	0.2 mg	0.5–1 mg
Syntometrine	0.5 mg—Ergometrine +	
(sandoz)	5 units—Syntocinon	

Table 15.7: Comparative study of onset and duration of action of different oxytocics onset of action

Routes	Ergometrine	Methergin	Syntometrine	Syntocinon on puerperal uterus
IV	1 min	1½ min	Not to be used	30 sec
IM	7 min	7 min	2½ min	2½ min
Oral	10 min	10 min	–	–
		Duration of action		
	3 hrs.	3 hrs.	3 hrs.	8 min

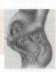

Table 15.8: Comparative study of ergot derivatives and oxytocin

	Ergot derivatives	Oxytocin
Mode of action	Acts directly on the myometrium producing tetanic contraction with complete loss of polarity	Acts on the physiological contractile system. Law of polarity is maintained.
Onset of action	Comparatively slower	Faster in action
Duration	Long sustained	Short lived
	• To stop haemorrhage from open uterine sinuses following delivery; abortion or expulsion of hydatidiform mole.	• In the induction of labour

Clinical uses	• Prophylactic use in second or in third stage, to hasten separation of placenta and to minimise blood loss	• To accelerate uterine contraction during labour
		  - Uterine inertia
		  - Judicious and selective use as a routine
		• As an haemostasis in adjunct with ergo-metrin or in isolation

Hazards	• Nausea and vomiting • Rise in blood pressure • Rarely grangrene of the toe	• Related more to injudicious use • Uterine rupture • Antidiuretic effect • Anginal pain or rarely shock

Limitations	• Should not be used prophylactically in
	  – Cardiac diseases
	  – Severe hypertensive disorders
	  – Rh negative mothers
	• Must not be used during pregnancy and labour prior to crowning of the head
		• As induction or acceleration of labour in
		  – Grand multipara
		  – Contracted pelvis
		  – Post caesarean section
		  – Malpresentation
		• As a haemostatic—rapid intravenous administration is contraindicated

useful drug not only for induction but also for acceleration of labour.

• It has got no antidiuretic effect.

Drawbacks

• It is costly and is not available widely.

• Unpleasant side effects caused by its stimulatory effect on the smooth muscles produce nausea, vomiting, diarrhoea, pyrexia or bronchospasm. If the drug accidentally, passes into the general circulation the side effects become intensified. But the symptoms subside promptly due to rapid metabolism of prostaglandins.

• When used as an abortifacient, extensive cervical lacerations may occur.

• The hyperactivity of the uterus, if occurs during induction, may continue for a variable period even after discontinuation of its administration.

Preparations

Prostaglandin E_2 is widely used because it is less toxic and more effective than $PGF_{2\alpha}$. It is, however, more costly. Some of the preparations are mentioned below:

• Tablet—contains 0.5 mg dinoprostone (Prostin E_2)

- Vaginal suppository—containing 20 PGE_2 or 50 mg $PGF_{2\alpha}$ in a lipid base
- Vaginal pessary containing 3 mg PGE_2
- Prostin E_2 (Dinoprostone) gel—500 µg into the cervical canal, below the level of internal os or 1–2 mg in the posterior fornix.

Injectable ampoules or vials

1. PGE_2—Prostin E_2 containing 1 mg/ml
2. $PGF_{2\alpha}$—Prostin $F_{2\alpha}$ (Dinoprost trometha-mine) containing 5 mg/ml
3. Methyl analogue of $PGF_{2\alpha}$ (Carboprost—containing 2.5 µg/10 ml vial)

Methyl ester of PGE_1 (Misoprostol) 50 mg 4 hourly schedule by oral, vaginal or rectal route is used. It is less expensive, can be stored at room temperature and has less side effects. It is rapidly absorbed and is more effective than oxytocin or dinoprostone for induction of labour.

Remarks about oxytocics

All the oxytocics have got their places in obstetrics.

- To stop bleeding from the open uterine sinuses following delivery or abortion, ergot preparation (ergometrine or mether-gin) is the life saving drug. In this respect, there is no second substitute, as yet in refractory cases of atonic PPH carboprost is an effective choice.
- For induction of labour—either prosta-glandins or oxytocin can be used. With favourable preinduction cervical score, there is very little to choose between oxytocin and prostaglandin. But when the score is unfavourable as in IUD, shorter period of gestation or in elderly primi-gravida prostaglandins have got a distinct advantage over oxytocin. However, prosta-glandins are costly with very restricted availability.
- For induction of abortion—prostaglandins have got a distinct advantage over oxyto-cin. Oxytocin alone is ineffective but can supplement the other methods used in induction of abortion without any conclu-sive proof of enhancing the efficacy.
- In augmentation or acceleration of labour, oxytocin still enjoys its popularity although prostaglandins are equally effective.

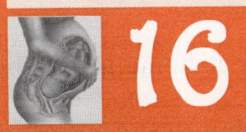

Home Birth

A home birth takes place in the woman's territory, to which the nurse-midwife goes. This is a fundamental difference which involves different responsibilities for the woman or couple and different planning, approaches and methods of providing care by the nurse-midwife.

The home is the birth setting in which the woman or couple can have the greatest amount of control over their childbirth experience. It is also the setting for which they must assume the greatest amount of responsibility for their own childbirth experience and for the care the mother and baby receive.

LEGAL ISSUES

The provision of home care services is not without risk of legal liability. Two types of legal liability can be faced by home care agencies and nursing staff. They are professional negligence and violation of state licensing laws. The nurse can be involved in a lawsuit for professional negligence when a patient is injured or dies and it is alleged that the nurse or other home health care team member's conduct was the direct, proximate cause of the injury or death. The nurse must have thorough understanding of the Nurse Practice Act related to his or her level of expertise and be careful to work within those guidelines, referring the patients as needed. Counselling and advice must be objective and have a sound rationale.

To reduce the risks of legal liability, consent forms and documentation are extremely important. Health care interventions must be established on a sound basis and backed up by a quality assurance program. In the home, the nurse must act as a member of the interdisciplinary health care team and maintain close communication with the team for proper client care.

Selection of mothers to visit

The following criterion for selecting mothers for one or more home visit is suggested:
1. Visit all expectant mothers at least once to gain an insight and understanding of the factors that may affect the pregnancy.
2. Mothers who have a history of stillbirths or who have lost babies during infancy.
3. Mothers who show signs of complications such as swelling, dizziness, headache, bleeding, etc.
4. Mothers who are anaemic and indicate that they do not have enough food.
5. Mothers who seem insecure or afraid and
6. Mothers who expect to have the delivery at home should be visited more frequently during the last two months ensuring safe delivery and engagement of a trained midwife or dai to help arrange for supplies and to help the mother understand the process of labour.

Under ideal conditions, the normal expectant mother should be observed every month either in the clinic or in the home up to 8 months, and every week in the 9th month. Any plan for visiting the expectant mother must be flexible

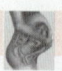

because her condition may change from month to month. It is essential that the mother should understand from the very beginning that she may call the nurse, or midwife at any time if she feels the need.

Factors which couples consider in making the decision to deliver at home include the following

1. Normalcy of the pregnancy
2. Previous hospital experience
3. Availability of alternatives both in and out of hospital.
4. Availability of preferred health care provider in different birth settings.
5. Safety for the woman in and out of hospital.
6. Safety for the baby in and out of hospital.
7. Availability of what they want in another setting, such as:
   - Presence of significant others
   - No restriction as to the number of others they want present.
   - Presence of siblings (no age restrictions) for birth as well as during labour and postpartum.
   - Ability to assume responsibility for their baby's birth.
   - No intravenous infusion
   - No restriction of activity
   - No electronic fetal monitoring
   - No artificial rupture of membranes
   - No analgesia or anaesthesia
   - No transfer to a delivery room
   - No restriction on birth position
   - Gentle birth
   - No separation of mother and baby
   - Early initiation of unlimited breastfeeding
8. Amount of control of the situation they perceive they will have.
9. Degree of participatory decision making they perceive they will have.
10. Amount of responsibility they perceive they will have.
11. Smells, noise and cleanliness of a setting.
12. Their desire to be at home in familiar surroundings.

Women and couples thus choose home birth for a variety of reasons.

ADVANTAGES OF HOME BASED ANTENATAL CARE

The following advantages of home visits should be considered:

1. The mother is generally more relaxed at home and there is more privacy than in the centre. The mother is likely to talk more freely and tell how she feels, what she eats and speak about other problems that may affect her family.
2. A home visit provides opportunity to understand the socioeconomic factors, the stress and strain as well as the positive factors that may affect the mother's attitude and action relative to the pregnancy and the instruction.
3. The home visit provides time for the nurse to listen, observe and learn. She listens and learns about what the family believes, she observes habits and health practices and uses this as a basis for learning. For example, a mother may say that water is not good for baby. Agree with her and explain that this water (unboiled) is very bad for the child but this water (boiled) is good and necessary for the child.
4. During the home visit, the nurses may meet and talk with the father-in-laws, and other relatives. The relatives must learn all that is said and done as they influence actions and attitudes.
5. Observations of the environment and health needs of other members of the family give rise to discussions and plan for improvement.

PREPARATION FOR BIRTH

More preparation on the part of the family is required when birth occurs out of hospital.

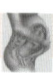

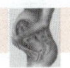

1. Teach the mother to wash, boil and dry in the sun an old sari, dhoti, skirt or any other old soft absorbent material to be used during the delivery.
2. The midwife or dai may bring scissors, flat cord ties, and boiler for sterilizing; she may bring the instruments already boiled or the mother may furnish a boiler.
3. The father or some other member of the family should whitewash the area set aside for delivery.
4. The mother and other members of the family should understand that only clean things and persons that are dressed in clean cloths should be allowed in the delivery area.
5. The family should understand that a trained midwife or dai should be engaged early.

MANAGEMENT OF LABOUR

The mother should be made to understand
1. When to call the trained midwife or trained dai.
2. That vaginal examination is made only when it is absolutely necessary.
3. No one should apply fundal pressure or push on the abdomen during labour.
4. The umbilical cord is cut with boiled scissors or boiled knife or new razor blade, to prevent tetanus.
5. No one pulls on the cord or pushes the placenta out. The placenta will come soon after the baby is born or within 20 minutes. If it does not come; doctor must be called at once or the mother must be taken to the hospital.

PREPARATION BEFORE CONFINEMENT FOR BABY AND MOTHER

Many mothers are averse to making any preparation before birth for superstitious reasons.

REQUIREMENTS OF BABY

1. *Enough clothes:* The custom of using old clothes has the advantage of being soft. It must, however, be adequate in quantity and collected beforehand so that it can be washed preferably by boiling, dried by hanging in the sun and ironed with a hot iron. After washing, the material should be folded and wrapped in thick clean cloth, and kept in a clean place as far as possible.
2. Katori (cup) for oil
3. Soda free soap
4. Cotton wool or small pieces of clean soft old rag
5. Cradle with firm bottom
6. Katori (cup) and spoon for boiled drinking water
7. Bottle with cork for boiled water.

PREPARATION FOR CONFINEMENT

1. Newspapers, clean banana leaves or jute sacks (well washed and dried in the sun).
2. Chula (stove)
3. Large container to be used as stabilizer.
4. Shallow mud pots about 8" diameter.
5. Linen—properly prepared and adequate in quantity.
6. For mothers—sanitary towels or old rags that have been washed, boiled and ironed.
7. Bed covering.
8. Specially scrubbed bed, floor canvas or clean mat.
9. Breast tray
10 Drinking vessel

The room to be used should be well cleaned. Any unnecessary furniture should be moved away from the delivery area as is the custom. The doors and windows should be left wide open to let in the sun and air.

When labour begins
1. Notify the trained midwife or *dai*
2. Bathe and take nourishment
3. Prepare boiling water

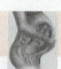

PREPARATION AND PROCEDURES FOR HOME BIRTH

In the centre

On receiving the call, take out the patients record read carefully. Check midwifery bag and add equipment at the time of call, time of leaving the office and address or required record of the mother. Leave call slip on supervisor's desk. Take record to home to be visited.

At home: first stage of labour

1. Greet the family and ascertain details regarding duration of labour pain, etc. and reassure mother and family.
2. Place midwifery bag on paper or banana leaves or on an elevated surface in confinement room.
3. Place your watch and other personal belongings at a convenient safe place.
4. Ask the family to prepare boiling water.
5. Take out soap and towel from midwifery bag.
6. Wash hands thoroughly under running water and dry.
7. Put on the apron. Prepare the mother for examination.
8. Examine the mother: Palpate abdomen and ascertain positions, watch nature of pain, enquire about bowel action, when urine was passed, etc. If the mother is in first stage give enema, examine the urine and check blood pressure.
9. Wash hands and take out the necessary equipments from bag and put them in a covered container and boil for 20 minutes.
   - Enamel bowls, 2 kidney trays, 2 covered basins.
   - A pair of artery forceps, scissors, 1 teaspoon, cord tie.
10. Boil eye dropper and syringe, and cotton swab (if required) separately.
11. Boil gloves and catheter (if used) separately.
12. Take mother's temperature.
13. Watch the progress of labour and give sufficient nourishment (milk, tea, etc.).
14. Prepare to receive baby.

Second stage

1. Wash hands and put on mask.
2. Set up articles for confinement on newspaper or clean banana leaf in order of use (Table 16.1).
3. Prepare about a pint of dettol lotion 2%.
4. Take a sterile bowl, artery forceps, sterile swab and prepare for perineal wash.
5. Place the mother in a comfortable position for delivery and bring mother down towards foot end of bed leaving enough space for delivering baby.
6. Scrub hand thoroughly for about three minutes.
7. Swab the perineal area with dettol lotion.
8. Support perineum with the sterile pad and deliver the baby.
9. Soon after the baby's head is delivered, clean the eyes, mouth and nose to remove mucus, and if necessary suck out mucus by a mucus catheter.
10. Tie the cord and separate the baby soon after the pulsation of the cord stops.

Third stage

1. Keep a kidney tray or mud pot ready to receive placenta.
2. Wash your hands thoroughly with soap.
3. Watch for the separation of placenta and deliver.
4. Rinse hands and clean perineum, examine the labia and perineum for lacerations or tears.
5. Apply sterile pad loosely and make the mother comfortable.
6. Examine the placenta.
7. Wash hands thoroughly.
8. Take the mother's temperature, pulse and respiration.

9. Assemble all the articles, wash them and, if possible, boil and replace in the mid-wifery bag.

10. Examine the mother carefully before leaving the home.

Table 16.1: Articles required for confinement

Item	Number
Plastic bag, containing plastic apron and sheet, with soap, nailbrush and towel in a water-proof bag	
Kidney tray	1
Bowls (lotion)	2
Artery forceps	2
Dissecting forceps	2
Scissors	2
Bowl-lifting forceps	1
Gloves	1 pair
Instrument box (containing syringe and needles)	1
Complete set of enema can with connection (tubing, catheter and clamp)	1
Uretheral catheter (rubber)	1
Mucus extractor	1
Spring balance	1
Oral thrmometer	1
Rectal thermometer	1
Stock of cotton for making boiled swabs	1
Sterile gauze pieces for cord dressing, mouth wipes, cord binders	
Dettol	1
Spirit	1 bottle
Bottle with antiseptic drops for baby's eye (to be used when advised)	1 bottle
Methergine or ergometrine	1
Fetoscope	1
Measuring tape	1
Notebook, pen/pencil, paper bags (not to be kept inside the kit)	

Immediate care of the newborn

1. Prepare equipment for the baby's bath in a protected corner of the room.
2. Wash hands; put on apron, take the baby in lap after protecting lap with a sheet.
3. Remove excess vernix, leave some vernix on the skin and do not bathe unless the family insists.
4. Inspect the cord for bleeding, religature and apply tincture of benzoin or iodine, dress the cord if required or if indicated. It is better to leave the cord without a dressing when home is clean and free from flies.
5. Inspect the baby thoroughly for abnor-malities.
6. Put on clean clothes for baby.
7. Place the baby in bed with head on one side without pillow and keep warm.
8. Remove apron, clean and replace equip-ments.

Instructions to family

1. Watch for abnormal bleeding of mother and report if unusual amount appears. Watch for any bleeding from the cord. If it bleeds, take child to the doctor or midwife at once.
2. Feeding—to place the baby to the breast immediately.
3. To follow proper perineal care as demons-trated by the nurse.
4. The nurse should urge the family to give the mother a full diet. She needs food to regain her strength.

The nurse or midwife should complete the birth report and give it to the health authority.

POSTNATAL VISIT

Steps to follow

1. Leave postnatal bag on a raised clean surface after greeting the mother.
2. Take out soap and towel and wash hands.

 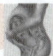

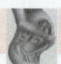

3. Put on the apron.

4. Take out the bowl, one dissecting forceps and cotton swabs.

5. Enquire regarding the condition of mother and child, nutrition, after pains, sleep lochial discharge, urine and motion. Take her temperature, pulse and respiration.

6. Prepare and place the perineal tray at the foot of the bed.

7. Bring the mother down towards the foot end of the bed and prepare her for perineal care.

8. Wash hands, inspect perineum and give perineal care.

9. Measure the height of fundus and note it down.

10. Demonstrate sponge bath and general care.

11. Wash the equipment and replace in the bag.

12. Advise the mother regarding her diet and baby's feeding.

13. Report any abnormality to the doctor.

14. Examine the nipples and give instruction regarding breast care.

15. Inspect the child and demonstrate infant care, and observe the child's ability to suckle. Demonstrate care, handling and position for nursing. Give baby-bath if permitted by family.

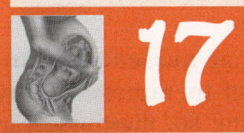

17

Complimentary and Alternative Therapies

COMPLEMENTARY AND ALTERNATIVE THERAPIES

- Historical context of complementary and alternative therapies
- Federal regulations
- Nursing acceptance of complementary and alternative therapies modalities
- Selected complementary/alternative therapies
  - Acupressure
  - Acupuncture
  - Aromatherapy
  - Biofeedback
  - Hypnosis
  - Transcutaneous electrical nerve stimulation
  - Visualization and guided imagery
  - Expressive therapy/Sound therapy
  - Reflexology
  - Yoga
  - Herbal medicine

Today, when consumer interest is increasing in self-care and responsibility for one's health, there is an upsurge of interest in complementary and alternative therapies. Complementary therapy means the therapy is used along with conventional treatments, e.g. treatment of hypertension using medication plus relaxation or biofeedback measures. Biofeedback assists or complements the medication so that it minim means an unorthodox or unconventional form of therapy. It includes therapies that generally replace or substitute a traditional or orthodox treatment. Mainstream (traditional) medicine follows a disease-oriented model with technology playing an important role in the care, whereas complementary and alternative therapies emphasize prevention, practising principles of healthy life styles, and developing the mental and spiritual healing power in the body's system. Consumers are becoming increasingly educated and are actively moving towards a holistic approach to health care. The role of the physician and the hospital are shifting from doing things for people to helping people to do things for themselves. The result is a rise of consumer driven, patient focused car. The growth of the wellness movement and increasing acceptance of such techniques, as acupuncture and biofeedback indicate the beginning of a change in health care in the western model of medicine. Many of the alternative and complementary therapies are based on the accepted theories of

1. Gate control theory of reduced pain
2. The fact that natural endorphins control pain and can be stimulated by drugs or alternative means.

HISTORICAL CONTEXT OF COMPLEMENTARY AND ALTERNATIVE THERAPIES

In ancient China a system of medical care was developed as a part of philosophical teaching. The normal activities of the human body resulted in the balance of yin and yang. A

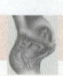

similar but distinct system, ayurveda, was developed in India centuries ago. Imbalance was the major explanation of disease. Complements to the lifestyle to restore balance included herbs, exercise and yoga. The Greek physician Galen's ideas influenced what would eventually become the beginning of modern medicine. During the Newtonian era of the eighteenth century, emphasis was placed on objective observations. By the Mid-1800s, medicine in the United States was a mix of many different contributions of Philosophies from various countries. Then a great change occurred in medicine with the advent of vaccines and antibiotics.

NURSING ACCEPTANCE OF COMPLEMENTARY AND ALTERNATIVE THERAPIES MODALITIES

In the United States, nursing has been promoting self-care for many years through Orem's self-care (Orem, 1995) framework and through Watson's theory of human caring, assessing and intervening on behalf of the whole person (Watson, 1996). The holistic approach has been a basic part of nursing since Nightingale. Modalities for self-care have increasingly been brought into nursing settings, such as the use of relaxation and imagery. Touch and massage have been therapeutic modalities of nursing care since the inception of modern American nursing. Today the importance of touch and massage have gained wide recognition as nursing interventions. Professional nursing associations have formed, such as the American Holistic Nursing, to educate nurses on self-care activities and treatment of the whole person.

Nurses neither advocate nor discourage the use of specific complementary/alternative therapies. Primarily, nurses need to become aware of herbal products and folk remedies to avoid potentially dangerous interactions and side effects in their patients.

The increasing demand by the consumer for alternative and complementary therapies makes it imperative that nurses acquaint themselves with types of therapies used by patients at home. In doing so, the nurse can collaborate with the patient, the family, the community, and the multidisciplinary health care team to provide holistic care. These practices enhance rather than inhibit or conflict with nursing care. Many patients from different cultures who have been using home remedies or folk medicine, conventional medicine, or traditional medicine are involved in alternative care. The 1980 social policy statement of the American Nurses Association states, "nursing helps to serve society's interests in the area of health. The nursing profession has made and continues to make a substantial contribution towards evolution of a health-oriented system of care."

SELECTED COMPLEMENTARY AND ALTERNATIVE THERAPIES

ACUPRESSURE

Definition

Acupressure is a traditional Chinese therapy that has been used for centuries. Acupressure is administered by a variety of practitioners, some of whom combine acupressure with other forms of Asian medicine, such as herbology.

According to traditional Chinese medicine, the body's healing energy flows along 12 to 14 meridians that connect vital organs throughout the body. The Chinese physicians have located hundreds of sensitive acupoints along these meridians. A blockage in the flow of one point on a meridian can, they believe, cause disease and discomfort in the organ or tissue. Western medical science has since shown that nerve trigger points coincide with these same acupressure points.

How the therapy is done

Acupressure is done without needles but uses finger, palm, or knuckle pressure at points

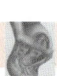

located along an invisible system of energy channels called meridians. The Chinese variation involves a more massage like kneading motion. It may be performed on a floor mat or massage table, and the person receiving the treatment usually wears comfortable, loose clothing. Practitioners may administer pressure to various points.

What the therapy hopes to accomplish

Acupressure, as a massage, can be relaxing. It may work by triggering the body to release natural pain-killing compounds such as endorphins. It can be regarded as a way of toning the body and promoting general health and wellbeing. Some studies showed a decrease in nausea and vomiting during pregnancy with acupressure.

Contraindications

The massage is administered in a slow and steady manner, although it can involve forceful pressure. Thus this may not be a choice for a person with brittle bones (osteoporosis) or a history of spinal or other orthopedic injury or those who bruise easily.

Acupressure is recommended to ease discomforts of pregnancy and childbirth. However, any pressure near or on the abdominal area should be avoided. It should also be avoided on the legs and feet, if the patient has circulation problems or varicose veins.

Possible side effects

After an acupressure treatment, some individuals report feeling light-headed or slightly groggy for a while. This feeling may be caused by build-up of endorphins.

ACUPUNCTURE

Definition

Acupuncture is promoted as a treatment for relieving pain. "There is no question that it does in fact provide short-term benefit for many of the people who try it. By some estimates, between 50 and 70 percent of patients who have chronic pain receive at least temporary relief when treated with acupuncture, and some experience long-term relief as well."

How the therapy is done

The "puncture" refers to insertion of tiny needles at very specific points on the surface of the body. The insertion of the disposable needles has been described as feeling like a place up to 20 to 30 minutes. In some cases a weak electrical current is sent through the acupressure needles to enhance the effect.

What the therapy hopes to accomplish

Both acupressure and acupuncture use meridians and some acupoints have been shown to coincide with nerve trigger points (dermatomes). The basis for the effectiveness of acupressure is the "gate control theory".

Acupuncture may trigger the release of natural pain killing substances within the body, called endorphins thus blunting the perception of pain. It may also alter the body's output of neurotransmitters, such as serotonin and norepinephrine. It is also useful for low back pain, menstrual cramps, and headaches.

Contraindications

People at risk of easy bruising or bleeding and those taking a blood-thinning medication should avoid acupuncture. Pregnant women should avoid needle insertion on or near the abdomen.

Possible side effects

Careless application or improperly sterilized needles can cause serious complications, if a blood vessel is punctured or injury to organs or nerves occurs. Therefore acupuncture should be done by a skilled and reputable practitioner.

As with acupressure, after treatment, individuals may feel light-headed for a while. This is usually attributed to the release of endorphins.

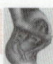

AROMATHERAPY

Definition

Aromatherapy can improve one's quality of life despite whether it has other benefits. Improvement is derived from an emotional response to pleasing scents rather than any physiologic effects. It may enhance relaxation and reduce stress, and for some people, it has helped to lessen insomnia.

How the therapy is done

The therapy relies on the use of concentrated essential oils extracted from various plants. Many oils are used as a form of a home remedy. The use of herbal teas and vapours is reported to have good effects on labour and pregnancy for some women. A few drops of lavender (diluted in a bathtub of warm water) is sometimes used to promote relaxation. Inhalation may improve respiratory conditions. Massage and rubbing aromatic oil into the skin may be calming or stimulating and may relieve muscle soreness. Some people have been able to reduce their intake of antiinflammatory drugs. *Never take aromatherapy oils internally.* Usually essential oils are very concentrated and extremely potent, and many can be toxic.

What the therapy hopes to accomplish

Fragrant oils have been used for thousands of years to lubricate the skin. For some, scented candles and potpourri have a relaxing effect. It is suggested that the vapour inhaled will have a medicinal and relaxing effect on the body.

Contraindications

During pregnancy, women should avoid many of the essential oils because of toxicity to their fetus. Also, pregnant women appear to have a particularly sensitive sense of smell, therefore aromatherapy mixtures, if used, should be very diluted.

Possible side effects

Some essential oils are contraindicated because of a possible increased risk of an abortion, preg-nancy induced hypertension or haemorrhage, therefore, oils should be administered by trained aromatherapists.

BIOFEEDBACK

Definition

Biofeedback is a technique that allows individuals to gain control over physiologic reactions that are ordinarily subconscious. Malfunctions in these automatic responses contribute to several medical problems. Biofeedback has shown the ability to help bring counterproductive reactions back into line, providing significant relief.

Biofeedback requires intensive focused concentration as one learns to control such normally involuntary (automatic) functions as heart rate, blood pressure, skin temperature, muscle tension, breathing, brain waves and digestion.

When modern instrumentation made it possible to identify subtle changes in unconscious physical reactions, Western medicine turned its attention to the mind-body connection Individual can be educated to recognize their own body responses, to learn how to relax, and through biofeedback, gain control over ordinary physiologic reactions.

Box 17.1: Pain management

- Evaluate the patient concerning her pain perceptions.
- Determine the patient's ability to manage her own pain.
- Help the patient recall positive coping techniques.
- Consider cultural factors regarding pain management.
- Empower the patient to make her own decisions concerning the pain management.
- Teach pain control techniques to the patient and family.
- Document the responses of the patient and family to interventions and teaching.

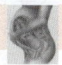

Table 17.1: Some essential oils contraindicated in pregnancy for aromatherapy

Oils	Contraindication
Pennyroyal, Rosemary, sage thyme, camphor	Can cause abortion Hypertensive can complicate PIH
Peppermint	Can cause adverse pregnancy outcome
Geranium	Has anticoagulant effect
Black pepper, caraway, cinnamon, hyssop, nutmeg, thyme	Causes cardiovascular adaptations contraindicated in pregnancy
Benzoin, cedarwood, garlic, camomile, eucalyptus, fennel, lavender, rose, sandalwood	Increases diuresis, contraindicated in severe blood loss

How the therapy is done

Biofeedback therapy applies noninvasive sensors to various points on the person's body. The location depends on the problem that needs attention. For example, to treat heart problems, the sensors are attached to monitor the heartbeat, and to treat muscle tension, the sensors are placed on the skin (electromyelogram). Some biofeedback machines signal changes on a computer display. The therapist teaches the individual mental and physical exercises that can help affect the function that is causing the problem. Once the individual has learned the pattern of actions, he or she can assert control without the aid of the feedback device.

What the therapy hopes to accomplish

Biofeedback seeks control over specific, measurable physiologic reactions that have gone astray by aggravated muscular tension or tightening. Through disciplined mental effort, biofeedback has shown the ability to reduce tension and anxiety and combat insomnia and fatigue. It has proved useful for any disorder caused or aggravated by involuntary muscular tension or tightening. Biofeedback is a relaxation technique that can be used for labour. A woman must be educated to become aware of her body and its responses and how to relax for biofeedback to be effective.

Contraindications

If a pregnant woman has an implanted pacemaker, the biofeedback technique that requires an electrical device, should not be used to gain control over physiologic reactions.

Possible side effects

Like other mind-body forms of therapy, biofeedback is notably free of side effects. Although biofeedback is harmless, it is not a substitute for medical care if a person has a serious medical problem, e.g. diabetes, heart disease or hypertension.

HYPNOSIS

Definition

Hypnosis is an altered state of consciousness, somewhat like daydreaming. The brain appears to "switch off" for a few seconds. Hypnosis seems to provide a link with the subconscious mind, with its ability to enhance the power of suggestion. Hypnosis has been found effective for a variety of problems that hinge on emotions, habits, and the body's involuntary responses. However, it does not work for everybody. Suggestions refer to the presentation of an idea to a person, and the person accepts the idea, which is influenced by motivation and expectation. The hypnotic state can be self-induced and can be implemented with regular practice. This may take 15 minutes a day to reproduce the feeling and concentrate on the images learned in the sessions with the therapist.

How the therapy is done

Commonly, individuals are asked to focus on a point and let their breathing become slow and regular. As the eyelids become heavy, the person is asked to close them and relax. As the individual feels deeply relaxed, the conscious mind will no longer control every thought and emotion as it does when awake. While the person is in a trancelike state the facilitator may make suggestions. The facilitator may tell the person how to make an unwanted symptom of habit disappear. A patient may be given a direct suggestion about pain relief, and on receiving the posthypnotic suggestion, she may, for example, increase her confidence to accept diminished sensation. Once the woman has been taught how to move into the self-hypnotic state, she can put her self-hypnosis suggestion on tape and respond to her own voice giving commands.

What the therapy hopes to accomplish

Although there seems to be a little doubt that hypnosis provided lasting benefits more many of those who try it, no one is quite certain of the reason. Some scientists speculate that it prompts the brain to release the chemicals enkephalins and endorphins, which are natural mood altering substances that can change the way we perceive pain and other physical symptoms. Many feel that hypnotherapy acts through the subconscious thereby placing the reaction under one's control.

One of hypnotherapy's greatest benefits may be its ability to reduce the effects of stress. Psychologists believe that the mind has a direct impact on physical well-being. Hypnosis can allay stress by putting one into a relaxed state, offering positive suggestions, and eliminating negative thoughts. As tension in one's muscles and blood vessels recedes, the circulation improves, and the person's entire body feels healthier. Hypnosis is associated with shorter labours and less need for analgesic medication. Hypnosis techniques used for labour and birth place an emphasis on relaxation. Some women are more susceptible to hypnosis, but it is not effective for everyone.

Contraindications

Hypnosis is considered safe for everyone although persons with a history of psychosis need careful evaluation.

Possible side effects

When offered by an appropriately qualified professional, hypnosis is considered safe under most conditions. Many people fear losing control to the therapist; however, the fact is that the hypnotist is never in control. A hypnotic suggestion works only if one accepts it. The therapist cannot make a person do something that he or she could not consciously do.

TRANSCUTANEOUS ELECTRICAL NERVE STIMULATION (TENS)

Definition

Transcutaneous electrical nerve stimulation is therapy promoted as energy medicine. It is used for all types of localized pain, such as chronic back pain, and can be used in combination with analgesic medication. It is advocated for conditions such as labour contractions, menstrual pain, jaw muscle pain, cancer pain, and nerve damage.

How the therapy is done

TENS is done with a small electronic unit that sends pulsed currents to a set of electrodes applied to the skin. When used for labour uterine contractions, TENS may involve the placement of two pairs of electrodes from a battery-operated device on either side of thoracic and sacral spine. Other electrode placement is done depending on the protocol

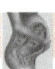

of the technician or institution. During the contraction the woman increases the stimulation by turning control knobs on the device. Women describe the sensation as a tingling or buzzing that provides pain relief.

What the therapy hopes to accomplish

The pulsed currents delivered by TENS are believed to drown out pain signals in the affected nerves, thus preventing the pain message from reaching the brain. This hypothesizes that pain must pass through a gate in the spinal cord. TENS units are also believed to stimulate the production of endorphins, the body's natural pain killers, thus the woman's discomfort is alleviated. TENS is credited with reducing the need for analgesia while increasing woman's perception of control over the experience.

Contraindications

TENS should only be used by women after full medical consultation. It should not be used if the individual has poorly controlled epilepsy or a pacemaker. The therapy should be discontinued if there is skin irritation from the electrode patches. TENS is not used before 37 weeks gestation.

Possible side effects

No harmful side effects have been reported in healthy women in labour, however, approval should be given by the physician. Benzodiazepine drugs and corticosteroids may reduce effectiveness of TENS. Application of electrodes at appropriate sites must be done by a competent, trained professional.

VISUALIZATION AND GUIDED IMAGERY

Definition

Visualization and guided imagery refer to concentration on images held in the mind's eye. Visualization is a form of mind-to-body technique that has been tested is used extensively in labour. Visualization and guided imagery work in connection between the brain and the involuntary system. Visual images can influence both the voluntary and involuntary nervous system.

How the therapy is done

Instruments or monitors are not used. Sometimes music is played in the background to aid relaxation. Sessions begin with general relaxation exercises, then move on to a specific visualization. The individual is asked to build a detailed image in her mind, using all five senses (touch, see, smell, feel and hear) and may repeat the exercise with a different image. If the person has a specific medical complaint (or discomfort), she will be asked to picture the affected organ(s) working properly. She may be asked to recall a scene from a book or some peaceful image from the past. Often, guided imagery asks the person to focus on a journey through several visualization, which may be described as a "focused daydream." Between sessions, the person is asked to use a book or audiotape to practise the visualization.

When used in preparation for childbirth classes, the woman is asked to focus on a pleasant memory using a favorite object, such as a photograph that she can take with her to the birth facility. During her labour she can focus her attention on the object. This will likely reduce her perception of pain.

What the therapy hopes to accomplish

Numerous studies have confirmed the ability of meditation training to lower blood pressure and control heart rate. Evidence shows that guided imagery can do so as well. One theory proposes that picturing something and actually experiencing it are equivalent as far as brain activity is concerned. Brain scans have verified this effect. Therefore, stimulating the brain through imagery can have a direct effect on both the nervous and endocrine systems, ultimately producing changes in the immune and other body systems.

 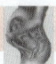

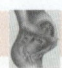

Contraindications

Guided imagery is generally considered safe for everyone.

Possible side effects

There are no known side effects unless memory of an unpleasant event occurs.

EXPRESSIVE THERAPY/SOUND THERAPY

Definition

Expressive therapy is a nonthreatening outlet for people to express their feelings that are difficult to put in words and is used as a coping strategy. Expressive therapy includes many forms of expression, such as music, puppetry, and personal diaries. Only music is discussed at this time.

Sound therapy (music) has had an impact on many people. Classical music is soothing to some, soft ballads soothe others, heavy metal music can be both enjoyable or anxiety provoking, and an anthem sung at the beginning of a ball game can stir people. In hospitals, music is used to improve patient's moods, counteract depression, promote rehabilitation, reduce muscle tension, and induce sleep.

What the therapy hopes to accomplish

Music can also enhance relaxation during labour. Sound has a profound influence on the nervous system. It has a special power to affect consciousness. Women are often encouraged to bring their musical preferences (with tape recorders or compact disc players) to the hospital and listen to music during their labour. If they have earphones on, the sounds around them will not be a distraction to others. Although scientific documentation is limited, music is known to decrease the amount of drugs required during labour.

Contraindications

Sound therapy is considered safe to use. If possible, the selection of the type of music should be made by the patient.

Possible side effects

The volume should be kept low when using a sound therapy device. With loud music, the client might suffer hearing loss. No other side effects are known.

HYDROTHERAPY

Definition

Hydrotherapy, or water therapy, by bathing, showering, or jet hydrotherapy, (whirlpool baths). Warm water may be used to promote comfort and relaxation. Water therapy can also reduce anxiety, which triggers a decrease in andrenaline production. This in turn can trigger an increase in endorphins, which reduces the pain such as labour. Pain relief associated with bathing, showering, or jet hydrotherapy has been proposed to be that of a distraction device or stimulation of large-diameter nerve fibers, as mentioned in the gate control theory. The warm water allows local vasodilatation and muscle relaxation. The water should be kept at a controlled temperature to prevent hyper-thermia or hypothermia.

How the therapy is done

Water therapy can be done by bathing, showe-ring, or jet hydrotherapy (whirlpool baths). Jet hydrotherapy or showering can stimulate the nipples and trigger more oxytocin production. If a tub bath is used, it must be extremely clean to prevent infection. If *Escherichia coli* gets in the water in the tub, the risk for infection is increased.

What the therapy hopes to accomplish

Using warm water can promote comfort and relaxation. Hydrotherapy can trigger an increase in endorphins, which reduces pain in labour and reduces need for analgesia during requirements. If the nipples are stimulated, more oxytocin production can be triggered, which is known to cause the cervix to dilate quicker when the woman is in active labour.

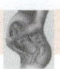

Water birth is a common practice in independent-based birthing centres.

Hydrotherapy is used for relaxation and comfort during labour, soft tissue injuries, musculoskeletal injuries, back pain, menstrual cramps and impaired circulation. The application of hot and cold water-soaked compressed to reduce swelling is used and has proven effective in research clinical trials.

Contraindications

Hot/Cold therapy is ill advised for patients with asthma, kidney disease, heart disease, and a bleeding disorder. Water births are contraindicated in women who have high-risk pregnancies and should be in a hospital-based centre where facilities are available for emergencies.

HOMEOPATHY

Definition

Homeopathy is based on premise that a small amount of a substance that causes a symptom can actually relieve the symptom. The remedies are very diluted solutions of herbs, animal products, and chemicals. Many people tend to think of homeopathic products as herbal remedies, when the products usually contain little of the desired herb.

What the therapy hopes to accomplish

Homeopathy is an approach designed to promote and improve health rather than reverse disease. Remedies are based upon individual symptoms rather than disease entities.

Possible side effects

Unlike vitamins and herbal remedies, which are sold as "dietary supplements" homeopathic remedies are sold as over the counter medication, with an exemption from standard regulatory procedures. The labels do include the ingredients, directions, and dilution. The smallest dose possible to stimulate a reaction is a basic principle of homeopathy, which should be guided by a professional.

Contraindications

Coffee, menthol and strong flavours such as peppermint should be avoided as they may reduce the effect of the homeopathic product. Many homeopathic tablets contain lactose which may be contraindicated in diabetic or allergic individuals.

MASSAGE/TOUCH THERAPY

Definition

Effleurage and counter pressure are two methods that have brought relief to many women during labour. *Massage* is not capable of curing any medical disorder, but it can provide relief from the symptom of tension, anxiety, insomnia, muscle pain, headache, and back pain. It is often recommended for minor sports injuries. Some individuals find that it relieves digestive disorders, such as constipation. Membership and licence in the American Massage Therapy Association means the therapist has graduated from an approved training program and has passed the membership or the National Certification Examination.

How the therapy is done

Many massage techniques are practised, but the most widespread modern variation builds on the basic strokes of Swedish massage. *Effleurage* is slow, rhythmic, gliding strokes, usually in the direction of blood flow towards the heart. Often the care provider uses the whole hand gradually applying an increasing amount of pressure. Variations of effleurage involves strokes applied with the fingertips, heel of the hand, or knuckles. Effleurage is a procedure taught in prenatal classes and is used when the woman is having labour contractions.

What the therapy hopes to accomplish

Massage is an application of pressure and movement to the soft tissue of the body. It

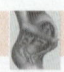

encourages healing by promoting the flow of blood and lymph, relieving tension, and loosening muscles and connective tissue. Before physical exercise, massage helps get blood moving to assist in the warm up. Massage after the exercise workout has been shown to reduce the buildup of waste products. When these build up in muscles after exercise, they cause cramping and discomfort. In addition to general health benefits, massage has shown to be of value in many special problems. During labour, massage provides the woman relaxation, comfort, and relief from painful contractions.

Contraindications

Massage is not advised for anyone who has an infectious skin disease, a rash, or an unhealed wound. If the person is prone to blood clots, it is unwise to have the therapy immediately after surgery. Circulatory problems such as varicose veins preclude the use of massage. It should never be done over bruises, infected injuries, areas of bleeding, or deep tissue damage. Massage should be avoided over any known tumour. In an unstable pregnancy, abdominal massage should not be done. It is also not advisable for the woman to have her legs massaged throughout pregnancy.

Possible side effects

Massage can aggravate existing swelling (edema). The pressure on the skin can be painful for someone who has nerve injury. It is advisable to avoid massage immediately after surgery, such as caesarean birth, because of the increased risk of a phlebitis or blood clot.

REFLEXOLOGY

Definition

Reflexology has been practised for thousands of years in China and Egypt. It was introduced in the West at the beginning of the twentieth century. Reflexology suggests that reflexes, zones, or pathways run along the body and terminate in the palms of the hands, soles of the feet, ears, tongue, and head. All systems and organs are said to be reflected on the surface of skin, in particular, the hands and the feet. Although some studies have been conducted and this therapy often helps with problems such as headaches and bladder control, no major clinical trials verify the theoretical effectiveness.

How the therapy is done

Unlike massage, which involves a generalized rubbing action, reflexologist use their hands to apply pressure on specific points of one's feet and hands. Usually one remains fully clothed, sitting with legs raised or lying on a treatment table. After gently massaging the feet, the reflexologist begins applying pressure to the reflex points thought to correspond to the reported health problems. No instruments are required, but some therapists use devices such as a rubber ball to apply some of the pressure. One can learn to do reflexology by having the practitioner demonstrate the techniques appropriate to the problem.

What the therapy hopes to accomplish

The idea that manipulating the feet can improve health has been an accepted philosophy for many years. Ancient Egyptians massaged feet, and illustrations show that people of many cultures applied massage to their feet to combat illness. Originally, reflexology was thought to work in much the same way as acupuncture. Practitioners believed that stimulation of reflex points in the foot could break up blockages in the flow further along the channel. Although none of the theories have been scientifically verified, reflexology appears to produce satisfactory results for a surprising number of people. Reflexology offers women in labour a gentle method of pain control. Gentle pressure applied to the feet and hands helps restore the body's natural equilibrium. Massage to the feet while the woman is in labour assists in relaxing her.

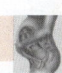

Contraindications

Reflexology has been considered safe. However, if one has a foot injury, ulcers, phlebitis, or any other vascular problems in the lower legs, reflexology should be discussed with the physician before having the procedure. The reflex zone related to the uterus should not have sustained pressure, and reflexology should not be used in unstable pregnancies.

YOGA

Definition

Yoga is a set of exercises that offers a variety of proven health benefits. It increases the efficiency of the heart and slows the respiratory rate, improves fitness, lowers blood pressure, promotes relaxation, and reduces stress and anxiety. It also serves to improve coordination, range of motion, posture, concentration, sleep, and digestion.

Although yoga, as we know it today, is practised mainly for health benefits, it is rooted in Hindu religious and mind body unity principles of some 5000 years ago.

How the therapy is done

Yoga exercises are usually conducted in group classes. People are asked to wear loose, comfortable clothing for the class and bring a mat to prevent slipping during the exercises. The typical session includes three disciplines, breathing exercises, body postures, and meditation. Advice about nutrition may also be given. Each session begins with warm-up exercises.

Some posture exercises may be complicated contorted.

What the therapy hopes to accomplish

The exercises are done to prepare the body by strengthening muscles and by encouraging relaxation and concentration. Through controlled breathing, prescribed postures, and meditation, yoga seeks to enhance the body and achieve a state of balance and harmony between body and mind. Exercises are practised in prenatal classes to prepare muscles for labour and birth. Regular yoga practice throughout pregnancy will help the pregnant woman to get "in tune" with her body. It can help to prevent headaches, morning sickness, fatigue, and back pain and help her be in good physical condition for labour.

Contraindications

Yoga should be avoided in patients who have had a recent back injury or surgery. Individuals should check with their physician if they have heart disease, arthritis, or hypertension before initiating this treatment. Some postures are not recommended during pregnancy, thus special classes are often available for expectant mothers. Some suggest that pregnancy is not the ideal time to begin yoga exercises.

Possible side effects

In the beginning, one may have some stiffness while the body adapts. However, yoga should not be stressful or tiring, and any stiffness should be temporary and minor.

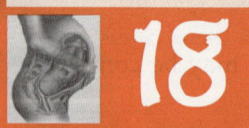

18

Contraception

CONTRACEPTIVE METHODS

Contraceptive methods are, by definition, preventive methods to help women to avoid unwanted pregnancies. They include all temporary and permanent measures to prevent pregnancy resulting from coitus.

Ideal contraceptive methods should fulfil the following criteria—widely acceptable, inexpensive, simple to use, safe, highly effective and requiring minimal motivation, maintenance and supervision. No one single universally acceptable method has yet been discovered.

The contraceptive methods may be broadly grouped into two classes, *spacing methods* and *terminal methods*, as shown below:

Spacing methods

1. Barrier methods
   - Physical methods
   - Chemical methods
   - Combined methods
2. Intrauterine devices
3. Hormonal methods
4. Post-conceptional methods
5. Miscellaneous

Terminal methods

1. Male sterilization
2. Female sterilization

PHYSICAL METHODS

1. Condom

Condom is most widely known and used barrier device by the males around the world. In India, it is better known by its trade name 'Nirodh', a Sanskrit word, meaning prevention.

The condom is fitted on the erect penis before intercourse. The air must be expelled from the teat end to make room for the ejaculate. The condom must be held carefully when withdrawing it from the vagina to avoid spilling seminal fluid into the vagina after intercourse. A new condom should be used for each sexual act.

Condom prevents the semen from being deposited in vagina. The effectiveness of a condom may be increased by using it in conjunction with a spermicidal jelly inserted into the vagina before intercourse.

The advantages of condom are
1. They are easily available
2. Safe and inexpensive
3. Easy to use, do not require medical supervision
4. No side effects
5. Light compact and disposable
6. Provide protection not only against pregnancy but also against sexually transmitted diseases.

The disadvantages are
1. It may slip off or tear during coitus due to incorrect use.

2. Interferes with sex sensation locally about which some complain while others get used to it.

Three types of condoms are available in India. *Dry Nirodh, Deluxe Nirodh and Super Deluxe Nirodh*. Besides commercial outlets, condoms are supplied under social marketing programme.

Female condom

The female condom is a pouch made of polyurethane, which lines the vagina. An internal ring in the close end of the pouch covers the cervix and an external ring remains outside the vagina. It is prelubricated with silicon and a spermicide need not be used. It is an effective barrier to STD infection.

2. Diaphragm

The diaphragm is a vaginal barrier. Also known as "Dutch cap", the diaphragm is a shallow cup made of synthetic rubber or plastic material. It ranges in diameter from 5–10 cm (2–4 inches). It has a flexible rim made of spring or metal. It is important that a woman be fitted with a diaphragm of the proper size. It is held in position partly by the spring tension and partly by the vaginal muscle tone.

The diaphragm is inserted before sexual intercourse and must remain in place for not less than 6 hours after sexual intercourse. A spermicidal jelly is always used along with the diaphragm. The diaphragm holds the spermicide over the cervix.

Advantages: The primary advantage of the diaphragm is the almost total absence of risks and medical contraindications.

Disadvantages: Initially a physician or other trained person will be needed to demonstrate the technique of inserting the diaphragm into the vagina and to ensure a proper fit.

3. Vaginal sponge

It is a small polyurethane foam sponge measuring 5 cm × 2.5 cm, saturated with the spermi-cide, nonoxynol - 9. The sponge is far less effective than the diaphragm.

CHEMICAL METHODS

They comprise four categories:
1. *Foams:* foam tablets, foam aerosols
2. *Creams, jellies and pastes:* squeezed from a tube
3. *Suppositories:* inserted manually
4. *Soluble films:* C-film inserted manually

The main drawbacks of spermicides are

1. They have a high failure rate.
2. They must be used almost immediately before intercourse and repeated before each sex act.
3. They must be introduced into those regions of the vagina where sperms are likely to be deposited.
4. They may cause mild burning or irritation, besides messiness.

INTRAUTERINE DEVICES (IUD)

Types of IUD

There are two types of IUD: Nonmedicated and medicated: Both are usually made of polyethylene or other polymers, in addition, the medicated or bioactive IUDs release either metal ions (copper) or hormones (progestogens).

The device may be nonmedicated. First generation IUD as Lippes loop or medicated (bioactive), second generation IUD by incorporating a metal copper, in devices like Cu T-200, Cu T-380A, multiload 375.

Hormone containing IUD third generation either releasing progesterone (progestasert) or levonorgestrel (LNG-IUS) has also been introduced. Now-a-days the following medicated intrauterine contraceptive devices are in use:

DESCRIPTION OF THE DEVICES

Copper T 200: The widely used medicated device is Copper T 200B. It carries 215 sq mm

 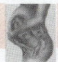

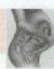

• Cu T 200	• Multiload 250	• Progestasert
• Cu T 380A	• Multiload 375	• LNG-IUS

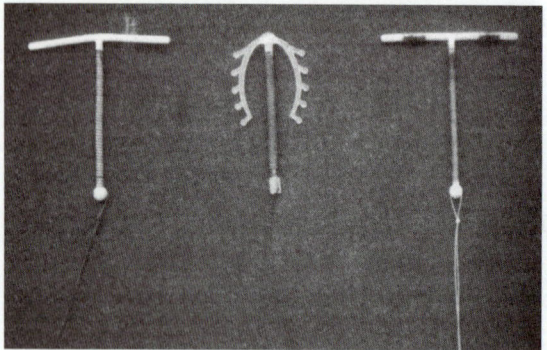

Fig. 18.1: Commonly used intrauterine devices

surface area of fine copper wire wound round the vertical stem of the device. Stem of the T-shaped device is made of a polyethylene frame. It has a polyethylene monofilament tied at the end of the vertical stem. These two threads are used for detection and removal. In spite of the copper being radio opaque, additional barium sulphate is incorporated in the device. The device contains 124 mg of copper. The copper is lost at the rate of about 50 mgm per 24 hours during a period of one year. It is supplied inside a sterilized sealed packet. The device is to be removed after 4 years. Cu T 200 carries 200 sq mm surface area of wire containing 120 mg of copper and is removed after 3 years.

Cu T 380A: Cu T 380A carrying 380 mm^2 surface area of copper wire around the stem (176 mg) and copper sleeves on the horizontal arms (66.5 mg). The frame contains barium sulphate and is radio opaque. Replacement is every 10 years.

Multiload Cu 250: The device is available in a sterilized sealed packet with an applicator. There are no introducer and plunger. The device emits 60–100 mg of copper per day during a period of one year. The device is to be replaced every 3 years.

Multiload 375: It has 375 mm^2 surface area of copper wire wound around its vertical stem. Replacement is every 5 years.

Levonorgestrel intrauterine system (LNG-IUG) (Fig. 18.2): This is a T shaped device, with polydimethylsiloxane membrane around the stem which acts as a steroid reservoir. The amount of levonorgestrel is 52 µg and is released at the rate of 20 µg/day. This device is to be replaced every 5 years.

Progestasert: It is a progesterone (38 mg) containing IUD that releases progesterone 65 µg/day in the uterine cavity. It is to be replaced after 1 year. Progestasert is no longer being manufactured.

Lippes loop: It is a nonmedicated open intra-uterine device. It is no longer used in India.

Mode of action

Mechanism of antifertility effect of all the IUDs is not yet clear. They act predominantly in the uterine cavity and do not inhibit ovulation. Probable factors are:

- ***Biochemical and histological changes in the endometrium:*** There is a nonspecific inflammatory reaction along with biochemical changes in the endometrium which have got gametotoxic and spermolytic effect.
- ***There may be increased tubal motility*** which results in quick migration of the fertilized ovum into the uterine cavity before the endometrium is receptive.

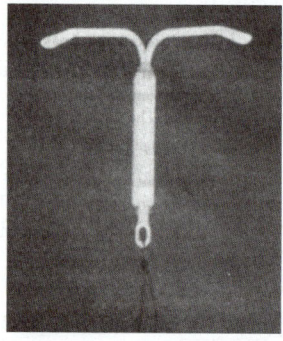

Fig. 18.2: Levonorgestrel containing intrauterine system

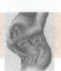

- *There may be impaired sperm ascent* probably due to local chemical effect affecting the sperm vitality and migration.
- *Copper devices:* Ionized copper has got an additional local antifertility effect by *preventing implantation through enzymatic interference.* Copper initiates the release of cytokines which are cytotoxic. Serum copper level is not increased. It seems that the progressive calcium deposition in the device prevents copper diffusion, if kept for longer period.
- *Levonorgestrel-IUS:* It induces strong and uniform suppression of endometrium. Cervical mucous becomes very scanty. Anovulation and insufficient luteal phase activity has also been mentioned. Serum progesterone level is not increased.

Contraindications for insertion

The contraindications are

1. Presence of pelvic infection
2. Dysfunctional uterine bleeding
3. Suspected pregnancy
4. Prolapse uterus because of chance of ascending infection
5. Distortion of the shape of the uterine cavity as in fibroid or congenital malformation. There is difficulty in insertion and contraceptive efficacy is diminished.
6. Severe dysmenorrhoea
7. Suspicious cervix with abnormal cytology
8. Past history of ectopic pregnancy
9. Nullipara
10. Within 6 weeks following caesarean section
11. HIV (STD) positive women.

Time of insertion

1. *Interval* (when the insertion is made in the interconceptional period beyond 6 weeks following childbirth or abortion): *It is preferable to insert 2–3 days after the period is over.* But it can be inserted any time during the cycle even during menstrual phase which has certain advantages (open cervical canal, distended uterine cavity, less cramp). However, during lactational amenorrhoea, it can be inserted at any time.
2. *Post abortal:* Following termination of pregnancy by suction evacuation or D and E, or following spontaneous abortion, the device may be inserted.
3. *Postpartum:* Insertion of the device can be done before the patients are discharged from the hospital. Because of high rate of expulsion, it is preferable to withhold insertion for 6 weeks when the uterus will be involuted to near normal size.
4. *Post placental delivery:* Insertion immediately following delivery of the placenta could be done. But the expulsion rate is high.

Methods of insertion

- Cu T 200
- Cu T 380A

1. Preliminaries

- History taking and examinations (general and pelvic) to exclude any contraindication of insertion.
- Patient is informed about the various problems, the device is shown to her and consent is obtained.
- *The insertion is done in the outpatient department,* taking aseptic precautions without sedation or anaesthesia. To reduce cramping pain Ibuprofen (NSAID) may be given 30 minutes before insertion.
- *Placement of the device inside the inserter:* The device is taken out of the sealed packet. The thread, the vertical stem and the horizontal stem folded to the vertical stem are introduced through the distal end of the inserter. The device is now ready for introduction.

2. Actual steps

- The patient empties her bladder and is placed in lithotomy position. Uterine size and position are ascertained by pelvic examination.

- Posterior vaginal speculum is introduced and the vagina and cervix are cleansed by antiseptic lotion.
- The anterior lip of the cervix is grasped by Allis forceps. A sound is passed through the cervical canal to note the position of the uterus and the length of the uterine cavity. The appropriate length of the inserter is adjusted depending on the length of the uterine cavity.
- The inserter with the device placed inside is then introduced through the cervical canal right up to the fundus and after positioning it by the guard, the inserter is withdrawn keeping the plunger in position. *Thus, the device is not pushed out of the tube but held in place by the plunger while the inserter is withdrawn (withdrawal technique)* (Fig. 18.3).
- The excess of the nylon thread beyond 2–3 cm from the external os is cut. Then the Allis forceps and the posterior vaginal speculum are taken off.

"No-touch" insertion technique includes:

- Loading the IUD in the inserter without opening the sterile package. The loaded inserter is now taken out of the package without touching the distal end.

- Not to touch the vaginal wall and the speculum while introducing the loaded IUD inserter through the cervical canal.

MULTILOAD CU 250

Multiload

The applicator with the device is just to be taken out of the sealed packet in a 'no-touch' method and *the same is pushed through the cervical canal up to the fundus of the uterus.* The applicator is then withdrawn (Fig. 18.4).

Instructions to the patient

The possible symptoms of pain and slight vaginal bleeding should be explained. The patient should be advised to feel the thread periodically by the finger. The patient is checked after 1 month and then annually.

Complications

Immediate

- *Cramp like pain:* It is transient but, at times, severe and usually lasts for ½ to 1 hour. It is relieved by analgesic or antispasmodic drugs.
- *Syncopal attack:* Pain and syncopal attack are more often found in nulliparous or when the device is large enough to distend the uterine cavity.
- *Partial or complete perforation:* It is due to faulty technique of insertion but liable

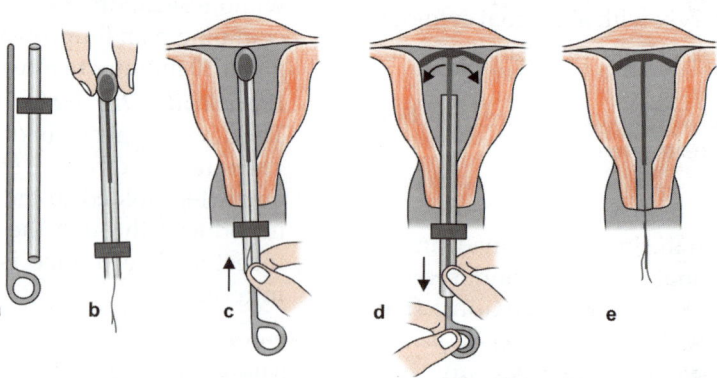

Fig. 18.3: Withdrawal technique of insertion of CuT

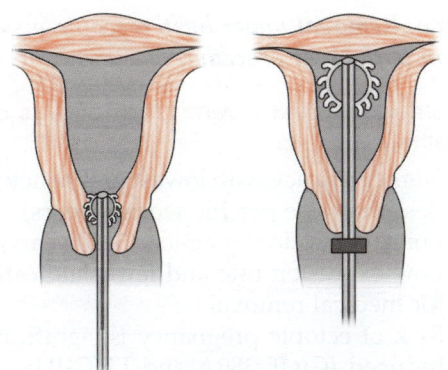

Fig. 18.4: Technique of insertion of multiload IUDs

to be met within lactational period when the uterus remains small and soft.

Remote

- *Pain:* The pain is more or less proportionate to the degree of myometrial distension. A proper size of the device may minimize the pain.
- *Abnormal menstrual bleeding:* The excessive bleeding involves increased menstrual blood loss, prolongation of duration of period and intermenstrual bleeding. The patient may become anaemic and is of concern in one who is already anaemic. Iron supplement is advocated.
- *Pelvic infection (PID):* The risk of developing PID is 2–10 times greater amongst IUD users. The chance is more in nullipara.

Pain, abnormal uterine bleeding and PID are the principal factors related to its discontinuation (10–15%).

- *Spontaneous expulsion:* Spontaneous expulsion usually occurs within a few months following insertion, more commonly during the period, at times unnoticed by the patient. Failure to palpate the thread which could be felt before, is an urgent ground to report to the physician. The expulsion rate is about 5%.
- *Perforation of the uterus:* The incidence of uterine perforation is difficult to estimate but should not be more than 1 in 1000 insertions. Most perforations occur at the time of insertion but the migration may also occur following initial partial perforation with subsequent myometrial contraction.

Diagnosis

Nonvisibility of the thread through the external os and the appearance of pelvic symptoms after a long asymptomatic period are suspicious. *Negative findings on exploration* of the uterine cavity by a probe is suggestive.

Ultrasonography can detect the IUD in abdominal cavity and is better than radiography. *Straight X-ray,* anteroposterior and lateral view, following insertion of another device or following introduction of radio opaque probe (uterine sound) into the uterine cavity, is conclusive. The device is found away from the

Table 18.1: Cu devices and hormone-releasing IUDs	
Advantages	**Disadvantages**
• Inexpensive: Cu T-distributed free of cost through Government channel.	• Require motivation
• Simplicity in technique of insertion.	• Limitation in its use
• Prolonged contraceptive protection after insertion and suitable for the rural population of developing countries.	• Adverse local reactions manifested by menstrual abnormalities, PID, pelvic pain and heavy periods.
• Systemic side effects are nil. Suitable for hypertensive and epileptics.	• Risk of ectopic pregnancy
• Reversibility to fertility is prompt.	

 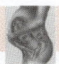

opaque shadow placed in the uterine cavity, if it has perforated the uterine wall.

Indications for removal

The indications for removal are

1. Persistent excessive regular or irregular uterine bleeding
2. Flaring up of salpingitis
3. Perforation of the uterus
4. IUD has come out of place (partial expulsion)
5. Pregnancy occurring with the device in situ
6. Patient desirous of a baby
7. Missing thread
8. One year after menopause
9. When effective life span of the device is over.

IUD removal is simple and can be done at any time. It is done by pulling the strings gently and slowly with a forceps.

Missing thread: The thread may not be visible through the cervical os due to:

1. Thread coiled inside
2. Thread torn through
3. Device expelled outside unnoticed by the patient
4. Device perforated the uterine wall and is lying in the peritoneal cavity.
5. Device pulled up by the growing uterus in pregnancy.

Methods of identification

Pregnancy is to be excluded first

1. *Sounding* the uterine cavity by a probe
2. If negative, *straight X-ray* after introducing radio opaque probe (uterine sound) into the uterine cavity. This will not only reveal the presence or absence of the device but also its existence outside the uterine cavity.
3. *Ultrasonography*
4. *Hysteroscopy*

Removal: If it remains inside the uterus, the device can be removed by a specially designed hook or by an artery forceps or by uterine curette. *Removal under hysteroscopic visualization is the best procedure.*

Advantages of third generation of IUDs over the others

- Higher efficacy with lowest pregnancy rate (less than one per 100 women years)
- Longer duration of action (5–10 years)
- Low expulsion rate and fewer indications for medical removal
- Risk of ectopic pregnancy is significantly reduced (Cu T 380A and LNG-IUS: 0.02 HWY).
- Risk of PID is reduced, anaemia is improved.
- *Significant reduction in:* Menstrual blood loss, menorrhagia, dysmenorrhoea and premenstrual tension syndrome (PMS).

Disadvantage of third generation of IUDs

Expensive

HORMONAL STEROIDAL CONTRACEPTIVES

Hormonal contraceptives when properly used are the most effective spacing methods of contraception.

COMBINED ORAL CONTRACEPTIVES (PILLS)

In the combination pill, the commonly used progestins are either levonorgestrel or norethisterone or desogestrel and the oestrogens are principally confined to either ethinyl-oestradiol or mestranol (3 methyl-ether of ethinyl-oestradiol).

Mode of action

The probable mechanism of contraception are:

- *Inhibition of ovulation:* Both the hormones synergistically act on the hypothalamo-pituitary axis. The release of gonadotrophic releasing hormones from the hypothalamus is prevented through a negative feedback mechanism. There is thus no peak release of FSH and LH from the anterior pituitary.

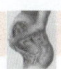

- *Producing static endometrial hypoplasia:* There is stromal oedema, decidual reaction and regression of the glands.
- *Alteration of the character of the cervical mucus* (thick, viscid and scanty) so as to prevent sperm penetration.
- *Probably interferes* with motility and secretions of the fallopian tubes.

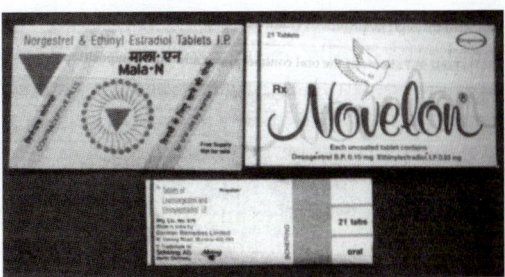

Fig. 18.5: Some commonly used oral contraceptives

Selection of the patient

History and general examination should be thorough, taking special care to screen cases for contraindications. Examination of the breasts for any nodules, weight and blood pressure are to be noted. Pelvic examination to exclude fibroid or cervical pathology, is mandatory. Pregnancy must be excluded. If the facilities are available, cervical cytology to exclude abnormal cells, is of help. Thus, any woman of reproductive age group without any systemic disease and contraindications listed, is a suitable candidate for combined pill therapy.

HOW TO PRESCRIBE A PILL

Instructions

New users should normally start their pill packet on day one of their cycle. One tablet is to be taken daily preferably at bed time for consecutive 21 days. It is continued for 21 days and then have a seven days break, with this routine there is contraceptive protection from the first pill. Next pack should be started on the eighth day, irrespective of bleeding (same day of the week, the pill finished). Thus, a simple regime of "3 weeks on and 1 week off" is to be followed. Packing of 28 tablets, there should be no break between packs. Seven of the pills are dummies and contain either iron or vitamin preparations. However, a woman can start the pill up to day 5 of the bleeding. In that case she is advised to use a condom for the next 7 days. The pill should be started on the day after abortion. Following childbirth in non-lactating woman, it is started after 3 weeks and in lactating woman it is to be withheld for 6 months.

Follow-up

The patient should be examined after 3 months, then after 6 months and then yearly. The patient above the age 35 should be checked more frequently.

Missed pills

Management: When a woman forgets to take one pill she should take the missed pill at once and continue the rest as schedule. There is nothing to worry.

Table 18.2: Some of the oral contraceptives and their composition

Commercial names	Composition		Number of tablets
	Progestins (mg)	Oestrogen (µg)	
• Mala N (Govt. of India) • Mala D • Femilon (Infar) • Loette (Wyeth)	Norgestrel 0.30 D-norgestrel 0.30 Desogestrel 0.15 Levonorgestrel 0.1 mg	Ethinyl oestradiol 30 - do - Ethinyl oestradiol 20 - do -	21 + 7 iron tablets 21 + 7 iron tablets 21 21

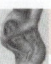

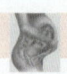

If she misses 2 pills in the first 2 weeks, she should take 2 pills on each of the next 2 days and then continue the rest as schedule. Extra precaution has to be taken for next 7 days either by using a condom or by avoiding sex. If 2 pills are missed in the 3rd week or if more than 2 active pills are missed at any time, another form of contraception should be used as back up for next 7 days as mentioned before.

INDICATIONS FOR WITHDRAWAL

The indications for withdrawal of the pill are
1. Severe migraine
2. Visual disturbances
3. Sudden chest pain
4. Severe cramps and pains in legs
5. Excessive weight gain
6. Severe depression
7. Prior to surgery (it should be withheld for at least 6 weeks to minimize postoperative vascular complications)
8. Patient wanting pregnancy

How long can the pill be continued

A woman who does not smoke and has no other risk factors for cardiovascular disease, may continue the pill (with careful monitoring) until the age of fifty. This offers the dual advantages of effective contraception and hormone replacement therapy. However, for spacing of births, use of 3 to 5 years is considered enough and safe.

Adverse effects: The minor complications or ailments are:

- *Nausea, vomiting, headache and leg cramps:* These are transient and often subside following continuous use for 2–3 cycles.
- *Mastalgia:* Heaviness or even tenderness in the breast is often transient.
- *Weight gain:* The progestins have got an anabolic effect due to its chemical relation to testosterone which results in a positive nitrogen balance and fat deposition. Oedema legs ascribed to retention of sodium, is due to increase in cortisol.
- *Chloasma and acne* are annoying for cosmetic reason.
- *Menstrual abnormalities*
  - Breakthrough bleeding is commonly due to subthreshold blood level of hormones
  - *Hypomenorrhoea:* It is due to the local endometrial changes
  - Menorrhagia
  - *Amenorrhoea:* Post pill amenorrhoea of more than 6 months of duration occurs in less than 1% cases. It is usually more in women with pre existing functional menstrual disorders.

Table 18.3: Contraindications of combined oral pills

Absolute			Relative
A. Circulatory diseases (past or present)	B. Diseases of the liver	C. Others	1. Obesity
• Arterial or venous thrombosis • Severe hypertension • Valvular heart disease, ischaemic heart disease, angina • Hyperlipidaemia • Focal migraine	• Active liver disease • History of cholestatic jaundice in pregnancy • Liver adenoma, carcinoma	• Pregnancy • Undiagnosed genital tract bleeding • Oestrogen dependent neoplasm, e.g. breast cancer	2. Varicosities 3. Epilepsy 4. Bronchial asthma 5. Depression and fluctuation of the mood 6. Age over 35 7. Nursing mothers in the 1st six months 8. Smoking 9. Gallbladder disease

- *Libido:* Libido may be diminished probably due to dryness of the vagina.
- *Leucorrhoea:* It may be due to excessive cervical mucus secretion or due to increased preponderancy of monilial infection.

The major complications are

- Depression, change of mood, sleep disturbances and psychotic manifestations.
- *Hypertension:* The effect on blood pressure is thought to involve the renin angiotension system. There is marked increase in plasma angiotensinogen.
- *Vascular complications*
  - Venous thromboembolism (VTE): The overall risk is to the extent of 4–6 times more than the non-users. Pre-existing hypertension, diabetes, obesity and elderly patient (over 35 especially with smoking habits) are some of the important risk factors.
  - Arterial thrombosis: The high-risk factors for myocardial infarction and stroke (ischaemic and haemorrhagic) are hypertension, smoking habit, age over 35 and high dose pills.
- *Cholestatic jaundice:* Susceptibility is increased in women with previous history of idiopathic recurrent jaundice in pregnancy or hepatitis.
- *Neoplasia:* Conclusions regarding association of combined oral contraceptives (COC) and cervical carcinoma are not definite. However, pill users should have regular cervical cytology screening. Hepatocellular adenomas have been found with high dose preparations over a long period of use.

Metabolic effects

A great deal of attention has been focused recently on the metabolic effects induced by oral contraceptives. These have included the elevation of blood pressure, the alteration in serum lipids with a particular effect on decreasing high density lipoproteins, blood clotting and the ability to modify carbohydrate metabolism with the resultant elevations of blood glucose and plasma insulin. These effects are positively related to the dose of the progestogen component.

Other adverse effects

1. *Liver disorders*: The use of the pill may lead to hepatocellular adenoma and gallbladder disease.
2. *Lactation:* Preparations containing a relatively high amount of oestrogen adversely affect the quantity and constituents of breast milk and less frequently cause premature cessation of lactation.
3. *Subsequent fertility:* In general, oral contraceptive use seems to be followed by a slight delay in conception. The proportion of women becoming pregnant within 2 months of discontinuing the pill may range from 15 to 35 percent.
4. *Ectopic pregnancies:* These are more likely to occur in women taking progestogen, only pills, but not in those taking combined pills.
5. *Foetal development:* Several reports have suggested that oral pills taken inadvertently during (or even just before) pregnancy might increase the incidence of birth defects of the foetus, but this is not yet substantiated.

TRIPHASIC FORMULATIONS OF COMBINED ORAL PILLS

In these preparations, the hormonal doses of each compound vary over the course of the cycle. It is an attempt to minimize undesirable side effects on lipid metabolism. This is due to low total amount of steroids and the balanced oestrogen-progestogen relationship.

Triquilar tablets (Shering-AG/German Remedies Ltd.)—First 6 tablets contain 0.05 mg levonorgestrel and 30 mg of ethinyl oestradiol, next 5 tablets contain 0.075 mg levonorgestrel and 40 mg ethinyl oestradiol, the last 10 tablets contain 0.125 mg levonorgestrel and 30 mg ethinyl oestradiol. It has to be taken like conventional pills.

PROGESTIN ONLY PILL (MINI PILL)

It contains very low dose of a progestin in any one of the following forms—levonorgestrel 75 mg, norethisterone 350 mg, desogestrel 75 mg, lynestrenol 500 mg or norgestrel 30 mg. It has to be taken daily from the first day of the cycle.

Mechanism of action: It works mainly by making cervical mucous thick and viscous, thereby prevents sperm penetration. Endometrium becomes atrophic, so blastocyst implantation is also hindered.

How to prescribe mini pill

The first pill has to be taken on the first day of the cycle and then continuously. It has to be taken regularly and at the same time of the day. There must be no break between the packs.

Advantages

1. Side effects attributed to oestrogen in the combined pill are totally eliminated.
2. No adverse effect on lactation and hence can be suitably prescribed in lactating women and as such it is often called "Lactation pill".
3. Easy to take as there is no On and off regime.

4. It may be prescribed in patient having hypertension, fibroid, diabetes, epilepsy, smoking and history of thromboembolism.
5. Reduces the risk of PID and endometrial cancer.

Drawbacks

1. There may be acne, breakthrough bleeding or, at times, amenorrhoea in about 20–30% cases.
2. All the side effects, attributed to progestins, may be evident.
3. Simple cysts of the ovary may be seen, but they do not require any surgery.
4. Failure rate is about 0.5–2 per 100 women years of use.

EMERGENCY CONTRACEPTION (SYN: POSTCOITAL CONTRACEPTION)

- Hormones
- IUD
- Antiprogesterone
- Others

Indications of emergency contraception

Unprotected intercourse, condom rupture, missed pill, sexual assault or rape and first time intercourse, as known to be always unplanned. Risk of pregnancy following a single act of unprotected coitus around the time of ovulation is 8 percent.

Table 18.4: Combined preparations

Advantages	Disadvantages
• Highly effective	• Requires education and motivation
• Good cycle control	• Limitation in its use
• Well tolerated in majority	• Requires initial check up and periodic supervision
• Additional non-contraceptive - benefits are many	• Inconvenience caused by daily schedule in its use
• Low dose pill with 'lipid friendly' progestins further reduces the risk	• Risk of drug interactions
• Reversibility rate is prompt	• Costly but free supply through government channel (Mala-N)

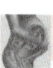

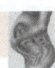

HORMONES

Morning-after pill: This is not true contraceptive, but has rightly been called interception, preventing conception in case of accidental unprotected exposure around the time of ovulation. Any of the following drugs is used—ethinyloestradiol 2.5 mg, premarin (conjugated oestrogen) 15 mg. The drug is taken orally twice daily for 5 days, beginning soon after the exposure but not later than 72 hours.

Combined hormonal regimen (Yuzpe method) is equally effective. Two tablets of Ovral (0.25 mg levo norgestrel and 50 mg ethinyl-oestradiol) should be taken as early as possible after coitus and two more tablets are to be taken 12 hours later.

Levonorgestrel (progestin only pill) 0.75 mg, two doses given at 12 hours interval (ECee2-German Remedies), is very successful and without any side effects. The first dose should be taken within 72 hours.

Mode of action: The exact mechanism of action of hormonal preparations remains unclear. The following are the possibilities:

- Ovulation is either prevented or delayed when the drug is taken in the beginning of the cycle.
- Fertilization is interfered.
- Implantation is prevented as the endometrium is rendered unfavourable.
- Interferes with the function of corpus luteum or may cause luteolysis.

Drawbacks: Nausea and vomiting are much more intense with oestrogen use.

INJECTABLE STEROIDS

The preparations commonly used are depo medroxy progesterone acetate (DMPA) and norethisterone enanthate (NET-EN). Both are administered intramuscularly, DMPA in a dose of 150 mg every three months or 300 mg every six months, NET-EN in a dose of 200 mg given at two-monthly intervals.

Mechanism of action

1. Inhibition of ovulation—by suppressing the mid cycle LH peak.
2. Cervical mucous becomes thick and viscid thereby prevents sperm penetration.
3. Endometrium is atrophic preventing blastocyst implantation.

Advantages

1. It eliminates regular medication as imposed by oral pill.
2. It can be used safely during lactation. It probably increases the milk secretion without altering its composition.
3. No oestrogen related side effects.
4. Menstrual symptoms, e.g. menorrhagia, dysmenorrhoea are reduced.
5. Protective against endometrial cancer.
6. Can be used as an interim contraception before vasectomy becomes effective.

Table 18.5: Post coital contraceptives

Drug	Dose	Pregnancy rate (%)
Ethinyl oestradiol	2.5 mg b.d. x 5 days	0–0.6
Conjugated oestrogen	15 mg b.d. x 5 days	0–0.6
Ethinyl oestradiol 50 µg + Norgestrel 0.25 mg	2 tab stat and 2 after 12 hours	0–2
Levonorgestrel	0.75 mg stat and after 12 hours	0–1
Mifepristone	600 mg single dose	0–1.6
Copper IUDs	Insertion within 5 days	0–1

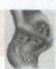

7. Reduction in PID, endometriosis, ectopic pregnancy and ovarian cancer.

Drawbacks: Failure rate for DMPA—(0–0.3) (HWY). There is chance of irregular bleeding and occasional phase of amenorrhoea. Return of fertility after their discontinuation is usually delayed for several months (4–8 months).

IMPLANT

Norplant is a progestin only delivery system containing levonorgestrel. It consists of six flexible closed capsules (made of poly dimethyl siloxane 34 mm × 2.4 mm) and each contains 36 mg of levonorgestrel. It initially releases 85 mg and later on reduced to 30 mgm levonorgestrel per day over 5 years.

Mechanism of action: It inhibits ovulation in 90% of the cycles for the first year. It has got its supplementary effect on endometrium (atrophy) and cervical mucous (thick) as well.

Insertion: The capsules are inserted subdermally, in the inner aspect of the nondominant arm, 6–8 cm above the elbow fold. It is done under local anaesthetic. It is ideally inserted on day one of a menstrual cycle, immediately after abortion and three weeks after postpartum.

Removal: Norplant should be removed within 5 years of insertion. Loss of contraceptive action is immediate.

Advantages are the same as with DMPA. Others are:

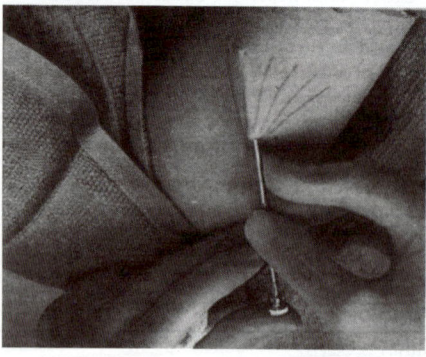

Fig. 18.6: Insertion of norplant

1. Highly effective for long term use and rapidly reversible.
2. Suited for women who have completed their family but do not desire permanent sterilization.

Efficacy is comparable to the combined pills.

Drawbacks: Frequent irregular menstrual bleeding, spotting and amenorrhoea are common. Difficulty in removal is felt occasionally.

Implanon: Single implant rod (4 cm long), containing 60 mg of 3-keto-desogestrel is used. It releases the hormone about 60 mg per day over 3 years. Use of single rod makes implanon easier for insertion and removal. Efficacy and side effects are the same as that of norplant.

POST-CONCEPTIONAL METHODS
(TERMINATION OF PREGNANCY)

Menstrual regulation

A relatively simple method of birth control is "menstrual regulation". It consists of aspiration of the uterine contents 6 to 14 days of a missed period, but before most pregnancy tests can accurately determine whether or not a woman is pregnant. Cervical dilatation is indicated only in nullipara or in apprehensive subjects.

The immediate complications are uterine perforation and trauma. Late complications (after 6 weeks) include a tendency to abortion or premature labour, infertility, menstrual disorders, increase in ectopic pregnancies and Rh immunization.

MENSTRUAL INDUCTION

This is based on disturbing the normal progesterone-prostaglandin balance by intrauterine application of 1–5 mg solution (or 2.5–5 mg pellet) of prostaglandin F_2. Within a few minutes of the prostaglandin impact, performed under sedation, the uterus responds with a sustained contraction lasting about 7 minutes, followed by cyclic contractions continuing for

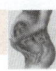

3–4 hours. The bleeding starts and continues for 7–8 days.

ABORTION

Abortion is theoretically defined as termination of pregnancy before the foetus becomes viable (capable of living independently).

Abortions are usually categorized as spontaneous and induced. Spontaneous abortions occur once in every 15 pregnancies. They may be considered "Nature's method of birth control". Induced abortions, on the other hand, are deliberately induced, they may be legal or illegal.

The Medical Termination of Pregnancy Act 1971 is a health care measure which helps to reduce maternal morbidity and mortality resulting from illegal abortions. It is also an opportunity for motivating such women to adopt some form of contraception.

MISCELLANEOUS

Abstinence

The only method of birth control which is completely effective is complete sexual abstinence. It is sound in theory, in practice, an oversimplification.

COITUS INTERRUPTUS

It continues to be a widely practised method. The male withdraws before ejaculation and thereby tries to prevent deposition of semen into the vagina. Some couples are able to practise this method successfully, while others find it difficult to manage. The chief drawback of this method is that the precoital secretion of the male may contain sperm and even a drop of semen is sufficient to cause pregnancy. Further, the slightest mistake in timing of withdrawal may lead to the deposition of a certain amount of semen. Therefore, the failure rate with this method may be as high as 25 percent.

SAFE PERIOD (RHYTHM METHOD)

This is also known as the "calendar method" first described by Ogino in 1930. The method is based on the fact that ovulation occurs from 12 to 16 days before the onset of menstruation. The days on which conception is likely to occur are calculated as follows:

The shortest cycle minus 18 days gives the first day of the fertile period. The longest cycle minus 10 days gives the last day of the fertile period. For example, if a woman's menstrual cycle varies from 26 to 31 days, the fertile period during which she should not have intercourse would be from 8th day to 21st day of menstrual cycle, counting day one as the first day of the menstrual period. Figure 18.7 shows the fertile period and the safe period in a 28 days cycle.

However, where such calculations are not possible, the couple can be advised to avoid intercourse from 8th to the 22nd day of the menstrual cycle, counting from the first day of the menstrual period.

The drawbacks of the calendar method

- A woman's menstrual cycles are not always regular. If the cycles are irregular, it is difficult to predict the safe period.

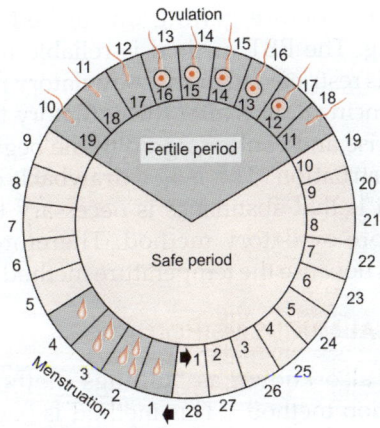

Fig. 18.7: Safe period in a 28 days cycle

- It is only possible for this method to be used by educated and responsible couples with a high degree of motivation and cooperation.
- Compulsory abstinence of sexual intercourse for nearly one half of every month—what may be called "programmed sex".
- This method is not applicable during the postnatal period.
- High failure rate 9 per 100 woman per years. The failures are due to wrong calculations, inability to follow calculations, irregular use and "taking chances".

NATURAL FAMILY PLANNING METHODS

The principle is the same as in the calendar method, but here the woman employs self-recognition of certain physiological signs and symptoms associated with ovulation as an aid to ascertain when the fertile period begins.

BASAL BODY TEMPERATURE (BBT) METHOD

The BBT method depends upon the identification of a specific physiological event—the rise of BBT at the time of ovulation, as a result of an increase in the production of progesterone. The rise of temperature is very small, 0.3 to 0.5 degree C. When no ovulation occurs, e.g. as after menarche, during lactation, the body temperature does not rise. The temperature is measured preferably before getting out of bed in the morning. The BBT method is reliable if intercourse is restricted to the post-ovulatory period, commencing 3 days after the ovulatory temperature rise and continuing up to the beginning of menstruation. The major drawback of this method is that abstinence is necessary for the entire pre-ovulatory method. Therefore, few couples now use the temperature method alone.

CERVICAL MUCUS METHOD

This is also known as "Billings method" or "ovulation method". This method is based on the observation of changes in the characteristics of cervical mucus. At the time of ovulation, cervical mucus becomes watery clear resembling raw egg white, smooth, slippery and profuse. After ovulation, under the influence of progesterone, the mucus thickens and lessens in quantity. It is recommended that the woman uses a tissue paper to wipe the inside of vagina to assess the quantity and characteristics of mucus.

BREASTFEEDING

Field and laboratory investigations have confirmed the traditional belief that lactation prolongs postpartum amenorrhoea and provides some degree of protection against pregnancy. No more than 5–10 percent of women conceive during lactational amenorrhoea and even this risk exists only during the month preceding the resumption of menstruation.

TERMINAL METHODS OR STERILIZATION

Permanent surgical contraception, also called voluntary sterilization, is a surgical method whereby the reproductive function of male or female is purposefully and permanently destroyed. The operation done on male is vasectomy and that on the female is tubal occlusion or tubectomy.

VASECTOMY

It is a permanent sterilization done in the male where a segment of vas deferens of both the sides are resected and the cut ends are ligated.

Advantages

1. The operative technique is simple and can be performed by one with minimal training.
2. The operation can be done as an outdoor procedure or in a mass camp even in remote villages.
3. Complications—immediate or late are few.

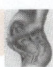

4. Failure rate is minimal—0.15% and there is a fair chance of success of reversal anastomosis operation (50%).
5. The overall expenditure is minimal in terms of equipment, hospital stay and doctor's training.

Drawbacks

1. Additional contraceptive protection is needed for about 2–3 months following operations, i.e. till the semen becomes free of sperm.
2. Frigidity or impotency, when occurs, is mostly psychological.

Selection of candidates: Sexually active and psychologically adjusted husband having the desired number of children is an ideal one.

TECHNIQUE

Written consent of a person is a must and the surgeon should be convinced about the family structure of the couple. The operation is done as an outdoor procedure in the camp. Premedication is usually not necessary. The local area is shaved and an antiseptic dressing is given with Savlon. Full surgical asepsis has to be maintained during operation.

The vas is palpated at the base of the scrotum and is fitted up by the thumb and index finger of the left hand. The area over the vas and the adjoining part are infiltrated with 1% lignocaine (5–10 cc). Small vertical incision ½"–3/4" is given over the vas. After dissecting the dartos muscle and cutting the sheath, the vas is reached and is separated from the surrounding structure and lifted up by an Allis forceps. The vas is ligated at two places 1 cm apart by No. '00' chromic catgut and the segment of the vas in between the ligatures is cut. Haemostasis is secured and the skin is sutured by interrupted catgut. The same procedure is repeated on the other side. A scrotal suspensory bandage is worn. The patient is allowed to go home after ½ an hour. If facilities are available, histological examination of the excised segment of the vas is done for confirmation (Fig. 18.8).

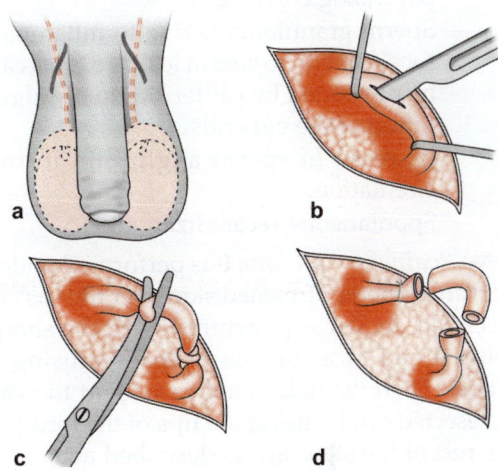

Fig. 18.8: Steps of vasectomy operation

Advices: Antibiotic (inj. Penidure LA 6 IM) is administered as a routine and an analgesic is prescribed. Weight lifting, heavy work or cycling is restricted for about two weeks, while usual activities can be resumed forthwith. For check up, the patient should report back after 1 week, or earlier, if complication arises. Additional contraceptive should be used for 2–3 months.

Precaution: The man does not become sterile soon after the operation as the semen is stored in the distal part of the vas channels for a varying period of about 2–3 months. It requires about 20 ejaculations to empty the stored semen. Semen should be examined once a month and then again at two months and if the two consecutive semen analyses show an absence of spermatozoa, the man is declared as sterile. Till then, additional contraceptive (condom or DMPA) should be advised.

Complications

- *Immediate*
  - Wound sepsis which may lead to scrotal cellulitis or abscess
  - Scrotal haematoma

 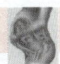

- *Remote*
  - Frigidity or impotency: It is mostly psychologic in origin.
  - Sperm granuloma is due to inflammatory reaction to sperm leakage. This can be prevented by cauterisation or fulguration of the cut ends.
  - Increase in sperm agglutinin in the circulation.
  - Spontaneous recanalization.

No-scalpel vasectomy: It is performed under local anaesthetic. Stretched skin over the vas (as described above) is punctured with the sharp pointed end of a forceps instead of using a scalpel. Then the hole is increased and the vas is dissected out by using the tips of the forceps. The rest of the steps are as described above.

Percutaneous vas occlusion (popular in China) is an effective and reversible method. Polyurethane elastomere is injected into the vas. It solidifies and forms a plug and blocks the sperm passage. The plugs can be removed under local anaesthetic.

Open ended vasectomy: The abdominal end of the resected vas is coagulated. The testicular end is left open. This will prevent congestive epididymitis.

FEMALE STERILIZATION

Occlusion of the fallopian tube in some form is the underlying principle to achieve female sterilization. It is the most popular method of terminal contraception all over the world.

Indications

1. *Family planning purpose:* This is the principal indication in most of the developing countries, India in particular. Intensive motivation is done and even cash incentives are provided to boost up the programme.
2. *Socioeconomic:* An individual is advised to accept the method after having the desired number of children.
3. *Medico-surgical indications (therapeutic):* Medical diseases such as heart disease, diabetes, chronic renal disease, hypertension are likely to worsen, if repeated pregnancies occur and hence sterilization is advisable.

Time of operation: the operation can be performed

1. *During puerperium (puerperal):* If the patient is otherwise healthy, the operation can be done 24–48 hours following delivery. Hospital stay and rest at home following delivery, are enough to help the patient to recover simultaneously from the two events, i.e. delivery and operation.
2. *Interval:* The operation is done beyond 3 months following delivery or abortion. The ideal time of operation is following the menstrual period in the proliferative phase.
3. *Concurrent with MTP:* Sterilization is performed along with termination of pregnancy. This is mostly done in the urban centres.

Methods of female sterilization: Occlusion by resection of a segment of both the fallopian tubes (commonly called tubectomy) is the widely accepted procedure. During recent years, occlusion of the tubes with rings or clips using a laparoscope is gaining popularity.

TUBECTOMY

It is an operation where resection of a segment of both the fallopian tubes is done to achieve permanent sterilization. The approach may be abdominal or vaginal.

Abdominal

- Conventional
- Minilaparotomy

CONVENTIONAL (LAPAROTOMY)

Steps

- *Anaesthesia:* The operation can be done under general or spinal or local anaesthesia.

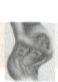

In mass camp, local anaesthesia is preferable. In case of local anaesthesia, premedication with inj. Morphine 15 mg or inj. Pethidine 100 mg with Phenergan 50 mg IM is to be administered at least 30–45 minutes prior to surgery. The incisional area is infiltrated with 1% lignocaine.

- *Incision:* In puerperal cases, where the uterus is felt abdomen, the incision is made two fingers breadth (1") below the fundal height and in interval cases, the incision is made 2 fingers breadth above the symphysis pubis. The incision may be either midline or paramedian or transverse. The abdomen is opened by the usual procedure.
- *Delivery of the tube:* The index finger is introduced through the incision. The finger is passed across the posterior surface of the uterus and then to the posterior leaf of the broad ligament from where the tube is hooked out. *The tube is identified by the fimbrial end and mesosalpinx containing utero-ovarian anastomotic vessels.*
- *Techniques* (Fig. 18.9)
  a. *Pomeroy's:* A loop is made by holding the tube by an Allis forceps in such a way that the major part of the loop consists mainly of isthmus and part of the ampullary part of the tube (at the junction of proximal and middle third). Through an avascular area in the mesosalpinx, a needle threaded with No. '0' chromic catgut is passed and both the limbs of the loop are firmly tied together. About 1–1.5 cm of the segment of the loop distal to the ligature is excised. The tube is so excised as to leave behind about 1.5 cm of intact tube adjacent to uterus. Segment of the loop removed is to be inspected to be sure that the wall has not been partially resected and to send it for histology. The same procedure is repeated on the other side. Because of the absorption of the absorbable ligature, the cut ends become independently sealed off and are separated after a few weeks.

Advantages: It is easy, safe and very effective in spite of the simplicity of the technique. The failure rate is 0.1–0.5%. The cut ends become independently sealed off and retract widely from each other.

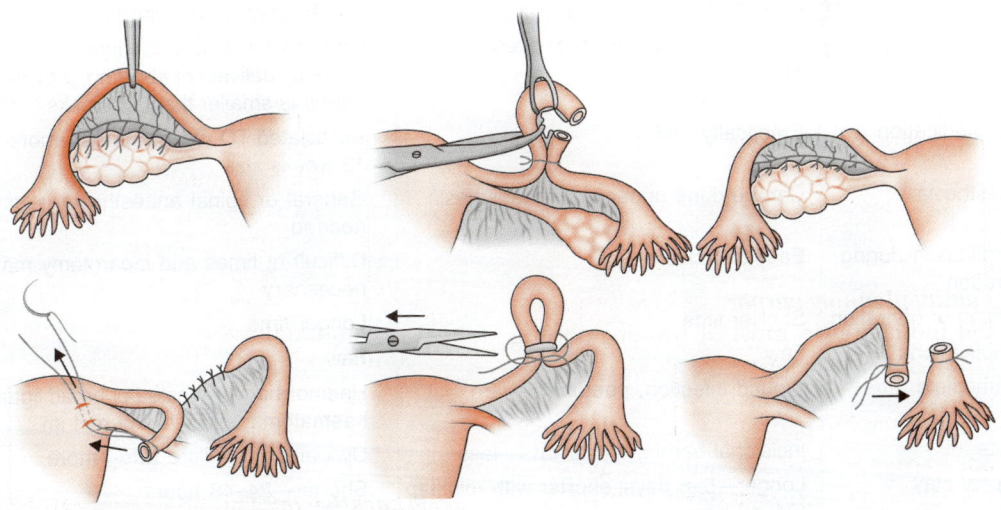

Fig. 18.9: Steps of tubectomy by Pomeroy's technique

b. *Madlener's technique:* It is the easiest method. The loop of the tube is crushed with an artery forceps. The crushed area is tied with black silk. The loop is not excised. The failure rate is very high to the extent of 3% and hence, it is abandoned in preference to the Pomeroy's technique.

The abdomen is closed in layers. Antibiotics are given routinely in the post operative period. The abdominal stitches are removed on the 5th day and the patient is discharged. However, if the patient is otherwise normal, passes flatus and urine normally, the patient may be discharged after 48 hours. The stitches may be removed in the outpatient department.

Minilaparotomy (mini-lap)

When the tubectomy is done through a small abdominal incision along with some device, the procedure is called mini-lap.

Steps

1. *Anaesthesia:* Always under local anaesthesia
2. *Plan of incision:* As described in conventional method but the incision should be ½"–¾".
3. Specially designed retractor may be introduced after the abdomen is opened.
4. Uterus is elevated or pushed to one side or the other by the elevator that has already been introduced transvaginally into the uterine cavity. This helps manipulation of the tube in bringing it close to the incisional area, when it is seized by artery forceps.
5. The appropriate technique of tubectomy is performed on one side and then repeated on the other side.
6. The peritoneum is closed by purse string suture.

Once conversant with the technique, it can be performed with satisfaction to the patient. It also benefits the organization (turn over of the

Table 18.6: Female sterilization		
	Abdominal approach	**Vaginal approach**
Surgeon	Can be performed by any one conversant with surgery	Can be done only by a surgeon conversant with vaginal plastic operation
Time of operation	Can be done at any time, puerperal or interval	Can only be done in the interval period or following delivery or abortion, provided the uterus is smaller than 12 weeks
Contraindication	Practically—nil	Associated TO mass, uterus—more than 12 weeks size
Anaesthesia	Can be done under local anaesthesia	General or spinal anaesthesia is usually needed
Complication during operation	Easy to tackle	Difficult at times and laparotomy may be necessary
Duration of operation	Shorter time	Longer time
Complications	Few	Few
• Immediate	Wound infection, peritonitis—rare	Haemorrhage, revealed or broad ligament haematoma, injury to the rectum
• Late	Incisional hernia, failure rate—less	Dyspareunia, failure rate—more
Hospital stay	Longer—5–6 days; shorter with mini-lap (24–48 hours)	Shorter—24–48 hours

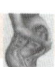

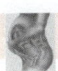

patient per bed is more than that in the conventional method). The patient is usually discharged within 24–48 hours.

Vaginal ligation: Tubectomy through the vaginal route may be done along with vaginal plastic operation or in isolation. When done in isolation, the approach to the tube is through posterior colpotomy. Its limitation and relative merits and demerits in contrast to that of abdominal approach are given in Table 18.6.

Laparoscopic sterilization (Fig. 18.7)

Laparoscopy is the commonly employed method of endoscopic sterilization. It is gradually becoming more popular—especially in the camps. The procedure is mostly done under local anaesthesia. The operation is done in the interval period, concurrent with vaginal termination of pregnancy or 6 weeks following delivery. It should not be done within 6 weeks following delivery.

The procedure can be done either with single puncture or double puncture technique. The tubes are occluded either by a silastic ring (silicone rubber with 5% barium sulphate) devised by Falope or by Filshie clip made of titanium lined with silicon rubber. Endothermic coagulation is not practised now, due to high failure rate. Bipolar cautery is safer than unipolar one.

Principal steps: (single puncture technique)

Premedication: Pethidine hydrochloride 75–100 mg with phenergan 25 mg and atropine sulphate 0.65 mg are given intramuscularly about half an hour prior to operation.

Local anaesthesia: Taking usual aseptic precautions about 10 ml of 1% lignocaine hydrochloride is to be infiltrated at the puncture site (just below the umbilicus) down up to the peritoneum. (If necessary, diazepam 10 mg is given intravenously slowly just prior to local anaesthesia).

Table 18.7: Mini-lap vis-a-vis Laparoscopic sterilization

	Mini-lap	Laparoscopic sterilization
1. Cost	Minimal	Expensive instrument and requires adequate maintenance
2. Personnel	Any medical personnel with little surgical skill	Should only be performed by persons with special training
3. Assistance	Minimal or nill	Requires a team work consisting of medical and para medical personnel
4. Selection of time	Any time—puerperium, Interval, with MTP	Should not be done within 6 weeks following delivery or with enlarged uterus
5. Contraindication	Practically none. Can be done in conditions contraindicated for laparoscopy	Lung lesions, organic heart diseases, anticipated intra abdominal adhesions, extreme obesity
6. Complication	Minimal but not life threatening	Minimal but at times fatal: injury to bowels, blood vessels, surgical emphysema
7. Hospital stay	3–5 days	3–4 hours
8. Failure rate	0.1–0.3%	0.2–0.6%
9. Reversibility	Difficult due to adhesion formation. Success depens on the length the tube left behind, after excision	Easier and effective. Only 4 mm of the tube is destroyed with the Filshie clip

Position of the patient: The patient is placed in lithotomy position. The operating table is tilted to approximately 15 degrees of Trendelen-burg position. Usual aseptic precaution is taken as in abdominal and vaginal operations. The bladder should be fully emptied by a metal catheter. Pelvic examination is done methodically. A uterine manipulator is introduced through the cervical canal for manipulation for visualization of tubes and uterus at a later step.

Producing pneumoperitoneum: A small skin incision (1.25 cm) just below the umbilicus. The Verres needle is introduced through the incision with 45° angulation into the peritoneal cavity. The abdomen is inflated with about 2 litres of gas (carbon dioxide or nitrous oxide or room air or oxygen).

Introduction of the trocar and laparoscope with ring loaded applicator: Two silastic rings are loaded one after the other on the applicator with the help of a loader and pusher. The trocar with canula is introduced through the incision previously made with a twisting movement. The trocar is removed and the laparoscope together with ring applicator is inserted through the cannula.

The ring loaded applicator approaches one side of the tube and grasps at about 2–3 cm from the uterotubal junction (Fig. 18.10). A loop of the tube (2.5 cm) is lifted up, drawn into the cylinder of the applicator and the ring is slipped into the base of the loop under direct vision. The procedure is to be repeated on the other side.

Removal of the laparoscope: After viewing that the rings are properly placed in position, the tubal loops looking white and there is no intraperitoneal bleeding, the laparoscope is removed. The gas or air is deflated from the abdominal cavity. The abdominal wound is sutured by a single chromic catgut suture.

Hazards of tubal sterilization

Immediate: These are related to general anaesthesia and to the particular method used in

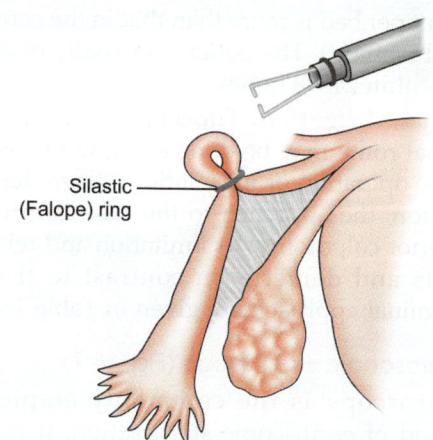

Silastic (Falope) ring

Fig. 18.10: Laparoscopic tubal sterilisation by silastic ring

sterilization. The related complications have already been discussed.

Remote

- Specific for the approach
- Related to the sterilization

The remote complications specific for the approach of the operation, abdominal or vaginal, have already been described.

The complications related to sterilization can be grouped into:

- *General complications:* These include occasional obesity, psychological upset.

- *Gynaecological*
  - Chronic pelvic pain
  - Congestive dysmenorrhoea
  - Menstrual abnormalities in the form of menorrhagia, hypomenorrhoea or irregular periods. Pelvic pain, menorrhagia along with cystic ovaries constitute a post ligation syndrome. It may be vascular in origin.
  - Alteration in libido

Failure rate: The failure rate in tubal sterilization is about 0.7%.

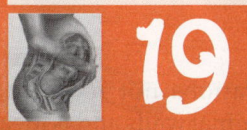

19

Instruments in Obstetrics and Gynaecology

OUTLINE

- Instruments used for the examination of a gynaecological and obstetric patient
- Instruments used in dilatation, curettage and evacuation operation
- Instruments used for destructive operations
- Specialized gynaecological instruments
- Common surgical instruments

INSTRUMENTS USED FOR THE EXAMINATION OF A GYNAECOLOGICAL AND OBSTETRIC PATIENT

SIMS DOUBLE BLADED POSTERIOR VAGINAL SPECULUM

It is a vaginal speculum used in all vaginal examinations and operations to retract the anterior, posterior or lateral vaginal walls. Two blades in each instruments are of two different sizes. The blades are at an angle to the shaft and point towards the same side. They are grooved which helps in drainage of secretions by slightly tilting the instruments and can also be used for collection of specimens from vagina.

Technique

The instrument is introduced in an antero posterior direction. The introitus being an antero-posterior slit, this causes least discomfort to the patient and she remains cooperative. The blade is then rotated by 90°. Only 2/3rds of the blade should go in to have maximum exposure.

Uses

It is used for retracting the vaginal walls in:

1. ***All gynaecological and obstetric examinations*** known as per speculum examinations
2. ***Operation on the perineum***
   - 1/3rd degree perineal tear
3. ***Operations on the vagina***
   - Vaginal examination in APH and PPH
   - Vaginal hysterectomy
   - Fothergill's repair
   - VVF repair and collection of urine for culture in VVF cases
   - Culdocentesis
   - Vaginal cytology
4. ***Operations on the cervix***
   - Stitching of cervical tears
   - Cervical biopsies and cytology
   - Conisation of cervix
   - Application of McDonald's stitches and Shirodhkar's operation for cervical incompetence
   - Dilatation of cervix
   - Cerviprime gel insertion

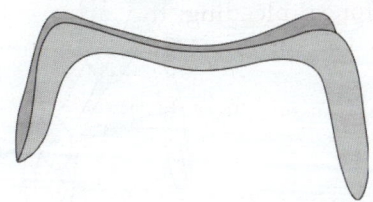

Fig. 19.1: Sim's double bladed posterior vaginal speculum (Sim's bivalved vaginal speculum)

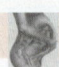

5. *Operations on the uterus*
   - Dilatation and curettage
   - Medical termination of pregnancy
   - Endometrial biopsy
   - Hysterosalpingography and tubal insufflation tests
   - IUCD insertion, follow-up and removal
   - Packing for PPH

Advantage

Gives a better field of view than self retaining speculums.

Disadvantage

An assistant is needed by the surgeon to hold the speculum during the operation.

CUSCO'S BIVALVED SELF-RETAINING SPECULUM

It is a self-retaining vaginal speculum consisting of two blades shaped like the beak of a duck which are hinged together. The blades can be opened up and fixed at the required angle by an arrangement which is adjustable.

Technique

The blades are closed and then introduced in an anteroposterior direction and rotated by 90° as in case of Sim's speculum to cause minimal discomfort to the patient. The fixation screw is tightened depending on amount of exposure needed.

Uses

It can be used in operations not requiring excessive retraction of vaginal walls and is ideal for operation on the cervix.
1. Cervical biopsy
2. Pap's smear
3. Cautery and cryosurgery of cervical lesions
4. IUCD insertions, removal and follow-up
5. Colposcopy
6. Used in destructive operation by Heilder's wire saw for decapitation

Advantages

1. No assistant is required by surgeon.
2. Gives a very good view of the cervix.
3. Causes lesser discomfort to the patient.

Disadvantage

1. Only a limited field of vision is available.

AUVARD'S VAGINAL SPECULUM

It is a heavy instrument used to retract the posterior vaginal wall. It consists of a curved blade at one end and a heavy lead weight at the other end and hence acts as a self retaining speculum with the advantages of both Sim's speculum and Cusco's speculum.

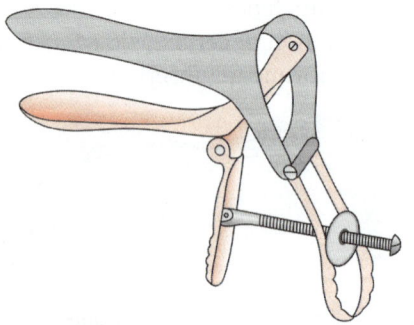

Fig. 19.2: Cusco's bivalved self-retaining speculum

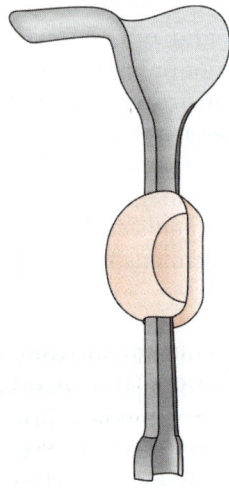

Fig. 19.3: Auvard's vaginal speculum

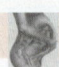

Technique
Similar to Sim's speculum

Uses
All operations on the vagina, cervix and uterus

Disadvantage
As it is heavy it is cumbersome to use.

SIM'S ANTERIOR VAGINAL WALL RETRACTOR

It is a long instrument with a shaft and two oval fenestrated ends. The oval ends have transverse serrations and are at an angle of 15° to the shaft, and face opposite directions. The transverse serrations prevent slipping of the instrument and the fenestrations make the instrument lighter.

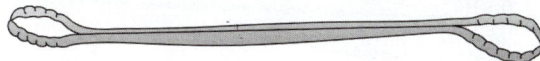

Fig. 19.4: Sim's anterior vaginal wall retractor

Technique
1. It is introduced into the vagina after the posterior vaginal wall has been retracted away by a Sim's speculum.
2. It helps in retracting the anterior vaginal wall.

Uses
1. In all gynaecological and obstetric operations requiring visualization of the cervix and anterior vaginal fornix.
2. It can be used as a blunt curette in case of postpartum haemorrhage just after delivery when the cervix is wide open as it can remove retained products of conception by curetting large areas with each stroke.

TEALE'S VULSELLUM

It is a long instrument consisting of two blades which are toothed, a joint, shank, handles and a lock. The teeth provide a firm grip and the curve helps by not blocking the field of vision and causing lesser discomfort to the patient.

Technique
The cervix is visualized after retracting the posterior vaginal wall with a Sim's speculum and anterior vaginal wall with anterior vaginal wall retractor. The anterior lip of the cervix is then grasped with the teeth and the instrument is locked after obtaining a firm grip of the cervix.

The curve should face upwards so that the instrument does not abut against the lower border of symphysis pubis.

Uses
To hold the anterior lip of the cervix in
1. All operations on the cervix, e.g.
   - Cervical biopsy
   - Laminaria tent insertion
2. All operations on the uterine cavity, e.g.
   - MTP
   - Endometrial biopsy
   - Dilatation and curettage
   - Insertion of IUCD and its removal
   - Polypectomy
   - Drainage of haematometra or pyometra
3. Assessment of a patient for the degree and type of prolapse
4. Vaginal hysterectomy
5. Anterior colporrhaphy in Fothergill's repair

To hold the posterior lip of the cervix
1. Culdocentesis
2. Culdoscopy
3. Colpotomy
4. In assessing a patient of prolapse to rule out the presence of an enterocele
5. Vaginal hysterectomy
6. Fothergill's repair and posterior colpoperineorrhaphy

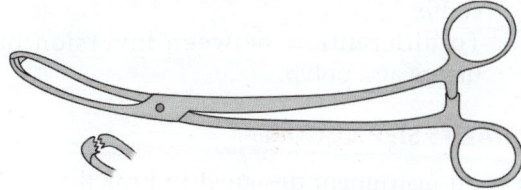

Fig. 19.5: Teale's vulsellum

It can be used to apply gentle traction on fetal head after craniotomy for its vaginal extraction or for extracting a collapsed head of an old IUD baby.

Disadvantage

It can sometimes cause damage to the cervix when it is soft and friable as it is a toothed instrument.

SIMPSON'S UTERINE SOUND

It is a long, slender instrument about 12 inches in length. It has an olive shaped distal end, a shaft and a handle. The tip is blunt so that it does not cause injuries when introduced inside. The whole instrument is graduated in inches from the tip. The angled tip prevents uterine perforation and fits well into an anteverted or retroverted uterus.

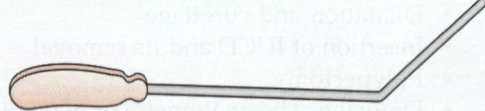

Fig. 19.6: Simpson's uterine sound

Technique

The sound is introduced in a pen holding manner keeping the angle anteriorly or posteriorly depending on whether the uterus is anteverted or retroverted.

Uses

1. Measuring uterocervical length
2. To confirm the direction of the uterus, i.e. whether it is anteverted or retroverted
3. Measuring the length of cervical canal
4. Prior to most operation on the uterus and cervix
5. To differentiate between inversion of uterus and polyp.

PINARD'S STETHOSCOPE

It is an instrument designed to hear the fetal heart sound. The instrument is simple in design consisting of a hollow tube with one wide end and another narrow end. The narrow end has a wide rim which is used as an ear piece.

Technique

The wide end is placed over the patient's abdomen such that it is at right angle to the abdominal wall. The ear piece is applied near the ear and the instrument should not be touched by the hand while listening to the fetal heart. The maternal pulse is palpated at the same time to confirm that one is listening to the fetal heart and any maternal pulsations are not being wrongly transmitted.

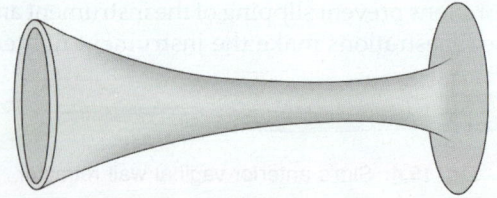

Fig. 19.7: Pinard's stethoscope

BOULDELOQUE'S PELVIMETER

It is an instrument consisting of a pair of calipers and a measuring scale. It is designed to measure the external pelvic diameters, i.e. the diameter of the false pelvis. The measurement of these diameters helps in the assessment of the pelvic outlet and indicates to some extent the presence of gross cephalopelvic disproportion. The following diameters are measured:

1. *External conjugate:* It is the distance from the depression below the 5th lumbar spine to the upper border of symphysis pubis. It usually measures 8 inches.
2. *Interspinous diameter:* It is the distance between the two anterior superior iliac spines and measures about 10 inches.
3. *Intercristal diameter:* It is the distance between the outermost parts of both iliac crests and is around 11 inches.
4. *Intertrochantric diameter:* It is the distance between the outer surfaces of the two

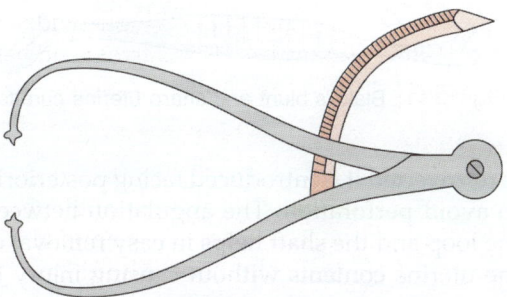

Fig. 19.8: Bouldeloque's pelvimeter

greater trochanters and measures 12.5 inches

5. *Obstetric conjugate:* Besides measuring the external diameters it can also predict the obstetric conjugate. The diagonal conjugate is the distance between the lower border of symphysis pubis and the upper border of sacral promontory.

Two fingers are introduced into the vagina and the sacral promontory is reached. The position where the lower border of symphysis pubis is falling on the hand is marked and the hand is withdrawn. The distance between the tip of the finger and the point marked on the hand is measured with the pelvimeter. This distance gives the diagonal conjugate. Substracting 1.5 cm from this gives the value of the obstetric conjugate. A distance of less than 10 cm of obstetric conjugate indicates probable dystocia due to pelvic contraction.

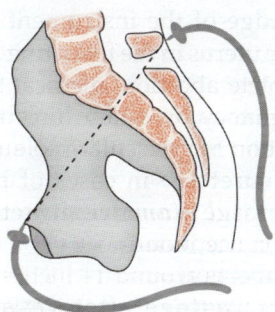

Fig. 19.9: Measurement of external conjugate

INSTRUMENTS USED IN DILATATION, CURETTAGE AND EVACUATION OPERATION

HEGAR'S DILATORS

These instruments are sinuously curved double ended instruments and have conical tips. Tips are arranged to the shaft and point in opposite directions. They are available in gradually increasing sizes ranging from a diameter of few millimetres to more than 2 cm. The dilators are numbered according to the diameter of the shaft. Two sizes are available in one double ended dilator with a difference of one mm in their diameters.

Technique

The dilator should be introduced keeping the tip directed anteriorly or posteriorly according to the direction of the uterus, whether anteverted or retroverted. The dilator should be introduced gently starting from a smaller size to gradually increasing sizes.

Uses

- Dilatation of the cervix is required in the following operations on uterine cavity in order to approach the uterine cavity:
  - In tubal insufflation test and HSG usually up to 5 mm dilatation is required.
  - IUCD insertion may also require some amount of dilatation with number 4 and 5 dilators.
  - Prior to removing an endometrial polyp, placental polyp and fibroid polyp.
  - To reach the uterine cavity in endometrial biopsy, D&C, S&E and MTP. In MTP the dilatation required should be enough to allow easy passage and rotation of suction cannula.
  - In Fothergill's repair to prevent cervical stenosis
- Only dilatation is required in:
  - Treatment of cervical stenosis
  - Draining of haematometra and pyometra

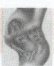

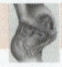

– Prior to operations on cervix, e.g. repair operations, cautery and amputation to prevent stenosis.
• Smaller sizes can also be used as urethral dilators.

Advantage

The angle makes the instrument less traumatic when used according to the direction of uterus. The gradually increasing sizes help in making the cervical canal patulous by stretching the muscle and fibrous tissue of the cervix without causing trauma and thus providing approach to the uterine cavity.

Disadvantages

The following complications may occur:
1. Sepsis, haemorrhage
2. Perforation
3. Cervical injuries
4. Incompetent cervical os leading to habitual abortion or premature labour
5. Injury to the bladder or rectum

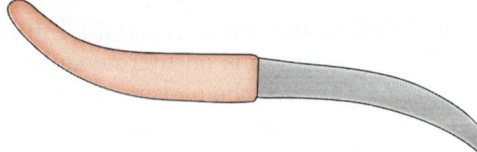

Fig. 19.10: Hegar's dilators

BLAKES' BLUNT AND SHARP UTERINE CURETTE

It is a long double ended instrument. The terminal ends have oval loops which are angled to the shaft. One end has a sharp cutting edge while the other has a blunt edge (compare with anterior vaginal wall retractor where the instrument is larger with transverse serrations on the loop). The sharp ends has a smaller sized loop while blunt end has a larger loop.

Technique

If the uterus is anteverted the curette is introduced with tip facing anteriorly while if it

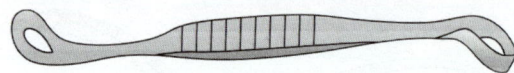

Fig. 19.11: Blake's blunt and sharp uterine curette

is retroverted it is introduced facing posteriorly to avoid perforation. The angulation between the loop and the shaft helps in easy removal of the uterine contents without causing injury to the uterus.

Uses

A small sized uterine curette can be used in all the indications where endometrial biopsy curette is used.

Gynaecological indications

Here the sharp end of the instrument is used:
1. Diagnosis of vaginal tuberculosis. The cornu should be specially curetted as genital tuberculosis starts from this area.
2. Infertility
3. Dysfunctional uterine bleeding
4. Primary and secondary amenorrhaea
5. For fractional curettage in cases of CA endometrium and to assess the extent of uterine involvement in carcinoma cervix
6. After removal of a uterine polyp and prior to myomectomy
7. To diagnose causes of postmenopausal bleeding
8. Diagnosis of choriocarcinoma

Obstetric indications

The blunt edge of the instrument is used for curetting the uterus in the following indications:
1. Incomplete abortion, medical termination of pregnancy by ovum forceps and after evacuation for vesicular mole
2. Check curettage in cases of postpartum haemorrhage to remove any retained products of conception
3. Septic abortion
4. Check curettage after vesicular mole evacuation may be done very gently

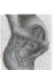

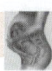

Disadvantages

1. Sepsis
2. Haemorrahage
3. Infertility
4. Cervical injuries

LAMINARIA TENT

These are used as slow cervical dilators. They are made from *Laminaria japonica,* a seaweed which is hygroscopic in nature. The stems of this weed are dried and cut into 6–8 cm pieces with diameters ranging from 2 to 10 mm. A string is looped one end for easy removal. The tents are sterilized prior to use. They swell up by 3–5 times of their size after absorbing the secretions of the cervical canal within 24 hours and thus dilate the cervix gradually. They are sterilized by ethylene oxide or by dipping in absolute alcohol.

Technique

The tent is passed to lie just beyond the internal os. One or more laminaria tents may be needed to fit snugly into the cervical canal. The vagina may be packed with sterile gauze after fixing the terminal ends of the tent to the gauze. This prevents premature expulsion and makes it easier to remove them. They may be removed after 24 hours and a second set may be inserted if dilatation is not adequate.

Uses

1. First trimester and second trimester pregnancy termination
2. Induction of labour

Advantage

They dilate the cervix gradually, so there are minimal chances of injury to the cervix and any

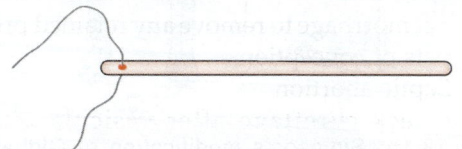

Fig. 19.12: Laminaria tent

late sequelae like incompetent cervical os is prevented.

Disadvantages

1. Infection
2. If tip lies below the os its purpose is wasted and the os remains undilated.
3. Migration upwards into the uterine cavity may occur.
4. False passage may be created during insertion.

LAMINARIA TENT INTRODUCING FORCEPS

It is a long forceps with 2 blades, a joint, shank and handles with a lock. The forceps is angled near the blades and the blades are deeply grooved to hold a tubular structure. When apposed together it is used to introduce the laminaria tents into the cervical canal.

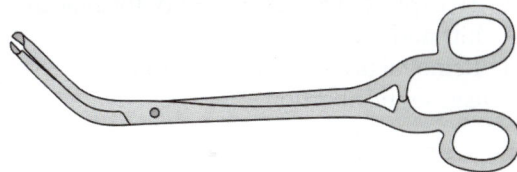

Fig. 19.13: Laminaria tent introducing forceps

HAYWOOD SMITH'S OVUM FORCEPS

It is a long straight instrument with 2 spoon shaped blades, a shank and a hand. There is no lock in this instrument. The blades can hold a good amount of tissue in between. The absence of a lock minimizes damage to any structure which may be accidently held in between the blades.

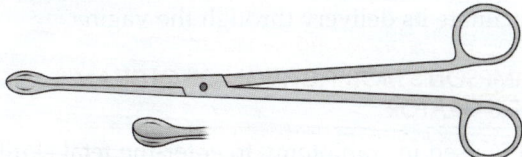

Fig. 19.14: Haywood Smith's ovum forceps

 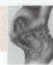

The forceps are available with varying sizes of blades used according to the necessity, the larger one for advanced pregnancies and smaller one for early pregnancies. The fenestrations allow part of the tissue to bulge out so that the grip is secure.

Technique

The ovum forceps is introduced with the blades closely approximated. Once inside the uterine cavity the blades are opened up and the products of conception are grasped. The forceps is withdrawn after a few gentle rotatory movements which help in detaching the products of conception from the uterus.

Uses

1. To remove the products of conception in:
   • Ist trimester pregnancy termination
   • Incomplete abortion
   • Septic abortion
2. To explore the uterine cavity for placental bits and membranes in PPH
3. Removal of a foreign body from the uterus, e.g. septic abortion

Disadvantages

1. Perforation
2. Sepsis
3. Injury to intra-abdominal structures like bowel, omentum, etc. secondary to uterine perforation
4. Incomplete evacuation

INSTRUMENTS USED FOR DESTRUCTIVE OPERATIONS

These instruments are designed to reduce the bulk of the fetal head or trunk in order to facilitate its delivery through the vagina.

SIMPSON'S MODIFICATION OF OLDHAM'S PERFORATOR

It is used in craniotomy to enter the fetal skull and collapse it by draining out the brain matter.

It consists of a blade about 1 inch in length having an inner blunt and an outer cutting edge, a shoulder just below the blades, a shank and a handle with metal bars. The metal bars help in maintaining a rigid fixation of the handles keeping the blades in close approximation when the head is being pierced.

Indication of craniotomy

1. Live baby with hydrocephalus
2. Dead baby with
   • Forecoming head with cephalopelvic disproportion
   • Aftercoming head of breech
   • Face presentation with obstructed labour
   • Failed forceps operation due to cephalo-pelvic disproportion

The parietal bones in case of the forecoming head, the occipital bone in aftercoming head and the orbits in brow presentation are the sites for perforation. Perforation is done only during a uterine contraction after fixing the presenting part from above. The blades of the perforator are closed and fixed and introduced after protecting the maternal tissues with a hand such that palms face the blades. Full asepsis is

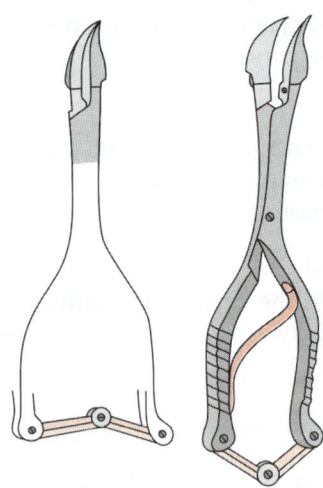

Fig. 19.15: Simpson's modification of Oldham's perforator

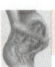

maintained. The blades are guided to skull by the right hand while left hand protects the maternal tissues. An assistant fixes the head suprapubically and the perforator is pushed in, till the level of the shoulder. It is then opened up and rotated by 90° after closing the blades. After rotation, the blades are again opened up and a cruciate incision is thus obtained and brain matter is crushed with it. Suprapubic pressure will now drain out the brain matter or it may be drained with the help of a flushing curette or suction cannula or a Drew Smythe's catheter.

Complications

Severe maternal lacerations and even uterine rupture may result.

DREW SMYTHE'S CATHETER

It is a long double curved instrument, sinusoidal in shape with a double opening. There is an inlet and an outlet and a double tube.

Uses

1. High rupture of membranes as in hydramnios to prevent cord prolapse and accidental haemorrhage due to sudden decompression.
2. For perforation of a hydrocephalic aftercoming head of breech through the foramen magnum or a spinal bifida or by dividing the vertebral canal in the cervical region.
3. For draining a forecoming hydrocephalic head after perforating it with scissors.

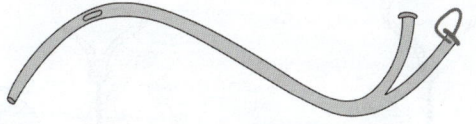

Fig. 19.16: Drew Smythe's catheter

FLUSHING CURETTE

It is a metallic spoon shaped cannula used to remove brain matter by flushing it out after attaching it to an enema can with a rubber tubing.

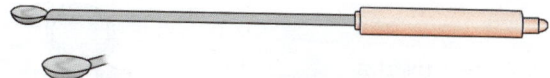

Fig. 19.17: Flushing curette

TWO-BLADED BRAXTON-HICK'S CRANIOCLAST

It consists of the central and the left outer blade of the Winter's cephalotribe. The smaller solid central blade is pointed and acts as a perforator while the large curved fenestrated outer blade acts as a crusher. The opposed surfaces of the blades are strongly serrated and the handles are firmly closed by a screw and locked. The pointed central blade perforates the skull and is screwed into the foramen magnum while the outer blade is placed outside between the scalp and the bones. The firm grip on the head and some amount of crushing action helps by negotiating cephalopelvic disproportion.

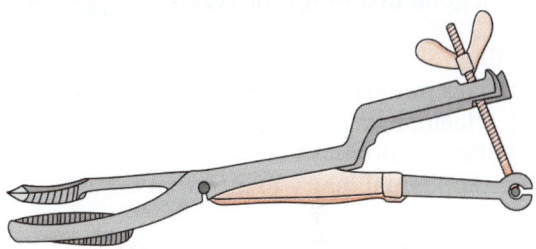

Fig. 19.18: Two-bladed Braxton-Hick's cranioclast

WILLET'S SCALP TRACTION FORCEPS

This forceps has 2 blades shaped like the letter T and a handle with a lock.
The spikes, transverse serrations and the lock provide a firm grip of the fetal scalp. The instrument has no role in modern obstetrics except when the baby is dead.

Uses

1. It is used in cases of placenta praevia when the patient is bleeding profusely and facilities for cessation are not available. To save the life of the mother a quick rupture

 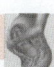

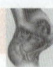

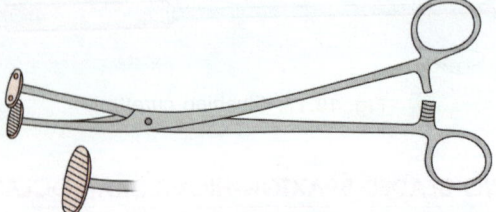

Fig. 19.19: Willet's scalp traction forceps

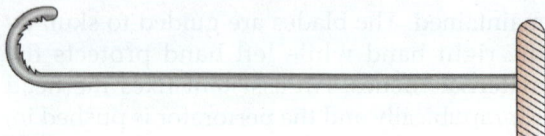

Fig. 19.20: Ramsbotham's decapitation saw

of the membranes is done and the fetal head is pulled down with the forceps. A small weight is applied to it for traction. The bleeding is controlled by the compression of the placental bed from the pressure exerted by the fetal head.

2. To extract the fetal head after perforation during a craniotomy operation.
3. To hasten the delivery of an IUD baby with a collapsed head which is unable to act as a good dilator for the cervix.

Complications

1. Lacerations and avulsion of the fetal scalp
2. Haemorrhage from fetal scalp injury
3. Fetal scalp infection
4. Accidental injury to maternal tissues

RAMSBOTHAM'S DECAPITATION SAW

It has a blade, shaped like a wide hook with a bent tip and a serrated inner edge.

The prolapsed hand in a transverse lie is pulled down or if not already prolapsed then it is made to prolapse. The saw is introduced under cover of the palmar surface of the left hand keeping the tip towards the occiput. When the neck of the baby is reached the saw is rotated by 90° to guide the cutting edge along the neck of the baby. The decapitation is started by gentle to and fro sawing movements until the bones are severed. The remaining soft tissues of the neck are cut with the embryotomy scissors. The baby is delivered by pulling on the arm after checking that no bony spicules are present which can

damage maternal tissues or it may be delivered by version. The severed head is delivered by:

1. Putting a finger in the mouth and applying traction
2. By forceps
3. By craniotomy
4. By crochet and hook

BLOND-HIEDLER'S DECAPITATION SAW WIRE WITH THIMBLE

It consists of a thimble with a ring, a 43 cm long wire, saw blade with a rubber sheath at each end and 2 handles. The rubber sheath covers about 1/3 of the length of the wire saw to prevent damage to the surrounding area. Each end has a small metal ball on which traction handles may be fitted. It is a safer and more effective instrument for decapitation. It is supplied with the aid of a metal thimble on the operators thumb which temporarily carries one end of the saw and is made to encircle the neck of the baby. The sawing is then done after applying traction handles.

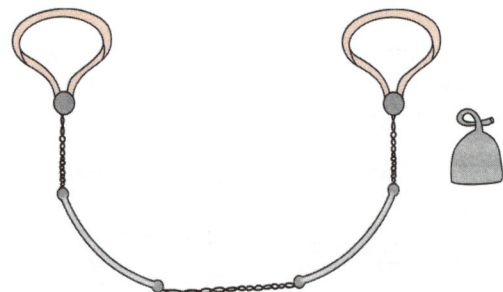

Fig. 19.21: Blond-Hiedler's decapitation saw with thimble

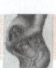

BREECH HOOK WITH CROCHET

The instrument has a hook on one end which is wider and gradually bent while the other end has an acutely bent hook known as the crochet. The curvatures face each other. The breech hook is used to put traction on the groin in case of impacted breech of a dead fetus. The crotchet part is used to hook down a decapitated head through the mouth or a hole in the skull.

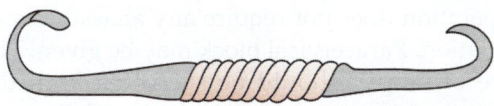

Fig. 19.22: Breech hook with crochet

SPECIALIZED GYNAECOLOGICAL INSTRUMENTS

UTERINE DRESSING FORCEPS

It is a long straight instrument with a lock and transverse serrations on the inner aspect. It is used to swab the uterine cavity.

Technique

A small piece of gauze is held between the blades and introduced inside the uterine cavity and all the walls and the fundal area of the uterus are cleaned by gently rotating it all around.

Uses

1. To swab the uterine cavity
2. Suction and evacuation
3. Draining of pyometra
4. Draining of haematometra

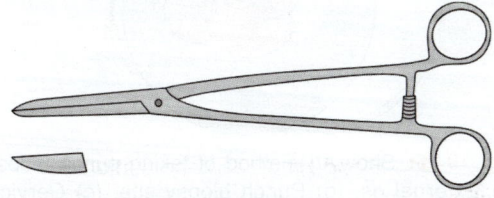

Fig. 19.23: Uterine dressing forceps

Disadvantages

1. Injury may occur in the vagina, uterus or cervix.
2. A small piece of swab or threads may be left behind and may serve as nidus for infections.

UTERUS PACKING FORCEPS

It is a long slender sinuously curved instrument having blades and handles. The blades have transverse serrations on the inside so a firm grip is obtained. It is used to pack the uterine cavity in cases of PPH to control bleeding.

Technique

A check curettage is done to rule out retained placental bits as a cause of postpartum haemorrhage. The cervix is grasped with a sponge holder after retracting the vaginal walls. A sterilized ribbon gauze is introduced and packing is started from one cornual end to the other and back again till the whole cavity is packed. The cervix and vagina should also be packed along with uterine packing. If one ribbon gauze is insufficient another may be attached to it with a firm knot and the number of ribbons used should be noted down. Care should be taken not to leave any dead space at the fundus or in between as bleeding will occur and defeat the purpose of packing. The patient is watched carefully for any deterioration of vitals, bleeding per vaginum or increase in fundal height. These events suggest continuing uterine bleed and failure of the procedure and decision for hysterectomy or internal iliac artery ligation be taken immediately.

Uses

- **It is used for uterine packing in**
    - Uncontrolled atonic postpartum hae-morrhage
    - Uncontrolled post abortal haemorrhage
    - Bleeding from the uterus after polypec-tomy, not controlled by curettage.

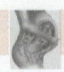
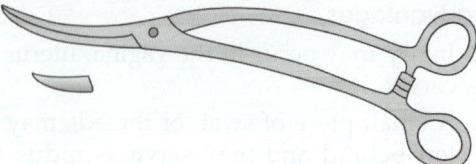

Fig. 19.24: Uterus packing forceps

- **For vaginal packing**
  - After vaginal hysterectomy to control oozing from vault
  - After cervical or vaginal biopsy
  - To control oozing from a ragged cervix after delivery
  - To control secondary hemorrhage after operations like vaginal hysterectomy, Fothergill's repair, conisation, etc.
  - After insertion of laminaria tents or intrauterine radium needles to prevent their expulsion.

Disadvantages

The following complications may occur:
1. Intrauterine collection of blood may be missed unless fundal height is carefully monitored.
2. Sepsis
3. Injury by the instrument
4. Asherman's syndrome especially if sepsis occurs.
5. Placental anomalies like placenta accreta in subsequent pregnancies.
6. Procedure may fail and patient may require a major operation with precious time being lost in between.

Advantages

1. It is a useful measure to control postpartum haemorrhage especially in cases where the patient wants to conserve her reproductive capability.
2. It also helps in avoiding major operations like a hysterectomy in a patient with poor general condition.

CERVICAL PUNCH BIOPSY FORCEPS

It is a strong instrument with two blades, handles with finger grips and a lock. The blades consist of one smaller blade with a sharp cutting edge that fits closely into the larger blade which holds the specimen like a basket. The handles are angulated to avoid obstruction of the field of vision while taking the biopsy.

Technique

Operation does not require any anaesthesia or sedation. Paracervical block may be given. The site of biopsy should be such that both the abnormal area and a part of normal area are included in the specimen for a proper comparison. The suspicious area can be demarcated by painting with Schiller's iodine or by a colpomicroscope. The raw area of biopsy may bleed and haemostasis can be done by taking one or two stitches or by packing the vagina.

Uses

1. Recurrent cervicitis with nonhealing erosions not responding to antibiotics, i.e. 'bad cervix'.

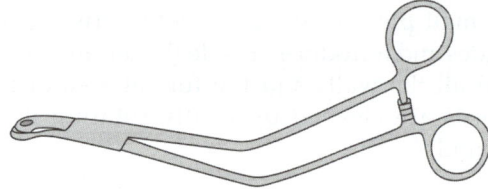

Fig. 19.25: Cervical punch biopsy forceps

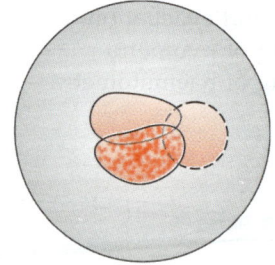

Fig. 19.26: Showing method of taking punch biopsy. (a) External os, (b) Punch biopsy site, (c) Cervical lesion, (d) Cervix

2. Postcoital bleeding
3. Abnormal Pap's smears
4. Nonhealing ulcers on the cervix
5. Abnormal finding on Schiller's test or colpomicroscopy

Disadvantages

The following complications can occur:
1. Sepsis
2. Haemorrhage

SHIRODKAR'S CERVICAL ENCIRCLAGE NEEDLES

These are two 5 cm long blunt tipped ½ circle needles each having an eye near the tip and attached to a handle at the other end. The needles are designed separately for the right and the left sides with opposite curves, i.e. they are mirror images of each other. They are used to pass a nonabsorbable encircling suture around the cervix at the level of the internal os. The suture operates by disturbing the uterine polarity and prevents the internal os and the adjacent uterine lower segment from being 'taken up'.

Technique

The suture is applied onto patients of habitual abortion due to incompetent cervical os. The suture is given around 14 weeks of pregnancy

or at least one week before the age of gestation at which the patient usually aborts.

Postoperative care after encirclage includes bed rest, prophylactic antibiotics, tocolytic drugs and progesterone. The suture is removed around 36 weeks of pregnancy or immediately if membranes rupture or if the patient goes into premature labour.

Contraindications

1. Rupture of the membranes
2. Uterine bleeding
3. Uterine contractions
4. Chorioamnionitis
5. Cervical dilatation more than 4 cm
6. Polyhydramnios
7. Fetal anomaly

Complications

The complications of encirclage operation range from mild to fatal. These include:
1. Haemorrhage
2. Rupture of membranes
3. Severe infections may occur
4. Cervical dystocia
5. Uterine rupture
6. Vesicovaginal fistula
7. Fetal death

GREEN ARMYTAGE CLAMP

The instrument consists of solid, triangular blades with transverse serrations, a shaft and a handle with a lock. The flattened broad blades achieve haemostasis over a wider area and can therefore occlude large bleeders.

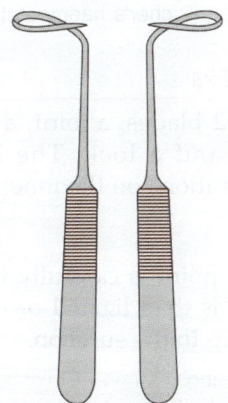

Fig. 19.27: Shirodkar's cervical encirclage needles

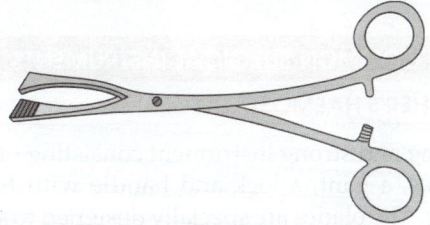

Fig. 19.28: Green Armytage clamp

Uses

1. To hold the cut edges of the uterine scar in caesarean section operation. It helps in compressing the large uterine sinuses and clearly defines the edges for suturing.
2. To hold the angles of the caesarean section scar while suturing.
3. To hold the cervix during its exploration for a cervical tear in place of a sponge holding forceps.

WERTHEIM'S VAGINAL CLAMP

It is an L-shaped instrument with oblique serrations both in the vertical and horizontal part of the blade. The clamp has a lock and a handle with finger grips. The clamp is applied on the vagina during Wertheim's hysterectomy after the uterus has been separated from its attachments and the cardinal and uterosacral ligaments have been divided.

Uses

During Wertheim's hysterectomy to prevent the spillage of malignant cells and infective material from the growth onto the raw areas in the pelvis resulting in further spread of the carcinoma.

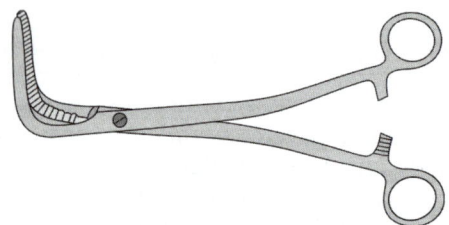

Fig. 19.29: Wertheim's vaginal clamp

COMMON SURGICAL INSTRUMENTS

KOCHER'S HAEMOSTATIC CLAMP

A long and strong instrument consisting of two blades, a joint, a lock and handle with finger grips. The blades are specially designed to serve the function of efficient haemostats. They have transverse serrations on the inner aspect and are toothed. There are transverse serrations on the inner aspect and are toothed. The transverse serrations, the tooth and the lock together provide a very firm grip of the structure held.

Technique

In gynaecological surgery the instrument finds special use in hysterectomy operation for clamping, cutting and ligating the pedicles. Wherever bleeding is expected, the structure is held in between two clamps and then cut and ligated.

Uses

1. To clamp, cut and ligate various pedicles like ovarian ligament, Mackenrodts ligament, uterine artery and ovarian pedicles in operations like abdominal hysterectomy, oophorectomy, salpingectomy, etc.
2. As a clamp for umbilical cord.
3. For doing an artificial rupture of membranes in labour.

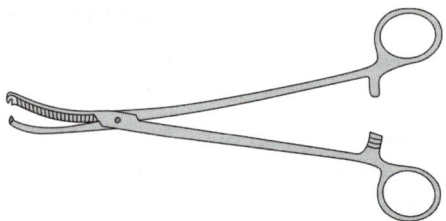

Fig. 19.30: Kocher's haemostatic clamp

ARTERY FORCEPS

It consists of 2 blades, a joint, a handle with finger grips and a lock. The blades have transverse serrations on the inner aspect.

Technique

Any bleeding point is carefully held between its tips which is than ligated or cauterized by showing the tip to the surgeon.

Uses

1. To hold the bleeders for ligating and cautery.

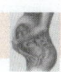

2. To hold the edges of a wound while suturing it.
3. To hold the free end of a suture.

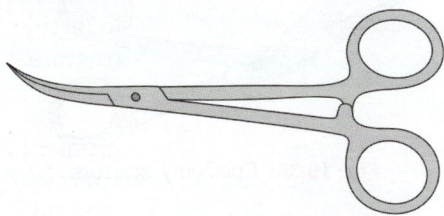

Fig. 19.31: Artery forceps

NEEDLE HOLDER

It is an instrument used to hold needles while passing sutures during surgery. The shape is similar to an artery forceps but with the difference that the blades are smaller and the serrations on the inner surface are criss-cross with a single longitudinal groove to prevent slipping and turning of the needle.

Technique

The needle should be held at the junction of anterior 2/3rds with posterior 1/3rd of its body. If held more posterior, the needle may break as this is its weakest point. If held more towards the middle of the needle there is a mechanical disadvantage and it deforms the shape of the needle.

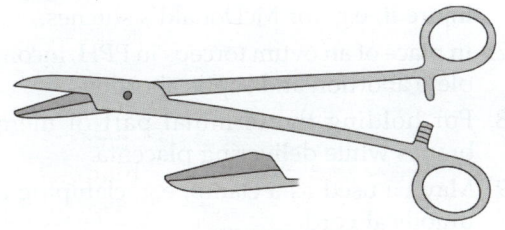

Fig. 19.32: Needle holder

ALLIS'S TISSUE HOLDING FORCEPS

It is a straight instrument with two blades and a handle with lock and finger bows. The blades have distance in between and come close together only at the tips and are toothed. The lock and toothed blades provide a firm grip. The teeth are multiple and fine. The space in between the blades prevents trauma and crushing of the structures held.

Uses

1. To hold thin but tough structures like skin and rectus sheath during opening and closure of abdomen.
2. To hold the bleeding edges of the vaginal vault after the uterus has been removed in an abdominal hysterectomy.
3. To hold any fibrous capsule for dissection.
4. To hold the cervix in D and C, HSG, etc.
5. In LSCS for holding the edges of the uterine incision in place of a Green Armytage forceps.
6. To hold the apex of any wound which is being repaired, e.g. episiotomy and perineal tear.
7. As a towel clip.

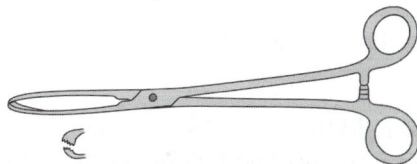

Fig. 19.33: Allis's tissue holding forceps

LANES'S TISSUE HOLDING FORCEPS

The blades of this forceps are curved like a spoon, longitudinally fenestrated and the tip is toothed. The handle has a lock. The toothed tip helps in providing a good grip while the fenestrated blade can hold tubular structures without damaging them.

Uses

1. To hold thick, tough structures like rectus sheath lymphnode, lining of a sac, etc.
2. To hold tubular structures like appendix fallopian tubes, ureters, etc. but one has to be careful as the sharp teeth can cause damage.

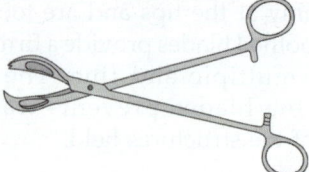

Fig. 19.34: Lanes's tissue holding forceps

BABCOCK'S TISSUE HOLDING FORCEPS

It is a light, small instrument with curved fenestrated blades having a transverse bar at the tip. The handles have a lock. The absence of teeth at the tip makes it an ideal instrument for holding delicate, soft tubular structures. The fenestrated and curved blades allow the tubular structures to bulge out preventing damage.

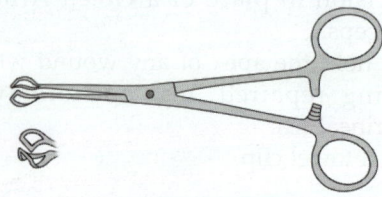

Fig. 19.35: Babcock's tissue holding forceps

Uses

1. To hold the appendix, intestine, spermatic cord, ureters and fallopian tubes, etc.
2. To hold two levator ani muscles in order to bring them to the centre for approximation in a third degree perineal tear repair operation and posterior colpoperineorrhaphy.

SCISSORS

EPISIOTOMY SCISSORS

This is a curved one angle type of scissors with blunt tips so that it cannot damage any structure. One blade has lateral serrations for a secured grip of the tissue to give a smooth and straight incision without ragged edges.

Uses

For blunt dissection in tissues containing lots of connective tissue. The scissors may be used here with closed blades which are opened up in various directions to break the connective tissue.

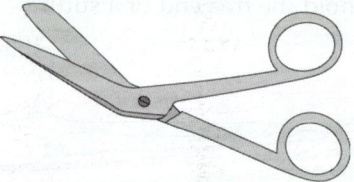

Fig. 19.36: Episitomy scissors

RAMPLEY'S SPONGE HOLDING FORCEPS

It is a long forceps with 2 blades, a handle with finger grips and a lock. The blades are ring like, fenestrated and have transverse serrations.

Uses

1. For cleaning and dressing of the patient.
2. For swabbing a cavity, e.g. the uterus in lower segment caesarean section and vaginal wash down.
3. The transverse serrations help in making the instrument a good haemostat so can be used for holding the angles in caesarean section.
4. For packing a cavity, e.g. vaginal in cervical tears.
5. For holding small rounded pieces of gauze for mopping the operative field.
6. Holding the cervix in pregnancy when the cervix is soft and the toothed volsellum can injure it, e.g. for McDonald's stitches.
7. In place of an ovum forceps in PPH, incomplete abortion and septic abortion.
8. For holding the terminal part of membranes while delivering placenta.
9. May be used as a clamp, e.g. clamping of umbilical cord.

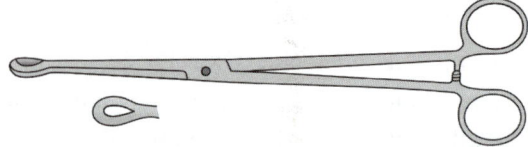

Fig. 19.37: Rampley's sponge holding forceps

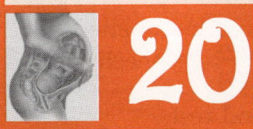

20

Gynaecological Disorders in Pregnancy

OUTLINE

- Uterine displacements
- Retroversion
  - Retroverted gravid uterus
- Genital prolapse in pregnancy
- Uterine fibroid in pregnancy
- Carcinoma of the cervix in pregnancy
- Ovarian tumours in pregnancy

UTERINE DISPLACEMENTS

Introduction

The elasticity of the supporting structures; the female pelvic organs are quite mobile and therefore very favourable for displacement. This is true not only of the uterus, but of the ovaries as well and very often there is an accompanying displacement of the abdominal viscera also.

The uterus may be displaced forward (or) backward, upward (or) downward or to the either side, but only two of these are of any great consequence viz. backward displacement/retroversion and downward displacement/prolapsus. Retroversion is known as "tipping of the womb" and of prolapsus as "Falling of the womb".

Definition

"Version" refers to the direction of the cervical canal, whereas flexion refers to the inclination of the body of the uterus on the cervix. A occurrence of combination of the above mentioned on an average (or) occurrence of any one is called uterine displacements.

The two types of displacements are

1. A change in the long axis of the uterus, for example, anteflexion, malposition and retroflexion and
2. A change in the direction of the long axis of the uterus in relation to the vaginal canal for example, lateral retroversion and retrocession.

Most positional differences are simple anatomic variations. They are asymptomatic and have no clinical significance. Retroversion is the most common simple displacement caused by factors that are congenital or acquired after childbirth. Cul-de-sac disease may be responsible and is of clinical significance.

Lateral displacement may signal adnexal disease such as large ovarian tumor on the opposite side.

The supporting ligaments that hold the uterus in anteversion are the round and uterosacral ligaments. The uterosacral ligaments pull the cervix backward and upward; the round ligaments hold the fundus in the anterior position. These ligaments gradually regain their length and return the uterus to anteversion in two-thirds of women within approximately 2 months after delivery; in one third of women the uterus remains retroverted.

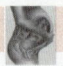

- *Anteflexion:* The abnormal bending forward of a part of the uterus at its body and neck.
- *Anteversion:* Tipping forward of the uterus as a whole.
- *Retroflexion:* A condition in which the body of the uterus is bent backward at an angle with the cervix, whose position usually remains unchanged.
- *Retrocession:* Backward displacement of the uterus.
- *Retroversion:* Backward displacement of the uterus with the cervix pointing forward toward the symphysis pubis. Normally the cervix points toward the lower end of the sacrum with the fundus toward the supra pubic region.

Retroversion is classified into 2 as:
1. Mobile retroversion
2. Fixed retroversion

Causes of uterine displacements
- Disclined girlhood activity
- Weak and flabby muscles (abdomen)
- Heavy eater
- Constipation prone
- Either very lean/very stout
- Wearing cossets to trim thus forcing the abdominal contents downwards.
- Heavy lifting, active exercises (jumping, dancing and swimming)
- Relaxation of the pelvic floor following laurations in childbirth.
- Habitual constipation
- Constant distension of the bladder
- Presence of pelvic/abdominal tumours.
- Getting up too soon after childbirth.
- Chronically overworked women
- Very poor posture in any case.

Clinical features
Symptoms of retroversion
A certain degree of displacement is possible without symptoms, but when there is a decided retroversion the patient may suffer considerably.

- Less vigour
- Easily tired
- Incomplete sleep and rest
- Dragging feel of the pelvic region
- Intense pain and ache at times in sacral region
- Unduly protracted pelvis accompanied with pain.
- Constipation
- Frequent micturition
- If there is pregnancy, a miscarriage may follow.

Symptoms of prolapses
- Prolapse (or) falling of the womb may be a slight (or) pronounced descent into the vagina or the entire uterus may even appear outside of the vulva, carrying the vaginal walls down with it
- In some cases it is simply an elongation of the cervix
- Prolapse is practically a more advanced stage of retroversion
- The uterus sinks gradually into the vagina until the cervix appears at the orifice
- If the tissues here are relaxed, the entire uterus is soon outside the vagina
- Continual dragging sensation incident to the stretching of ligaments
- Sense of foreign body between the thighs.
- Discomfort ceases when full descent has occurred
- Thickening and hardening of vaginal wall
- Erosion and ulceration of vaginal wall.

Treatment of uterine displacements
- If there are no symptoms and the condition is discovered on examination, no treatment is required
- Put back uterus into original position by manual means
- Pack this uterus with gauze (or) pledgets of cotton, but these must be removed after twenty-four hours and are therefore not effective.

- Pessary is often used and is useful temporarily when the woman is obliged to be on her feet continually. Pessary may be a cause of inflammation, leucorrhea and ulceration may occur from pressure. Therefore, it should not be worn continuously.
- Frequent douches are necessary during the time the pessary is used.
- Before any permanent cure can be expected, the tone of the entire muscular system must be improved through exercising including use of all the muscles.
- Knee-chest position
- Sleeping chest downward
- Cold sitz bath
- Complete prolapse or complete bed rest, preferably in prone position, with large pledgets of cotton attached to a string may be introduced into the vagina to prevent the uterus from descending again. The woman is encouraged to do exercises on bed.

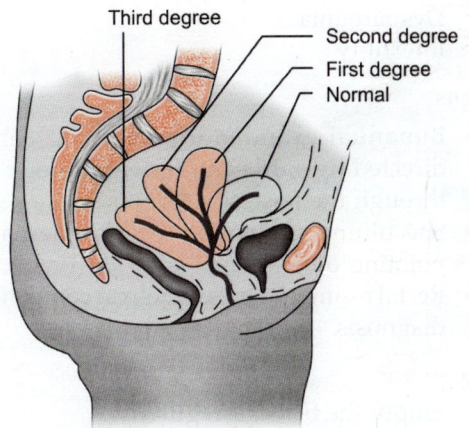

Fig. 20.1: Degrees of retroversion

RETROVERSION

Definition

A term used when the axes of the corpus and cervix are in line and the whole organ turns backwards in relation to the long axis of the birth canal.

Degrees (Fig. 20.1)

1. First degree
   Fundus is vertical and pointing towards the sacral promontory.
2. Second degree
   Fundus lies in the sacral hollow, not below the internal os.
3. Third degree
   Fundus lies below the level of the internal os in the pouch of the Douglas.

Causes

1. Developmental
2. Acquired

Developmental

- Due to developmental defect there is lack of tone of the uterine muscles.
- Infantile position is retained

Acquired

- *Puerperal:* Childbirth fails to keep the uterus in its normal position.
- *Prolapse:* Mechanically caused by traction following cystocele.
- *Tumour:* Either in the anterior or posterior wall produces heaviness of the uterus and hence it falls behind.
- *Pelvic adhesions:* Adhesions either inflammatory or operative pull the uterus posteriorly.

Incidence

15–20% of normal women.

Clinical presentation

The condition is classified as mobile and fixed or complicated and uncomplicated.
Symptoms: Mobile retroverted uterus is quite common and almost always remains asymptomatic.

- Chronic premenstrual pelvic pain
- Backache

- Dyspareunia
- Infertility

Signs

- Bimanual examination showing cervix directed upwards and forwards, body felt through the posterior fornix.
- Speculum examination reveals external os pointing outwards.
- Rectal examination is of help to confirm the diagnosis.

Prevention

- Empty the bladder regularly.
- Regular exercise.
- To lie in prone position for half to one hour once or twice daily between 2 and 4 weeks during postpartum.

Corrective treatment

- Pessary
- Surgical

Pessary

Hodge Smith pessary is used usually. The pessary stretches the uterosacral ligaments so as to pull the cervix backwards.

Surgical treatment

The principle of surgical correction is ventro suspension of the uterus by plicating the round ligaments of both the sides extra peritoneally to the under surface of the anterior rectus sheath. This will pull the uterus forwards and maintains it permanently.

RETROVERTED GRAVID UTERUS

Definition

A retroverted gravid uterus results from pregnancy occurring in a retroverted uterus. Retroflexion may accompany retroversion of the uterus.

Clinical features

As a rule, retroverted gravid uterus does not produce any symptom up to twelve weeks after

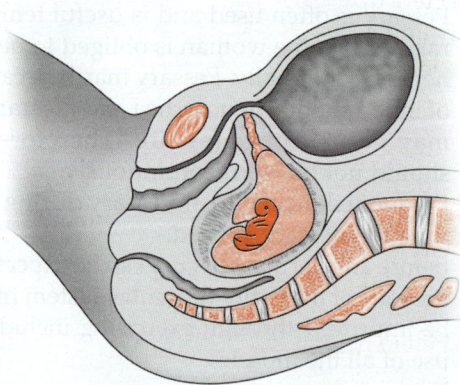

Fig. 20.2: Retroverted gravid uterus causing retention of urine

which the majority correct spontaneously to be an abdominal organ. *Rarely, retroverted gravid uterus may be incarcerated or imprisoned in the sacral hollow to produce symptoms during 12–16 weeks of pregnancy.*

Symptoms of incarcerated retroverted gravid uterus

1. Retention of urine due to elongation of the urethra by the upwardly pushed cervix is the most characteristic symptom (Fig. 20.2). Following overdistention of bladder, incontinence of urine occurs. Very rarely in the untreated cases, the infection of the urinary tract may lead to cystitis, pyelonephritis, uraemia, and passage of bits of mucous membranes per urethra and even rupture of the bladder due to necrosis following obstruction in circulation. Now even with a days' neglect cases with such extreme fatal complications are not encountered.
2. Abortion may follow.
3. There may be pain in the back and a bearing down feeling in the pelvis.
4. Constipation due to pressure on the rectum by the uterus.

Very rarely, an imprisoned retroverted gravid uterus may grow with the anterior wall

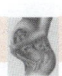

projected upwards in the general abdominal cavity and a sacculation occurs in the pouch of Douglas.

Obstetrical issues related to incarceration of the gravid retroverted uterus

- Additional technical difficulty in chorionic villus sampling
- Greater likelihood of failure with endo-metrial resection and thermal balloon ablation
- Pelvic pain and dyspareunia
- Increased difficulties with embryo transfer
- Difficulties regarding IUD insertion and diaphragm insertions
- Sonography
- Infertility issues

Effects on pregnancy

- Retroversion actually has got practically no adverse effect either on fertility (or) on early pregnancy wastage.
- In pregnancy spontaneous correction usually occurs by 12–14 weeks.
- Cause of infertility is mechanical (because the external os is away from the seminal pool at the posterior fornix during coitus (or) it may be occluded by the anterior vaginal wall.
- Repeated pregnancy wastage may be due to disturbance in uterine vascularity (or) due to thrust during intercourse especially on abortion prone women.

Signs

1. Patient may be in distress due to acute retention of urine.
2. Per abdomen, a cystic swelling in the hypogastric region up to the umbilicus can be felt due to full bladder.
3. On vaginal examination, a soft cystic globular swelling (pregnant uterus) is felt through the posterior fornix. The cervix lies high up behind the pubis and is directed upwards and forwards; the vaginal fingers

can reach the high up cervix with difficulty. After the bladder is emptied, no abdominal swelling is felt, and the uterus is also felt in the pelvis.

4. Per rectal examination, the gravid uterus in the pouch of Douglas can be better defined.

Treatment

1. Symptomless retroverted gravid uterus during 8 to 10 weeks pregnancy requires no treatment but expectant observations; she is advised to lie on her face for 15 minutes twice a day for one month and is re-examined at about 12th week.

2. Retroverted gravid uterus with retention of urine is treated as follows:
   - *Expectant treatment:* Inj. Voveran 50 mg IM if there is pelvic pain. Patient is put to bed and continuous drainage by Foley's catheter is set up for 7–10 days. Urine is sent for culture and sensitivity test. Suitable antibiotic or chemotherapy is then administered. She should lie on her face as much as possible or in Sim's position. Bowel is to be evacuated regularly by milk of magnesia or cremaffin. Spontaneous correction of retroverted gravid uterus happens within 24–48 hours following emptying of the bladder. On removal of catheter, prolonged 14 days course of furadantin 100 mg daily at bed time is given orally given.
   - *Catheter care is given regularly.*
   - *Manual reposition:* Very rarely, if above treatment fails, manual reposition should be tried by pushing the uterus upwards and forwards with two fingers in the vagina while the patient is placed in the Sim's, or knee-chest position. If the uterus can be displaced forwards, the cervix should be pressed backwards towards the hollow of the sacrum. After manual reposition, a Hodge-Smith pessary is inserted immediately, which

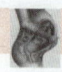

is to be kept till the uterus becomes an abdominal organ (i.e. until 16 weeks of pregnancy) (Fig. 20.3).

- In a rare case of anterior sacculation where pregnancy goes to term, caesarean section becomes necessary for delivery.

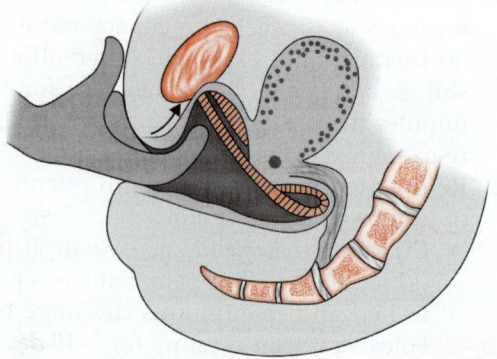

Fig. 20.3: Pessary to correct the position of a retroverted uterus

GENITAL PROLAPSE IN PREGNANCY

Pregnancy can occur in women with cystocele, rectocele and uterine prolapse.

Clinical features

Symptoms

The symptoms become distressing mainly during early months. The symptoms are fall of womb, white discharge per vagina, pelvic pain, backache, bladder symptoms, frequency of urination, inability to pass urine completely and stress incontinence, and rectal symptoms, difficulty in completing defaecation and constipation.

Signs

Locally they are those for genital prolapse - cystocele, rectocele, uterine prolapse with ulcerated hypertrophic elongated cervix and urethrocele.

Clinical course

1. The uterine descent gradually recedes up as the pregnant uterus becomes an abdominal organ after 12 weeks of pregnancy. Premature labour often occurs.
2. During labour, cervix may show improper dilatation, oedema, and improper effacement, early rupture of membranes, early bearing down pains at the first stage due to descent of the cervix on the pelvic floor, delayed second stage due to obstruction by the cystocele and rectocele. Puerperal sepsis is common.

Treatment

1. Early pregnancy with uterine prolapse producing distressing symptoms. Rest in bed is essential; ring pessary for a few weeks should be applied. After 16 weeks, gravid uterus grows up out of the pelvis and thus pulls up the cervix.
2. *During labour:* During first stage, rest in bed with plugging of the vagina with roller gauze soaked in glycerine and acriflavine to lift up the cervix helps in dilatation of the cervix. Head being high up with oedematous tubular nondilating cervix with premature rupture of membranes and foetal distress lower uterine caesarean section is advisable.

UTERINE FIBROID IN PREGNANCY

Uterine fibroid complicates pregnancy in an elderly primigravida commonly following a period of infertile marriage.

Effects of uterine fibroid on pregnancy and labour

Uterine fibroid does not produce any difficulty in pregnancy or labour in majority cases. In others, the effects observed are higher incidence of the following:

1. Abortion and premature labour.
2. Painful fibroid and pelvic pain.

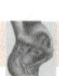

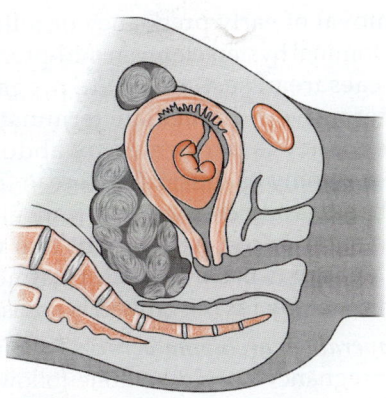

Fig. 20.4: Uterine fibroid in pregnancy

3. Malpresentation and nonengagement of foetal head.
4. Uterine inertia, nondilatation of cervix in cervical fibroid.
5. Obstructed labour especially in posterior cervical fibroid.
6. Third stage complications—postpartum haemorrhage and puerperal sepsis.

Effects of pregnancy on uterine fibroid

The changes in fibroid produced by pregnancy are:

1. Increased in size with softness due to hypertrophy and oedema; the tumour tends to be flattened.
2. Upward displacement of fibroid in position.
3. Rupture of subserous vein in the fibroid.
4. Red degeneration during second half of pregnancy or puerperium.
5. Torsion of a pedunculated subserous fibroid after delivery.

Clinical features

Symptoms

1. It may remain asymptomatic.
2. Undue enlargement of the abdomen, dyspnoea, pressure symptoms—on the bladder, retention of urine or on the rectum, constipation, rectal pain. Retention of urine is an important symptom during early

pregnancy due to incarceration of posterior fibroid into the pelvic cavity.
3. Symptoms of red degenerations—pain in abdomen, nausea, vomiting, fever. In severe cases, all these symptoms may be acute producing symptoms of acute abdomen. Twisted subserous fibroid can also cause acute abdominal symptoms.

Signs

1. During early pregnancy, the external uterine wall is felt nodular. Ultrasonography can diagnose gestation sac in the uterine cavity and uterine fibroid.
2. During late pregnancy, feeling of separate solid fixed lumps attached with uterus. Ultrasonography can diagnose foetus and uterine fibroid.
3. In complicated cases of red degeneration there are evidences of tachycardia, rise of temperature, coated tongue; per abdomen-rigidity and tenderness on the abdomen overlying the tumour, in a severe case; fibroid is felt as a tender lump.

Treatment

During pregnancy

1. Uncomplicated cases—close antenatal supervision is provided till labour.
2. Complicated cases
   - Cervical fibroid causing retention of urine—bladder is catheterized; manual reposition is attempted, if spontaneous correction does not occur.
   - Red degeneration—conservative treatment by bed rest, pethidine and oral aspirin (Disprin) and gelusil MPS twice daily for 5 days; this invariably relieves the condition.
   - Acute abdomen due to twisted subserous fibroid or intraperitoneal haemorrhage from vein need also laparotomy.

All cases should have vaginal examination about at 38th week of pregnancy to exclude any fibroid in the pelvis which might cause obstructed labour. All pregnant women with uterine fibroids must have hospital confinement since this is a high risk pregnancy.

During labour

1. Tumour not lying in the pelvis—spontaneous delivery is awaited followed by appropriate treatment of fibroid after puerperium. Prophylactic ergometrine should be given.
2. Tumour lying in the pelvis causing obstruction—caesarean section is performed.

CARCINOMA OF CERVIX IN PREGNANCY

Carcinoma of cervix is a rare association with pregnancy.

Effects of carcinoma cervix on pregnancy and labour

During pregnancy, the effects are abortion and premature labour. The baby becomes growth restricted. During labour, the effects are those of nondilatation of the cervix, its tear, rupture of the lower uterine segment and puerperal sepsis.

Effects of pregnancy on carcinoma cervix

Opinions suggest that pregnancy does neither hasten nor retard the growth of the carcinoma cervix.

Clinical features

Symptoms

Scanty, irregular vaginal bleeding; blood-stained white discharge per vagina.

Signs

Signs of carcinoma of the cervix can be detected on vaginal speculum and pelvic examination in addition to evidences of pregnancy. Biopsy and histological section confirm the diagnosis.

Treatment

During pregnancy

1. *Operable early carcinoma cervix:* radical surgery (Wertheim's operation) with removal of early pregnancy or following abdominal hysterectomy in mid-pregnancy or caesarean section in late pregnancy. Alternatively, immediate termination of pregnancy is performed by abdominal hysterotomy or classical caesarean section; antibiotics and chemotherapy are given in adequate doses. After about two weeks when sepsis is controlled, treatment by radiotherapy for the growth is advisable.
2. *Inoperable carcinoma cervix:* Termination of pregnancy should be done followed by palliative radiotherapy.

During labour

For cervical growth appearing to cause non-dilatation of the cervix, classical caesarean section followed by appropriate treatment of the carcinoma is advisable.

OVARIAN TUMOURS IN PREGNANCY

This can be rarely associated with pregnancy. These tumours are largely benign neoplasms. Malignant ovarian tumour may very rarely complicate pregnancy.

Effects of ovarian tumours on pregnancy and labour

Pregnancy usually continues undisturbed but the following upsets may develop

1. Increased ailments of pregnancy—abdominal pain, undue enlargement of abdomen, dyspnoea.
2. Abortion and premature labour may develop.
3. Non-engagement and malpresentations
4. Obstructed labour.

Effects of pregnancy on ovarian tumour

There are possibilities of all complications of ovarian tumour, torsion of pedicle, rupture, intracystic haemorrhage, infection and malignant change.

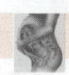

However, the rate of torsion runs at least double than that of non-pregnant state and it commonly develops at 13–14th week of pregnancy and after delivery. This is the commonest complication. Infection occurs more commonly after delivery.

Clinical features of ovarian tumour in pregnancy

Symptoms

There may be pain, undue enlargement of the abdomen and dyspnoea, bladder and rectal symptoms. There may be acute abdomen due to complications.

Signs

During early pregnancy, the palpation of a separate commonly cystic mass apart from the pregnant uterus during bimanual palpation gives the diagnosis.

Treatment

1. *During first half of pregnancy:* Ovariotomy is immediately performed in complicated tumours. The operation should preferably be performed between 15 and 20th week of pregnancy even if it lies uncomplicated and asymptomatic. There is postoperative risk of abortion. Bed rest is mandatory.

2. *During second half of pregnancy:* Ovariotomy is immediately performed, if the tumour shows evidences of complications. Asymptomatic abdominal tumour is left alone and is kept under observation up to term. With such abdominal tumour, spontaneous labour is awaited followed by ovariotomy after labour.

3. *Ovarian tumour in labour:* If the tumour lies above the pelvic brim and is not likely to obstruct labour, spontaneous vaginal delivery is awaited followed by ovariotomy soon after labour. For tumour obstructing labour, caesarean section followed by ovariotomy should be performed. Ovarian tumour detected after labour be removed without delay.

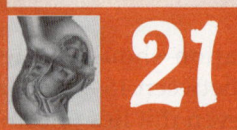

21

Social and Preventive Obstetrics

OUTLINE

- Family welfare programme in India
- Maternal mortality, morbidity, perinatal mortality
- Infertility and assisted reproductive technology
- Legal aspects in obstetrics
- Menopause

The concept of social obstetrics has gained currency in recent years. It may be defined as the study of the interplay of social and environmental factors and human reproduction going back to the preconceptional or even premarital period. The social and environmental factors which influence human reproduction are a legion, viz. age at marriage, childbearing, child spacing, family size fertility patterns, level of education, economic status, customs and beliefs, role of women in society etc. A study of these factors is an important aspect of social obstetrics. The social obstetric problems in the developed countries, because of various differing social, economic, cultural an other factors. While accepting the influence of environmental and social factors of human reproduction, social obstetrics has yet another dimension, that is the influence of these factors on the organization, delivery and utilization of obstetrics is concerned with the delivery of comprehensive maternity and child health care services including family planning so that they can be brought within the reach of the total community.

FAMILY WELFARE PROGRAMME IN INDIA

National Family Welfare Programme in India has been started from 1975. National Family Planning programme was launched in India in 1952.

National Family Welfare Programme in India has five components

1. Maternal and child health RCH care
2. Immunization of pregnant women by tetanus toxoid and that of children-infant of 1 year age and pre-school age up to 5 years by BCG, oral polio, diphtheria, tetanus, pertussis, measles.
   National pulse polio programme (2 doses)—another booster polio programme for 5 years old children.
3. Nutritional supplement—iron folic acid (tablet folifer) to pregnant women and children and vitamin A in oil to children for prevention of blindness.
4. Contraceptive education and distribution—(free and social marketing, i.e. contraceptive on sale) of spacing contraceptives (Nirodh, oral contraceptives, Mala D, copper device and that of voluntary surgical contraception (tubectomy, vasectomy)—VSC.
5. Health education on primary health care particularly motivation to accept contraception. Emphasis on VSC was made in the

national programme. Currently spacing contraception is promoted.

Medical termination of pregnancy (MTP)

This service is also available from 1972 throughout the country as a health measure for protection of woman's health against criminal abortion. This follows MTP Act passed by Indian Parliament 1971; MTP service is followed by acceptance of contraception.

Reproductive and child health (RCH) care

RCH care is an integrated and composite approach to improve the health status of women and children in India.

The aims of RCH care are to prevent malnutrition, infection and unregulated fertility. Obstetric complications, e.g. anaemia, pre-eclampsia, IUGR, preterm birth, PPH, rupture of uterus could be prevented to a large extent, once the above mentioned triad are taken care of. The main objectives are—(i) reduction of maternal and perinatal morality and morbidity and (ii) promotion of health for the mother, child and the adolescent.

RCH INTERVENTIONS

1. Safe Motherhood

- **Antenatal care**
  - **Early registration of pregnancy**.
  - **A minimum of 4 antenatal visits** (1st at 16 weeks, 2nd at 24–28 weeks, 3rd at 32 weeks and 4th at 36 weeks) should be carried out.
  - **Risk approach to identify high-risk cases during pregnancy** labour or puerperium and appropriate referral to an equipped centre through an efficient referral system.
  - **Routine immunization** with tetanus toxoid and **supplementary iron folic acid (IFA)** therapy daily for at least 100 days after the first trimester

- **Intranatal care**
  - Institutional deliveries in 80% cases and 100% delivery by skilled persons
  - Three cleans (hands, perineal area) and umbilical area must be maintained
- **Postnatal care**
  - Support to restore the health of mother and care of the newborn.
  - Breast feeding—early and exclusive. Ten baby friendly hospital initiatives.
  - Family planning services to prevent unplanned pregnancy and unsafe abortion.

2. Adolescent and reproductive health

20% of the total population in India are adolescent (age group of 10–19 years), of which half are either sexually active or married.

Problems to overcome are

(i) Early mother–risk of the motherhood and her newborn.
(ii) Undernutrition and anaemia.
(iii) Psychological immaturity and vulnerability.
(iv) Consequences of unprotected sex– unwanted pregnancy, unsafe abortion, STIs and RTIs.

3. Reproductive tract infections (RTIs) and sexually transmitted infections (STIs)

RTIs are mainly due to unsafe abortion, uncleaned delivery, poor menstrual hygiene and unhygienic IUD insertion. All these are avoidable by proper preventive and curative measures at the FRU, under the RCH programme.

4. Gender issue

Gender inequality unfavourable to woman and girl child is an important hindrance to social development. This is evident in terms of food, education, medical care, access to financial resources and decision making. Gender discrimination is to be removed.

 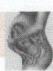

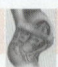

5. Others—safe abortion, child health care and universal immunization to children

Levels of RCH care

In India, RCH services are available at three levels to reach the target "Health for All". Each level provides care up to a certain limit.

1. *Primary care (Level I):* Essential health care to low risk mother and neonate (75%). Primary health centres, sub-centres and municipality hospitals provide such care.
2. *Secondary care (Level II):* is the next higher level where high-risk mother and neonate (20%) are managed. District and sub-divisional hospitals and rural hospitals with obstetric, anaesthetic and paediatric specialities provide such care.
3. *Tertiary care (Level III):* Provides highly specialized care for high-risk mother and neonate (5%). Medical College Hospital, Regional Centres and All India Institutes provide such care. These centres are equipped with highly specialized units covering all the discipline.

MATERNAL MORTALITY AND MORBIDITY AND PERINATAL MORTALITY

Maternal mortality rate

It indicates the number of maternal deaths divided by the number of women of reproductive age (15–49). It is expressed per 100,000 women of reproductive age per year. In India it is about 120 as compared to 0.5 of United States.

Definition

As per World Health Organization (WHO) and approved by International Federation of Gynaecology and Obstetrics (IFGO) 1976.

Maternal death is defined as the death of a woman while pregnant or within 42 days of termination of pregnancy, irrespective of the duration and the site of pregnancy, due to obstetric complications and diseases in pregnancy. Maternal death is subdivided into two groups:

1. *Direct obstetric death:* Those resulting from obstetric complications of pregnant state (pregnancy, labour and puerperium).
2. *Indirect obstetric deaths:* Those resulting from previous existing disease or disease that developed during pregnancy. This group is also called "Associated deaths".

Causes of maternal mortality

Predisposing causes of MM are

1. *Biological factors*
   (i) Woman's poor health
   (ii) Teenage pregnancy, elderly pregnancy at 35 years or more
   (iii) Parity risk slightly more in primigravida, 3–4 times more at grand multipara (above para 4),
   (iv) Poor birth spacing.
2. *Social factors*
   (i) Poverty
   (ii) Illiteracy
   (iii) Poor woman's status
   (iv) Religious backwardness
   (v) Evil social customs and beliefs
   (vi) Poor habitation, sanitation and unclean drinking water
   (vii) Poor roads and transports for attendance of antenatal clinic and also delay in transport of high-risk clinic and also delay in transport of high-risk pregnancy and labour " to referral centre in emergency.
   (viii) Poorer MCH services
   (ix) Unavailable MTP services
   (x) Poor community participation–ignorant community in RCH care. Predisposing factors operate more in rural and urban slums.

The precipitating causes given in the box. They are the tip of iceberg in MM while poor biological and social factors are the main iceberg.

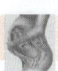

SUDDEN COLLAPSE FOLLOWING CHILDBIRTH OR ABORTION

Causes

1. *Haemorrhage:* Mainly postpartum haemorrhage. Other causes are antepartum haemorrhage, ectopic gestation, spontaneous abortion, hydatidiform mole, MTP, rupture uterus.
2. *Shock* following caesarean section, operative delivery. Septic shock in criminal abortion, puerperal sepsis.
3. *Pulmonary embolism* in thromboembolism. Liquor amnii embolism.
4. *Anaesthetic accidents:* During and following anaesthesia, aspiration of vomitus or regurgitation of stomach contents leads to chemical pneumonia (Mendelson's syndrome) cardiac arrest on operating or delivery table.
5. *Medical diseases and conditions*: Acute heart failure, renal failure in accidental haemorrhage, septic abortion, mismatched blood transfusion, hepatic coma in jaundice, diabetic coma, cerebral vascular accidents.

FACTORS INFLUENCING MATERNAL MORTALITY

- *Age and parity:* It is a well known fact that maternal mortality increases with increasing age and parity. Mortality is lowest in the second and third deliveries, and shows a significant rise after the fourth. In fact, the greater the parity after four, the greater is the mortality. This is not only due to obstetric factors but also because diseases like hypertension, diabetes, renal and vascular diseases complicate pregnancy with advancing age.

- *Socioeconomic standards* influence maternal health significantly. In the developed countries due to their high socioeconomic levels, maternal mortality has been reduced to negligible, proportions. Malnutrition, anemia, infectious diseases and other allied conditions seldom complicate a pregnancy in these countries while they are still rampant in the developing countries contributing significantly to maternal mortality.

- *Efficient antenatal and intranatal care:* Availability of such care to the vast majority, if not to all pregnant women, and highly specialized care being made available to all who require it, have contributed in significantly decreasing the mortality rates in developed countries. On the other hand, in the developing regions, efficient antenatal care is available to only a fraction of those who need it; specialized care is available to only a few.

- *Place of delivery and the presence of a skilled birth attendant:* More than 50% of pregnant mothers are not given skilled attention of any sort from medical or paramedical personnel. In India, a large proportion of deliveries take place at home. In most of the developed areas of the world, the majority of the deliveries take place in well equipped hospitals.

- *Integration between domiciliary and hospital services:* In some countries, excellent domiciliary service is provided with close integration of the domiciliary and hospital

---

Box 21.1: Causes of maternal mortality in India

A. **Direct causes**–70%
- **Eclampsia**, severe PIH– 24%
- **Haemorrhage** (**PPH**, retained placenta, APH, ectopic pregnancy etc.)–23%
- **Abortions**–10%
- **Sepsis** (puerperal, septic abortion)–7%
- **Obstructed labour**–3%
- **Operative complications** (thromboembolism, anaesthetic accidents)–3%

B. **Indirect causes**–30%
- Anaemia–11%
- Viral hepatitis–7%
- Heart disease and others–12%

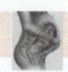

services. Such an integration results in excellent obstetric service. In the developing areas, on the other hand, hospital facilities cannot meet even a fraction of the requirements, domiciliary services are not properly organized and there is no integration between domiciliary and hospital services.

- *Availability of blood transfusion and transport services:* These are extremely important for both hospital and domiciliary services.

Needless to say, well trained doctors, nurses and midwives form the backbone of any efficient obstetric service and all these factors along with creating awareness to utilize such services influence the maternal mortality rate.

During the last three decades, significant changes have taken place in medicine. The birth of chemotherapy and antibiotics, establishment of blood transfusion services, improvements in anesthesia and surgical techniques were some of significant breakthroughs in medicine. The impact of such advances had been significant in all fields of medicine including obstetrics and this is reflected in the reduction of the maternal mortality rate.

Preventive and social measures

High maternal mortality reflects not only inadequacy of health care services for mothers, but also a low standard of living and socio-economic status of the community.

1. Early registration of pregnancy
2. At least three antenatal check-ups
3. Dietary supplementation, including correction of anaemia
4. Prevention of infection and haemorrhage during puerperium.
5. Prevention of complications, e.g., eclampsia, malpresentations, ruptured uterus.
6. Treatment of medical conditions, e.g. hypertension, diabetes, tuberculosis.
7. Anti-malaria and tetanus prophylaxis.

8. Clean delivery practice.
9. A large number of maternal deaths could be prevented with the help of trained local Dias and female health workers.
10. Institutional deliveries for women with bad obstetric history and risk factors.
11. Promotion of family planning — to control the number of children to not more than two, and spacing of births.
12. Identification of every maternal death, and searching for its cause.

MATERNAL MORBIDITY

Definition

Obstetric morbidity originates from any cause related to pregnancy or its management any time during antepartum, intrapartum and postpartum period usually up to 42 days after confinement. The parameters of maternal morbidity are:

Box. 21.2: High-risk pregnancy

1. Maternal height below 145 cm.
2. Grande Multipara with more than 4 previous viable pregnancies.
3. Pregnancy in teenage between 10–19 years or at above 35 years
4. Bad obstetric history—dead baby (stillbirth), repeated pregnancy loss, previous caesarean section and operative procedures.
5. Malpresentations and twin pregnancy, unengaged foetal head in primigravida.
6. Haemorrhage in pregnancy
7. Anaemia, diabetes, heart disease, jaundice, other medical diseases in pregnancy
8. High Blood pressure in pregnancy at and above 40/90 mm Hg—previous or present. Any convulsion.
9. Intrauterine growth restricted baby and overdated pregnancy. Pregnancy in Rh negative woman, foetal malformation.
10. Pregnancy in unwed or unplanned pregnancy seeking MTP. All the rest of pregnancy are considered low-risk pregnancies.

---

1. Fever more than 100.4°F or 38°C and continuing more than 24 hours.
2. Blood pressure more than 140/90 mm Hg.
3. Recurrent vaginal bleeding.
4. Hb% less than 10.5 gm irrespective of gestational period.
5. Asymptomatic bacteriuria of pregnancy.

Causes

1. *Maternal injuries:* (other than well healed episiotomy and caesarean section). These are badly healed episiotomy, complete perineal tear, pelvic floor injury (genital prolapse, genital fistula) cervical incompetence, low back pain due to sacroiliac joint sprain, caesarean section scar hernia, keloid, endometriosis.
2. *Maternal infection:* Urinary tract infection, puerperal infection (pelvic abscess, episiotomy and caesarean section wound infection), secondary infertility, menorrhagia, leucorrhoea, breast infection (breast abscess).
3. *Maternal ill health*
   - Anaemia due to haemorrhage.
   - Loss of weight due to prolonged breast feeding.

- Hypertensive disorder following improper care, emotional disturbances.
- Medical diseases like anemia, cardiac disease, pulmonary tuberculosis, etc. get aggravated when left uncared for.

PERINATAL MORTALITY

Perinatal mortality is defined as deaths among fetuses weighing 1000 gm or more at birth (28 weeks gestation) who die before or during delivery or within the first 7 days of delivery.

Predisposing factors of perinatal mortality

Many factors influence the perinatal survival

- *Epidemiological:* Age over 30 years, parity above 5, low socioeconomic condition, poor maternal nutritional status—all adversely affect the pregnancy outcome.
- *Medical disorders:* Anemia (Hb< 8 gm/dl), hypertensive disorders of pregnancy, diabetes mellitus, syphilis, acute fever (malaria) and infection (HIV) are often associated. Perinatal deaths increase due to hypoxia, intrauterine growth restriction, prematurity and infection.
- *Obstetric complications*
  - Antepartum haemorrhage particularly abruption placenta is responsible for about 10 percent of perinatal deaths due to severe hypoxia.
  - *Pre-eclampsia:* Eclampsia is associated with high perinatal loss either due to placental insufficiency or prematurity—spontaneous or induced.
  - *Cervical incompetence:* Premature effacement and dilatation of cervix between 24 and 36 weeks is responsible for significant perinatal deaths from prematurity.
- *Fetoplacental factors*
  - Multiple pregnancy most often leads to pre term delivery and usual complications
  - Congenital malformation is responsible for 8–10 perinatal deaths

- Intrauterine growth restriction and low birth weight babies
- Preterm labour and preterm rupture of the membranes are the known leading causes of prematurity.

Prevention

As every mother has the right to conclude her pregnancy safely so also has the baby got a right to be born alive safe and healthy.

The following measures are helpful in reducing the perinatal mortality

- Prepregnancy health care and counseling
- Genetic counseling in high risk cases and prenatal diagnosis to detect genetic, chromosomal or structural abnormalities are essential. Termination of an affected fetus is a positive step in reduction of deaths due to congenital malformations.
- Regular antenatal care, with advice regarding health, diet and rest.
- Detection and correction of anemia an prevention of pre-eclampsia, eclampsia. Immunisation against tetanus should be dine as a routine.
- Screening of high-risk patients those of poor socioeconomic status of high parity, extremes of age, and twins, etc. and their mandatory hospital delivery. Risk approach to RCH care essential.
- Careful monitoring in labour and avoidance of traumatic vaginal delivery.
- Skilled birth attendant—to minimize sepsis, at least three cleans are to be

maintained—clean hands, clean surface where delivery takes place and to cut the cord clean.

- Provision of referral neonatal service specially to look after the preterm babies.
- Health care education of the mother about the care of the newborn. Early and exclusive breastfeeding, prevention of hypothermia.
- Educating the community to utilize family planning services and also to utilize the available maternity and child health care services. Family planning services can prevent unwanted pregnancies.
- Autopsy studies of all perinatal deaths.
- Continued study of perinatal mortality problems.
- Perinatal morbidity: It implies major illness of the neonate from birth to first four weeks of life. Important causes of morbidity are due to:
  - Prematurity and growth restriction
  - Birth asphyxia and birth trauma
  - Congenital malformations

INFERTILITY AND ASSISTED REPRODUCTIVE TECHNOLOGY

Infertility or inability to conceive a child or sustain a pregnancy to childbirth affects as many as 10 to 15% of couples who desire children. One of the national health goals identified by the healthy people 2010 directly addresses the problems of infertility. "Reduce the portion of married couples whose ability to conceive or maintain a pregnancy is impaired from a baseline of 13% to a target of 13% nurses play key roles in educating the couple about the variety of tests and procedures that may be performed. They are important members of fertility health care teams often assuming responsibility for health assessment, client education and counseling.

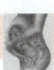

Definition

Infertility is strictly defined as the inability to conceive after one year of unprotected regular sexual intercourse. The definition is commonly extended to include those couples who conceive but repeatedly lose a pregnancy before the fetus is old enough to survive.

Types of infertility

1. Primary infertility–there have been no previous conceptions.
2. Secondary infertility–there has been a previous viable pregnancy but the couples is unable to conceive at present.

Incidence of infertility

About 13% to 20% couples in United States are infertile. In about 40% of couples with infertility cause is multifactor. In about 30% of couples, it is man who is unfertile 20–30% of couple experience ovulatory failure, 20–40% experience tubal, vaginal or uterine problems as cause of their infertility.

Factors contributing to infertility

- Disturbance is spermatogenesis (production of sperm cells).
- Obstruction in seminiferous tubules, duezor vessels preventing movement of spermatozoa.
- Qualitative and quantitative changes in the seminal fluid preventing sperm motility.
- Development of autoimmunity that mobilizes sperm.
- Problems in ejaculation or deposition preventing spermatozoa from being placed close enough to the woman's cervix to allow ready perpetration and fertilization.

1. Problems with the sperm

Many factors may impair the number, structure or function of sperm. Some conditions are temporary such as acute illness other conditions are permanent such as genetic disorder. Evaluation of semen may reveal that the man has azoospermia or oligospermia. The average number of sperm released at ejaculation is 400 million. Twenty million sperm per milliliter of semen is considered to be the minimum number adequate for fertilization.

Many factors can impair the number and function such as

- Acute or chronic illness.
- Infections of the genital tract.
- Anatomical abnormalities such as varicocele or obstruction of the ducts that carry sperm to penis.
- Expose to toxins such as lead, pesticides or other chemicals.
- Therapeutic treatments such as antineoplastic drugs or radiation for cancer.
- Excessive alcohol intake.
- Use of illicit drugs such as marijuana or cocaine.
- An elevated scrotal temperature resulting from febrile illness or repeated use saunas or hot tubs, varicosity.
- Immunological factors produced by the man against his own sperm (autoantibodies) or by the women causing the sperm to clump or to be unable to penetrate the ovum.
- Congenital abnormality such as cryptachidism (undecended testis).

2. Abnormalities of seminal fluid

The seminal fluid nourishes, protects and caries sperm into the vagina until they enter cervix. The specific abnormality found in the seminal fluid suggests the cause of the abnormality, such as obstruction or infection in a specific area of genital tract. Seminal fluid that the abnormal in amount, consistency or chemical composition suggest obstruction inflammation or infection. The presence of large number of leukocytes suggests infection.

3. Abnormal ejaculation

- Abnormal ejaculation prevents deposition of the sperm in the ideal place to achieve

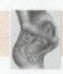

pregnancy. Retrograde ejaculation is the release of semen backward into bladder, rather than forward through the tip of penis.

- Conditions that cause retrograde ejaculation are diabetes, neurological disorder, and anti-hypertensive psychotropics.
- Men who suffer spinal cord injury may retain the ability to ejaculate depending on the level of cord damage.
- Excessive alcohol intake or use of illicit drugs affect ejaculation.
- Erectile dysfunction.

Factors in the women

A women's fertility depends on
- Regular production of normal ova.
- An open receptive path from her cervix to the fallopian tube to promote fertilization and movement of embryo into uterus for implantation.
- An endometrium that supports the pregnancy after conception.

1. Anovulation: (absence of ovulation)

The most common cause of infertility in women, it occurs from a genetic abnormality such as Turner's syndrome. In which there are no ovaries to produce ova.

- Ovarian tumors may produce anovulation due to feedback stimulation on the pituitary.
- Chronic or excessive exposure to X-rays or radioactive substances, general ill health, poor diet or stress may all contribute to poor ovarian function.
- Decreased body weight or body fat ratio of less than 10% as in female athletics or in women such are excessive lean or anorexia can reduce pituitary hormones such as FSH and LH and half ovulation.
- A recent study has shown that ova released from right ovary may favour fertilization more that left sided ones.

2. Abnormalities of the fallopian tube

At least one patent tube is needed for conception and implantation to occur. Tubal obstruction commonly occurs because of scarring and adhesions following reproductive tract infection.

- STD is responsible for infertility.
- Endometriosis may cause tubal adhesions, painful menstrual periods and painful intercourse; large lesions may significantly distort tubal anatomy and lead to infertility.
- Tubal obstruction after pelvic surgery, ruptured appendix, or peritonitis or some ovarian cysts.
- Congenital abnormalities in fallopian tube obstruct the normal function.
- Poor movement of the fabricated end of the tube may prevent pick up of the ovum from the ovarian surface after ovulation .
- Complete blockage prevents fertilization.

3. Abnormalities of the cervix

- Polyps or scaring from post surgical procedures such as cauterization or conization may obstruct woman's cervix.
- Cervical damage secondary to infection or other factors prevents normal movement of the sperm into the uterus and fallopian tubes for fertilization.

Repeated pregnancy loss

1. *Abnormalities of the fetal chromosomes:* Errors in fetal chromosomes may result in spontaneous abortion usually in the first trimester. Chromosomal abnormalities often severely disrupts growth and development during prenatal life and embryo or fetus cannot survive to live birth.

2. *Abnormalities of the cervix or uterus*
   - Stenosis or congenital malformations of cervix or uterine cavity causes repeated loss of normal fetus.
   - Women who were prenatally exposed to diethyl stilbestrol are more likely to have uterine myomas and adhesions

inside the uterine cavity may cause repeated fetal losses. These problems alter blood supply to the developing fetus or may cause uterine irritability that results in preterm labour and birth.

3. *Endocrine abnormalities*

- Inadequate progesterone secretion by the corpus luteum prevents normal implantation and establishment of placenta. The embryo may not implant or it may implant poorly . In other cases corpus luteum may develop and function properly but the woman's endometrium may not respond to its progesterone recreation.
- Hypothyroidism and hyperthyroidism may be associated with inability to conceive and with recurrent pregnancy loss.
- Poorly controlled diabetes can result in repeated pregnancy loss.

4. *Immunological factors*

- Women with autoimmune diseases such as lupus erythematous are more likely to experience spontaneous abortion:
- The embryo has antigens different from those of mother and would ordinarily be rejected as any other foreign tissue would be rejected.

5. *Environmental agents*

- Radiation exposure in the form of chest X-ray.
- Alcohol, cigarette smoke
- Anesthetic gas
- Chemicals such as solvents or pesticides, lead and mercury in occupational settings.

These agents may be directly toxic to the embryo or fetus causing the death or may interfere with normal placental function that is necessary to sustain pregnancy.

6. *Infections*: Infections of the reproductive tract are associated with poor pregnancy

outcomes in general they be related to early pregnancy losses as well.

DIAGNOSTIC EVALUATION OF INFERTILITY

History

Nurses often assume the responsibility for initial history taking with the infertile couple. A minimum history for the man should include:

- General health
- Nutrition
- Use of alcohol, drug, tobacco
- Congenital health problems such as hypospadias or cryptorchidism.
- Illness such as mumps orchitis, urinary tract infection or sexually transmitted diseases.
- Operations such as surgical repair of a hernia, which could have resulted in a blood compromise to the testes.
- Current illness, particularly endocrine illness or low-grade infections.
- Past and current occupation and work habits (e.g., does his job involve sitting at a desk all day or exposure to X-rays or other forms of radiation?)

It is important to document sexual practices such as the frequency of coitus and masturbation, failure to achieve ejaculation, premature ejaculation, coital positions used, use of lubricants and past contraceptive measures, and existence of any children produced from a previous relationship.

History for woman

- Current or past reproductive tract problems, such as infections
- Endocrine problems such as galactorrhea or symptoms of thyroid dysfunction; and any abdominal or pelvic operations
- Frequency of using douches or intravaginal medication or sprays (these may interfere with vaginal pH)
- Exposure to occupational hazards such as X-rays or toxic substances; and nutrition especially folic acid intake.

 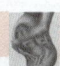

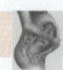
Also obtain information from the woman about whether she can detect ovulation. Pay particular attention to the typical symptoms, such as breast tenderness and midcycle "wetness" that indicate ovulation.

To determine the woman's general state of health, laboratory tests a Pap smear, rubella titer and HIV evaluation may be done. Serum or urine hormone levels and a serologic test for syphilis may be necessary. If the client has symptoms of thyroid dysfunction, a thyroid uptake determination and thyroid dysfunction, a thyroid uptake determination and thyroid stimulating hormone levels may be ordered. If the woman has a history of menstrual irregularities, blood will be assayed for FSH, estrogen, LH and progesterone levels. If the client has galactorrhea, a serum prolactin level will be obtained. A pelvic sonogram may be performed to rule out ovarian, tubal, or uterine structural disorders.

Semen analysis

For a semen analysis, after 2 to 4 days of sexual abstinence, the man ejaculates by masturbation into a clean, dry specimen jar, and the spermatozoa are examined under a microscope within 1 hour. The numbers of spermatozoa in the specimen are counted, and their appearance and motility are noted. An average ejaculation should produce 2.5 go 5.0 ml of semen and should contain a minimum of 20 million spermatozoa per milliliter of fluid. The analysis may need to be repeated in 2 to 3 more moths because spermatogenesis is an ongoing process, requiring 30 to 90 days for new sperm to reach maturity.

Sperm penetration assay and antisperm antibody testing

One reason for poor sperm mobility may be the presence of antisperm antibodies, which tend to cause agglutination to sperm. These sperms, when deposited, are agglutinated in vagina and cannot travel to the fallopian tubes for fertilization of the ovum.

Sperm penetration studies are laboratory tests to determine whether sperm, once they reach the ova, can penetrate the ova. Using an artificial reproductive technique such as *in vitro* fertilization, poorly mobile sperm or those with poor penetration can be injected into the woman's ovum under laboratory conditions bypassing the need for sperm to be fully mobile.

In addition to the above, a menstrual history should be obtained including:
- Age of menarche
- Length, regularity, and frequency of menstrual periods.
- Amount of flow
- Any difficulties experienced, such as dysmenorrhea or premenstrual dysphonic disorder.
- History of contraceptive use
- History of any previous pregnancies or abortions.

After a thorough history, both men and women need a complete physical examination. Inspect, in particular, for secondary sexual characteristics and genital abnormalities, such as the absence of a vas deferens or the presence of undescended tests or a varicocele. The presence of a hydrocele is rarely associated with infertility but should be documented if present.

For the woman, a through physical assessment including breast and thyroid examination is necessary to rule out current illness. Of particular importance are secondary sex characteristics, which indicate maturity and good pituitary function. A complete pelvic examination is needed to rule out anatomic defects and infection.

Fertility testing

Typically, laboratory testing for men includes a semen analysis, urinalysis, and some blood tests and other testing such as a complete blood count; blood typing, including Rh factor; a serologic test for syphilis, sedimentation rate protein—bound iodine cholesterol level and

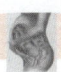

gonadotropin, prolactin and testosterone levels may be obtained. Testing for the presence of human immunodeficiency virus (HIV) infections is also crucial.

Women ovulation determination by basal body temperature

One of the first tests ordered for women is the recording of basal body temperatures, a simple test for ovulation. It documents the slight temperature increase that normally occurs with the release of progesterone following ovulation. If, not, a luteal phase defect is suggested.

Ovulation determination by test strip

Various brands of commercial kits are available for assessing the upsurge of LH that occurs just before ovulation. These can be used in place of obtaining BBT. The woman dips a test strip into a midmorning urine specimen and then compares it with the kit instruction for a color change. Such kits are purchased over the counter, are easy to use, and have the advantage of marking the point just before ovulation occurs rather than after ovulation, as is the case with BBT. They are not as economical as simple temperature recording but are advantages for women with irregular work or daily schedules.

Ovulation determination by cervical mucus assessment

At the height of estrogen stimulation, cervical mucus is copious and thin and has a low viscosity and cellularity. It "ferns" or forms a distinct pattern when allowed to dry. This easy test of hormonal influences.

Fern test

When high levels of estrogen are present in the body, as they are just before ovulation, the cervical mucus forms fernlike patterns when it is placed on a glass slide and allowed to dry. Women who do not ovulate continue to show the fern pattern throughout the menstrual cycle (progesterone levels never become dominant),

or they never demonstrate it because their estrogen levels never rise.

Spinnbarkeit test

At the height of estrogen secretion, the cervical mucus not only becomes thin and watery, but it also can be stretched into long strands. This stretch ability is in contrast to its thick, viscous state when progesterone is the dominant hormone. Performing this test, known as spinbarkeit, at the midpoint of a menstrual cycle is another way to demonstrate that high levels of estrogen are being produced and, by implication that ovulation is about to water, or it can be tested in an examining room by smearing a cervical mucus specimen on a side and stretching the mucus between the slide and cove slip.

Postcoital test

A postcoital test combines both ovulation detection and semen analysis. The couple has coitus at this time, and then the woman reports to the health care facility within 2 to 8 hours. With the woman in a lithotomy position, a specimen of cervical mucus is removed and examined microscopically for ferning, Spinnbarkeit, cell count and viable spermatozoa. The postcoital test shows the presence of sperm and how that interact with the woman's vaginal and cervical environment.

A good result shows abundant, elastic mucus with a high number of motile sperm. If sperm are found to be clumped and immobile or if the mucus is very thick, this may indicate a problem with timing or possibly point to a sperm antibody problem. A finding of no sperm could indicate azoospermia. If white blood cells are preset in the cervical mucus, an endocervical or endometrial infection is suggested, requiring treatment with an appropriate antibiotic.

Ultrasonography and X-ray imaging

Ultrasound and X-ray imaging can be used to determine the patency of fallopian tubes and assess the depth and consistency of the endometrial lining.

Sonohysterography I

It is an ultrasound technique designed for inspecting the uterus. The uterus is filled with sterile saline introduced through a narrow catheter inserted into the uterine cervix. A transvaginal ultrasound transducer is then inserted into the vagina to inspect the uterus for abnormalities such as septal deviation or the presence of a myoma. Because, this is a minimally invasive technique, it can be done any time during the menstrual cycle.

Hysterosalpinography

It (uterosalpinography) is a radiologic examination of the fallopian tubes using a radioopaque medium. It is done immediately after the menstrual flow to avoid reflux of menstrual debris up the tubes and unintentional irradiation of a growing zygote.

Surgical evaluation

If the above assessments do not reveal the cause of infertility, a number of surgical procedures may be scheduled.

Uterine endometrial biopsy

Uterine Endometrial Biopsy may be used as a test for ovulation or to reveal an endometrial problem such as a luteal phase defect. The biopsy is usually done 2 or 3 days before the expected menstrual flow. After a paracervical block, a thin probe and biopsy forceps are introduced through the cervix. This procedure is contraindicated if pregnancy is suspected. And, also, if an infection such as acute PID or cervicitis is present. She should be instructed to call her primary case provider if she develops a temperature of more than 101°F, has a large amount of bleeding, or passes clots.

Hysteroscopy

Hysteroscopy is visual inspection of the uterus through the insertion of a hysteroscope, a thin hollow tube, through the cervix. This is helpful if uterine adhesions or other abnormalities were discovered on the hysterosalpingogram.

Laparoscopy

Laparoscopy is the introduction of a thin, hollow, lighted tube through a small incision in the abdomen just under the umbilicus to examine the position and state of the fallopian tubes and ovaries. Typically, it is rarely done except when uterosalpingography is abnormal.

MANAGEMENT OF INFERTILITY

Management of infertility focuses on correction of the underlying problems.

Correction of the underlying problem

The overall management of infertility involves treating such underlying causes as chronic disease, inadequate hormone production, endometriosis, or infection: If correcting these problems does not yield success, infertility management focuses on achieving conception through assisted reproductive techniques such as *in vitro* fertilization or sperm donation.

Increasing sperm count and motility

If spermatozoa are present but the total count is low, a man might be advised to abstain from coitus for 7 to 10 days to increase the count. Ligation of a varicocele and advising changes in lifestyle, such as wearing looser clothing, avoiding long periods of sitting, and avoiding prolonged hot baths, may be helpful to reduce scrotal heat and increase the sperm count.

Administration of clomiphene citrate, an estrogen antagonist, may successfully increase an in adequate sperm count. If spermatozoa appear to be immobilized by vaginal secretions due to an immunologic factor, the response can be reduced by abstinence or condom use for about 6 months. However, to avoid this prolonged time interval, washing of the spermatozoa and intrauterine insemination may be preferred.

Reducing the presence of infection

If a vaginal infection is present, the infection will be treated according to the causative organism based on culture reports. Women who are prescribe metronidazole for a trichomonal infection should be cautioned that it may be teratogenic early in pregnancy and so should not be continued if a pregnancy is suspected.

Hormone therapy

If the problem appears to be disturbance of ovulation, hormone therapy with clomiphene citrate is the treatment of choice to stimulate ovulation. In other women, ovarian follicular growth can be stimulated by the administration of human menopausal gonadotropin (HCG) to product ovulation. Human menopausal gonadotropins are combination of FSH and LH. If increased prolactin levels are identified, bromocriptine is added to the medication regimen to reduce prolactin levels and allow for the rise of gonadotropins.

Administration of either clomiphene citrate or human menopausal gonadotropins may over stimulate an ovary causing multiple ova to come to maturity and possibly resulting in multiple births.

Surgery

If a myoma is interfering with fertility, a myomectomy, or removal of the tumor by surgery, may be necessary. Myomectomy may be done by a hysteroscopic ambulatory procedure if the growth is small. Uterine adhesions may also be lysed by hysteroscopy. After this procedure, and IUD may be inserted foe 3 months to prevent the uterine sides from touching and estrogen is administered to prevent adhesions from reforming.

For problems of abnormal uterine formation, such as a septate uterus, surgery is also available. These defects, however, are generally related to early pregnancy loss, not infertility. If the problem is tubal insufficiency from

inflammation, diathermy or steroid administration may be helpful in reducing adhesions.

Assisted reproductive techniques

If ovulation, sperm production, or sperm mobility problems cannot be corrected, assisted reproductive strategies are available.

Artificial insemination

Artificial insemination is the installation of sperm into the female reproductive tract to aid conception. The sperm can be instilled into the cervix or into the uterus. Either the husband's sperm or donor sperm can be used. These techniques may be used.

- Inadequate sperm count.
- The woman has a vaginal or cervical factor interfering with sperm motility.
- Man has a known genetic disorder he does not want transmitted to offspring or the woman has no male partner.
- It is useful for men who underwent a vasectomy now wish to have children.
- Today, sperm can be cryopreserved in a sperm bank before radiation or chemotherapy, and then used for insemination afterwards.

One disadvantage of using frozen sperm is that it tends to have slower motility than unfrozen specimens. An advantage of cryopreserved sperm is that it can be used even after years of storage. On the day after ovulation, the seminal fluid is delivered to the cervix using a device similar to a cervical cap or diaphragm or injected directly into the uterus using a flexible catheter.

If therapeutic donor insemination is selected, the donors are usually volunteers who have no history of disease and no family history of possible inheritable disorders. The blood type or at least the Rh factor, can be matched with the woman's to prevent Rh incompatibility. If, a woman desires frozen sperm from sperm banks can be selected according to desires. Frozen sperm from sperm banks can be selected

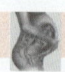

according to desired physical or mental characteristics.

With artificial insemination, especially therapeutic donor insemination, legal issues must be considered. Some states have specific laws regarding inheritance, child support, and responsibility concerning children conceived by this method.

In vitro fertilization and embryo transfer

In vitro fertilization refers to removing one or more mature oocytes from a woman's ovary by laparoscopy and then fertilizing them by exposing them sperm under laboratory conditions outside the woman's body. Embryo transfer (ET, also called ova transfer) refers to the insertion of the laboratory-grown fertilized ovum into the woman's uterus approximately 40 hours after fertilization, where ideally one or more of them will implant and grow.

Indications

- IVF-ET is most often used for
- Woman has blocked or damaged fallopian tubes.
- Man has oligospermia or a low sperm count, absence of cervical mucus prevents sperm from traveling to or entering the cervix, or antisperm antibodies cause immobilization of sperm.
- In addition, couples with unexplained infertility of long duration may be helped by IVF-ET.

Before the procedure, the woman is given an ovulation agent such clomiphene citrate or human menopausal gonadopin. Beginning about the 10th day of the menstrual cycle, the ovaries are examined daily by sonography to assess the number and size of developing ovarian follicles. When a follicle appears to be a mature, the woman is given an injection of HCG hormone. Causing ovulation in 28–42 hours.

A needle is then introduced intravaginally, guided by ultrasound, and the oocyte is aspirated through a sterile tube from its follicle. Often many oocyts ripen at once, and perhaps as many as 3–12 can be removed. The oocytes are incubated for at least 8 hours to ensure viability. In the meantime, the husband or donor supplies a fresh semen specimen. The sperm cells and oocytes are mixed and allowed to incubate in a growth medium.

When fertilization of the chosen oocytes occurs, the zygotes formed almost immediately begin to divide and grow. By 40 hours after fertilization they will have undergone their first cell division. The fertilized eggs are examined and, if normal, a chosen number are transferred back to the uterine cavity through the cervix using a thin catheter.

However, the overall pregnancy rate by IVF-ET is as low as 20% to 30% per treatment cycle. Once a pregnancy has been successfully implanted, the woman's prenatal care is the same as that for any pregnancy.

Gamete intrafallopian transfer (GIFT)

In gamete intrafallopian transfer procedures; ova are obtained from ovaries exactly as in IVF-ET. Instead of waiting for fertilization to occur in the laboratory, however, both ova and sperm are instilled with a matter of hours using a laparoscopic technique into the open end of a patient fallopian tube. Some centers are opting to perform this procedure using ultrasound to guide the collection and instillation of ova and sperm rather than using laparoscopic surgery. Fertilization then occurs in the tube, and the zygote moves to the uterus for implantation. This procedure has a pregnancy rate slightly higher than that of IVF-ET. The procedure is contraindicated if the woman's fallopian tubes are blocked because this could lead of ectopic pregnancy.

Zygote intrafallopian transfer (ZIFT)

Zygote intrafallopian transfer involves oocyte retrieval by transvaginal, ultrasound-guided aspiration, followed by culture and insemi-

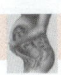

nation of the oocytes in the laboratory. Within 24 hours the fertilized eggs are transferred by laparoscopic technique into the end of a waiting fallopian tube. ZIFT differs from GIFT in that fertilization takes place outside the body, allowing health care providers to be certain that impregnation has occurred before the growth structure is reintroduced. As in GIFT, a woman must have one functioning fallopian tube for the technique to be successful because the zygotes are implanted into the fimbriated end of a tube rather than into the uterus.

Intracytoplasmic sperm injection (ICSI)

One single spermatozoon or even a spermatid is injected directly into the cytoplasm of an oocyte by micro puncture of zona pellucida. Micro pipette is used to hold the oocyte while spermatozoon is deposited inside the ooplasm.

Indications

- Azoospermia
- Severe oligospermia
- Anti sperm antibody
- Obstruction of efferent ductus system
- Failure of fertilization in IVF
- Unexplained infertility

Surrogate embryo transfer

Surrogate embryo transfer is an assisted reproductive technique for the woman who does not ovulate. The process involves an oocyte donated by a friend or provided by an anonymous oocyte donor. At the time of ovulation, the donor's ovum is removed by a transvaginal ultrasound guided procedure. The oocyte is then fertilized by the recipient woman's male partner's sperm and placed in the recipient woman's uterus by ET or GIFT. Once pregnancy occurs, it will progress the same as an unassisted pregnancy.

Intravaginal culture

Intravaginal culture is another reproductive technique that uses the woman's own body as an incubator-live device. Ova are obtained from the woman and placed with the sperm in a sterile, hermetically sealed container of culture medium. This container is then placed inside the woman's vagina, being held there by a diaphragm. As a result, the ova and sperm are maintained at normal body temperatures. After approximately 48 hours, the container is opened and any fertilized dividing eggs are transferred to the uterus.

ALTERNATIVES TO CHILDBIRTH

For some couples, even treatment for infertility with procedures such as IVF-ET will not be successful. These couples need to consider sill other options.

Surrogate mothers

A surrogate mother is a woman who agrees to carry a pregnancy to term for infertile couples. The surrogate may provide the ova and be impregnated by the man's sperm. In other instances, the infertile couple may donate the ova and sperm both, or donor ova and sperm may be used. Surrogate mothers are often friends or family members who assume the role out of friendship or compassion, or they can be referred to the couple through an agency or attorney and receive monetary reimbursement for their service. The infertile couple can enjoy the pregnancy as they watch it progress in the surrogate.

A number of ethical and legal problems can arise with surrogate motherhood if the surrogate mother decides at the end of pregnancy that she has formed an attachment to the fetus and wants to keep the baby despite the pre-pregnancy agreement she signed. Another potential problem occurs if the child is born imperfect and the infertile couple then no longer wants the child.

Adoption

Adoptions, once a ready alternative for infertile couples is still a viable alternative, although there are fewer children available for adoption today from official agencies than formerly. Often, it takes longer to find a child for adoption than it once did unless the couple considers foreign-born or physically or cognitively challenged children.

Childfree living

Childfree living is an alternative lifestyle available to both fertile and infertile couples. For many infertile couples who have been through the rigors and frustrations of infertility testing and unsuccessful treatment regimens, childfree living may emerge as the option they finally wish to pursue.

Nursing management

- *Nursing diagnosis:* Situational low self–esteem disturbance related to inability to conceive.
- *Outcome identification:* Client will express positive feelings about herself.
- *Outcome evaluation:* Client verbalizes feelings about possible infertility and effect on self-esteem; participates activity in care and treatment decisions; states she has some control over situation and required treatment.

Interventions

1. Attempt to identify the meaning of fertility to the client.
2. Encourage client to express feelings and thoughts about self, fertility and infertility.
3. Review and reinforce with client positive attributes about self.
4. Clarify any misconceptions client may have about fertility and infertility.
5. Assist with measures to increase independent role functioning and encourage active participation in decision-making.
6. Discuss possible support persons and groups; include spouse appropriate.

- *Nursing diagnosis:* Deficient knowledge related to reproductive functions and infertility.

- *Outcome identification:* Client will express accurate information about reproductive functioning and infertility.
- *Outcome evaluation:* Client verbalizes information about reproductive structures and normal function, fertilization, and conception; discusses possible factors associated with infertility; exhibits understanding of measures involved with evaluation of and treatment for infertility.

Interventions

1. Assess client's current knowledge level about reproductive functioning and infertility.
2. Review structure and function of male and female reproductive systems, including fertile periods, fertilization, and conception; clarify and misconceptions.
3. Discuss possible factors associated with fertility and infertility; include spouse in discussion as appropriate.
4. Instruct the client and spouse about recommended tests and possible long-term treatment.
5. Provide ample time for questions and concerns.

Conclusion

Infertility is said to exist when a pregnancy has not occurred after one year of unprotected coitus. Sterility refers to the inability to conceive because of a known condition. About 10 to 15% of couple today experience infertility. The incidence increases with the age of the couple. Artificial insemination, donor egg transfer, *in vitro* fertilization, adoption, surrogate mother, and child free living are all possible solutions for infertility.

LEGAL ASPECTS IN OBSTETRICS

Today nursing profession has set standards to as a professional nurse independently. The main aim of nursing is to provide "Quality Care",

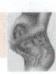

which demands the nurse to co-ordinate and collaborate within nursing profession as well as with others agencies. This challenges the professional nurse to view nursing as health-oriented system of care, and not as disease-oriented system of care. To achieve the goal of health for all by 2000 AD, the nurse should adapt to the changing health needs of the society and modify the care accordingly.

Whenever people live together, there is a tendency to develop certain rules of conduct to settle disputes among themselves, to organize government and state effort, to raise morals of the people and to build human character. The main objective is to discipline and control those activities which are likely to cause legal complications.

Law

Law is a set of rules enforced by the government from time to time through its courts, police and similar agencies. In short, it is a rule of conduct laid down by the controlling authority to be practiced by the members of the society and is enforced by certain means.

The legal foundations for the practice of nursing provides safeguards for health care and sets standards by which nurse's are evaluated. Nurses need to understand how the law applies specifically to them. When the nurse's do not meet the standards expected, they are at risk for being involved in legal action.

CURRENT LEGAL CONTROVERSIES IN OBSTETRICAL NURSING

The fetal right to fetal amendment

The nurse in the perinatal practice should be familiar with the regulations regarding abortion in her state, e.g. the medical termination of pregnancy act 1971. The five conditions being identified in this act are:

- *Medical:* Where continuation of pregnancy might endanger the mother's life or cause grave injury to her physical or mental health.

- *Eugenic:* Risk of the child being born with serious handicaps due to physical or mental abnormalities.
- *Humanitarian:* Where pregnancy is the result of rape.
- Socioeconomic
- Failure of contraceptive devices

The written consent is essential before MTP. The act provides safeguard to the mother by authorizing only a registered medical practitioner having experience in gynaecology and obstetrics. Abortion services are provided in Government hospitals in strict confidence.

THE CENTRAL BIRTHS AND DEATH REGISTRATION ACT, 1969

In an effort to improve the civil registration system, the government of India, promulgated the central birth and death registration act 1969. The act came into force on 1 April 1970. The time limit for registering the events of birth is 14 days and that of deaths is 7 days. In case of default a fine up to Rs.50/- can be imposed. The act makes the beginning of a new era in the history of vital statistics registration in India.

Safeguards for health care

Three categories of safeguards determine how the law views nursing practice.
1. Nurse practice acts
2. Standards of care set by professional organization
3. Rules and policies set by the institution employing the nurse.

NURSE PRACTICE ACTS

Every state has a nurse practice act that determines the scope of practice act that determines the scope of practice of registered nurses in that state nurse practice defines "what the nurse is and is not allowed to do in caring for clients." Some parts of the law may be very specific others are stated broadly enough to allow interpretation of the law that permits

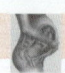

flexibility in the role of the nurse. Nurse practice act vary from one state to another and nurses must be knowledgeable about these laws wherever they practice.

In India the existing legislative regulation of nursing and nurses associations comprised mainly of the Indian Nursing Council Act 1947 as amended by ACT LXXV of 1950 and by ACT NO. XLV of 1957 (Daniel Latifi, 1997).

Laws relating to nursing practice also delineate methods, called standardized procedures by which nurses may assume certain duties commonly considered part of medical practice.

STANDARD OF CARE

Although courts do not have the force of laws, they have generally held that nurses practice according to established standards and hospital policies. Standards of care are set by professional association and describe the level of care that can be expected from practitioners.

Example

Maternity nurses are held to the standards published by the association of women's health obstetrics and neonatal nurses. Since it is widely respected organization for nurses in this field, formerly known as the organization for obstetrics and gynecologic and neonatal nurses.

AGENCY POLICIES

Each of the health care agency sets specific policies applying to nurses working for the agency, others applying only to those working on certain units or with certain types of clients.

Example: Policies for nurses working in labour and delivery units differ from those for nurses in the neonatal intensive care unit. All nurses should be familiar with the policies of agencies in which they work. Nurses are frequently involved in writing policies and changing them when necessary.

Legal issues

1. *Torts and crimes:* A tort is a legal wrong committed by one person against another person or the property of another. The injured party may sue for the damage and if the suit is successful, he is usually paid compensation.

2. *Negligence and malpractice:* Negligence is defined as the failure to exercise that degree of skill, care exercised by professional nurses in the light of the present state of nursing sciences in comparable situations. It usually means failure by the nurse to take the appropriate action to protect the safety of the patient. The common acts of negligence are:
   - Overlooked sponges, instruments, needles and the like inside the surgical wound, e.g. LSCS
   - Burns by hot water bottles, enema
   - Falls due to slippery floors
   - Injury to dependent patients by falls, e.g. leaving a baby alone on the table, improper handling of the newborns
   - Injury due to defective apparatus
   - Injury to patients as a result of wrong medication, wrong dosage, wrong patient and wrong concentration.
   - Injury due to administration of injection, e.g. abscess
   - Injury due to administration of blood
   - Injury due to hospital infections.
   - Failure to report to superior if any accidents occur.

Prevention of malpractice

Malpractice claims have been escalated in recent years. As a result of awards from such claims malpractice insurance has risen from all health care workers practice defensively accumulating evidence that they are acting in the clients best interest. Physicians may order for more diagnostic test and nurses are careful to include detailed data when they chart. This is especially true in maternity care, since this is the area in which most suits occur.

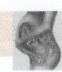

Health care agency and individual nurses have reason to try to prevent malpractice claims. Hospitals have paid for lawsuits claiming malpractice. Although nurses are not often used, there has been increase in the number of nurses named in lawsuits. Prevention of claims is sometimes referred to as risk management or quality assurance. Nurses can help prevent malpractice claims by following guidelines for informed consent, refusal of care and documentation and by maintaining their level of expertise.

1. *Informed consent:* Informed consent is an ethical concept that has enacted into law. Clients have the right to decide wisely, clients needful information about the treatment offered.

2. *Competence:* Certain requirement must be met before consent can be considered "informed". The first is that the client must be competent, or able to think through a situation and make rational decisions. A client who is comatose or severely mentally retarded or who is a newborn is incapable of making decisions. A client who has been medicated with drugs that interfere with the ability to think is temporarily in competent. In these cases, another person would be appointed to make decisions for the client.

3. *Full disclosure:* The second requirement is that of full disclosure of information, including what the treatment entails the expected results. The risks 'side effects and benefits' as well as other treatment options must also be informed as to what would happen if no treatment were chosen.

4. *Understanding of information:* The client must comprehend information about proposed treatment. Health professionals must explain the facts in terms the person can understand. If client does not speak English an entrepreneur may be necessary. Nurses may find that a client does not fully understand a treatment or has questions about it. The nurse must be a client advocate in such cases. If it is a minor point, the nurse may be able to clarify otherwise, the nurse must inform the physician so that the clients misconceptions can be clarified.

5. *Voluntary consent:* Clients must be allowed to make choices voluntarily without undue influence or coercion from others. Although others can give information the client alone makes the decision. Clients should not feel pressured to choose in a certain way or that their future care is dependent on the their decision.

6. *Refusal of care:* Sometimes clients decline treatment offered by the health care workers. This may be more serious, such as declining to take needed medication or to have surgery. Clients refuse treatment when they believe that the benefits of treatment or the life they will have after that treatment. Clients do have this right and they can withdraw agreement to treatment at any time. When this occur a number of steps should be taken. Some of them involve the physician.

First, it should be established by the physician or nurse that the client understands the treatment and the results of refusal. The physician if unaware of the clients decision, should be notified by the nurse. The nurse documents the refusal explanations given by the client and the notification of the physician on the chart. If the treatment is considered vital to the clients well being, the physician discusses the need with the client and documents the results. Opinions by other physicians may be offered to the client as well.

Client may be asked to sign a form indicating that they understand the possible results of rejecting treatment. This is to prevent a later lawsuit in which the client claims lack of knowledge of the possible, results in decision.

Example: When a woman refuses for the cesarean birth is likely to cause grave harm to the fetus and the mother.

Coercion is illegal (as well as unethical) in obtaining consent. Even though the nurse may strongly believe that the client should receive the treatment, the clients should not feel forced to submit to unwanted procedures. Nurse must be sure that personal feeling do not adversely affect the care they give. Clients have the right to good nursing care regardless of their decision to accept or reject treatment.

Documentation: It is the best evidence that a standard of care. This has been maintained. All the information records about the client should reflect the standard of care. This includes not only nurses notes but also fetal monitoring strips, flow sheets, nursing care plans and other data recorded in the chart. In many instances, notations on hospital record such as the charts or fetal monitor strips are the only proof that cares has been given. Statutes of limitations vary in different states. However, in regard to newborns, more than 20 year could be elapse before a suit is brought. Charting must be specific enough so that nurses do not have to rely on memory.

Fetal monitor strips are important sources of information about the mother and fetus during labour and delivery: Nurses record a great deal of information about nursing care on the monitor strip. Sometimes the clients require the nurses full attention and completion of charting must be temporarily delayed. In this situation, the nurses note on the monitor strips provide the basis for later charting.

Although monitor strips of a legal part of the chart, they may become lost. This makes it particularly important that all information from the strip is recorded in the nurses notes. Complete detailed charting ensures that the nurses actions will be clear many years later in the court of law, even without the monitor strip.

Another form of documentation is the incident report. Sometimes called as "quality assurance report" or an "unusual occurrence report". The nurse completes a report whenever something has occurred that might result in injury to the client. The report warns the hospital legal department that there may be a problem. The incident report also provides that there may be a problem. The incident report also provides a way of keeping track of situations that might endanger clients in the future. Finding a remedy to such a situation can prevent future problems. Incident reports are not a part of the clients chart and should be referred to on the chart should include the same type of factual information on the clients condition that would be records in any other situation.

Continuing education: It is the duty of the nurses to maintain their knowledge and skills at the level necessary to ensure that nurses are performing in the way reasonably prudent peer would perform include attending classes or conferences and reading nursing journals. These activities serve to update nurses and keep them breast of new developments. Most states require proof of continuing education for renewal of nursing licences.

Employers often provide continuing education classes for their nurses. There are also many workshops and seminars available on a variety of nursing subjects. Membership is a professional nursing organization such as state branches of the American Nurses Association and in a professional nursing organization, such as state branches like AWHONN, gives nurses access to new information through publications as well as educational offerings.

The nurse as a client advocate

Nurses are ethically and legally bound to act as the client advocate. This means that the nurse must act in clients best interests are not being served, they are obligated to seek help for the patient from appropriate sources. This usually involves taking the problem through the normal chain of command. The nurse consults a supervisor and the clients physician. If results are not satisfactory, the nurse continues through administrative channels to the director of nurses and the chief of medical staff is necessary.

In seeking help for clients, nurses must document their efforts. For example, when postpartum patients are experiencing excessive bleeding, nurses document what they have done to control the bleeding they call the physician, what information was given by the physician and the response received. When nurses can not contact the physician and the response received. When nurses cannot contact the physician or do not receive adequate instructions, they should document their efforts to seek instructions, from others, such as the supervisor. They should also complete an incident report.

Consumer protection

There has been other laws enacted to deal with such matters. Apart from the civil and criminal liabilities, the new legislation under the name of "consumer protection act of 1986" provides for action against deficient services are paid for action against deficient services if hired on payment basis come with in the preview of this act. Free services however are not within this limit. Therefore, the nurses working in government or charitable hospitals giving free services are relatively safer than so far as the new act is concerned. However, the liability under tortes or penal code remains keeping in view the facts and circumstances in a given situation.

The supreme court is a recent judgement has confirmed that the patients who received deficient services from the medical practitioners and hospital are entitled to claim damage under the consumer protection act, 1986. The services from the medical practitioners also include the services rendered by the nurse at the borderline depend on the control of the practitioners by the large nurses duties and responsibilities are

an integral part of the services receive in the hospital and therefore, they are subject to the disciplinary control of the Indian nursing council as well as the hospital authorities in which a nurse is working.

In the development of professional ethics and values, we must remember that there are implications I in exercising them. For example, what is the legal responsibility for causing harm and how far does one's moral responsibility go in protections of patient's safety?

A nurse during her career, comes to many a cross roads where she constantly debates to weigh between ethical and legal issues. The modernization has ushered in a tremendous change and development in the field of medicine and surgery. Along with the doctors, the nurses are also required to keep abreast of such development, and keep pace with information on the modern trend and requirement. Today we talk of computerization in hospitals, organ transplantation, and genetic manipulation. Artificial insemination, aminosynthesis which call for ethical attention with a tilt towards legal complications.

Recommendations

- Nursing procedures in practice must be periodically reviewed by the competent authorities in the institute.
- The nurse must have complete knowledge of all the rules and regulations.
- Written instructions must be put up an all nursing units of the institute for the necessary guidance and protection of the staff.
- All hospitals must have rules and codes of practice laid down to ensure the safety and well being of the patient and nurses. These may vary from dressing procedures to procedures related to care and safety.

MENOPAUSE

Menopause is the time of cession of ovarian function resulting in permanent amenorrhea. It takes 12 months of amenorrhea to confirm that menopause has set in and therefore it is a retrospective diagnosis.

The Menopause is defined as "ovarian failure due to loss of ovarian follicular function accompanied by oestrogen deficiency resulting in permanent cessation of menstruation and loss of reproductive function" (Utian, 1990).

Age

Menopause normally occurs between the ages of 45 and 50 years; the average age being 47 years. Menopause setting before the age of 40 is known as premature menopause. Menopausal age is not related to menarche, race and socioeconomic status, number of pregnancies and lactation, or taking of oral contraceptives. It is however directly associated with smoking and genetic disposition. Smoking induces premature menopause.

Pathophysiology

During climacteric, ovarian activity declines. Initially, ovulation fails, no corpus luteum forms, and no progesterone is secreted by the ovary. Therefore, the premenopausal menstrual cycles are often anovulatory and irregular. Later, graafian follicles also fail to develop, oestrogenic activity is reduced, and endometrial atrophy leads to amenorrhoea. Cessation of ovarian activity and a fall in the oestrogen level as well as inhibin level cause a rebound increase in the secretion of FSH and LH by the anterior pituitary gland. The FSH level may rise as much as 50-fold and LH 3-4 fold. Gonadotropin activity of the pituitary gland also ceases, and a fall in FSH level eventually occurs.

Hormone levels in a menopausal woman

- E2 : 5–25 pg/ml
- Oestrogen: 20–70 pg/ml—more in obese women
- FSH >40 mIU/ml
- Androgen: 0.3–1.0 ng/ml

- Testosterone: 0.1–0.5 ng/ml
- LH: 50–100 mIU/ml

There is 50% reduction in androgen production and 66% reduction in oestrogen at menopause. The Oestrogen level may remain low at 10 to 20 pg/ml. The ovary also secretes a small amount of testosterone which causes mild hirsutism at menopause. Oestrogen level of over 40 pg/ml exerts bone and cardiotrophic effect, but the level below 20 pg/ml may predispose to osteroprosis and ischaemic heart disease.

Risk factors for menopause related diseases

- Early menopause
- Surgical menopause or radiation
- Chemotherapy especially alkalytic agents
- Smoking, caffeine, alcohol
- Family history of menopausal diseases
- Drugs related like GnRh, heparin, corticosteroids and clomiphene when given over a prolonged period (over 6 months)—can lead to oestrogen deficiency.

Anatomical changes

The **genital organs** undergo atrophy and retrogression. The ovaries shrink and their surfaces become grooved and furrowed. The tunica albuginea thickens. The menopausal ovary measures less 2 × 1.5 × 1 cm in size (8 ml in volume) as seen on ultrasound. Fifteen years later, it should not measure more than 2 ml. The plain muscle in the fallopian tube undergoes atrophy, cilia disappear from the tubal epithelium, and the tubal plicae are no longer prominent.

The **uterus** becomes smaller through atrophy of its plain muscle. The endometrium is represented by only the basal layer with its compact deeply stained stroma, and a few simple tubular glands. It is common for the endometrial glands to dilate before menopause sets in and cystic glandular hyperplasia reported in some premenopausal women causes metropathia haemorrhagia, with irregular heavy bleeding.

The **cervix** becomes smaller and its vaginal portion is represented by a small prominence at the vaginal vault. The vaginal fornices gradually disappear as the cervix shrinks after the menopause. The vagina becomes narrow and its epithelium becomes pale, thin and dry and gets easily infected causing senile vaginitis.

The **vulva** atrophies and the vaginal orifice narrows and this can cause dyspareunia. The skin of the labia minora and vestibule becomes thin, pale and dry, and there is considerable reduction in the amount of fat contained in the labia majora. The pubic hair is reduced and becomes grey.

The **pelvic** cellular tissue becomes lax and the ligaments that support the uterus and vagina lose their tone, and predispose to prolapse of the genital organs.

Apart from the atrophy of the **genital organs** fat is deposited around the breasts, hips and abdomen. Although the mammary glandular tissue atrophies, disposition of fat often makes the breasts more pendulous. The skin wrinkles, and hair grow around the chin and lips. Hypertension, cardiac irregularities, and tachycardia are at times noticed after menopause. Arthritis, osteoporosis of the vertebral bones, upper end of the hip joint, and wrist are all related to oestrogen deficiency after menopause.

Menopausal symptoms

Menstrual: The three classical ways in which the menstrual period ceases are:
- Sudden cessation
- Gradual diminution in the amount of blood loss with each regular period until menstruation stops.
- Gradual increase in the spacing of the periods until they cease for at least a period of 1 year.

Other symptoms

Almost 60 to 70% women go through menopausal period without problems. Rest needs guidance and treatment. The most common and the most noticeable symptoms of hot flushes and sweating are the hallmark of the climacteric in 85% women. Hot flushes are the waves of vasodilatation affecting the face and the neck and these last for 2–5 minutes each. These are followed by severe sweating. Several of these flushes occur in a day, but are more severe during the night, and can disturb sleep or otherwise, irritability and lack of concentration are noticed. With passage of time, the frequency and severity of flushes diminish over a period of 1 to 2 years.

Some women develop a condition of pseudocyesis, when they fear pregnancy and attribute amenorrhoea and increased abdominal girth to pregnancy.

Cancer phobia may also develop, and the woman starts worrying over her looks.

Neurological: Vasomotor symptoms, paraesthesia takes the form of sensations of pins and needles in the extremities.

Libido: Sexual feeling and libido may increase in some, if they feel happy to get rid of menstruation and fear of pregnancy. Many however notice decreased libido after menopause. *The symptoms which develop little later are:*
- Urinary–dysuria, stress incontinence and urge, recurrent infection.
- Genital–atropic vagina reduces the vaginal secretion, and dry vagina can cause dyspareunia. Loss of libido adds to sexual dysfunction. Rarely senile vaginitis can cause vaginal bleeding. Prolapse of genital tract, stress incontinence of urine and faeces are mostly menopausal related.

Late sequelae: Menopausal women through chronic oestrogen deficiency are liable to develop.
- Arthritis, osteoporosis and fracture
- Cardiovascular accidents—ischaemic heart disease, myocardial infraction and atherosclerosis
- Stroke

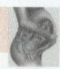

- Skin changes
- Alzheimer disease
- Anocolonic cancer
- Tooth decay

Locomotor system: Menopausal arthropathy, osteoarthritis, fibrositis, backache may be age related.

Osteoporosis: It is an incipient slowly progressing skeletal disorder characterized by microarchitectural deterioration of bone mass resulting in increased fragility and predilection to fracture in the absence of significant trauma. About 15% of elderly women suffer from osteoporosis and almost three times as many suffer from both osteopenia and osteoporosis predispose to fractures. These constitute a significant cause of morbidity like pain, deformity, and impaired respiratory and other bodily functions. Hip fractures are often associated with a high rate of mortality.

With increasing longevity in India , the medical practitioners will be called upon more often to care for osteoporosis related problems.

Pathophysiology

Bone is not an inert supporting tissue. Bone remodeling takes place constantly. At the cellular level, bone remodeling is a balance between bone resorption (osteoclastic activity) and bone formation (osteoblastic activity) whilst the main functions of the osteocytes and lining cells are metabolic subserving bone nutrition and maintenance of calcium homeostasis.

Cardiovascular disease

Oestrogen is cardio protective by maintaining a high level of high density lipoprotein (HDL), and lowering the low density lipoprotein (LDL) and triglycerides, ischaemic heart disease and myocardial infraction. Obese women, with hypertension, previous thromboembolic episodes are liable to cardiovascular accidents. Oestrogen prevents atherosclerosis through its antioxidant property.

Stroke: The incidence of stroke also increases in menopausal women.

Skin: Collagen content is reduced, causing skin to wrinkle.

Alzheimer disease: Lately it is reported that Alzheimer disease is precipitated by oestrogen deficiency at menopause.

Anocolonic cancer and teeth decay are known to increase after menopause.

Endocrine system: Mild virilization as seen in form of hirsutism is probably adrenal in origin, as also is obesity, especially the deposit of fat around the hips. Hypothyroidism with low BMR, high cholesterol level, dryness of skin, brittleness of hair, lack of concentration are noticed in a few menopausal women.

Investigations

Investigatory procedure is as follows

- History of various symptoms
- General examination–include blood pressure recording, palpation of the breasts, weight, hirsutism
- Pelvic examination–Pap smear
- Blood sugar, lipid profile, ECG
- Mammography, pelvic ultrasound
- Bone density study. DEXA (dual energy X-ray absorptiometry) is a quick test with less radiation
- Ostetrogen (E_2) level, FSH to decide on the need of hormone replacement therapy (HRT).

Management of menopause

The clinician should adopt a holistic approach towards management of health problems of menopausal women and selectively prescribe hormone therapy according to the requirement.

Counseling: The woman often develops pregnancy and cancer phobia. It is the duty of the gynecologists to convince her, after thorough examination and investigation that all is well with her. Regular counseling may be required until the woman is well settled in

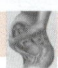

menopause. The advice on contraceptives is necessary. Until menopause is well established and amenorrhea has lasted for 12 months, couple is advised to use barrier method.

Diet should include at least 1.2 gm of calcium, vitamins A, C and E. Vitamin D 400 mg. Soya beans are good. Weight bearing exercises (walking and aerobic) prevent or delay osteoporosis. Yoga, meditation, social work can reduce mental stress

Mild tranquillizers: These relieve the woman's anxiety, sleeplessness and depression.

Hormone replacement therapy (HRT) is not required in all menopausal women. Besides, this therapy does not suit all. The question is who needs HRT?

These are women who are

- Symptomatic
- High-risk cases for cardiovascular disease, osteoporosis, Alzheimer syndrome and colonic cancer.
- Following surgical oophorectomy in premenopausal women and premature menopause.
- Those who demand HRT as prophylaxis.

Certain contraindications to be noted for oestrogen therapy are

- Breast cancer, uterine cancer or family history of cancer.
- Previous history of thromboembolic episode.
- Liver and gallbladder disease.

Osteoporosis

The benefit of HRT is proved beyond doubt in preventing or delaying bone resorption. When to start HRT remains a controversial point.

Oestrogen, progestogen, tibolone and raloxifene are beneficial in osteoporosis.

Cardioprotective effect of HRT

Oestrogen deficiency increases the risk of atherosclerosis, ischaemic heart disease and angina in a postmenopausal woman. Oestrogen is therefore, cardioprotective in prevention of cardiovascular disease. It also increases HDL and decrease LDL, cholesterol and triglycerides. Oestrogen is most effective when taken orally as far as its effect on lipid profile is concerned. Oestrogen and tibolone are strongly cardioprotective in menopausal women. Drugs, dosage and route of administration.

Oestrogen therapy: Oral Premarin in the dose of 0.625 mg daily, increasing to 1.25 mg if necessary. Progestogen like Primolut N 2.5 mg daily for 10 to 12 days each month should be added to prevent endometrial hyperplasia and carcinoma. Some prefer to give a combined hormone therapy (Femet) containing 2 mg 17 betaoestradiol and 1mg of norethisterone acetate.

Long-term therapy: Long-term oestrogen therapy is beneficial in delaying osteoporosis and reducing the risk of cardiovascular disease in a post-menopausal woman. However, it is observed that extending the medication beyond 8 to 10 years does not confer any future benefit.

Oral route: Oral administration of oestradiol undergoes extensive metabolism in the intestine and the liver to oestrone, so that only 10% reaches the systematic circulation as oestradiol. Larger doses therefore, need to be given orally as compared to the non-oral route. This metabolism in the gut and the liver is known as 'first pass' effect, and this also increases certain liver proteins, alters the clotting factors and increases the secretion of renin.

Transdermal patch: It avoids the first pass effect of liver metabolism, and the hormone reaches the systematic circulation as oestradiol. The risk of thromboembolic episode and probable hypertension is eliminated.

ADVANTAGES AND DISADVANTAGES OF ORAL AND TRANSDERMAL ROUTE OF OESTROGEN

Oral

Advantages

- Cheap
- Easy to take

Disadvantages

- High dose required
- First pass effect in the liver
- Daily intake
- Tablet contains lactose, and not suited to women who are allergic to lactose

Transdermal

Advantages

- Low dose oestradiol
- Avoids first pass effect and liver metabolism
- Reduces triglycerides
- No thromboembolic risk or hypertension

Disadvantages

- Costly
- Not tolerated in warm climates
- Variable absorption

Progestogens

Progestogens are used for 10 to 12 days in each cycle to avoid the risk of endometrial hyperplasia and cancer.

The drugs used are Primolut N 2.5 mg, medroxyprogesterone and Duphaston, 10 mg. To avoid the systematic side effects and poor compliance with oral progestogen, Mirena IUCD containing levonorgestrel is inserted for 5 years in HR programme.

Testosterone implant and combined tablet with oestrogen are used to improve libido controversial at present.

Other drugs

1. *Tibolone* (Livial) is a synthetic derivative of 19 nortestosterone, and has a weak oestrogenic, progestogenic and androgenic action. With a tablet containing 2.5 mg, it does not cause endometrial hyperplasis, but causes irregular bleeding in 15%. It also elevates the mood, relieves the vasomotor symptoms, improves the sex dry, and reduces bone resorption. Its main action is cardioprotection by reducing the level of triglycerides. Side effects include weight gain, oedema, tenderness in the breast, gastrointestinal symptoms, vaginal bleed (15%). The greasy skin and increased hair growth are due to androgenic action. It should be initiated only after 1 year of menopause to avoid vaginal bleeding. It may perhaps increase the risk of breast cancer.

2. *Raloxifene* (Evista) is a selective oestrogen receptor modulator (SERM), which reduces the risk of fracture by 50%, especially vertebra by increasing bone mineral density by 2 to 3%. It causes 10% reduction in total and low density lipoprotein and raises HDL level. It does not raise the level of triglycerides. It is therefore, cardioprotective in long-term. It has a very low risk of endometrial and breast cancer. It is mainly beneficial in reducing osteoporosis, and is given 60 mg daily with calcium and vitamin D. It is absorbed from the gastrointestinal tract (60%), glucuronidation occurs in the liver, and excreted in the faeces.

Side effects: Hot flushes, cramps, and increased incidence of venous thrombosis, retinopathy. It does not control vasomotor symptoms.

Contraindications are

- Venous thrombosis
- It should not given with oestrogen
- Hepatic dysfunction
- Stop the drug 72 hours before surgery
- Not to be given with drugs like indomethacin, naproxen, ibuprofen, diazepam.

3. *Soya:* Soya beans contain isoflavone which is strongly oestrogenic, through it is a nonsteroidal plant product. 45–60 mg soya daily is protective without the potential risk of breast cancer. It is a safe alternative to hormonal therapy. It also deceases cholesterol, LDL and triglycerides with a marginal

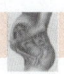

increase in HDL. It also has antiviral, antifungal and anticarcinogenic effects.

4. *Clonidine therapy:* Clonidine is an imidazoline derivative used to treat hot flushes. Clonidine lowers the blood pressure in addition to reliving hot flushes. Dose is 0.2 to 0.4 mg daily.

Androgens improve libido, but the risk of hirsutism has to be remembered.

Complementary approaches: (Reducing the impact of symptoms).

There are a number of simple measures that may reduce the impact of some symptoms of the menopause. Women have found the following measures helpful:

- Hot flushes may be triggered by particular activities such as smoking , eating spicy foods, and drinking alcohol and caffeine. Avoiding or modifying a known trigger may help. Wearing natural fabrics that can 'breathe' and using light-weight cotton bedding may also help.
- Exercise can help general well-being and mood as well as improving stamina and fitness.
- Relaxation or stress reduction techniques will improve coping strategies.
- Counselling may help to deal with life events that are causing anxiety.
- Vaginal symptoms: may be relieved by regular use of vaginal moistures, or non-systematic oestrogen.

Lifestyle advice at menopause

Many women only see health care practitioners for advice about their health when they are approaching or are at the menopause. They have concerns about living well for the rest of their lives.

Women want sensitive, unbiased and upto date information and an explanation of normal menopausal changes. General health advices is the same throughout a woman's life, but there is a particular emphasis on certain factors for menopausal woman; mainly the effects that the menopause has on cardiovascular and bone health as well as the day-to-day symptoms.

The key areas to cover are

- Smoking status
- Diet and nutrition
- Exercise
- Alcohol
- Weight control
- Psychological aspects of the menopause
- Breast and cervical screening

SMOKING

Smoking has many negative effects

- Cigarette smoking can increase the risk of having a heart attack by two or three times. Coronary heart disease (CHD) is the most common cause of death in women.
- Smokers are 1.5 times more likely to have a stroke.
- Smoking tends to increase blood cholesterol levels and adversely effects the HDL/LDL ratio.
- Smokers have an increased level of atherosclerosis in their coronary arteries.
- Smoking leads to an earlier menopause–up to two years earlier when compared with non-smokers.
- Smokers are at greater risk of developing osteoporosis.
- Smokers are more likely to experience vasomotor symptoms.

Diet and nutrition

Nutrition is important for all women around the time of the menopause, and a healthy, balanced diet should be low in fat, low in salt and rich in calcium.

Facts about nutritional health—calcium and salt

- High salt intake is linked with the development of high blood pressure.

- Hypertensives excrete higher amounts of calcium in their urine than people with low blood pressure.
- It is thought that calcium lost in the urine is replaced through calcium stripped from the bone, and that salt plays an important role in speeding calcium loss.
- Vitamin D is necessary for the effective absorption of calcium from the gut, most being obtained from direct sunlight; a smaller amount is obtained from direct sunlight; a smaller amount is obtained from the diet. Supplements of 10 mcg vitamin D may be necessary for elderly and house-bound people, those on a restricted diet, and where there is little exposure to sunlight.

Facts about nutritional health (general)

- Diet should be high in fruit and vegetables, containing at least five portions daily.
- Fruit and vegetables contain antioxidant vitamins and minerals which are crucial in preventing the damaging effects of free radicals.
- Smokers use antioxidants faster.
- You should aim for at least two portions of fish a week, one of which should be oily fish.
- Maintaining a healthy weight is important. Obesity is a major risk factor for CHD and is associated with high blood pressure, heart attacks, heart failure and diabetes. Women should aim for a healthy body mass index (BMI) of 20–25.

Exercise

Regular exercise is necessary to remain active, healthy and independent.

- Physical activity reduces the both the risk of developing CHD and of having a stroke by lowering blood pressure.
- Exercise increases energy levels, muscle strength and bone density.

- Exercise can reduce stress, anxiety and likelihood of depression.
- Exercise helps weight loss and improves sleep.
- Weight-bearing exercise such as brisk walking, dancing, skipping, aerobics, tennis and running stimulate bone to strengthen itself.
- Cycling and swinging are both good cardiovascular exercises.
- Exercise should be varied and should be taken for at least 30 minutes on five or more days of the week for maximum benefit.

Alcohol/Caffeine

It is recommended that women drink no more than 3 units of alcohol a day, with a weekly consumption of fewer than 14 units. The following are useful facts about alcohol:

- Keeping alcohol levels low can lower the risk of heart disease and stroke.
- Too much alcohol is damaging to bone turnover.
- Heavy drinking increases the risk of heart disease and stroke, and raises blood pressure, which can lead to depression, stress, difficulty in sleeping and relationship problems. It can also cause dementia.
- 1–2 alcohol – free days per week are recommended
- Alcohol can trigger vasomotor symptoms at menopause.

Weight control

It is not inevitable that women will put on weight at the menopause, but many do. This is in part due to a decline in muscle mass and a subsequent slow-down in the basal metabolic rate, without reducing the amount of food and alcohol and while taking little or no exercise. *Women should be advised to*

- Eat a healthy diet
- Exercise regularly; start slowly and gradually increase
- Lose extra weight slowly and steadily.

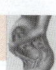

Psychological aspects

Depression, anxiety, tiredness, loss of concentration and memory problems are all common experiences during or after the menopause. To help these aspects, note that:

- Regular exercise can make sleeping easier.
- A balanced diet will ensure an adequate intake of essential minerals and vitamins.
- Social activity improves mental function.
- Concentration can be improved with crosswords, puzzles, quizzes, etc.
- Learning new skills or languages improves mental function.
- Moderating alcohol intake is important for good memory function.

Health screening

It is important to encourage women to attend breast and cervical screening. Women should also be encouraged to be aware of any changes in their breasts, seeking help promptly if they occur.

Breast awareness five point plan

1. Know what is normal for you
2. Look and feel
3. Know what changes to look for
4. Report any changes without delay
5. Attend for breast screening if aged 50 or over.

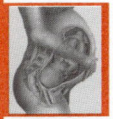

References

- Arlene Burroughs, Gloria Leifer. Maternity Nursing an Introductory Text. W.B. Saunders Company, Philadelphia, 2001.
- Bennet RV, Linda KB. Myles Textbook of Midwives. 13th Ed., Churchill Livingstone, Edinburgh, 1999.
- Bobak IM, Jenson MD. Maternity and Gynaecological Care. 4th Ed., CV Mosby, 1993.
- Datta AK. Essentials of Human Embryology. 5th Ed. CBS Publishers, Kolkata, 2005.
- Dawn C.S. Textbook of Gynaecology including Contraception and Demography. 14th Ed., Dawn Books, Kolkata, 2003.
- Diane M Fraser, Margaret A Cooper. Textbook for Midwives. 14th Ed., Churchill Livingstone, New York, 2003.
- Dutta DC. Textbook of Gynaecology including Contraception. 4th Ed., New Central Book Company, Kolkata, 2005.
- Hurlock Elizabeth B. Child Growth and Development. Tata McGraw-Hill, New Delhi, 2004.
- James DK, B Gonik. High-Risk Pregnancy Management Options. 3rd Ed., Saunders An Imprint Elsevier, Philadelphia, 2006.
- K. Park, Parks Textbook of Preventive and Social Medicine. 19th Ed., M/s Banarsidas Bhanot Publishers, Jabalpur, 2007.
- May KA, Mahlmeister LR. Maternal and Neonatal Nursing. 3rd Ed., Philadelphia, JB Lippincott Company, 1994.
- Mohan Harsh. Textbook of Pathology 2nd Ed., Jaypee Brothers, New Delhi, 1994.
- Parulekar VS. Textbook for Midwives. 2nd Ed., New Central Book Company, Kolkata, 2001.
- Pilleteri A. Maternal and Child Health Nursing, JB Lippincott Company, Philadelphia, 1992.
- Rabbani Tamkin. Instruments in Obstetrics and Gynaecology. 2nd Ed., CBS Publishers & Distributors, New Delhi, 2003.
- Sandra M Nettina. Lippincott Manual of Nursing Practice. 8th Ed., Indian, Lippincott Williams and Wilkins, Philadelphia, 2006.
- Varney Helen. Nurse Midwifery. 2nd Ed., Blackwell Scientific Publications, USA, 1987.
- Stafford I, Shiffield J. "Aamniotic fluid embolism, Obestrics and Gynecological Clinics of North America, Elsevier Saunders.

BIBLIOGRAPHY

1. Chattopadhayay K.S, Narayanaswamy M "Gynaecology for undergraduates" B1 Publications -2006 page 93–96.

JOURNALS

1. Hannah Patricia "Uterine Displacement: what exactly are retroversion and prolapse" Associated content, Nov 12, 2008.

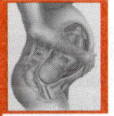

Index

Abdominal examination 57, 190, 264
Abdominal findings 285
Abnormal uterine action 314
Abnormalities in volume 29
Abnormalities of placenta and cord 202
Abortion 139, 473
Abruptio placentae 174
Actual management 114
Actual steps 362, 378, 379
Acupressure 450
Acupuncture 451
Acute DIC 344
Acute
  ectopic 156
  mastitis 388
  polyhydramnios 192
Advantages and disadvantages of oral and transdermal route of oestrogen 531
Advantages of home based antenatal care 444
Aftercare 374
Agency policies 524
Alimentary disorders 422
Allis's tissue holding forceps 495
Alternatives to childbirth 521
Amenorrhoea 31
Amniotic
  fluid 27
  fluid embolism (AFE) 318
Analgesics and antispasmodics in pregnancy and labour 427
Analgesics for pain relief during labour 428
Anatomical consideration 127
Anemia in pregnancy 221

Anoxic 416
Antenatal
  management 186, 275
  advice 65
  exercise 83
  period 419
Antepartum haemorrhage 170
Anterior fontanelle 88
Anticonvulsants 432
Antiemetics in pregnancy 428
Antiseptics and asepsis 112
Areas of skull 87
Aromatherapy 452
Arrest of the aftercoming head 282
Artery forceps 494
Asphyxia neonatorum 410
Assessment and screening of high-risk pregnancy 253
Assessment
  of labour contractions 102
  of physical characteristics 398
Assisted breech delivery 278
Asymmetrical or obliquely contracted pelvis 333
Auvard's vaginal speculum 482

Babcock's tissue holding forceps 496
Basal body temperature (BBT) method 474
Biofeedback 452
Birth
  injuries 414
  trauma 411
Blakes' blunt and sharp uterine curette 486
Blond-Hiedler's decapitation saw wire with thimble 490

Blood
  coagulation disorders 320
  transfusion 226
Bouldeloque's pelvimeter 484
Breast 9, 49
  abscess 389
  complications 387
  engorgement 387
  feeding 474
Breech
  hook with crochet 491
  presentation 271
Brow presentation 287

Caesarean section 217, 371
Carcinoma of cervix in pregnancy 504
Care
  and examination of the newborn 397
  of the preterm neonate 404
Carneous mole (Syn: blood mole, fleshy mole or tuberous mole) 145
Causes of onset of labour 97
Cephalhaematoma 414
Cervical
  dystocia 342
  mucus method 474
  punch biopsy forceps 492
Cervix 48
Changes of the fetal circulation at birth 41
Chemical methods 461
Chronic
  DIC 344
  ectopic 160
  or old ectopic 157

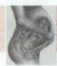

polyhydramnios 189
Chronological appearance of specific
symptoms and signs of
pregnancy 60
Circumferences 90
Classical caesarean section 375
Cleidotomy 380
Clinical
course of labour 290
features of primary
dysmenorrhoea 33
picture 354
types 210
Coitus interruptus 473
Combined method 311
Combined oral contraceptives
(pills) 466
Common surgical instruments 494
Compensated (reversible)
shock 326
Complementary and alternative
therapies 449
Complete abortion 144
Complications associated with
occipitoposterior positions 269
Complications 173
Compound presentation (Syn:
complex presentation) 294
Confirmation of diagnosis 172
Congenital anaemia of the
newborn 242
Constipation 70
Constriction ring 315
Contraceptive methods 460
Contracted pelvis 333
Controlled intravenous
infusion 435
Conventional (laparotomy) 476
Convulsions (seizure) in
newborn 424
Cord
abnormalities 204
prolapse 298
Cracked and retracted nipple 387
Craniotomy 378
Current legal controversies in
obstetrical nursing 523
Cusco's bivalved self-retaining
speculum 482
Cutaneous changes 50

Cytomegalovirus (CMV)
infection 247

Dangers of D and E operation 359
Decapitation 379
Decidua 19
Decompensated (irreversible)
shock 327
Deep vein thrombosis 390
of DIC (minimal acceptable
criteria) 343
Degrees of asphyxia 411
Denominator 76
Dependent oedema 71
Description of the devices 461
Destructive operations 378
Development of placenta 19
Diabetes mellitus in pregnancy 231
Diagnosis
of contracted pelvis 335
of ectopic pregnancy 158
of pregnancy 54
Diagnostic evaluation of
infertility 515
Diameters of skull 89
Dilatation and evacuation 357
Disorders of blood coagulation and
fibrinolysis in obstetrics 320
Disproportion 336
Disseminated intravascular
coagulation (DIC) in
obstetrics 343
Diuretics 431
Do's and don'ts 84
Drew Smythe's catheter 489
Drugs in asthama (during
pregnancy) 429
Drugs used in pregnancy, labour
and puerperium 428
Dysfunctional uterine bleeding
(DUB) 36
Dysmenorrhoea 33
Dyspareunia 72

Eclampsia 217
Ectopic pregnancy 152
Effects
of contracted pelvis on
pregnancy and labour 337
of diabetes on pregnancy 233

on pregnancy 248, 249
of pregnancy on blood
coagulation and fibrinolysis
systems 321
on the mother and fetus 315
Emergency contraception (Syn:
postcoital contraception) 470
Endotoxic shock 330
Episiotomy 363
scissors 496
Ergot derivatives 439
Etiology 322
Events
in first stage of labour 103
in second stage of labour 106
Events in third stage of labour 110
Evidences of foetal distress 115
Evisceration 380
Examination 63, 65
Exercises for muscle strengthening
and relaxation 83
Expressive therapy/sound
therapy 456
External
cardiac massage 414
cephalic version 361

Face presentation 282
Factors
influencing labour 101
influencing maternal
mortality 509
Failing lactation 389
Family welfare programme in
India 506
Fatigue 68
Favourable events (very rare) 291
Features of preterm baby 402
Female sterilization 476
Fertilization 17
Fetal 186
and neonatal infections 247
assessment during labour 85
circulation 40
development 42
skull 87
well-being assessment 85
Fetopelvic relationship 101
Fetus in utero 74
Fibrinolysis 321

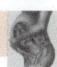

First trimester (first 12 weeks)   54
  pelvis   334
Flatulence   70
Flushing curette   489
Foetal distress   324
Fontanelles   87
Forceps   365
Formation of chorionic villi   20
Formulation of the line of
  treatment   293
Fracture skull   416
Functions   90
Further development of the
  placenta   23

General
  aches, pain and discomfort   427
  changes in shock (with special
    reference to hypovolaemic
    shock)   327
  appearance   397
  organs   45
  physiological changes   130
  prolapse in pregnancy 502
  tonic contraction (Syn: uterine
    tetany)   316
Gestational
  diabetes mellitus   232
  trophoblastic diseases
    (GTDs)   162
Green Armytage clamp   493

Haematological changes   51
Haemorrhagic
  anaemia   226
  disease in newborn   425
  shock   328
Haemorrhoids   70
Haywood smith's ovum
  forceps   487
Heart
  and circulation   52
  disease in pregnancy   228
  lungs, liver and spleen   64
Heartburn   69
Heavy menstruation and abnormal
  uterine haemorrhage   35
Hegar's dilators   485
HELLP syndrome   346
Herpes simplex virus infection   248

High rupture of the membranes
  (HRM)   310
Historical context of complementary
  and alternative therapies   449
History taking   61
Homeopathy   457
Hormonal steroidal
  contraceptives   466
Hormones   471
How to prescribe a pill   467
Human immunodeficiency virus
  (HIV) infection and acquired
    immunodeficiency syndrome
      (AIDS)   250
Human oogenesis   15
Hydatidiform mole (Syn: vesicular
  mole)   163
Hydrops foetalis is oedematous
  stillborn baby   422
Hydrotherapy   456
Hyperbilirubinaemia   421
Hyperemesis gravidarum   238
Hypertensive disorders in
  pregnancy   206
Hypnosis   453
Hysterotomy   360

Iatrogenic or traumatic   340
Icterus gravis neonatorum   241
Idiopathic thrombocytopenic
  purpura in pregnancy   323
Immediate care of the newborn   118
Implant   472
Incidence and effects during
  pregnancy   246
Incidence during pregnancy   244
Incidence   402
Incoordinate uterine action   315
Indications
  for withdrawal   468
  of vaginal examination   113
Induction of labour   307
Infections in pregnancy   244
Infertility and assisted reproductive
  technology   512
Initial screening   260
Injectable steroids   471
Injuries of head   414
Insomnia   72

Instruments
  used for destructive
    operations   488
  used for the examination of a
    gynaecological and obstetric
      patient   481
  used in dilatation, curettage and
    evacuation operation   485
Internal version   363
Interstitial pregnancy   159
Intracranial haemorrhage   416
Intramuscular   437
Intrauterine
  devices (IUD)   461
  fetal death (IUD)   198
  growth restriction (IUGR)   407
Investigation of puerperal
  pyrexia   383
Involution of other pelvic
  structures   128
Iron deficiency anaemia   223
Ivolution of the uterus   127

Jaundice in newborn   420

Kangaroo care for preterm
  infants   406
Kielland's forceps   367
Kocher's haemostatic clamp   494

Lactation   131
Laminaria tent introducing
  forceps   487
Laminaria tent   487
Lanes's tissue holding forceps   495
Laparotomy   342
Large placenta (more than
  500 gm)   202
Last trimester (29–40 weeks)   58
Leg cramps   71
Legal
  aspects in obstetrics   522
  issues   443
Leukorrhoea   69
Local infection   383
Lochia   129
Long curved obstetric forceps   366
Low back pain (nonpathological)   72

Low rupture of the membrane (LRM)   310
Lower segment caesarean section (LSCS)   373

Main movements   108
Major variables in the birth process   101
Management
    during labour   187
    of ailments   137
    of complicated breech delivery   280
    of contracted pelvis (inlet contraction)   338
    of ectopic pregnancy   160
    of infertility   518
    of labour   268, 287, 445
    of normal labour   112
    of normal puerperium   133
    of preterm labour   303
    of the first stage   114
    of the second stage   115
    of the third stage   120
    of vaginal breech delivery   277
Manifestations of the haemolytic disease   241
Manipulative procedures   296
Massage/touch therapy   457
Maternal
    and perinatal mortality   376
    factors (15%)   139
    morbidity   510
    mortality and morbidity and perinatal mortality   508
    pelvis   90
Mechanical factors   106
Mechanism
    of a left mentoanterior position   283
    of labour in contracted pelvis with vertex presentation   334
    of labour   288
    of left sacroanterior position   272
    of normal labour   108
Medical induction   309
Menopause   527
Menorrhagia   36

Menstrual cycle   11, 14
    disorders   31
    induction   472
Metabolic changes   52
Methods
    of induction   309
    of obstetrical examination   76
Metropathia haemorrhagia (Schroder disease)   36
Metrorrhagia   35
Microscopic appearance   164
Minor ailments
    in pregnancy   68
    of newborn   401
Miscellaneous   473
Missed abortion (silent miscarriage)   145
Mode of termination   154
Morbid anatomy   154
Multiload Cu 250   464
Multiple pregnancy   180

Naked eye appearance   164
Natural family planning methods   474
Nausea   68
Needle holder   495
Nerve supply   9
Neurogenic shock   332
Nocturia   72
Nonpathological hyperventilation and shortness of breath   73
Nonsuppurative thrombophlebitis   391
Normal
    delivery   419
    menstrual cycle   11
Nurse practice acts   523
Nursing
    acceptance of complementary and alternative therapies modalities   450
    management   253

Obstetric management   232
Obstructed labour   306
Occipitoposterior position   263
Oligohydramnios (Syn: Oligamnios)   194
One stage operation   357

Oral route   224
Osteomalacic pelvis   333
Other
    injuries   417
    organs   49
Outcomes following shoulder dystocia   298
Ovarian
    changes   164
    cycle   12
    tumours in pregnancy   504
Ovaries   6
Overt diabetes   233
Ovo-fetal factors   139
Ovulation   16
Oxytocic effect   440
Oxytocics in obstetrics   433
Oxytocin   434
    challenge test (oct)   438
    sensitivity test (ost)   438

Parasitic and protozoal infestations in pregnancy   253
Parasitologic considerations   244
Parenteral therapy   224
Partograph   123
Passenger   101
Pathophysiology   209
Patient seen in labour   293
Pelvic
    bones   91
    floor during pregnancy and parturition   9
    floor   7
    ligaments   92
Pelvis   101
Perinatal mortality   511
Perineum   6
Persistent mild diarrhoea   424
Physical methods   460
Physiological changes during pregnancy   45
Physiological jaundice in newborn and jaundice in prematurity   421
Physiology of lactation   131
Pinard's stethoscope   484
Placenta
    accreta and increta   204
    accreta   353
    extrachorialis   203

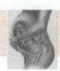

membranecae   203
praevia   170
succenturiata   202
Placental membrane   24
Placentography   172
Planned parenthood   79
Polyhydramnios (Syn: hydramnios)   188
Post-conceptional methods (termination of pregnancy)   472
Posterior fontanelle   89
Postmaturity (Syn: post-term pregnancy)   195
Postnatal visit   447
Postoperative care   365
Postpartum
    exercise   137
    haemorrhage   347
Powers: Uterine contractions   102
Precipitate labour   316
Prediction and prevention   213
Pre-eclampsia   206
Pregnancy
    and CMV infection   247
    and diabetes   231
    induced hypertension (PIH)   206
Preinduction scoring   308
Prelabour (Syn: premonitory stage)   99
Preliminaries   113, 114
Prenatal fetal assessment   85
Preparation
    and procedures for home birth   446
    before confinement for baby and mother   445
    for birth   444
    for confinement   445
Preterm
    baby   402
    labour (Syn: premature labour)   301
    rupture of the membranes (prom)   304
Prevention   302
Primary
    amenorrhoea   32
    or initial shock   325
Principles   114
Problems of the newborn   410

Procedures   310, 378, 379
Procedure
    at the first visit   61
    at the subsequent visits   65
Progestin only pill (mini pill)   470
Prognosis   173, 213, 219, 275, 286, 299
    of tubal pregnancy   162
Progressive decompensated shock   326
Prolonged labour   311
Prophylaxis   342, 384
Prostaglandins (PGs)   440
Psychiatric illness in pregnancy   392
Pueperium   226
Puerperal pyrexia   382
Puerperal sepsis (Syn: puerperal infection)   382
Puerperal venous thrombosis and pulmonary embolism   389
Pulmonary embolism   392

Rachitic flat pelvis   333
Rampley's sponge holding forceps   496
Ramsbotham's decapitation saw   490
RCH interventions   507
Reflexology   458
Requirements of baby   445
Retroversion   499
Retroverted gravid uterus   500
Rh incompatability   241
Right mentoanterior (RMA), left mentoposterior (RMP or LMP)   284
Risk
    approach of obstetric nursing care   253
    factors   244
Rubella   246
Rupture of the uterus   339

Safe period (rhythm method)   473
Sagittal fontanelle   89
Scalp injuries   416
Scar rupture   339
Scissors   496
Second trimester (13–28 weeks)   57
Secondary
    amenorrhoea   32

dysmenorrhoea   34
or true shock   325
Selected complementary and alternative therapies   450
Separation   25
Sex   182
Shirodkar's cervical encirclage needles   493
Shock in obstetrics   325
Short curved obstetric forceps   367
Shoulder dystocia   294
Sickle cell haemoglobinopathies   227
Signs   120
Simpson's modification of Oldham's perforator   488
Simpson's uterine sound   484
Sim's anterior vaginal wall retractor   483
Sims double bladed posterior vaginal speculum   481
Smoking   533
Specialized gynaecological instruments   491
Specific
    therapy   224
    treatment   32
Spontaneous   339
Spreading infection   383
Stages of labour   100
Standard of care   524
Steps of mediolateral episiotomy   364
Steroids during pregnancy   428
Stillbirth   201
Stripping the membranes   311
Subacute (chronic) ectopic   158
Subaponeurotic haemorrhage   415
Subinvolution   385
Sudden collapse following childbirth or abortion   509
Superficial vein thrombosis   390
Supine hypotensive syndrome   74
Supportive therapy   168
Suppurative thrombophlebitis   391
Surgical induction   309

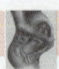

Sutures 87
Symphysiotomy 378
Syphilis 248
Systemic
    changes 53
    steroids in clinical use 429

Teale's vulsellum 483
Technique 475
Terminal methods or
    sterilization 474
Tests
    for coagulation failure 323
    to assess fetal well-being 86
Thalassaemia in pregnancy 227
The central births and death
The registration act, 1969 523
The fallopian tubes 6
The fetal membranes 26
The four types of pelvis 95
The normal female pelvis 91
The placenta and fetal
    membranes 24
The placenta at term 24
The true pelvis 92
The uterus 4
The vagina 2
The vulva 1
Theories 238
Tingling and numbness of
    fingers 74
To arrest preterm labour 302
To prevent or minimise
        fetomaternal bleed 244

Tocolytics in obstetrics for the
    next 12 to 48 hours, at the end
        of which the therapy can be
            switched over to oral
                medication 432
Tonic uterine contraction and
    retraction 317
Toxoplasmosis 244
Transcutaneous electrical nerve
    stimulation (TENS) 454
Transmission cycle 245
Transverse lie 289
Traumatic 249, 323, 385, 416
Trial labour 338
Triphasic formulations of combined
    oral pills 469
Tubectomy 476
Twin transfusion syndrome 186
Twins 180
Two
    stage operation 358
    bladed Braxton-Hick's
        cranioclast 489

Unfavourable events (most
    common) 291
Unruptured tubal pregnancy 161
Unstable lie 293
Upper backache
    (nonpathological) 69
Urinary
    complications in
        puerperium 386
    frequency (nonpathological) 69

Uterine
    action 103
    displacements 497
    dressing forceps 491
    fibroid in pregnancy 502
    inertia (hypotonic activity) 315
    infection 383
    malformations 5
Uterus 45
    packing forceps 491

Vagina 128
Vaginal
    examination in labour 113
    examination 264, 285
Varicose veins in pregnancy 231
Varicosities 71
Varieties 271
Vasectomy 474
Velamentous insertion of the
    umbilical cord 356
Ventouse 369
Version 361
Visualization and guided
    imagery 455
Vomiting 424

Weight gain and water
    metabolism 50
Wertheim's vaginal clamp 494
What causes AFE? 318
Willet's scalp traction forceps 489

Yoga 459